AF841563

The Springer Series on Human Exceptionality

Series Editors

Donald H. Saklofske, Ph.D.
Department of Psychology
Western University, Canada

Moshe Zeidner, Ph.D.
Center for Interdisciplinary Research on Emotions
Department of Human Development and Counseling
Haifa University, Israel

For further volumes:
http://www.springer.com/series/6450

Sandra Prince-Embury
Donald H. Saklofske
Editors

Resilience in Children, Adolescents, and Adults

Translating Research into Practice

Springer

Editors
Sandra Prince-Embury
Resiliency Institute of Allenhurst, LLC.
W. Allenhurst, NJ, USA

Donald H. Saklofske
Department of Psychology
The University of Western Ontario
London, ON, Canada

ISSN 1572-5642
ISBN 978-1-4614-4938-6 ISBN 978-1-4614-4939-3 (eBook)
DOI 10.1007/978-1-4614-4939-3
Springer New York Heidelberg Dordrecht London

Library of Congress Control Number: 2012950029

© Springer Science+Business Media New York 2013
This work is subject to copyright. All rights are reserved by the Publisher, whether the whole or part of the material is concerned, specifically the rights of translation, reprinting, reuse of illustrations, recitation, broadcasting, reproduction on microfilms or in any other physical way, and transmission or information storage and retrieval, electronic adaptation, computer software, or by similar or dissimilar methodology now known or hereafter developed. Exempted from this legal reservation are brief excerpts in connection with reviews or scholarly analysis or material supplied specifically for the purpose of being entered and executed on a computer system, for exclusive use by the purchaser of the work. Duplication of this publication or parts thereof is permitted only under the provisions of the Copyright Law of the Publisher's location, in its current version, and permission for use must always be obtained from Springer. Permissions for use may be obtained through RightsLink at the Copyright Clearance Center. Violations are liable to prosecution under the respective Copyright Law.
The use of general descriptive names, registered names, trademarks, service marks, etc. in this publication does not imply, even in the absence of a specific statement, that such names are exempt from the relevant protective laws and regulations and therefore free for general use.
While the advice and information in this book are believed to be true and accurate at the date of publication, neither the authors nor the editors nor the publisher can accept any legal responsibility for any errors or omissions that may be made. The publisher makes no warranty, express or implied, with respect to the material contained herein.

Printed on acid-free paper

Springer is part of Springer Science+Business Media (www.springer.com)

My mother, Katherine Lardner, and father, Matthew Prince, both resourceful individuals who weathered much adversity; my grandmothers, Marie Brannigan and Olga Frankel, who migrated to the United States alone as teenagers and reared families with very few resources; my husband Dennis, whose kind heart and humorous spirit have provided inspiration and support; and my clients who have shared their life stories of resiliency with me over the years.

Sandra Prince-Embury

My beautiful mother, Frances Annette, who passed away on October 30, 2011, and my devoted father, Harold.

Donald H. Saklofske

Preface

The study of resilience or the ability to "stay the course" or "bounce back" in the face of adversity has been a topic of investigation by developmental theorists for the past 50 years. Earlier researchers had observed that some persons, whether children or adults, managed to survive exposure to adversity and even thrive in later life while others succumbed to psychological disorders and physical illness that could either be acute or longer term. This observation has been repeated numerous times under conditions ranging from large natural disasters and war to the loss of a parent or child. The human result can also vary from the manifestation of increased capacity and will to "live and learn" or to anxiety, posttraumatic stress disorder, and suicide.

The study of resilience has gone through many rich phases of discovery, identifying aspects of both the person and environment that appeared to serve as protective or mitigating variables to the impact of adversity. Several outstanding researchers and theorists have attempted to integrate the many research findings and their implications for practical application. However, the understanding that resilience is a product of complex interactions of personal attributes and environmental circumstances, mediated by internal mechanisms, has presented an assessment challenge to developmental researchers (Luthar, Cicchetti, and Becker, 2000).

On the other hand, the past few years have been witness to a plethora of self-help books and interventions that have not been systematically linked to sound core developmental constructs nor empirically tested for effectiveness. Some interventions that are found to be effective are explained on the basis that they increase resiliency while this implied mediating process is not documented. Thus there is a disconnect between the complex theory and body of research on resiliency and the abundant self-help products employing this term.

There is a need in the study of resiliency for construct clarification and research grounded translation for practical application. Furthermore, links between constructs, assessments, interventions, and outcomes need to be made more transparent and hence more easily understood and applied. In particular, this volume presents a thorough discussion of the tools and techniques developed by leading experts for assessing resilience along with evidence for their psychometric rigor and practical application. Eleven of the twenty-one chapters link underlying definitions of resilience with assessment and application using well-known tools for assessing resilience. Embedded in the "science of test development" is the rigor of construct identification, operational definition of the construct, and psychometric analysis to determine the reliability, validity, and potential usefulness of the respective assessment. In this way, examination of carefully designed assessment tools allows comparison of different definitions of resilience.

This volume is divided into four parts which combine specific definitions and assessments with broad brushstrokes of application: Introduction and Conceptual Issues; Resilience and Children; Resilience, Youth, and Adults; and Resilience, Cultural, and Systemic Considerations. One intention of this volume is to present a diversity of specific definitions of resilience to the reader for the purpose of informed application with children, adolescents, and adults in ways that are theoretically sound, empirically supported, practical, and need specific. A second intention of this volume is to present a few broader contexts in which the resilience construct may be meaningfully understood and integrated in diverse human contexts.

We begin this book with an acknowledgement of the authors of the chapters to follow. The knowledge and expertise they bring to the study of resilience and their capacity to write informed, critical, and readable chapters have more than accomplished the task we set out when beginning this book. We also are grateful to Judy Jones and Garth Haller who provided the editorial support needed to bring this book to completion. We thank them and Springer.

W. Allenhurst, NJ, USA Sandra Prince-Embury
London, ON, Canada Donald H. Saklofske

About the Editors

Sandra Prince-Embury, Ph.D., is a licensed clinical psychologist and family therapist serving children, adolescents, and families for 30 years. In addition to clinical work, Dr. Prince-Embury taught at Pennsylvania State University and engaged in research on community response to technical disaster. Her work with residents of the Three Mile Island community is housed at the Dickenson College Archives in PA. Currently director of the Resiliency Institute of Allenhurst, LLC, she is engaged in research, writing, and consultation associated with her recently authored *Resiliency Scales for Children and Adolescents (RSCA).*

Donald H. Saklofske, Ph.D., is a Professor in the Department of Psychology, The University of Western Ontario, Canada. His main research interests include intelligence, personality, and individual differences. He is a Fellow of the Canadian Psychological Association and the Association for Psychological Science.

Contents

List of Contributors

Phillip J. Bowman, Ph.D. National Center for Institutional Diversity (NCID), The University of Michigan, Ann Arbor, MI, USA

Robert Brooks, Ph.D. Harvard University, Assistant Clinical Professor of Psychology, Department of Psychiatry, Needham, MA, USA

Jeremy Burrus, Ph.D. Educational Testing Service, Center for Academic and Workplace Readiness and Success, Princeton, NJ, USA

Paulette J. Christopher Department of Psychology, University of New Mexico, Albuquerque, NM, USA

Emmy A. Climie, Ph.D. Education Tower – University of Calgary, Calgary, Canada

Tara Crumpler Strengths in ADHD, University of Calgary, Calgary, AB, Canada

Melissa DeVries, Ph.D. Neurology, Learning and Behavior Center, Salt Lake City, UT, USA

Beth Doll, Ph.D. College of Education and Human Sciences, University of Nebraska Lincoln, Lincoln, NE, USA

Diane Cardenas Elliott Educational Testing Service, Center for Academic and Workforce Readiness and Success, Princeton, NJ, USA

Emerson M. Epstein Department of Psychology, University of New Mexico, Albuquerque, NM, USA

Jennifer L. Fleming, M.S. Devereux Center for Resilient Children, Villanova, PA, USA

Sam Goldstein, Ph.D. Neurology, Learning and Behavior Center, Salt Lake City, UT, USA

Raymond F. Hanbury, Ph.D., A.B.P.P. Department of Psychiatry, Jersey Shore University Medical Center, Private Practice, Behavioral Medicine, Trauma and Police Psychology, Manasquan, NJ, USA

Yvonne Hindes, Ph.D. University of Calgary, Calgary, AB, Canada

Monica J. Indart, Ph.D. Department of Clinical Psychology, Rutgers University Graduate School of Applied and Professional Psychology, Piscataway, NJ, USA

Private Practice, Maplewood, NJ, USA

Pamela Kaliski, Ph.D. The College Board, Newtown, PA, USA

Mark Kitzie, Psy.D. Youth Development Clinic, Newark, NJ, USA

Paul A. LeBuffe, M.A. Devereux Center for Resilient Children, Villanova, PA, USA

Benjamin Levin, Ph.D. Theory and Policy Studies, Ontario Institute for Studies in Education, University of Toronto, Toronto, ON, Canada

Linda Liebenberg, Ph.D. Resilience Research Centre, Dalhousie University, Halifax, NS, Canada

Barry Mallin, Ph.D. Department of Psychology, Faculty of Arts, University of Manitoba, Winnipeg, MB, Canada

Kelly Marth Counseling & School Psychology Department, Seattle University, Seattle, WA, USA

Sarah M. Mastoras Education Tower – University of Calgary, Calgary, AB, Canada

Adam W. McCrimmon, Ph.D. Education Tower – University of Calgary, Calgary, AB, Canada

Jack A. Naglieri, Ph.D. Devereux Center for Resilient Children, Villanova, PA, USA

University of Virginia, Charlottesville, VA, USA

David W. Nordstokke, Ph.D. School and Applied Psychology Program, University of Calgary, Calgary, AB, Canada

Sarah Nugent Foothills Academy, Calgary, AB, Canada

Geraldine V. Oades-Sese, Ph.D. Institute for the Study of Child Development, Department of Pediatrics, Robert Wood Johnson Medical School, Rutgers University, New Brunswick, NJ, USA

J. Alexis Ortiz Department of Psychology, University of New Mexico, Albuquerque, NM, USA

Sandra Prince-Embury, Ph.D. Resiliency Institute of Allenhurst, LLC, West Allenhurst, NJ, USA

Richard D. Roberts, Ph.D. Educational Testing Service, Center for Academic and Workforce Readiness and Success, Princeton, NJ, USA

Katherine M. Ross, B.S. Devereux Center for Resilient Children, Villanova, PA, USA

Wai-Ling Rubic, M.S. Head Start Serving Northern San Diego, Community Development Institute, San Diego, CA, USA

Sarah Rutstein Graduate School of Applied and Professional Psychology, Rutgers University, Piscataway, NJ, USA

Donald H. Saklofske, Ph.D. Department of Psychology, Social Science Centre, The University of Western Ontario, London, ON, Canada

Ralf Schwarzer, Ph.D. Freie Universität Berlin Psychology, Berlin, Germany

Vicki L. Schwean, Ph.D. Faculty of Education, The University of Western Ontario, London, ON, Canada

Bruce W. Smith, Ph.D. Department of Psychology, University of New Mexico, Albuquerque, NM, USA

Samuel Y. Song, Ph.D., N.C.S.P. Counseling & School Psychology Department, Seattle University, Seattle, WA, USA

Beverly Tignor, Ph.D. Private Practice, Menham, NJ, USA

Erin M. Tooley Department of Psychology, University of New Mexico, Albuquerque, NM, USA

Michael Ungar, Ph.D. Resilience Research Centre, Dalhousie University, Halifax, NS, Canada

Christopher Velderman Graduate School of Applied and Professional Psychology, Rutgers University, Piscataway, NJ, USA

Ashley Vesely Department of Psychology, Social Science Centre, The University of Western Ontario, London, ON, Canada

Gail Wagnild, R.N., Ph.D. The Resilience Center, Billings, MT, USA

John R. Walker, Ph.D. Department of Clinical Health Psychology, St. Boniface Hospital, University of Manitoba, Winnipeg, MB, Canada

Miles Waltuck Graduate School of Applied and Professional Psychology, Rutgers University, Piscataway, NJ, USA

Lisa Marie Warner, Ph.D. Freie Universität Berlin Psychology, Berlin, Germany

Part I

Introduction

1 Translating Resilience Theory for Application: Introduction

Sandra Prince-Embury and Donald H. Saklofske

The study of resiliency or the ability to "bounce back" in the face of adversity has been a topic of investigation by developmental psychology theorists for the past 50 years. Earlier researchers had observed that some youth managed to survive exposure to adversity and even thrive in later life, while others were less successful even to the point of developing various physical and psychological disorders. As discussed in the chapters of this volume, the study of resilience and resilient children and adults has gone through many rich phases of discovery, identifying aspects of both the person and environment that appear to serve as protective or mitigating variables to the impact of adversity. While much of previous resilience research examined the interaction of protective factors and risk in high risk populations, the particular focus of this work has been the identification of factors that were present in the lives of those who both survived and thrived in the face of adversity compared to those who did not (Garmezy, Masten, & Tellegen, 1984; Luthar, 1991, 2003, 2006; Masten, 2001; Rutter, Harrington, Quinton, & Pickles, 1994; Werner & Smith, 1982, 1992, 2001; Luthar & Zelazo, 2003; Luthar & Zigler, 1992; Masten, 2007; Masten & Coatsworth, 1998; Masten & Curtis, 2000; Masten & Powell, 2003; Masten et al., 1999; Masten & Wright, 2009).

Several outstanding researchers and theorists have attempted to integrate the many research findings and their implications for practical application. However, the understanding that resilience is a product of complex interactions of personal attributes and environmental circumstances, mediated by internal mechanisms, has presented an assessment challenge to developmental researchers (Luthar, Cicchetti, & Becker, 2000). Some longitudinal studies from a developmental psychopathology perspective have tried to capture contextual aspects of resilience specific to the group and sets of circumstances (Masten, 2001, 2006; Werner, 1997, 2005). These studies have employed extensive batteries of preexisting tests, along with measures of achievement, to assess personal resiliency. Research has used different measures across studies and across populations, making it difficult to compare findings across studies and across groups. The research based tools employed in previous studies have often been impractical for widespread use in the schools and communities because they are too labor intensive, expensive, or focused on presence or absence of psychiatric symptoms. Consequently, the lack of a common metric for measuring resiliency has

S. Prince-Embury, Ph.D. (✉)
Resiliency Institute of Allenhurst, LLC,
625 North Edgemere Drive, West Allenhurst,
NJ 07711, USA
e-mail: sandraprince-embury@earthlink.net

D.H. Saklofske, Ph.D.
Department of Psychology, Social Science Centre,
The University of Western Ontario, 7th Floor, London,
ON, Canada N6A 5C2
e-mail: dsaklofs@uwo.ca

S. Prince-Embury and D.H. Saklofske (eds.), *Resilience in Children, Adolescents, and Adults: Translating Research into Practice*, The Springer Series on Human Exceptionality,
DOI 10.1007/978-1-4614-4939-3_1, © Springer Science+Business Media New York 2013

resulted in difficulty in assessing the need for, choice of, and effectiveness of preventive intervention strategies in a way that allows comparison across methods and populations.

Controversy Over Usefulness of the Resilience/Resiliency Construct

In light of the definitional diversity and research complexity, those with a more rigorous bent have challenged the utility and conceptual integrity of the resilience construct (Kaplan, 1999, 2005). Kaplan (1999) concluded that resilience is a once useful construct whose time has passed. He concluded that conceptualizations of resilience as a trait did not pass scrutiny in that there were no common defining features across all instances of resilience. Kaplan defined resilience as an aberration—a failure in the predictive model, causes for which being infinite (Kaplan, 1999). Kaplan suggests that resilience is not a phenomenon per se, but rather a conceptual tool in the development of increasingly refined predictive models. These criticisms, although perhaps understandable from the perspective of a researcher and statistician, may leave practitioners without working tools to use while the refined predictive models are being worked out.

Some have claimed that in spite of conceptual complexity, the phenomenon of resilience has too much heuristic power to be abandoned, (Luthar et al., 2000). Elias, Parker, & Rosenblatt (2005) propose the use of working definitions of resilience/resiliency that satisfy two criteria: (1) does the definition add value to existing constructs in understanding circumstances? (2) does the definition inform the design of interventions? Kaplan in his 2005 review conceded that concepts are not by their nature true or false but may be evaluated with regard to their usefulness.

The Current Volume

This volume on Resilience is written in the spirit of those who suggest that the construct has too much heuristic power to be abandoned (Luthar et al., 2000). The emphasis of this volume is not to identify the one true definition of the term with the purpose of excluding applications that lack conceptual purity. The major goal of this volume is to enhance practical usefulness of the "resilience" construct. In this pursuit, the first goal of the volume is to identify constructs of resilience that have practical usefulness, across contexts and to demonstrate this usefulness. The second goal of the volume is the examination of tools developed for the assessment of resilience for practical application. Embedded in the science of test development is the rigor of construct identification, development of tools for assessment and psychometric analysis to determine the reliability, validity, and potential usefulness of the respective assessment. The third purpose of the volume is to present cultural considerations in the discussion and application of resilience and related constructs. It is the hope of this volume's editors that the volume will be a valuable reference contribution to the growing literature on the construct of resilience as well as a practical guide for the application of this construct.

Organization of this volume begins with this introduction and a consideration of "Conceptual Issues" by Prince-Embury in Chap. 2. This chapter will touch upon some of the conceptual issues associated with the "resilience" construct and together with this introduction, constitute Section 1. Chapter 2 will also touch on but not claim to comprehensively explore all conceptual issues related to resilience. For this purpose, references presented in this introduction and in Chap. 2 are offered for the reader who wants to read more extensively. Following these introductory chapters, the volume is divided into three broad sections: Resilience and Children, Resilience, Youth and adults, and Resilience, Cultural and Systemic Issues.

Section 2 contains six chapters on resilience in children representing different perspectives: the subjective experience of the child, the ratings of teachers and parents, and the assessment of aspects of the classroom. Chapter 3 describes the underlying theoretical constructs, research with and application of the Resiliency Scales for Children and Adolescents (RSCA) (Prince-Embury, 2007). The RSCA is designed to reflect the child's experience of core aspects of personal resiliency: sense of mastery, sense of relatedness, and emotional reactivity for use in preventive screening, treatment planning, and outcome monitoring. Chapter 4 presents the Devereux Suite of Assessments (DECA-Infant, DECA-Toddler, DECA-Preschool, and DESSA) (LeBuffe, Shapiro, & Naglieri, 2009), discussing how these reflect the growing emphasis on strength-based assessment, how they are designed to advance professional practice, and how they (and other strength-based measures) can influence professional attitudes and practices. Chapter 5 by Song et al., describes an ecological approach to assessing resilience of classroom environments using "ClassMaps" a tool developed by Doll et al. (2010). This assessment is proposed as a tool for providing feedback to teachers on ways to modify their classroom environments to be more supportive of resilience. Section 1 then moves toward intervention. Chapter 6 discusses the principle of training parents and teachers in the attitudes supportive of a resilient mind-set in children presented by Goldstein, Brooks, and DeVries. In Chap. 7, Mallin, Walker, and Levin overview prevention programs aimed at screening for and enhancement of resiliency in children. In Chap. 8 Climie et al. discuss the integration of resilience into the study of childhood disorders.

Section 3 focuses on the assessment of resilience in youth and adults as well as interventions. Chapters 9–13 present assessment tools that are designed to assess resilience and related constructs. Each of these assessment tools reflects a different assessment approach. Chapter 9 presents the work of Jack Block, focusing on his "Ego Resiliency Scale (Block & Kremen, 1996)." The "Ego-Resiliency Scale" is based on a psychodynamic view of ego-resiliency as a personality trait that allows the individual to adjust ego control of emotion appropriate to presenting circumstances.

Chapter 10 by Schwarzer and Warner presents the General Self-Efficacy Scale (Schwarzer & Jerusalem, 1995). Schwarzer presents validity information for the Self-Efficacy Scale and differentiates the construct of self-efficacy from resilience and other constructs. Chapter 11 by Gail Wagnild presents her Resilience Scale designed to tap constructs of resilience in middle and older adults. Wagnild identified the "resilience core" as Purpose, Equanimity, Self-Reliance, Perseverance, and Existential Aloneness and aimed to tap these attributes in the RS (Wagnild & Young, 1993).

Chapters 12 and 13 present the CD-RISC, the Connors–Davidson Resilience Scale (Connor & Davidson, 2003) and the Brief Resilience Scale (Smith et al., 2008). Both of these assessment tools have been used with medical populations and with specific disorders. The CD-RISC is discussed as an instrument that has shown sensitivity to medication response in patients with PTSD. Chapter 13 presents the BRS which defines resilience more narrowly as a quick response to upset.

Chapters 14 and 15 expand past the basic assessment of resilience. In Chap. 14 Saklofske et al., employ the adult versions of the RSCA-A in relation to other measures of well-being and emotional intelligence to gain a further understanding of the construct of resilience in adults. Chapter 15 by Eliot, Kaliski, Burrus, and Roberts explores the importance of self-evaluation as an important component of personal resilience.

Chapters 16 and 17 examine resilience in the face of disaster. Chapter 16, written by psychologist first responders Hanbury and Indart, discusses response to disaster immediately after it has occurred. Chapter 17 by Prince-Embury applies principles of resilience retroactively to the design of a community level intervention under remaining conditions of uncertainty in the aftermath of technological disaster.

Chapters 18–22 explore some cultural and systemic considerations of resiliency. In Chap. 18 Michael Unger and Linda Libenberg (Ungar & Liebenberg, 2011) discuss the cultural relativity of resilience, the CYRM-28 and caution against generalizing assumptions across cultures. Chapter 19 by Tignor and Prince-Embury, tests the applicability of the RSCA to youth in the slums of Nairobi, Kenya. In Chap. 20, Oades-Sese et al. look at bilingualism and language development as sources of educational resilience in Hispanic children. In Chap. 21, Bowman looks at role strain as a chronic risk factor for African Americans and explores protective factors at many levels including public policy. In Chap. 22, Prince-Embury introduces Bowen Family Systems Theory as a framework for considering resilience at multiple levels of human systems.

In all, we trust that this collection of original papers will shed new light on both theoretical and assessment issues of relevance to understanding and measuring resiliency.

References

Block, J., & Kremen, A. M. (1996). IQ and ego-resiliency: Conceptual and empirical connections and separateness. *Journal of Personality and Social Psychology, 70*, 349–361.

Connor, K. M., & Davidson, J. R. (2003). Development of a new resilience scale: the Connor-Davidson Resilience Scale (CD-RISC). *Depression and Anxiety, 18*, 76–82.

Doll, B., Spies, R. A., Champion, A., Guerrero, C., Dooley, K., & Turner, A. (2010). The ClassMaps Survey: A measure of students' perceptions of classroom resilience. *Journal of Psychoeducational Assessment, 28*, 338–348.

Elias, M. J., Parker, S. R., & Rosenblatt, J. L. (2005). Building educational opportunity. In R. B. Brooks & S. Goldstein (Eds.), *Handbook of resilience in children* (pp. 315–336). New York: Kluwer Academic/Plenum.

Garmezy, N., Masten, A. S., & Tellegen, A. (1984). The study of stress and competence in children: A building block for developmental psychopathology. *Child Development, 55*, 97–111.

Kaplan, H. B. (1999). Toward an understanding of resilience: A critical review of definitions and models. In M. D. Glantz & J. L. Johnson (Eds.), *Resilience and development: Positive life adaptations* (pp. 17–83). New York: Kluwer Academic/Plenum.

Kaplan, H. B. (2005). Understanding the concept of resilience. In S. Goldstein & R. Brooks (Eds.), *Handbook of resilience in children*. New York: Kluwer Academic/Plenum.

LeBuffe, P. A., Shapiro, V. B., & Naglieri, J. A. (2009). *The Devereux student strengths assessment (DESSA), technical manual, and User's guide*. Lewisville: Kaplan.

Luthar, S. S. (1991). Vulnerability and resilience: A study of high-risk adolescents. *Child Development, 62*, 600–616.

Luthar, S. S. (2003). *Resilience and vulnerability: Adaptation in the context of childhood adversities*. Cambridge: Cambridge University Press.

Luthar, S. S. (2006). Resilience in development: A synthesis of research across five decades. In D. Cicchetti & D. J. Cohen (Eds.), *Developmental psychopathology: Risk, disorder, and adaptation* (2nd ed., Vol. 3, pp. 739–795). Hoboken: Wiley.

Luthar, S. S., Cicchetti, D., & Becker, B. (2000). The construct of resilience: A critical evaluation and guidelines for future work. *Child Development, 71*(3), 543–562.

Luthar, S. S., & Zelazo, L. B. (2003). Research on resilience: An integrative review. In S. S. Luthar (Ed.), *Resilience and vulnerability: Adaptation in the context of childhood adversities* (pp. 510–549). Cambridge: Cambridge University Press.

Luthar, S. S., & Zigler, E. (1991). Vulnerability and competence: A review of research on resilience in childhood. *The American Journal of Orthopsychiatry, 61*(1), 6–22.

Luthar, S. S., & Zigler, E. (1992). Intelligence and social competence among high-risk adolescents. *Development and Psychopathology, 4*, 287–299.

Masten, A. S. (2001). Ordinary magic: Resilience processes in development. *American Psychologist, 56*(3), 227–238.

Masten, A. S. (2006). Developmental psychopathology: Pathways to the future. *International Journal of Behavioral Development, 31*, 47–54.

Masten, A. S. (2007). Resilience in developing systems: Progress and promise as the fourth wave rises. *Development and Psychopathology, 19*, 921–930.

Masten, A. S., & Coatsworth, J. D. (1998). The development of competence in favorable and unfavorable environments: Lessons from research on successful children. *American Psychologist, 53*(2), 205–220.

Masten, A. S., & Curtis, W. J. (2000). Integrating competence and psychopathology: Pathways toward a comprehensive science of adaptation in development [Special issue]. *Development and Psychopathology, 12*, 529–550.

Masten, A., Hubbard, J., Gest, S., Tellegen, A., Garmezy, N., & Ramirez, M. (1999). Competence in the context of adversity: Pathways to resilience and maladaptation from childhood to late adolescence. *Development and Psychopathology, 11*, 143–169.

Masten, A. S., & Powell, J. L. (2003). A resilience framework for research, policy, and practice. In S. S. Luthar (Ed.), *Resilience and vulnerability: Adaptation in the context of childhood adversities* (pp. 1–25). Cambridge: Cambridge University Press.

Masten, W., & Wright, M. O. (2009). Resilience over the lifespan. In J. W. Reich (Ed.), *Handbook of adult resilience* (pp. 213–237). New York: Guilford.

Prince-Embury, S. (2007). *The resiliency scales for children and adolescents: Profiles of personal strength*. San Antonio: The Psychological Corporation.

Rutter, M., Harrington, R., Quinton, D., & Pickles, A. (1994). Adult outcome of conduct disorder in childhood: Implications for concepts and definitions of patterns of psychopathology. In R. D. Ketterlinus & M. E. Lamb (Eds.), *Adolescent problem behaviors: Issues and research* (pp. 57–80). Hillsdale: Lawrence Erlbaum Associates.

Schwarzer, R., & Jerusalem, M. (1995). General self-efficacy scale. In J. Weinman, S. Wright, & M. Johnston (Eds.), *Measures in health psychology: A user's portfolio. Causal and control beliefs* (pp. 35–37). Windsor: NFER-Nelson.

Smith, B. W., Dalen, J., Wiggins, K., Tooley, E., Christopher, P., & Bernard, J. (2008). The brief resilience scale: Assessing the ability to bounce back. *International Journal of Behavioral Medicine, 15*, 194–200.

Ungar, M., & Liebenberg, L. (2011). Assessing resilience across cultures using mixed-methods: Construction of the child and youth resilience measure-28. *Journal of Mixed Methods Research, 5*(2), 126–149.

Wagnild, G., & Young, H. M. (1993). Development and psychometric evaluation of the resilience scale. *Journal of Nursing Measurement, 1*, 165–177.

Werner, E. E. (1997). Vulnerable but invincible: High-risk children from birth to adulthood. *Acta Paediatrica Supplement, 422*, 103–105.

Werner, E. E. (2005). What can we learn about resilience from large-scale longitudinal studies? In S. Goldstein & R. Brooks (Eds.), *Handbook of resilience in children* (pp. 91–206). New York: Kluwer Academic/Plenum.

Werner, E. E., & Smith, R. S. (1982). *Vulnerable but invincible: A longitudinal study of resilient children and youth*. New York: McGraw-Hill.

Werner, E. E., & Smith, R. S. (1992). *Overcoming the odds: High risk children from birth to adulthood*. Ithaca: Cornell University Press.

Werner, E. E., & Smith, R. S. (2001). *Journeys from childhood to midlife: Risk, resilience, and recovery*. Ithaca: Cornell University Press.

2 Translating Resilience Theory for Assessment and Application with Children, Adolescents, and Adults: Conceptual Issues

Sandra Prince-Embury

Complex aspects of human functioning are not always neatly deconstructed by researchers or neatly reconstructed for intentional application. Such is the case for the construct of "resilience." Over the past 50+ years, definitions of resiliency have been numerous and research has operated at different levels of analysis, each with its own language and caveats. This complexity has made standardized use and application of the construct more difficult. According to a critical review by (Wald, Taylor, Asmundson, Jang, & Stapleton, 2006) there are several existing definitions of resilience that share in common a number of features all relating to human strengths, some type of disruption and growth, adaptive coping, and positive outcomes following exposure to adversity (e.g., Bonanno, 2004; Connor & Davidson, 2003; Friborg, Hjemdal, Rosenvinge, & Martinussen, 2003; Masten et al., 1999; Richardson, 2002). There are also a number of distinctions made in attempts to define this construct. For example, some investigators assume that resilience is located "within the person" (e.g., Block & Block, 1980; Davidson et al., 2005). Other investigators (e.g., Friborg et al., 2003; Luthar, Cicchetti, & Becker, 2000; Masten, 2001) propose that there are multiple sources and pathways to resiliency, including social context (e.g., family, external support systems). Luthar et al. (2000) have provided clarification by distinguishing between "resilience" as a dynamic developmental process that involves the interaction of personal attributes with environmental circumstances and "resiliency" (Block & Block, 1980) as a personality characteristic of the individual.

There has been considerable divergence in the literature with regard to the definition, criteria, or standards for resiliency; whether it is a trait, process, or an outcome variable; whether it is enduring or situation specific; whether survival in the face of adversity is required and the nature of the adversity required for resiliency to be demonstrated (e.g., what is a sufficient exposure risk factor?). The following are just a few examples of definitions of resilience.

> Resilience is a dynamic process wherein individuals display positive adaptation despite experiences of significant adversity or trauma. This term does not represent a personality trait or an attribute of the individual … Rather, it is a two-dimensional construct that implies exposure to adversity and the manifestation of positive adjustment outcomes. (Luthar et al., 2000, p. 858).
>
> Resilience refers to a class of phenomena characterized by good outcomes in spite of serious threats to adaptation or development. (Masten, 2001, p. 228).
>
> Resilience embodies the personal qualities that enable one to thrive in the face of adversity. … Resilience is a multidimensional characteristic that varies with context, time, age, gender, and cultural origin, as well as within an individual subjected to different life circumstances. (Connor & Davidson, 2003, p. 76).

S. Prince-Embury, Ph.D. (✉)
Resiliency Institute of Allenhurst, LLC, 625 North Edgemere Drive, West Allenhurst, NJ 07711, USA
e-mail: sandraprince-embury@earthlink.net

S. Prince-Embury and D.H. Saklofske (eds.), *Resilience in Children, Adolescents, and Adults: Translating Research into Practice*, The Springer Series on Human Exceptionality,
DOI 10.1007/978-1-4614-4939-3_2, © Springer Science+Business Media New York 2013

> Resilience may be briefly defined as the capacity to recover or bounce back, as is inherent in its etymological origins, wherein 'resilience' derives from the Latin words salire (to leap or jump), and resilire (to spring back). (Davidson et al., 2005, p. 43).
>
> Psychological resilience has been characterized by the ability to bounce back from negative emotional experiences and by flexible adaptation to the changing demands of stressful experiences (Tugade & Fredrickson, 2004, p. 320).

Resilience in the face of adversity has been studied extensively by developmental psychopathologists for the past 50 years. Consistent with the definitions above this body of work has generally defined resilience as the ability to weather adversity or to bounce back from negative experience. Much of resilience research has examined the interaction of protective factors and risk in high-risk populations. As developmental research most of this work focused on children, sometimes in longitudinal studies of factors in the lives of youth that predicted positive outcomes in adulthood (Werner & Smith, 1982, 1992, 2001).

The earliest focus of this developmental work was the identification of factors that were present in the lives of those who thrived in the face of adversity as compared to those who did not (Garmezy, Masten, & Tellegen, 1984; Luthar, 1991, 2003; Masten, 2001; Rutter, Harrington, Quinton, & Pickles, 1994; Werner & Smith, 1982, 1992, 2001). Protective factors identified in previous research include personal qualities of the child that may have allowed them to cope with various types of adversity. The personal qualities identified include, intellectual ability (Baldwin et al., 1993; Brooks, 1994; Jacelon, 1997; Luthar & Zigler, 1991, 1992; Masten & Coatsworth, 1998; Rutter, 1987; Wolff, 1995; Wright & Masten, 1997), easy temperament (Jacelon, 1997; Luthar & Zigler, 1991; Rende & Plomin, 1993; Werner & Smith, 1982; Wright & Masten, 1997; Wyman, Cowen, Work, & Parker, 1991), autonomy (Jacelon, 1997; Werner & Smith, 1982), self-reliance (Polk, 1997), sociability (Brooks, 1994; Luthar & Zigler, 1991), effective coping strategies (Brooks, 1994; Luthar & Zigler, 1991), and communication skills (Werner & Smith, 1982).

Another group of protective factors identified in previous research pertained to the child's social environment, including family. Included in this group of factors are family warmth, cohesion, structure, emotional support, positive styles of attachment, and a close bond with *at least one* caregiver (Baldwin et al., 1993; Brooks, 1994; Cowen & Work, 1988; Garmezy, 1991; Gribble et al., 1993; Luthar & Zigler, 1991; Luthar & Zelazo, 2003; Masten & Coatsworth, 1998; Rutter, 1987; Werner & Smith, 1982; Wolff, 1995; Wright & Masten, 1997; Wyman et al., 1991, 1992).

Environmental protective factors outside the immediate family have been identified and include positive school experiences (Brooks, 1994; Rutter, 1987; Werner & Smith, 1982; Wright & Masten, 1997), good peer relations (Cowen & Work, 1988; Jacelon, 1997; Werner & Smith, 1982; Wright & Masten, 1997), and positive relationships with other adults (Brooks, 1994; Conrad & Hammen, 1993; Garmezy, 1991; Werner, 1997; Wright & Masten, 1997).

Examining the evolution of the construct and study of resilience, Masten and Wright (2009) describe four waves of research undergone primarily by developmental researchers that approached the study of this construct from different perspectives across time (Masten, 2007; Wright & Masten, 1997). The first wave focused on description, defining and measuring resilience, and in the identification of differences between those who did well and poorly in the context of adversity or risk of various kinds. This first wave of research revealed consistency in qualities of people, relationships, and resources that predicted resilience, and these potential protective factors were found to be robust in later research.

The second wave moved beyond description of the factors or variables associated with resilience to a focus on processes, the "how" questions, aiming to identify and understand specific processes that might lead to resilience. These studies led to new labels for processes as protective, moderating, compensatory, etc. Two of the most basic models described compensatory and moderating influences of explanatory factors. In compensatory models, factors that neutralize or counterbalance exposure to risk or stress have direct, independent, and positive effects on the outcome of interest, regardless of risk level. These compensatory factors have been termed *assets*, *resources*, and *promotive factors* in the literature. Good intelligence or an outgoing personality might be considered assets or resources that are helpful regardless of exposure to adversity. In protective or "moderating effect" models, a theoretical factor or process has effects that vary depending on the level of risk. A classic "protective factor" shows stronger effects at higher levels of risk. Access to a strong support system might be considered protective in that its protective influence is more noticeable in the face of adversity.

The third wave began with efforts to test ideas about resilience processes through intervention designed to promote resilience such as the promotion of positive parenting as advocated by Brooks and Goldstein (2001). Brooks and Goldstein translated basic principles of promoting a healthy mindset in children and disseminated this information to professionals, teachers and parents in a variety of venues. Beth Doll employed an ecological model of resilience by creating the ClassMaps system for helping teachers modify the educational experience to enhance resilience in the classroom environment.

The fourth wave of resilience includes discussion of genes, neurobehavioral development, and statistics for a better understanding of the complex processes that led to resilience (Masten, 2007). These studies often focus at a more molecular level examining how processes may interact at the biological level. Some of this work has led to concepts of "differential susceptibility" and "sensitivity to context" to explore the possibility that some children are more susceptible or sensitive to the influence of positive or negative contexts.

Although the study of early development is often viewed as the intellectual home of the construct, "resilience" has also been described as an aspect of adult personality. Block's conception of ego-resiliency in adults was distinct from the developmental conceptions of resilience that focused on bouncing back in the face of adversity. Block conceived of "Ego-resiliency" as a meta-level personality trait associated with the conception of "ego" as a complex integrative mechanism. The basic process underlying ego-resiliency according to Block may be described as flexibility in the control of emotion. According to Block, ego-resiliency is the ability to adapt ones level of emotion control temporarily up or down as circumstances dictate (Block, 2002; Block & Block, 1980). The related assumption is that this flexibility in controlling emotion is a relatively enduring trait which impacts a variety of other abilities including but not limited to survival in the face of adversity. As a result of this adaptive flexibility, individuals with a high level of resiliency are more likely to experience positive affect, and have higher levels of self confidence and better psychological adjustment than individuals with a low level of resiliency (Block & Kremen, 1996). When confronted by stressful circumstances, individuals with a low level of resiliency may act in a stiff and perseverative manner or chaotically and diffusely, and in either case, the resulting behavior is likely to be maladaptive (Block & Kremen, 1996).

Other theorists have identified traits in adults that overlap with the notion of "resilience." One such construct was that of "hardiness" defined and studied by Kobasa and others (Kobasa, 1979; Maddi, 2002). Hardiness as defined by Kobasa was characterized by three general assumptions about self and the world (Kobasa, 1979, 1982; Maddi, 2002, 2005). These include (a) a sense of control over one's life (e.g., believing that life experiences are predictable and that one has some influence in outcomes through one's efforts); (b) commitment and seeing life activities as important (e.g., believing that you can find meaning in, and learn from, whatever happens, whether events be negative or positive); and (c) viewing change as a challenge (e.g., believing that change, positive or negative, is an expected part of life and that stressful life experiences are opportunities).

A related construct was coined by Albert Bandura "Self-Efficacy," (1997). The construct of perceived self-efficacy is the belief that one can perform novel or difficult tasks and attain desired outcomes, as spelled out in Bandura's Social Cognitive Theory (Bandura, 1997). This "can do"-cognition reflects a sense of control over one's environment and an optimistic belief of being able to alter challenging environmental demands by means of one's own behavior. Hence, it represents a self-confident view of one's capability to deal with certain stressors in life. Although not conceptually the same as resiliency, self-efficacy may be viewed as a resource component of resiliency with or without the presence of adversity.

The importance of sense of meaning in adult resilience was highlighted in the life and work of Victor Frankl (1979). According to Frankl, one's sense of meaning can facilitate resiliency in adults in a number of ways. A sense of meaning in the context of religion, or other belief system can act as a buffer to negative affect in the face of adversity by allowing the individual to pray and thus find support in God, or understand within the context of a belief system. The belief that one still has choice in the face of adversity can provide strength as illustrated by Victor Frankl's *Man's Search for Meaning*, (1979).

Findings of earlier phases of developmental research of resilience as well as constructs such as "ego-resiliency" seemed to imply that resilient individuals are extraordinary and that this quality is not accessible to everyone. Later research or phase two suggested that resilience was largely a product of a complex interaction of factors in which the individual's environment played a significant part. Along with this shift in emphasis came a questioning of whether "resilience" is extraordinary. The emergence of resilience as "ordinary magic" by Masten identified the process as characteristic of normal development and not applicable in adverse circumstances only (Masten, 2001; Masten & Powell, 2003). Masten (2001) suggested that fundamental systems, already identified as characteristic of human functioning, have great adaptive significance across diverse stressors and threatening situations. This shift in emphasis had significant implications. The "ordinary magic" framework suggested by Masten extends application of resilience theory to a broader range of individuals in varied contexts.

Masten and Wright (2009) expanding this thinking to consideration of resilience as protective systems important across the lifespan. These include attachment relationships and social support; intelligence or problem-solving skills; self-regulation skills involved in directing or inhibiting attention, emotion, and action; agency, mastery motivation, and self-efficacy; *meaning making* (constructing meaning and a sense of coherence in life); and cultural traditions, particularly as engaged through religion. This shift of frameworks is accompanied by the possibility that resilience may be modified through interventions with individuals and the life circumstances in which they find themselves.

In more recent times examination of resilience in adults has crossed paths with the study of "positive psychology." Martin Seligman (2000) has written on the need for developing a systematic science of positive psychology to offset the prevailing focus on pathology. He points out that the major strides in prevention have come from a perspective of systematically building competency, not on correcting weakness. Seligman's approach, based in cognitive theory, is to provide structured interventions designed to build resilient attitudes that will then buffer against symptoms of depression.

Also in recent times, clinicians have expressed a need for a further shift toward clinical application. Goldstein and Brooks (2005) and Brooks and Goldstein (2001) have called for a clinical psychology of resiliency. These authors focus on the interaction between the child and the child's social environment. Goldstein has written on the importance of the mindset of a resilient parent in raising a child with a resiliency mindset and the importance of teaching parents how to identify and foster these qualities. These authors focus on changing the family and academic environments to be more supportive of the child's resiliency.

Controversy Over Usefulness of the Resilience/Resiliency Construct

In light of the definitional diversity, research complexity and evolution of the resilience construct described above, those with a more rigorous bent have challenged the utility and conceptual integrity of the construct (Kaplan, 1999, 2005).

Kaplan (1999) concluded that resilience is a once useful construct whose time has passed. He concluded that conceptualizations of resilience as a trait did not pass scrutiny in that there were no common defining features across all instances of resilience. Kaplan defined resilience as an aberration—a failure in the predictive model, causes for which being infinite (Kaplan, 1999). Kaplan suggests that resilience is not a phenomenon per se, but rather a conceptual tool in the development of increasingly refined predictive models. These criticisms, although perhaps understandable from the perspective of a researcher and statistician, may leave practitioners without working tools to use while the refined predictive models are being worked out. Similar criticisms have been made of the other similarly complex constructs of *hardiness*, *sense of meaning*, and *ego-resiliency* mentioned above.

Some have claimed that in spite of conceptual complexity, the phenomenon of resilience has too much heuristic power to be abandoned, (Luthar et al., 2000). Elias, Parker, and Rosenblatt (2005) propose the use of working definitions of resilience/resiliency that satisfy two criteria; (1) does the definition add value to existing constructs in understanding circumstances; (2) does the definition inform the design of interventions. Kaplan in his 2005 review conceded that concepts are not by their nature true or false but may be evaluated with regard to their usefulness.

Assessment Challenge

If we suggest that working definitions of resilience that pass utility criteria are of value, we are then left with the question of assessment. How do we assess the presence or absence of resiliency? Early researchers employed absence of pathology in the face of adversity as their essential yardstick that resilience was present. However, the understanding that resilience is a product of complex interactions of personal attributes and environmental circumstances, mediated by internal mechanisms, has presented additional assessment challenges to developmental researchers (Luthar et al., 2000). Kaplan (1999) has pointed out the difficulty of achieving statistically significant interaction effects. Kaplan asks "Can one ever adequately account for sufficient amounts of predictive variance from retroactive assessment?"

Studies from a developmental perspective have been longitudinal and have tried to capture contextual aspects of resilience specific to the group and sets of circumstances. Assessment of resilience in children has often focused on *assets* defined as the achievement of positive outcomes such as reaching developmental milestones. This approach has been useful in longitudinal studies in which researchers could examine risk and protective factors retrospectively from the numerous pieces of information carefully gathered about study participants (Werner & Smith, 1982, 1992).

These studies have employed extensive batteries of preexisting tests, along with measures of achievement, to assess personal resiliency. Research has used different measures across studies and across populations, making it difficult to compare across studies and across groups. The research-based tools employed in previous research have often been impractical for widespread use in the schools and communities because they are too labor intensive, expensive, or focused on presence or absence of psychiatric symptoms. In addition, identification of assets and developmental milestones occurs after the fact and are not useful in prevention of negative outcome. This leaves the identification of risk conditions regardless of individual differences as the source of preventive identification. Consequently, the lack of a screening tool has resulted in difficulty in assessing the need for and choice of preventive intervention strategies.

Assessment tools have been developed in an attempt to tap resilience/resiliency. These tools have most commonly been constructed for adults, each focusing on different aspects of the construct. These instruments have undergone some scrutiny. For example, some critics claim that resilience/resiliency cannot be assessed in the absence of adversity. Ahern, Kiehl, Sole, and Byers (2006) reviewed some instruments that were designed to measure resilience. They focused on six measures, and the range of constructs measured included "protective factors that support resiliency," "successful stress-coping ability," "central protective resources of health adjustment," "resilient coping behavior," and "resilience as a positive personality characteristic that enhances individual adaptation" (p. 110). These authors concluded that rather than specifically assessing resilience as the ability to bounce back, resist illness, adapt to stress, or thrive in the face of adversity, previous measures have generally assessed protective factors or resources that involve personal characteristics and coping styles. These authors thus suggest that assessment has not captured the process of resilience or bouncing back from adversity.

It should be noted that assessment tools for resilience/resiliency are more prevalent for adults than for children although much of the research on resilience has emerged from the study of early development. There are many reasons for this circumstance. First, developmental psychologists are keenly aware of the reliance of children on their parents and environmental circumstances. Therefore focusing on the child could run the risk of blaming the child for failure to thrive in the face of adverse circumstances. Similarly, focus on the child might run the risk of assuming that a "resiliency child" is invulnerable and therefore would not need special attention in the face of adversity. One might argue that in an effort to protect the child from blame, there has been a dismissal of the child's personal experience that would ultimately be the mediating process between protective factors and good outcomes.

Definition and assessment problems notwithstanding, there has in the past few years been a plethora of self-help books and interventions published that have not been systematically linked to sound core developmental constructs. These interventions are not often tested for effectiveness. Some interventions that are found to be effective are explained on the basis that they increase resiliency while this implied mediating process is not documented. Thus there is a disconnection between the complex theory and body of research on resiliency and the abundant self-help products employing this term.

In summary, there is a need in the field for construct clarification for practical application and evaluation. Furthermore links between constructs, assessments, interventions and outcomes need to be made more transparent and hence more easily understood and applied. The intention of this volume is to describe diverse efforts at translating resilience theory for assessment and application with children, adolescents, and adults. It is the mission of the volume to allow the readers to make their own judgments on the soundness, practicality and usefulness of these constructs and related assessments, informed by exposure to diverse perspectives on the topic.

References

Ahern, N. R., Kiehl, E. M., Sole, M. L., & Byers, J. (2006). A review of instruments measuring resilience. *Issues in Comprehensive Pediatric Nursing, 29*, 103–125.

Baldwin, A. L., Baldwin, C. P., Kasser, T., Zax, M., Sameroff, A., & Seifer, R. (1993). Contextual risk and resiliency during late adolescence [Special issue]. *Development and Psychopathology, 5*(4), 741–761.

Bandura, A. (1997). *Self-efficacy: The exercise of control*. New York: Freeman.

Block, J. (2002). *Personality as an affect-processing system*. Mahwah: Erlbaum.

Block, J. H., & Block, J. (1980). The role of ego-control and ego-resiliency in the organization of behavior. In W. A. Collins (Ed.), *Development of cognition, affect, and social relations. The Minnesota symposia on child psychology* (Vol. 13, pp. 39–101). Hillsdale: Lawrence Erlbaum.

Block, J., & Kremen, A. M. (1996). IQ and ego-resiliency: Conceptual and empirical connections and separateness. *Journal of Personality and Social Psychology, 70*, 349–361.

Bonanno, G. A. (2004). Loss, trauma, and human resilience: Have we underestimated the human capacity to thrive after extremely aversive events? *American Psychologist, 59*, 20–28.

Brooks, R. B. (1994). Children at risk: Fostering resilience and hope. *The American Journal of Orthopsychiatry, 64*(4), 545–553.

Brooks, R., & Goldstein, S. (2001). *Raising resilient children: Fostering strength, hope, and optimism in your child*. New York: Contemporary Books. San Antonio: The Psychological Corporation.

Connor, K. M., & Davidson, J. R. T. (2003). Development of a new resilience scale: The Connor-Davidson resilience scale (CD-RISC). *Depression and Anxiety, 18*, 76–82.

Conrad, M., & Hammen, C. (1993). Protective and resource factors in high- and low-risk children:

A comparison of children with unipolar, bipolar, medically ill, and normal mothers [Special issue]. *Development and Psychopathology, 5*(4), 593–607.
Cowen, E. L., & Work, W. C. (1988). Resilient children, psychological wellness, and primary prevention. *American Journal of Community Psychology, 16*(4), 591–607.
Davidson, J. R. T., Payne, V. M., Connor, K. M., Foa, E. B., Rothbaum, B. O., Hertzberg, M. A., et al. (2005). Trauma, resilience, and saliostasis: Effects of treatment in post-traumatic stress disorder. *International Clinical Psychopharmacology, 20*, 43–48.
Elias, M. J., Parker, S. R., & Rosenblatt, J. L. (2005). Building educational opportunity. In R. B. Brooks & S. Goldstein (Eds.), *Handbook of resilience in children* (pp. 315–336). New York: Kluwer Academic/ Plenum.
Frankl, V. (1979). *Man's search for meaning*. New York: Simon & Schuster.
Friborg, O., Hjemdal, O., Rosenvinge, J. H., & Martinussen, M. (2003). A new rating scale for adult resilience: what are the central protective resources behind healthy adjustment? *International Journal of Methods in Psychiatric Research, 12*, 65–76.
Garmezy, N. (1991). Resiliency and vulnerability to adverse developmental outcomes associated with poverty. *American Behavioral Scientist, 34*(4), 416–430.
Garmezy, N., Masten, A. S., & Tellegen, A. (1984). The study of stress and competence in children: A building block for developmental psychopathology. *Child Development, 55*, 97–111.
Goldstein, S., & Brooks, R. B. (Eds.). (2005). *Handbook of resilience in children*. New York: Kluwer Academic/ Plenum Publishers.
Gribble, P. A., Cowen, E. L., Wyman, P. A., Work, W. C., Wannon, M., & Raoof, A. (1993). Parent and child views of parent-child relationship qualities and resilient outcomes among urban children. *Journal of Child Psychology and Psychiatry, 34*(4), 507–519.
Jacelon, C. S. (1997). The trait and process of resilience. *Journal of Advanced Nursing, 25*, 123–129.
Kaplan, H. B. (1999). Toward an understanding of resilience: A critical review of definitions and models. In M. D. Glantz & J. L. Johnson (Eds.), *Resilience and development; positive life adaptations* (pp. 17–83). New York: Kluwer Academic/Plenum.
Kaplan, H. B. (2005). Understanding the concept of resilience. In S. Goldstein & R. Brooks (Eds.), *Handbook of resilience in children*. New York: Kluwer Academic/ Plenum.
Kobasa, S. C. (1979). Stressful life events, personality, and health: An inquiry into hardiness. *Journal of Personality and Social Psychology, 37*, 1–11.
Kobasa, S. C. (1982). Commitment and coping in stress resistance among lawyers. *Journal of Personality and Social Psychology, 42*, 707–717.
Luthar, S. S. (1991). Vulnerability and resilience: A study of high-risk adolescents. *Child Development, 62*, 600–616.
Luthar, S. S. (2003). *Resilience and vulnerability: Adaptation in the context of childhood adversities*. Cambridge: Cambridge University Press.
Luthar, S. S., Cicchetti, D., & Becker, B. (2000). The construct of resilience: A critical evaluation and guidelines for future work. *Child Development, 71*(3), 543–562.
Luthar, S. S., & Zelazo, L. B. (2003). Research on resilience: An integrative review. In S. S. Luthar (Ed.), *Resilience and vulnerability: Adaptation in the context of childhood adversities* (pp. 510–549). Cambridge: Cambridge University Press.
Luthar, S. S., & Zigler, E. (1991). Vulnerability and competence: A review of research on resilience in childhood. *The American Journal of Orthopsychiatry, 61*(1), 6–22.
Luthar, S. S., & Zigler, E. (1992). Intelligence and social competence among high-risk adolescents. *Development and Psychopathology, 4*, 287–299.
Maddi, S. R. (2002). The story of hardiness: Twenty years of theorizing, research, and practice. *Consulting Psychology Journal, 54*, 173–185.
Maddi, S. R. (2005). On hardiness and other pathways to resilience. *American Psychologist, 60*, 261–262.
Masten, A. S. (2001). Ordinary magic: Resilience processes in development. *American Psychologist, 56*(3), 227–238.
Masten, A. S. (2007). Resilience in developing systems: Progress and promise as the fourth wave rises. *Development and Psychopathology, 19*, 921–930.
Masten, A. S., & Coatsworth, J. D. (1998). The development of competence in favorable and unfavorable environments: Lessons from research on successful children. *American Psychologist, 53*(2), 205–220.
Masten, A., Hubbard, J., Gest, S., Tellegen, A., Garmezy, N., & Ramirez, M. (1999). Competence in the context of adversity: Pathways to resilience and maladaptation from childhood to late adolescence. *Development and Psychopathology, 11*, 143–169.
Masten, A. S., & Powell, J. L. (2003). A resilience framework for research, policy, and practice. In S. S. Luthar (Ed.), *Resilience and vulnerability: Adaptation in the context of childhood adversities* (pp. 1–25). Cambridge: Cambridge University Press.
Masten, W., & Wright, M. O. (2009). Resilience over the lifespan. In J. W. Reich (Ed.), *Handbook of adult resilience* (pp. 213–237). New York: Guilford Publications.
Polk, L. V. (1997). Toward a middle-range theory of resilience. *Advances in Nursing Science, 19*(3), 1–13.
Rende, R., & Plomin, R. (1993). Families at risk for psychopathology: Who becomes affected and why? [Special issue]. *Development and Psychopathology, 5*(4), 529–540.
Richardson, G. E. (2002). The metatheory of resilience and resiliency. *Journal of Clinical Psychology, 58*, 307–321.
Rutter, M. (1987). Psychosocial resilience and protective mechanisms [Special report]. *The American Journal of Orthopsychiatry, 57*(3), 316–331.

Rutter, M., Harrington, R., Quinton, D., & Pickles, A. (1994). Adult outcome of conduct disorder in childhood: Implications for concepts and definitions of patterns of psychopathology. In R. D. Ketterlinus & M. E. Lamb (Eds.), *Adolescent problem behaviors: Issues and research* (pp. 57–80). Hillsdale: Lawrence Erlbaum Associates.

Seligman, M. E. P. (2000). Positive psychology. In J. E. Gillham (Ed.), *Science of optimism and hope: Research essays in honor of Martin E. P. Seligman* (pp. 415–429). Philadelphia: Templeton Foundation Press.

Tugade, M. M., & Fredrickson, B. L. (2004). Resilient individuals use positive emotions to bounce back from negative emotional experiences. *Journal of Personality and Social Psychology, 86*, 320–333.

Wald, J., Taylor, S., Asmundson, G. J. G., Jang, K. L., & Stapleton, J. (2006). *Literature review of concepts final report: Psychological resilience*. Toronto: DRDC.

Werner, E. E. (1997). Vulnerable but invincible: High-risk children from birth to adulthood. *Acta Paediatr Suppl, 422*, 103–105.

Werner, E. E., & Smith, R. S. (1982). *Vulnerable but invincible: A longitudinal study of resilient children and youth*. New York: McGraw-Hill.

Werner, E. E., & Smith, R. S. (1992). *Overcoming the odds: High risk children from birth to adulthood*. Ithaca: Cornell University Press.

Werner, E. E., & Smith, R. S. (2001). *Journeys from childhood to midlife: Risk, resilience, and recovery*. Ithaca: Cornell University Press.

Wolff, S. (1995). The concept of resilience. *The Australian and New Zealand Journal of Psychiatry, 29*(4), 565–574.

Wright, M. O., & Masten, A. S. (1997). Vulnerability and resilience in young children. In J. S. Greenspan, S. Weider, & J. Osofsky (Eds.), *Handbook of Child and Adolescent Psychiatry and Preschooler Development and Syndromes* (pp. 202–224). New York: Wiley.

Wyman, P. A., Cowen, E. L., Work, W. C., & Parker, G. R. (1991). Developmental and family milieu correlates of resilience in urban children who have experienced major life stress. *American Journal of Community Psychology, 19*(3), 405–426.

Wyman, P. A., Cowen, E. L., Work, W. C., Raoof, A., Gribble, P. A., Parker, G. R., et al. (1992). Interviews with children who experienced major life stress: Family and child attributes that predict resilient outcomes. *Journal of the American Academy of Child and Adolescent Psychiatry, 31*(5), 904–910.

Part II

Resilience and Children

Resiliency Scales for Children and Adolescents: Theory, Research, and Clinical Application

3

Sandra Prince-Embury

This chapter will describe the Resiliency Scales for Children and Adolescents (RSCA) (Prince-Embury, 2006a, 2006b, 2006c, 2007) as an assessment of personal resiliency that is based on three core developmental systems commonly associated with adaptive functioning. In addition, this chapter will summarize and integrate the developmental theory underlying the RSCA, present research including reliability and validity evidence and discuss clinical application of the RSCA for preventive screening and clinical intervention.

Broad-Based Resilience Assessment Issues

The definition of resilience as a product of complex interactions of personal attributes and environmental circumstances, mediated by internal mechanisms, has presented an assessment challenge to developmental researchers in the past (Luthar, Cicchetti, & Becker, 2000). In an effort to clarify constructs, theorists have distinguished "resilience" from "resiliency" in that the former is defined as interactive and contextual and the latter addresses personal attributes of the individual (Luthar et al., 2000; Luthar & Zelazo, 2003; Masten, 1994). Studies of resilience have been longitudinal, have employed a developmental-psychopathology perspective and have tried to capture contextual aspects of resilience specific to groups and sets of circumstances. Studies assessing personal resiliency, in an effort to be comprehensive, have employed extensive batteries of preexisting tests, along with various criteria of competence, achievement or successful adaptation. Researchers of both resilience and resiliency have used different measures across studies and across populations, making it difficult to compare results across studies and across groups. In addition, these measures employed in research have often been impractical for widespread use because they are too labor intensive or expensive and in some cases require longitudinal research. In summary, there has been a lack of common metrics across different studies of resilience/resiliency and across research and practice.

On a practical level, Masten has suggested that there is work to be done to make resiliency assessment tools more field-friendly (Masten, 2001; Masten & Powell, 2003). In this pursuit measures should be brief, easily administered, simple to score and interpret and applicable across populations, bias free with respect to gender and ethnicity and worded so that they might be used with a broad range of age and reading levels while retaining core meaning. In addition,

S. Prince-Embury, Ph.D. (✉)
Resiliency Institute of Allenhurst, LLC.,
625 North Edgemere Drive, West Allenhurst,
NJ 07711, USA
e-mail: Sandraprince-embury@earthlink.net

S. Prince-Embury and D.H. Saklofske (eds.), *Resilience in Children, Adolescents, and Adults: Translating Research into Practice*, The Springer Series on Human Exceptionality,
DOI 10.1007/978-1-4614-4939-3_3, © Springer Science+Business Media New York 2013

for widespread application such as universal screening, a measure assessing resiliency needs to be strength-based and informative while at the same time not stigmatizing or "pathologizing" of groups or individuals.

Developmental Systems of Personal Resiliency

The first step in the assessment of resiliency is to define what aspect to assess. A criticism in the field has been that there has not been consensus on a definition of the construct (Kaplan, 2005). Resilience research has identified lengthy lists of protective factors present in the child's family, school, and community as well as in personal characteristics of the child. An ecological perspective also considers the complex interaction of these factors and their effect on the child. Selecting what factors to assess or determining how to assess complex interactions presents a measurement challenge. First researchers must decide whether to focus on the context or environmental factors (resilience), personal attributes of the youth (resiliency), or the interaction between the two. Assessment of the interaction that underlies resilience requires multiple measures and specific plans on how to assess them in conjunction with each other. Alternatively, assessment of personal attributes must be based on developmental research and research showing that these attributes are correlated with protective factors and successful behavioral outcome.

The RSCA provides an assessment of three previously identified attributes of personal resiliency and is based on personal experience reflective of three core developmental systems: Sense of Mastery, Sense of Relatedness, and Emotional Reactivity and the relationship of these factors to one another (Prince-Embury, 2006a, 2006b, 2006c, 2007). Focus on the personal experience of the child assumes that this experience mediates between external protective factors and positive behavioral outcomes. The developmental research that demonstrates the relevance of these three constructs to children's subsequent coping and success is discussed below.

Sense of Mastery

Core mechanism that have been consistently identified as important for resiliency in developmental and resilience research are Sense of Mastery and self-efficacy. White (1959) suggested that children's sense of competence or efficacy provides them with the opportunity to interact with and enjoy cause and affect relationships in the environment. According to White, a sense of competence, mastery, or efficacy is driven by an innate curiosity, which is intrinsically rewarding and is the source of problem solving skills. Bandura (1977, 1993) suggested that students' self-efficacy beliefs for regulating their own learning and mastering academic activities determine their aspirations, level of motivation, and academic accomplishments. The construct of competence also found its way into what has been termed the third wave of resilience research. This work examined competence as a strategy for preventing or ameliorating behavioral and emotional problems (Masten & Curtis, 2000; Masten, Burt, & Coatsworth, 2006; Masten, Roisman, Long, Burt, Obradovic, Riley, et al., 2005; Masten & Coatsworth, 1998). Consistent with this, the Project Competence group (Masten & Obradovic, 2006), focused on competence criteria for positive adaptation in age-salient developmental tasks (Masten & Powell, 2003). Several studies conducted as part of the Rochester Child Resilience Project supported the hypothesis that positive expectation is related to resilience. Positive efficacy expectations in 10–12 year-olds predicted better behavioral adaptation and resilience to stress (Cowen, Pryor-Brown, Hightower, & Lotyczewski, 1991). Positive expectations about their future predicted lower anxiety, higher school achievement and better classroom behavior control (Wyman, Cowen, Work, & Kerley, 1993). In summary, previous research and theory suggests that children and youth who have a greater sense of competence/efficacy may be more likely to succeed in a school environment and less likely to develop pathological symptoms. Consistent with these findings, Sense of Mastery, which includes perception of self-efficacy, along with optimism and adaptability, was selected as a core construct underlying personal resiliency for the RSCA.

Sense of Relatedness

Reviewing five decades of resilience research in child development, Luthar (2006, p. 780) concluded, "Resilience rests, fundamentally, on relationships." The importance of relationships for human resilience has been noted in every major review of protective factors for resilience (see Masten & Obradovic, 2006). The importance of relationships and relational ability as mediators of resilience has been supported in research by developmental psychopathologists such as Werner and Smith (1982). Throughout their writing, Werner and Smith have stressed the importance of children having relationships with caring adults other than, or in addition to, their parents. Werner and Smith (1982) noted that resilient youth sought support from non-parental adults (especially teachers, ministers, and neighbors) more often than non-resilient youth. These supportive relationships were influential in fostering resilience.

The implication from this body of literature is that social relatedness is important but the mechanism by which this occurs is explained in a variety of ways. Youth may view relationships as providing specific supports in specific situations. In addition, internal mechanisms that emerge from youths' cumulative experience of previous support may shield youth from negative psychological impact by providing an internalized expectation of support. This expectation might lead to a youth's ability to find and use support when needed. Previous research has indicated that perceived support, as distinguished from actual support, is the dimension of social support that is most strongly related to psychological well-being in adults and children (Barrera, 1986; Cohen & Wills, 1985; Jackson & Warren, 2000; Sarason, Shearon, Pierce, & Sarason, 1987).

Developmental theorists have worked throughout the twentieth century to identify and label internal mechanisms of relatedness. Psychosocial theories of development, such as that of Erikson (1963), identified the first developmental psychosocial process that occurred in infancy through interaction between the child and the primary caregiver as the development of trust versus distrust. The significance of trust was identified by Erikson as the first stage of social-emotional development, upon which all other social development is built. Erikson defined basic trust as the ability to receive and accept what is given. Another theorist, Bowlby (1969), observing the interaction between the infant and primary caregiver, conceptualized this early social interactive process as the development of attachment, which has implications for the individual's ability to relate to others throughout their lifetime. The attachment system was originally described by John Bowlby in three volumes on attachment and loss (1969) and later examined in many studies of attachment in human development (Ainsworth, 1989; Bolby, 1982, 1988; Bretherton & Munholland, 1999; Sroufe, Carlson, Levy, & Egeland, 1999; Thompson, 2000). Consistent with this extensive body of research, the RSCA Sense of Relatedness Scales was designed to tap some aspects of youth's relational experience.

Emotional Reactivity

Developmental research has demonstrated that children's development of pathology in the presence of adversity is related to their Emotional Reactivity and their ability to regulate this reactivity. Specifically, strong Emotional Reactivity and related difficulty with regulation of this reactivity have been associated with behavioral maladjustment and vulnerability to pathology. Emotional Reactivity is the child's arousability or the threshold of tolerance that exists prior to the occurrence of adverse events or circumstances. Rothbart and Derryberry (1981) have defined Emotional Reactivity as the speed and intensity of a child's negative emotional response. Children's reactivity varies in its intensity, sensitivity, specificity, windows of tolerance, and recovery (Siegel, 1999). Conversely, emotional regulation, or the ability to modulate emotional responses is a significant factor in fostering resilience (Cicchetti, Ganiban, & Barnett, 1991; Cicchetti & Tucker, 1994; Eisenberg, Champion, & Ma, 2004). Regulation and redirection of emotional arousal is necessary for children to function adaptively in emotionally challenging situations (Cicchetti et al., 1991; Thompson, 1990).

Consistent with previous research, the RSCA assumes that the degree of a child's Emotional Reactivity potentially aroused by adversity would be important in determining relative vulnerability or risk. Specifically, Emotional Reactivity is defined in the RSCA in terms of the child's self-perceived relative sensitivity or intensity of reaction, recovery or length of time it takes for the child to recover and the degree to which the emotion interferes with functioning.

Description of the Resiliency Scales for Children and Adolescents

The RSCA is a self-report instrument designed to tap the three core developmental systems defined above as experienced and expressed by a child or adolescent. The RSCA consists of three global scales designed to reflect the three designated underlying systems: Sense of Mastery, Sense of Relatedness, and Emotional Reactivity. *T*-Scores on these three global scales comprise a Personal Resilience Profile which graphically displays the child's relative strengths and vulnerabilities. Two composite scores, the Resource Index and the Vulnerability Index, are summary scores that quantify the child's relative strength and vulnerability for use in preventive screening. The three global scales are comprised of ten subscales that can be used to understand the child's specific strengths and vulnerabilities in more depth. All scores are standardized on age and gender based normative samples that are stratified by race/ethnicity and parent education level to match the US Census for 2003 (Prince-Embury, 2007, 2008).

The *Sense of Mastery* Scale is a 20-item self-report questionnaire written at a third-grade reading level. Response options are ordered on a 5-point Likert scale: 0 (Never), 1 (Rarely), 2 (Sometimes), 3 (Often), and 4 (Almost Always). The *Sense of Mastery* Scale consists of three conceptually related content areas: *optimism* about life and one's own competence; *self-efficacy* associated with developing problem-solving attitudes and strategies; and *adaptability*, being personally receptive to criticism, and learning from one's mistakes. Higher scores on this global scale or subscales suggest higher personal resiliency in this developmental system. Internal consistencies for the Sense of Mastery Scale are good with an alpha of 0.85 for youth ages 9–11, 0.89 for youth ages 12–14 and 0.95 for youth ages 15–18. Test–retest reliability coefficients were 0.79 for youth ages 9–14 and 0.86 for youth ages 15–18 (Prince-Embury, 2007).

The *Sense of Relatedness* Scale is a 24-item self-report questionnaire written at a third-grade reading level. Response options are frequency-based, ordered on a 5-point Likert scale: 0 (Never), 1 (Rarely), 2 (Sometimes), 3 (Often), and 4 (Almost Always). Within this scale, a Sense of Relatedness refers to *comfort* with others, *trust* in others, perceived access to *support* by others when in need, and *tolerance* of differences with others. Higher scores on this global scale or subscales suggest higher personal resiliency in this developmental system. Internal consistency is good to excellent for the Sense of Relatedness Scale: 0.89 for children ages 9–11, 0.91 for children ages 12–14, and 0.95 for youth ages 15–18. Test–retest reliability coefficients were good; 0.84 for youth ages 9–14 and 0.86 for youth ages 15–18 (Prince-Embury, 2008).

The *Emotional Reactivity* Scale is a 20-item self-report questionnaire written at the third grade reading level. Response options are ordered on a 5-point Likert scale: 0 (Never), 1 (Rarely), 2 (Sometimes), 3 (Often), and 4 (Almost Always). Unlike the Sense of Mastery and Sense of Relatedness Scales, lower scores on the Emotional Reactivity Scale are indicative of low reactivity and high scores suggest higher vulnerability in this developmental area and consequently less personal resiliency. This scale consists of three related content areas: the *Sensitivity* subscale assesses the child's threshold for emotional reaction and the intensity of the reaction, the *Recovery* subscale describes the length of time required for recovering from emotional upset, and the *Impairment* subscale describes the child's experience of disrupted functioning while upset. Internal consistency for the Emotional Reactivity Scale is excellent with alphas of 0.90 for youth ages 9–11, 0.91 for youth ages 12–14 and 0.94 for youth ages 15–18. Test–retest reliability coefficient was 0.88 for youth ages 9–14 and youth ages 15–18 (Prince-Embury, 2007).

Summary Index Scores

The RSCA Summary Index scores combine information into two scores, which may be unfolded to provide more detailed information at the global and subscale levels. The Index scores were developed based on empirical analyses of RSCA Scale score profiles, factor analytic studies and validity studies (Prince-Embury, 2006a, 2006b, 2006c, 2007; Prince-Embury & Courville, 2008a, 2008b). Resilience theory traditionally divided factors of resilience into those that were protective versus those that increased risk. Protective factors were viewed as characteristics that buffered the negative effect of adversity on the individual. Risk factors were viewed as increasing the potential for negative outcome in the face of adversity. Within this framework, higher Sense of Mastery and Sense of Relatedness may be viewed as protective, while higher Emotional Reactivity may be viewed as a personal risk factor.

Factor analytic studies indicate that although the three RSCA Scales represent three distinct factors, two of these factors, Sense of Mastery and Sense of Relatedness, are highly correlated consistent with the assumption that both represent protective factors of resiliency (Prince-Embury & Courville, 2008a). Thus theory and analyses of empirical data suggested the first index score, the *Resource Index*, which is calculated as the standardized average of the Sense of Mastery and Sense of Relatedness Scale scores. This average is an estimate of students' personal strength or resources, weighting *Sense of Mastery* and *Sense of Relatedness* equally. It must be emphasized that equal weighting of these factors is an estimate for simplification and that more precise weights of these factors in protective significance may differ across groups and/or individuals. Internal consistency for the *Resource Index* was excellent with alpha coefficients of 0.93 for youth ages 9–11, 0.94 for youth ages 12–14 and 0.97 for youth ages 15–18. Test–retest reliability coefficient was 0.90 for youth ages 9–14 and 0.85 for youth ages 15–18 (Prince-Embury, 2007). Resilience theory suggests that youth who perceive themselves as having sufficient personal Resources will be more resilient and less likely to develop psychopathology as a consequence of adversity than those who experience themselves as having insufficient personal resources.

Developmental theory suggests that an individual's resiliency relates to whether the individual has sufficient resources and whether these resources are sufficient to offset the amount of personal risk experienced by the individual. The *Vulnerability Index* is designed to estimate the discrepancy between an individual's personal risk and perceived available personal resources. The *Vulnerability Index* score is calculated as the standardized difference between the *Emotional Reactivity* *T*-score and the *Resource Index* *T*-score. It quantifies children's personal vulnerability as the relative discrepancy between their combined self-perceived resources (the *Resource Index*) and their fragility as described by Emotional Reactivity the *Emotional Reactivity Scale* (Prince-Embury, 2007). Internal consistency for the *Vulnerability Index* score is excellent with alpha coefficients of 0.93 for youth ages 9–11, 0.94 for youth ages 12–14, and 0.97 for youth ages 15–18. Test–retest reliability coefficient was 0.83 for youth ages 9–14 and 0.93 for youth ages 15–18. Personal vulnerability would be indicated by a high *Vulnerability Index* score which would indicate that students' personal resources were significantly below their level of Emotional Reactivity.

Psychometric Adequacy of the RCSA

Reliability

Cicchetti (1994) suggests that coefficient alphas at or above 0.70 are adequate, at or above 0.80 are good, and at or above 0.90 are excellent.

Table 3.1 Alpha coefficients for the RSCA Global Scales across six countries

Scale	Canada 2009 (543)	Canada 2010 (390)	China (726)	Brazil (1,226)	Lebanon (599)	Nairobi, Kenya (83)	South Africa (487)
Mastery	0.90	0.92	0.95	0.83	0.78	0.70	0.74
Relatedness	0.92	0.93	0.94	0.90	0.86	0.74	0.83
Emotional Reactivity	0.90	0.91	0.89	0.87	0.87	0.80	0.76

Alpha coefficients of 0.90 are thought of as adequate for tracking individual scores over time. Alpha coefficients of 0.80 or more are considered adequate for tracking group scores over time. Using these criteria, reliability evidence was excellent for the RSCA Index scores, good for the Global Score, and adequate for most subscales. The RSCA Index and global scale scores show good or excellent internal consistency across age and gender groups and, as expected, greater internal consistency was evidenced with increased age (Prince-Embury, 2007). For children ages 9–11, the *RSCA Index* scores and the *Emotional Reactivity Scale* score meet the criterion of alpha coefficient >0.90 for individual-level tracking. The *Sense of Mastery* and *Sense of Relatedness Scale* scores meet the criterion of alpha coefficient >0.80 for group level tracking. For children ages 12–14, the *RSCA Index* scores and all three Global Scores meet the criterion for individual level tracking. Six of the *RSCA* subscales met criterion for group level tracking. For youth ages 15–18, both Index scores, three global scale scores, and three subscale scores meet the criterion for individual level tracking. For this age group all scores meet the criterion for group-level tracking. Hence the RSCA demonstrates good internal consistency, supporting the conceptual and theoretical derivation of the scale, subscales and indices. Cross-cultural studies indicate adequate to excellent internal consistency for the three global RSCA Scale Scores (see Table 3.1). The RSCA has been employed previously with youth in Canada (Saklofske & Nordstatt, 2011), South Africa (Van Wyk, 2011), Kenya (Tignor & Prince-Embury, 2013), China (Cui, Teng, & Oei, 2010), Brazil (Jordani, 2008), and Lebanon (Ayyash-Abdo & Sanchez-Ruiz, 2011).

Research and Validity Evidence

Establishing validity evidence for the RSCA is a conceptually complex process because the construct has been approached in many ways and has raised many conceptual questions. A few of these questions are the following. Is resiliency operable only in adverse circumstances or do these factors operate under normal circumstances as well? Are adverse circumstances required to identify resiliency? Does resiliency operate across circumstances or is it situation specific? Is resiliency a state or a trait and if a trait is it modifiable? Is resiliency one-dimensional or multidimensional?

The RSCA design assumes that resiliency is multidimensional, that these dimensions are relevant across circumstances but vary in relative salience depending on the validity question being asked. Therefore, validity evidence below will be presented with respect to protective factors first; Sense of Mastery, Sense of Relatedness and the summary Resource Index. Secondly validity evidence will be provided pertaining to risk facts; Emotional Reactivity and the summary Vulnerability Index. The RSCA design assumes that personal resiliency is based on core developmental processes that exist in normative as well as populations exposed to adversity. Therefore much of the validity evidence presented below is based on the presence of protective and risk factors in normative samples, as well as in the comparison of normative and clinical samples.

Protective Factors: Self-Concept

Validity evidence for the RSCA as a reflection of protective factors may be explored in the relationship between RSCA scores and measures of Self-concept. Previous theorists have suggested that resiliency is associated with positive Self-concept or self-esteem (see Rutter, 1987, 1993), Luthar, & Brooks). Research by Dumont and Provost (1999) and others have previously provided support for this relationship. Prince-Embury (2007) described the relationship between the positive Self-concept score of the BYI-II and the RSCA protective factor scores for children and adolescents (see Table 3.2). Significant positive correlations were found for both child and adolescent samples, between a positive BYI Self-concept score and the RSCA Resource Index score (0.78, 0.79), the Sense of Mastery Scale score (0.74, 0.80), and the Sense of Relatedness Scale score (0.70, 0.70), suggesting convergent validity for these scores as reflective of positive Self-concept as a protective factor. At the subscale level the RSCA Self-efficacy subscale was most significantly related to positive Self-concept as assessed by the BYI-II for both children (0.75) and adolescents (0.77) suggesting that perceived Self-efficacy is an area of overlap between a positive Self-concept and personal resiliency.

These Self-concept findings were supported in a separate study using the Pier-Harris Children's Self-concept Scale, Second Edition (Piers-Harris 2; Piers, 2002) (see Table 3.2 and Prince-Embury, 2007). The RSCA Sense of Mastery, Sense of Relatedness and Resource Index scores were positively correlated with the Pier Harris 2 Total Score (0.60, 0.55, 0.59). The Behavior Adjustment Domain subscale of the Piers Harris 2 was most strongly related to the RSCA scores (0.70, 0.61, 0.69). The RSCA subscale most strongly correlated with Piers Harris 2 Total and Domain scores was the optimism subscale of the Sense of Mastery Scale.

Emotional Intelligence

Emotional Intelligence defined as awareness of and understanding of emotions has been defined as a protective factor. Total score on the Self-reported Emotional Intelligence Test (SSEIT; Schutte et al., 1998) was positively correlated with the RSCA Resource Index score (0.59), Sense of Mastery (0.54), and Sense of Relatedness (0.46) Scale scores, for 157 adolescents attending a charter school located in a low income area of a New England city (Luthar, 2006, unpublished study). The fact that the RSCA Resource Index score correlates more strongly than either the Sense of Mastery or Sense of Relatedness scores with emotional intelligence suggests that the combination of these protective factors is more salient than either of these considered separately for this variable.

Protective Factor: Parent Attachment

As discussed above in the introduction section of this chapter, most formulations of resiliency include positive relationships with others as a significant protective factor. Developmental theory has identified quality of Parent Attachment as a major variable underlying all attachments. Construct validity of the RSCA and the Sense of Relatedness Scale in particular may be explored in relation to parental attachment as examined by the Inventory of Parent and Peer Attachment (IPPA; Armsten & Greenberg, 1987). One study of 157 adolescents attending high school in a low SES area of Connecticut correlated overall attachment scores for mother and father with RSCA Index and global scale scores (Luthar, 2006) (see Table 3.2). Overall attachment score with mother was significantly and positively correlated with the RSCA Resource Index score (0.52), Sense of Mastery Scale score (0.48), and Sense of Relatedness Scale score (0.50). Overall attachment with father was related to a lesser extent to the three RSCA protective scores (0.36, 0.29, and 0.33). Convergent validity evidence was provided by the positive and significant relationships between RSCA protective scores and mother and father attachment scores. Correlations between Sense of Relatedness scores and attachment scores are slightly but not significantly higher than those between Sense of Mastery scores and attachment. The Resource Index score correlates most strongly with parental attachment suggesting that combined resources of Sense of Relatedness and Mastery are related to strength of Parent Attachment.

Table 3.2 Correlations of RSCA Index and Global Scale Scales with Self-Concept, Parent Attachment, and Emotional Intelligence scores

RSCA Index and Global Scale Scores	Piers-Harris Self-Concept Total Score (49)	Piers-Harris Self-Concept Behavior Adjustment (49)	BYI-II Self-Concept (46)[a]	BYI-II Self-Concept (200)[a]	IPPA Mother Attachment (157)[b]	IPPA Father Attachment (157)[b]	Emotional Intelligence (SREIT) (157)[b]
Vulnerability	−0.61	−0.62	−0.64	−0.76	−0.48	−0.37	−0.47
Resource	0.59	0.69	0.78	0.79	0.52	0.36	0.59
Mastery	0.60	0.70	0.74	0.80	0.48	0.29	0.54
Relatedness	0.55	0.61	0.70	0.70	0.50	0.33	0.50
Emotional Reactivity	−0.49	−0.43	−0.31	−0.58	−0.27	−0.22	−0.24
Age Range	(9–14)	(15–18)	(9–14)	(15–18)	(15–18)	(15–18)	(15–18)

All correlations were statistically significant at $p<0.05$
[a]Stratified sample, (Prince-Embury, 2007)
[b]Luthar Bridgeport sample

Risk Factors and Measures of Negative Affect and Behavior

As stated earlier, the RSCA assumes that personal risk would be reflected by higher Emotional Reactivity Scale scores and higher Vulnerability Index scores. Convergent validity for these variables may be assessed by strength of their correlations with measures of negative affect and behavior. Strong positive correlations were found between the Emotional Reactivity Scale score and all Beck Youth Inventory—Second Edition (BYI-II; Beck, Beck, Jolly, & Steer, 2005) scores in non-clinical samples of children and adolescents; (0.43, 0.65) with Anxiety, (0.70, 0.67) with Disruptive Behavior, (0.44, 0.74) with Depression and (0.59, 0.76) with Anger (see Table 3.3 below). The Vulnerability Index score was also associated with the BYI-II scores; (0.36, 0.65) with Anxiety, (0.71, 0.66) with Disruptive Behavior, (0.51, 0.75) with Depression, and (0.59, 0.77) with Anger (see Table 3.3 below). These strong correlations suggest that higher Emotional Reactivity and associated higher Vulnerability are associated with more negative affect and behavior for children and adolescents. These relationships appears to be stronger for adolescents than for children although this finding would need to be replicated in studies of larger groups of children.

It should also be noted that the RSCA Resource Index, Sense of Mastery, and Sense of Relatedness scores were negatively correlated with all of the BYI-II scores of negative affect and behavior. These negative correlations are consistent with the notion that personal resources have a buffering effect against negative affect and behavior. This buffering effect is suggested more strongly for adolescents than for children (see Table 3.3).

Similar results were found in correlational studies of the RSCA with other assessments of problem behaviors such as the Connors Adolescent Symptom Scale: Short Form (CASS; Connors, 1997) (see Prince-Embury, 2007). In a sample of 89 youth ages 15–18, conduct, cognitive, and ADHD problems as assessed by the CASS:S were associated with higher Emotional Reactivity Scale scores (0.48–0.65) and higher Vulnerability Index score (0.48–0.68) providing additional support for the Emotional Reactivity Scale score and associated Vulnerability Index as risk variables. In addition, lower Resource Index, Sense of Mastery and Relatedness Scale score were associated with higher CASS scores (–0.37 to –0.64) indicating that lower personal resources are associated with more behavioral difficulties (see Table 3.4).

Personal Resiliency, Bullying, and Victimization

A study correlating RSCA scores with Bullying and Victimization Scale scores of the *Reynolds Bully Victimization Scales* (Reynolds, 2004) for 47 children ages 9–14 suggested some gender differences between the relationship of these behaviors with vulnerability and resources in children (see Table 3.4 below and Prince-Embury, 2007). For boys, Vulnerability and Emotional Reactivity were significantly positively related to self-reported bullying (0.60, 0.60) and victimization (0.54, 0.45). Resource scores were inversely and less significantly related to bullying (–0.21 to –0.38) and victimization (0.02 to –0.21) for boys. For girls on the other hand, lower perceived personal resources were inversely and significantly related to both bullying and victimization. The Resource Index, Sense of Mastery and Sense of Relatedness Scale scores were negatively correlated with self-reported bullying and victimization in the following manner (Resource Index, –0.75, –0.57), (Sense of Mastery, –0.77, –0.44), (Sense of Relatedness, –0.63, –0.61). Emotional Reactivity was less related to bullying and victimization for girls (0.26, 0.08). It must be noted that these results are preliminary and should be replicated and expanded upon in larger studies of bullying and victimization. However, if replicated these results would suggest that bullying prevention programs might differ for males and females. Interventions might focus more on managing Emotional Reactivity for males and on enhancing Sense of Mastery and Relatedness for females (Table 3.5).

Table 3.3 Correlations of RSCA Global Scale and Index Scores with BYI-II scores of negative affect and behavior for children and adolescents

	BYI-II Anxiety (46) (9–11)	BYI-II Anxiety (200) (15–18)	BYI-II Depress (46) (9–11)	BYI-II Depress (200) (15–18)	BYI-II Anger (46) (9–11)	BYI-II Anger (200) (15–18)	BYI Disruptive Behavior (46) (9–11)	BYI Disruptive Behavior (200) (15–18)
Vulnerability	0.36	0.65	0.51	0.75	0.59	0.77	0.71	0.66
Resource	–0.11	–0.53	–0.38	–0.61	–0.36	–0.62	–0.43	–0.51
Mastery	–0.07	–0.51	–0.31	–0.59	–0.32	–0.61	–0.42	–0.53
Relatedness	–0.13	–0.50	–0.38	–0.56	–0.34	–0.57	–0.37	–0.45
Emotional Reactivity	0.43	0.65	0.44	0.74	0.59	0.76	0.70	0.67

Table 3.4 Correlations between RSCA Index and Global Scale scores CASS: S scores of ADHD, conduct and cognitive problems

	CASS:S Conduct Problems (89)	CASS:S Cognitive Problems (89)	CASS:S Hyperact (89)	CASS:S ADHD Index (89)
Vulnerability	0.62	0.59	0.48	0.68
Resource	–0.56	–0.51	–0.43	–0.63
Mastery	–0.57	–0.45	–0.37	–0.60
Relatedness	–0.51	–0.54	–0.48	–0.64
Emotional Reactivity	0.59	0.59	0.48	0.65
Age Range	(15–18)	(15–18)	(15–18)	(15–18)

All correlations significant at the $p<0.05$

Table 3.5 Correlations of Reynolds Bully/Victimization Scale scores with RSCA Global, Index and subscale scores (Table reprinted from RSCA Technical Manual, Prince-Embury, 2007)

	Male ($n=24$)		Female ($n=23$)		Total ($n=47$)	
Scale/Subscale/Index	Bully	Victim	Bully	Victim	Bully	Victim
Sense of Mastery	–0.21	0.02	–0.77	–0.44	–0.44	–0.16
Optimism	0.08	0.01	–0.58	–0.44	–0.20	–0.16
Self-efficacy	–0.27	0.03	–0.65	–0.33	–0.41	–0.10
Adaptability	–0.38	–0.28	–0.76	–0.45	–0.52	–0.32
Sense of Relatedness	–0.38	–0.21	–0.63	–0.61	–0.40	–0.29
Trust	–0.26	–0.29	–0.58	–0.62	–0.33	–0.34
Support	–0.09	–0.14	–0.51	–0.61	–0.21	–0.25
Comfort	–0.28	0.03	–0.66	–0.65	–0.45	–0.21
Tolerance	–0.55	–0.27	–0.49	–0.27	–0.36	–0.16
Emotional Reactivity	0.60	0.54	0.26	0.08	0.49	0.42
Sensitivity	0.64	0.50	0.02	–0.15	0.40	0.31
Recovery	0.23	0.34	0.14	–0.06	0.09	0.08
Impairment	0.53	0.48	0.34	0.21	0.51	0.44
Resource Index	–0.32	–0.10	–0.75	–0.57	–0.46	–0.24
Vulnerability Index	0.60	0.45	0.59	0.38	0.58	0.41
Reynolds BVS						
Mean	51.17	52.21	46.00	47.48	48.64	49.89
SD	8.09	10.79	5.74	5.62	7.44	8.89

Personal Resiliency and Risk Behavior

Risk behavior was assessed by the *Adolescent Risk Behavior Inventory* (ARBS; Prince-Embury, 2006a) which consists of item clusters tapping self-reported frequency of alcohol and drug abuse, sexual behavior, self-harm ideation, and sensation seeking. The sample which comprised the normative adolescent sample for the RSCA was stratified by race/ethnicity and parent education level within gender and age (see Prince-Embury, 2007, for details of the sample). Results were the following. The Emotional Reactivity Scale and Vulnerability Index scores were positively correlated with self-reported frequency of substance use (0.51, 0.50), sexual behavior (0.42, 0.39), self-harm ideation (0.67, 0.68), and sensation seeking (0.33, 0.31). These findings suggest that higher Emotional Reactivity and associated Vulnerability

Table 3.6 Correlations of frequency of risk behaviors and negative life outcomes with RSCA Index and Global Scale Scores (all correlations significant at $p<0.05$)

	Substance use (200)	Sexual behavior (200)	Self-harm (200)	Sensation seeking (200)	Negative life outcomes (200)
Vulnerability	0.50	0.39	0.68	0.31	0.54
Resource	–0.40	–0.29	–0.55	–0.23	–0.48
Mastery	–0.40	–0.23	–0.52	–0.19	–0.47
Relatedness	–0.40	–0.29	–0.53	–0.24	–0.44
Emotional Reactivity	0.51	0.42	0.67	0.33	0.49

are related to higher frequency of risk behaviors in adolescents.

On the other hand, the Resource Index, Sense of Mastery and Sense of Relatedness Scale scores were negatively correlated with frequency of risk behaviors suggestive of a slight buffering effect. Sense of Relatedness was negatively correlated with frequency of substance use (–0.40), sexual behavior (–0.29), self-harm ideation and behavior (–0.53), and sensation seeking (–0.24). Sense of Mastery was negatively correlated with frequency of substance use (–0.40), sexual behavior (–0.23), self-harm ideation and behavior (–0.52), and sensation seeking (–0.19). Correlations above 0.30 were significant at the $p<0.001$ level and correlations above 0.20 were significant at the $p<0.05$ level. Overall, these findings suggest that Emotional Reactivity is more strongly related to risk behavior than protective factors.

Personal Resiliency and Negative Life Events

(Frequency of Negative Life Events was assessed by *The Negative Life Events Inventory*, Prince-Embury, 2006b). The sample of 200 was split by gender and stratified by race/ethnicity and parent education level to match the US Census. Negative Life Events were divided into Negative Life Events (NLE) that occurred to the teen over which he or she had no control, such as the death of a loved one or parental loss of job. Negative outcomes (NLO) were events over which the youth might have some control, such as dropping out of school or trouble with the law. Correlational analysis shown in Table 3.6 illustrates that the number of negative life outcomes is moderately correlated with RSCA global scale scores and index scores, particularly the Emotional Reactivity Scale score (0.49) and the Vulnerability Index score (0.54). Additional analyses suggested a possible gender difference. For males the Emotional Reactivity Scale score was correlated with Negative Life Outcomes (0.53) more than were the Sense of Mastery Scale (–0.41) or Sense of Relatedness Scale scores (–0.35).

For females on the other hand, the Sense of Mastery Scale (–0.52) and the Sense of Relatedness Scale (–0.53) were slightly more correlated with Negative Life Outcomes in a negative direction than was the Emotional Reactivity Scale score (0.46) in a positive direction. These possible gender differences are consistent with those found for the relationship between resiliency and bullying and victimization behavior.

Evidence of Criterion Group Differences

The relationship between RSCA scores and presence or absence of clinical pathology has been supported by analyses of criterion group differences. Prince-Embury (2007) reported significant differences between mean scores of ten clinical groups and matched control groups for children and adolescents (Depression Disorder, Anxiety Disorder, Conduct Disorder, ADHD, Bipolar Disorder). Overall, the non-clinical groups scored significantly higher than the clinical groups on self-reported protective factors; the Resource

Table 3.7 Mean *T* scores and SD of the Child Depressive Disorder sample and matched control group

	Clinical sample		Matched control					
Scale/Subscale	Mean	SD	Mean	SD	Diff	*t*	Significance	d^a
Sense of Mastery	42.2	10.8	52.1	9.3	9.90	3.51	0.0024	0.98
Optimism	6.9	3.3	10.9	2.8	4.00	4.41	0.0003	1.30
Self-efficacy	8.7	3.6	10.3	3.0	1.60	1.70	0.1055	0.48
Adaptability	8.3	2.7	10.5	3.4	2.20	2.16	0.0435	0.71
Sense of Relatedness	37.9	11.7	52.2	9.9	14.30	4.68	0.0002	1.33
Trust	6.5	3.2	10.7	3.3	4.25	4.82	0.0001	1.29
Support	6.9	3.7	10.6	2.9	3.70	3.40	0.0030	1.13
Comfort	7.8	3.5	10.4	2.6	2.60	3.04	0.0068	0.85
Tolerance	7.3	3.4	10.5	2.7	3.25	3.61	0.0019	1.05
Emotional Reactivity	63.0	7.3	47.7	10.1	−15.30	−6.60	<0.0001	−1.74
Sensitivity	13.5	2.3	9.9	2.4	−3.65	−6.32	<0.0001	−1.55
Recovery	11.9	3.0	9.7	3.2	−2.20	−2.45	0.0239	−0.72
Impairment	13.6	2.4	9.0	3.1	−4.55	−6.86	<0.0001	−1.66
Resource Index	39.0	10.0	52.4	9.6	13.45	4.64	0.0002	1.37
Vulnerability Index	64.5	8.9	47.2	9.9	−17.35	−7.15	<0.0001	−1.84

Note. Clinical sample $n=20$, matched control $n=20$. Using the Bonferroni correction (Hays, 1994, p. 450): $\alpha^{PC} \geq \alpha^{PW}/k = 0.05/15 = 0.0033$, differences between groups are significant where $p \leq 0.0033$
[a]*d* is the difference of the two test means divided by the square root of the people variance computed using Cohen's (1996) Formula 10.4 (table from Prince-Embury, 2007, RSCA technical manual)

Index score, Sense of Mastery, Sense of Relatedness Scales, and subscales. On the other hand, the clinical groups scored significantly higher on the Vulnerability Index, Emotional Reactivity Scale, and subscale scores. Effect sizes were large for all differences and in most cases significant. Tables 3.7 and 3.8 demonstrate differences in resiliency factors between youth diagnosed with Depressive Disorder and matched control group.

Table 3.7 reports RSCA scores for a sample of 20 depressed children and a matched sample of children ages 9–14 from the normative sample. The RSCA Index Scores and global scale scores for the clinical sample are significantly different from those of the matched control in the direction that would be expected. The depressed group differed from the control group most in Vulnerability (*T*65 versus *T*47), next in higher Emotional Reactivity (*T*63 versus *T*48) and then in Sense of Relatedness (*T*38 versus *T*52) and Sense of Mastery (*T*42 versus *T*52). Examination of subscale scores suggests that the clinically depressed group differs most in self-reported impairment, sensitivity, optimism, and trust. These findings are consistent with the diagnosis of Depressive Disorder.

Table 3.8 reports RSCA scores for a sample of 45 depressed adolescents and a matched sample of youth ages 15–18 from a normative sample. The RSCA Index Scores and global scale scores for the clinical sample are significantly different from those of the matched control in the direction that would be expected. The depressed group differed significantly from the matched control group on all measures with large effect sizes. The biggest differences were on the Vulnerability (*T*65 versus *T*47) and Resource Index (*T*35 versus *T*52) scores, Sense of Mastery Scale (*T*35 versus *T*53), Sense of Relatedness (*T*36 versus *T*51), and Emotional Reactivity Scale score (*T*62 versus *T*48). Similar to the sample of depressed children Vulnerability and Emotional Reactivity were in the high range for the clinical group while Resource, Mastery and Relatedness scores were in the low range. The matched control groups reported all scores within the average range.

Table 3.8 Mean *T* scores and SD of the Adolescent Depressive Disorder sample and matched control group

	Clinical sample		Matched control					
Scale/Subscale	Mean	SD	Mean	SD	Diff	*t*	Significance	d^a
Sense of Mastery	35.4	8.2	53.2	8.5	17.82	10.82	<0.0001	2.14
Optimism	5.7	2.7	10.6	2.8	4.93	9.22	<0.0001	1.81
Self-efficacy	6.1	2.6	11.2	2.4	5.09	9.42	<0.0001	2.00
Adaptability	6.9	2.5	10.6	2.4	3.71	8.41	<0.0001	1.53
Sense of Relatedness	35.7	10.7	51.3	7.9	15.53	8.71	<0.0001	1.66
Trust	5.7	2.9	10.4	2.5	4.71	8.98	<0.0001	1.73
Support	6.5	3.3	10.5	2.5	3.98	6.66	<0.0001	1.38
Comfort	6.6	3.3	9.8	2.7	3.24	5.31	<0.0001	1.07
Tolerance	6.7	3.3	10.6	2.4	3.69	7.15	<0.0001	1.33
Emotional Reactivity	61.6	8.6	47.7	7.2	−13.84	−7.04	<0.0001	−1.75
Sensitivity	13.0	3.3	9.5	2.3	−3.47	−5.23	<0.0001	−1.22
Recovery	12.9	3.2	10.2	2.8	−2.73	−3.88	0.0003	−0.91
Impairment	13.2	2.7	9.2	2.3	−4.00	−6.87	<0.0001	−1.62
Resource Index	34.8	9.5	52.4	8.2	17.62	10.30	<0.0001	2.00
Vulnerability Index	64.9	8.2	47.4	7.2	−17.53	−10.25	<0.0001	−2.27

Note: Clinical sample $n=45$; matched control $n=45$. Using the Bonferroni correction (Hays, 1994, p. 450): $\alpha^{PC} \geq \alpha^{PW}/k = 0.05/15 = 0.0033$, difference between groups are significant where $p \leq 0.0033$
[a]*d* is the difference of the two means divided by the square root of the pooled variance computed using Cohen's (1996) Formula 10.4 (table from Prince-Embury, 2007, technical manual)

Predicting Clinical Status

Additional analysis suggested that the RSCA Vulnerability Index score was a good predictor of clinical status in adolescents; in some cases predicting better than the presence of psychological symptoms. Discriminant function analysis (Prince-Embury, 2008) was employed to examine the relative predictive validity of the RSCA Index and scale scores, demographic variables, and the psychological symptoms assessed by the BYI-II (Beck et al., 2005). Variables entered as independent variable included the following: (1) parent level of education, (2) gender, and (3) RSCA Scale scores (Sense of Mastery, Sense of Relatedness, and Emotional Reactivity *T*-scores), Index scores (Vulnerability and Resource), and the Beck Youth Inventory II scores for Anxiety, Depression, Anger, and Disruptive Behavior. Groups to be discriminated were coded according to clinical status as 0 (non-clinical) or 1 (clinical). The classification sensitivity was 73% and specificity was 81% with the RSCA Vulnerability Index score emerging as the predictor of the most variance followed by the BYI-II Anxiety score accounting for a small part of the remaining unique variance.

In summary, validity evidence relating RSCA scores and psychological symptoms, risk behavior and clinical pathology included the following. Significant and high correlations were found between Negative Affect and Behavior (BYI-II scores) and all of the RSCA Scale and Index scores. The strongest correlations were between the RSCA Vulnerability Index and Emotional Reactivity scores and the BYI-II scores on Depression, Anger, Disruptive Behavior, Anxiety; as well as self-reported self-harm ideation and behavior and Substance Abuse. Some gender differences are suggested in aspects of vulnerability/resiliency that are most salient for bully/victimization and negative life outcomes. For males higher Emotional Reactivity appears to be a salient risk factor for bullying behavior and negative life outcomes. For females higher Sense of Relatedness and Sense of Mastery appear to be more salient protective factors against bullying, victimization, and negative life outcomes.

Discriminant function analysis using gender, parent education level, Resilience Scale and

Index scores, and BYI-II Negative Affect and Behavior scores to predict membership in the clinical versus non-clinical sample indicated the RSCA Vulnerability Index was the best single predictor. These findings suggest that high Emotional Reactivity in combination with low personal resources is associated with the development of psychological symptoms in youth.

Personal Resiliency Profiles: Normative

The Personal Resiliency Profile, based on RSCA global scale scores (Sense of Mastery, Sense of Relatedness, and Emotional Reactivity) when graphed provides a visual tool for better understanding the relative strengths of multiple aspects of personal resiliency. The profile presents the three global scale scores standardized using the same *T* metric, which when viewed together, emphasize relative perceived resources and vulnerabilities of children and adolescents. Personal Resiliency Profiles may be examined for individuals or in aggregate. Characteristic Personal Resiliency Profiles in the RSCA normative standardization sample ages 9–18 (stratified by race/ethnicity and parent education level to match the US census) were identified using cluster analysis, a statistical technique for summarizing the variability of profiles into those that most characterize the sample (Prince-Embury & Steer, 2010). This method produced three Personal Resiliency Profiles that most characterize the normative sample of children and adolescents in the USA. These profiles are displayed in Fig. 3.1. Profile A may be characterized as a high Personal Resiliency Profile characterized by high Sense of Mastery and Sense of Relatedness Scale scores (higher than *T*55) and a lower Emotional Reactivity Scale score (lower than *T*50). This high Personal Resiliency Profile cluster represented 31% of the normative sample. Profile B may be characterized as sufficiently resilient, characterized by Sense of Mastery, Sense of Relatedness, and Emotional Reactivity Scale scores within the average range (between *T*45 and *T*55). Profile B represented 44% of the normative sample. Profile C may be characterized as a Vulnerable Personal Resiliency Profile and was characterized by lower than average Sense of Mastery and Sense of Relatedness Scale scores (below *T*45) along with a higher than average Emotional Reactivity Scale Score (above *T*55). Profile C represented 25% of the normative sample. These normative resiliency profiles raise interesting issues. High resiliency group A supports the claim of Masten (2001) of resiliency as "ordinary magic" which is not unusual but characteristic of many children. The existence of Profile C in the normative sample raises questions in that it is similar to the resiliency profiles found in clinical samples (see Fig. 3.2). Are these youth who are vulnerable but who have not developed psychological symptoms or are they youth who have psychological symptoms but who have not been formally diagnosed? These and other questions await future research for illumination.

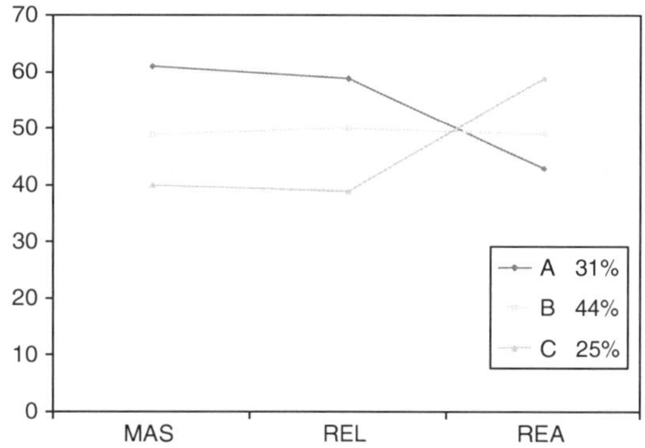

Fig. 3.1 RSCA Profiles of personal resiliency in a normative sample. $n=641$

It must be noted that these characteristic profiles represent statistical summaries which may be used as guides, but that the individual profiles within each group varied. Youth whose profiles were characterized by Profiles A and B demonstrated more within group similarity while youth whose profiles were characterized by Profile C were most varied from each other. Also, these profiles were based on a normative sample stratified by parent education level, race/ethnicity to match the US census. Characteristic profiles may differ for groups that differ demographically or which are representative of unique settings

Fig. 3.2 RSCA resiliency profiles for adolescent clinical groups (reproduced from RSCA Technical Manual, Prince-Embury, 2007)

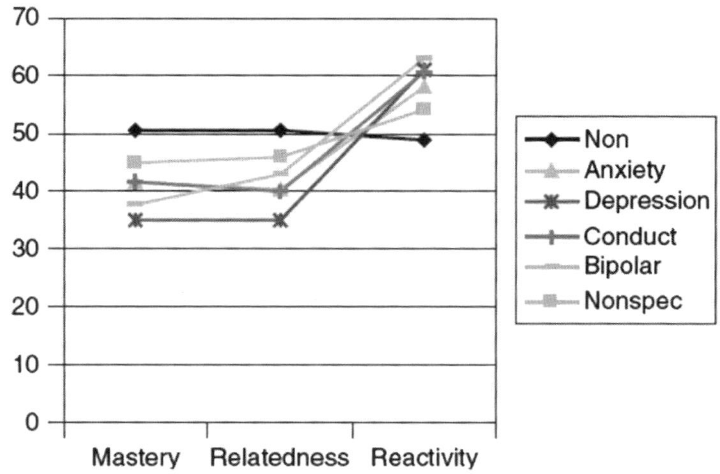

(see Kumar, Steer, & Gulab, 2010; Mowder, Cummings, & McKinney, 2010 for examples). The identification of characteristic Personal Resiliency Profiles in a normative sample have implications for preventive intervention. For example preventive screening might focus on youth whose individual profiles are most characterized by Profile C which suggests low personal resources and higher Emotional Reactivity.

Personal Resiliency Profiles: Clinical

Figure 3.2 displays aggregate Resiliency Profiles for six groups of adolescents: non-clinical, Anxiety Disorder, Depression, Conduct Disorder, Bipolar Disorder, and a group that had been in therapy previously (Prince-Embury, 2007). The Personal Resiliency Profile of the non-clinical group approximates a straight line around a *T*-score of 50 which is most similar to Profile B identified in the normative sample. The Resiliency Profiles of the four clinical groups vary somewhat but share these characteristics in common: high Emotional Reactivity Scale scores (above *T*55), low Sense of Mastery, and Sense of Relatedness Scale scores (below *T*45). These similarities suggest that in spite of differences in disorder, there are overarching themes of higher Emotional Reactivity and lower personal resources. It must be noted that the global scale scores in Fig. 3.2 represented aggregated means and that there is considerable variability within diagnostic groups (see Prince-Embury & Steer, 2010).

Preventive Screening Using the RSCA Index Scores

The relationships between the three global RSCA Scale scores illustrated in the profiles above may be quantified and expressed in the two Index scores described earlier in this chapter. The Resource Index combines the Sense of Mastery and Sense of Relatedness Scale scores. The Vulnerability Index score quantifies the difference between the Emotional Reactivity Scale score and the Resource Index score. As illustrated in Fig. 3.2, the graphic presentation of the Personal Resiliency Profile allows us to view this discrepancy across clinical groups. Validity evidence discussed earlier in this chapter suggests that the Vulnerability Index is correlated with negative affect and discriminates significantly between clinical and non-clinical samples (Prince-Embury, 2008). Therefore, preventive screening may use the Vulnerability Index to identify students who may be at-risk for developing clinical symptoms and other difficulties. Students who have Vulnerability Index *T*-scores in the above-average or higher ranges (*T*60 or above) may be screened for further examination and intervention (see Prince-Embury, 2010a, 2010b for additional information).

Resiliency-Based Interventions

According to the RSCA screening framework provided above, resiliency based interventions start with identifying children or adolescents who are the most Vulnerable according to the Vulnerability Index score (*T*60 or greater). Once vulnerability is identified then the RSCA scores may be examined further to determine whether the vulnerability is due to high Emotional Reactivity or low Resources, or both. Based on the research findings presented above and the clinical experience of the author, Emotional Reactivity is most related to the presence of and strength of psychological symptoms and risk behaviors. For these reasons, in the event of an elevated Emotional Reactivity Scale score, interventions to reduce Emotional Reactivity may be addressed first. The clinical experience of the author suggests that high Emotional Reactivity has a negative effect on relatedness and mastery and interferes with interventions to address these issues unless Emotional Reactivity is below *T*60. The presence of high Emotional Reactivity ($\geq T60$) suggests the application of interventions that are known to address this issue early in the treatment process.

Interventions to Reduce Personal Vulnerability: Emotional Reactivity

Interventions designed to reduce Emotional Reactivity should be informed by an understanding of the developmental underpinnings of high reactivity. Developmental researchers have informed us that a predisposition for high Emotional Reactivity may be related to temperament and may be exacerbated by many factors including intrauterine contamination, and early traumatic experiences that have been shown to alter the nervous system. Research of various psychiatric disorders suggest a "kindling" effect through which triggering of the nervous system that occurs in the initiation of a symptom event lowers the threshold at which this symptom event may occur in the future. In this respect the negative impact of heightened Emotional Reactivity may be cumulative. A temperament based predisposition to high Emotional Reactivity, may be exacerbated by early traumatic events, which may increase the likelihood of a triggered symptom event, which in turn may increase the likelihood of future symptom events. This series of circumstances suggests the value of prevention at any point along the way including, pre-natal care, parent education, and good public health policy decisions. Once high Emotional Reactivity is present, intervention may include increased awareness, education, emotion regulation training, and medication.

For youth who have higher-than-average Emotional Reactivity, (*T*60 or above), preventive intervention may focus initially on intentional management of Emotional Reactivity. This preventive strategy might start by helping the youth to identify Emotional Reactivity as a potential source of vulnerability. Some youth may already be aware of this, but others may need time to fully understand the connection. Awareness may be enhanced by breaking Emotional Reactivity down into the more discrete and observable components of sensitivity, recovery, and impairment (subscales of the Emotional Reactivity Scale). Once these constructs are understood by the youth in terms of his or her experience, strategies for self-monitoring and eventual self-management are possible. Interventions may focus on identifying triggers for Emotional Reactivity and helping youth quantify and communicate the difficulty they have in various types of situations.

Sensitivity

Interventions for reducing sensitivity may involve introducing the notion that everyone has triggers that upset him or her and that some people are more reactive than others. The youth's scores can be compared to others for the purpose of better understanding his or her own sensitivity. The counselor can explain that although Emotional Reactivity is to some extent automatic, it is possible to manage it by identifying triggers, learning to anticipate them, and learning better strategies for calming down, such as self-relaxation or systematic desensitization.

Work on reducing sensitivity might begin by generating a list of specific circumstances, hot spots, or trigger events that are upsetting to the youth. Such a list may be used to work on anticipating and managing response to triggering events.

Recovery

Recovery time reflects the time that it takes to recover from emotional upset which varies across youth. Recovery time is important because the longer the time to recover, the longer that the youth must experience discomfort and the longer the youth is exposed to possible impairment associated with the Emotional Reactivity. Questioning about a youth's ability to recover from emotional upset can introduce the notion that recovery from upset is within the control of the upset individual. Techniques for calming down or self-soothing may be introduced. The inquiry can also uncover self-strategies that the youth employs for self-calming intentionally and unintentionally. These self-calming behaviors may be positive, such as removing himself or herself from the situation or calling a friend. On the other hand, there can be negative coping strategies, such as use of drugs or alcohol, that may further increase the possibility of impairment. The negative impact of using negative strategies should be discussed with the youth and positive self-calming strategies introduced.

Impairment

Emotional Reactivity is known to have a potentially impairing effect on the functioning of children, adolescents, and adults. The impairment may affect any of the developmental systems such as cognitive or executive functioning, behavioral functioning, and relationship functioning. The RSCA attempts to tap several areas where such impairment might occur as well as the frequency with which this impairment occurs. Interventions might seek to help the youth further understand the potentially impairing effect of Emotional Reactivity, types of impairment that occur, and strategies to ameliorate this impairment. For example, a youth may also be asked to write down where he or she makes the most mistakes, get most confused, and gets into the most trouble and then to describe what is happening is these situations. The youth may discover that a common theme is that he or she cannot think clearly when upset. Positive intervention strategies might be introduced such as delaying decisions or actions while upset and not thinking clearly and waiting until more clear thinking prevails. Pros and cons of various strategies may then be discussed.

Interventions to Enhance Resources

Youth for whom personal resiliency is compromised by low personal resources may be characterized by low self-esteem, low motivation to achieve, and low expectation of success. Low personal resources may be the result of many factors including socio-economic circumstances that have not provided enriching experiences (Prince-Embury, 2009). These factors may be associated with lower parent educational level, a difficult personal history of neglect, abuse, failure, and lack of success. Interventions targeting Resource Enhancement would be implemented when Resource Index scores are below average (*T*44 or lower). The specific type of intervention implemented would be determined by whether low resources are associated with lower Sense of Mastery, lower Sense of Relatedness, or both (*T*44 or lower).

Interventions Targeting Sense of Mastery

Earlier research, theory, and interventions for children dealing with Sense of Mastery have focused on the constructs of optimism and Self-efficacy (i.e., Seligman's *Optimistic Child*, 1995). Seligman initially identified "learned helplessness" as the process by which failure experiences may lead to expectations of failure and decreased efforts to succeed. Consequently Seligman and others suggested "learned optimism" as a way of increasing expectations that may lead to more efforts and more success experiences (Seligman, Reivich, Jaycox, & Gillham, 1995). The Resilience program at the University of Pennsylvania grew out of this earlier work employing cognitive behavioral techniques to overcome depression and enhance resiliency in children (Reivich, Gilham, Chaplin, & Seligman, 2005). Cognitive behavior treatments for depression are based on the belief that depression is based in part on a triad of hopelessness about the future, oneself, and the world in general. Consistent with this assumption, many cognitive behavioral treatments focus on challenging negative assumptions and encouraging more positive reframing of beliefs.

Preparing for Mastery

For younger children, strength-based interventions may begin by preparing the child to experience a Sense of Mastery. Brooks and Goldstein (2001) advise parents and teachers to help youth to develop a "resilient mindset." Three examples of preparing children for mastery are presented below.

The power of "I think I can." Positive self-expectation may be discussed and the importance of whether or not you think you can do something. Research shows that whether you think you can do something or not makes a big difference in whether you do it.

Using baby steps. Mastery and self-determination may be introduced with the idea of baby steps, or breaking tasks down into smaller steps and tackling one at a time: step 1, step 2, step 3. Sometimes it helps to write the steps down or to remind oneself by saying baby step 1, baby step 2, etc.

Praising yourself. Mastery involves the ability to recognize and reward oneself when something is accomplished. Children lose their innate sense of pleasure in competence when they enter into social circumstances when not all of their acts are rewarded by teachers and parents. The ability to reward oneself for accomplishments should be nurtured by asking the children to keep a journal and each night before they go to bed to write down a list of things that they did and were proud of that day.

Mining for Mastery and Strength Identification

Children and adolescents who have experienced more failure than success in their lives may have lost the ability to identify their own strengths. For such youth, it is helpful to provide interventions that help them remember and identify positive experiences associated with hidden, forgotten, buried, or uncultivated strengths. For most youth, there is something that they can recall having done well.

Block and Block (1980) originally coined the term "islands of competence" and Brooks and Goldstein (2001, 2008) have recently expanded this concept with numerous clinical examples of identifying islands of competence to enhance resilience in youth. In addition, once areas of strength are identified, preventive intervention may further identify, elaborate, enhance, and generalize these strengths. These interventions can help youth generalize their strengths to other areas where they may not feel as successful. Structured interventions might help youth learn specific skills and how these skills could be employed in a variety of arenas.

Self-Praise and Self-Acknowledgment

As indicated above recognizing mastery experiences is important in developing a Sense of Mastery. Children seem to develop this ability early in life as recognized by White in motive for competence. The ability to experience competence becomes inextricably linked to acceptance and approval by significant others. In some cases parents are active in acknowledging and praising their children for mastery. In other cases this acknowledgement is not forthcoming or is replaced by censure by busy parents whose attention is captured only by negative behavior. In the latter case children and teens may experience both the lack of praise for mastery experiences and the loss of the ability for self-praise. Behavior therapy with children often focuses on helping parents to accurately identify and reward mastery experiences in their children.

Identifying Strength Distracters

Once strengths are identified and understood, the discussion may turn to distracters or reasons why the youth cannot appreciate or expand on a particular strength. Distracters may include many factors such as poverty, limited resources, lack of parental support, or an already internalized expectation that "it is not going to work anyway." Clinical intervention can then focus on identifying the strength distracters that are operating in the youth's life and developing strategies for deffusing them. Cognitive behavioral therapy techniques may be very useful in this regard.

Interventions Targeting Sense of Relationship

As mentioned previously, there is consensus among developmental theorists on the importance of relationship for resiliency in youth and adults alike. The ability to relate to others and to gain strength and resilience from these relationships is a multi-faceted and complex process. Subscales of the Sense of Relatedness Scale were designed to tap and target specific aspects of relatedness for the purpose of identifying strengths and weaknesses of relatedness as experienced and reported by the child or adolescent.

Perceived Social Support

Developmental theorists have acknowledged the significance of perceived support for resiliency in dealing with adversity. Research has indicated that an individual's perception that social support is available and accessible is the most important dimension of social support. This perception is predictive of psychological well-being and is not directly or strongly linked with enacted social support (see Hogan, Linden, & Najarian, 2002). Thompson, Flood, & Goodvin (2006) suggest that it is sometimes more important to focus on the person's subjective experience of supportiveness by carefully examining their expectations of support in relation to what they perceive to be provided by those around them. These authors also suggest that (1) troubled individuals may be less capable of viewing others as sources of available support because of their emotional turmoil and (2) individuals in difficulty may be less able to mobilize supportive networks when they are needed. These ideas highlight the need to explore with children and adolescents what their supports are, before a time of crisis, so that the youth can think about it objectively and think of how they might ask for help in difficult circumstances. Also, family therapy increasing positive communication between parents and their children might facilitate the child's ability to ask for help and the parent's ability to encourage this process.

Developing Possible "What If" Support Networks

With younger children the idea of support networks can be explained as a list of people that you can turn to for help when you need to. The clinician may initiate a list of people who might provide support when needed. The list can include family members, teachers, friends, neighbors, church members, etc. Then several types of situations may be discussed. For each situation the child may be asked to identify people who they could ask for help, how they would approach them, and what they would say. With young children, parents should be involved in this process, emphasizing the importance of a child's perception of support networks and parents support in this process.

Exploring Trust

Developmental theories suggest that the establishment of basic trust begins very early and is built upon throughout development. The implication is that basic trust is established as a core experience and is not easily modified. Enhancing a youth's experience of trust has been the subject of much therapeutic interest beyond the scope of this chapter. Traditional therapy approaches have often focused on providing supportive therapeutic relationships for youth as emotionally corrective experiences. Some clinicians work within the context of family, coaching parents in providing a more nurturing experience for youth within the home (Brooks & Goldstein, 2001). Other programs take a skills enhancement approach which assumes that increasing a youth's social skills will increase the likelihood of positive relationships with others, which in turn may enhance the youth's overall Sense of Relatedness. School psychologist, such as Doll et al. (2004), focus on ecological methods of changing classrooms to be more supportive environments.

The Trust subscale of the RSCA Sense of Relatedness Scale does not reflect basic trust in all of its complexity but rather, allows exploration of how the youth experiences trust or mistrust. Understanding of a youth's conceptualization and experience of trust may allow better understanding of how the youth experiences his or her relationships. The discussion may increase understanding of previous loss and or experiences of perceived betrayal. Therapeutic intervention might include revisiting these experiences and exploring the potential for trusting others in the future.

RSCA Use in Treatment Planning and Treatment Monitoring

This section illustrates the use of the RSCA Profile for treatment planning and monitoring with repeated administrations of the RSCA. An understanding of clinical use of the RSCA Profile requires understanding of the clinical ranges for the global scale scores (see Table 3.9). Of particular clinical note are Resource Index, Sense of Mastery or Sense of Relatedness Scale scores *T*40 or below, and/or Vulnerability Index and Emotional Reactivity Scale scores *T*60 or above. Also, a change of five *T* score points or half a standard deviation is conservatively considered a statistically significant change for the three RSCA Global Scores.

Table 3.9 Clinical ranges for RSCA Global Scale Scores and Index Scores

Ranking	*T* score ranges
High	≥60
Above average	56–59
Average	46–55
Below average	41–45
Low	≤40

Erik, is a 9 year old male, oldest of two siblings and son of a highly educated family. Erik was referred because of intense anger outbursts at home and during recess at school and complaints that he was being bullied in his third grade class. Erik had recently transferred from another school as the result of a family move. The first task of treatment was defined as helping Eric control his extreme angry outbursts. This work began by helping Eric identify triggers that set off the anger and the development of self-calming strategies. Triggers included his perception that he was being bullied by peers. This was exaggerated by Erik's recent transfer to a new school and associated aggressive testing behavior frequently experienced by children who have recently transferred. During this time, Erik's Emotional Reactivity interfered with his relating to peers and with his functioning well academically.

Erik's first profile 2.16.2011, portrayed in Fig. 3.3, represents his intake session RSCA scores. It may be observed that all three global scale scores are out of the average range; Emotional Reactivity was in the high range (*T*62), Sense of Mastery was below average (*T*41), and Sense of Relatedness is in the low range (*T*34). These scores and the overall profile are similar to profiles of other children characterized by

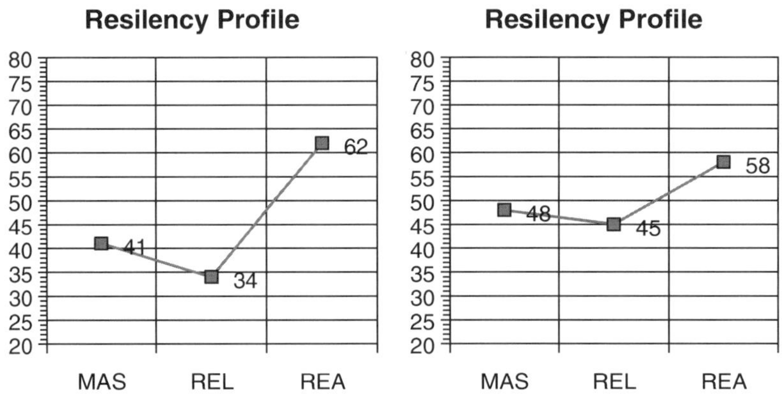

Fig. 3.3 RSCA profiles for Erik at intake (2.16.11) and 2 weeks later (3.03.11)

psychological symptoms and formal diagnosis (Prince-Embury, 2007). This similarity was highlighted by Erik's elevated Anxiety, Anger, and Depression scores on the BYI-II (Beck et al., 2005) scales administered at the same time and was consistent with the initial presenting problems.

Erik's second RSCA Profile 2 weeks later (3.03.2011) (Fig. 3.3) showed improvement in all areas related to new coping skills of anger management and a parental reinforcement system that had been introduced. Erik's Sense of Mastery had increased seven points and was now in the average range. His Sense of Relatedness score had increased 11 points and was also now in the average range. Erik's Emotional Reactivity Score had reduced four points and was now in the above average range. It is interesting to note that Erik showed more improvement in Sense of Mastery and Sense of Relatedness than Emotional Reactivity which was the targeted area of intervention. This is most likely common in therapy interventions but not detectable without an appropriate assessment tool. It is likely that the interventions helped Erik to experience an initial feeling of increased efficacy and greater parental support (Fig. 3.3).

Examination of Erik's scores 2 weeks (3.17.2011) and 4 weeks later (3.31.2011) (Fig. 3.4) indicated that Erik's increased Sense of Mastery had been sustained (*T*55, *T*52) and his Emotional Reactivity continued to decrease (*T*52, *T*48). On the other hand his earlier increase in Sense of Relatedness had not been sustained but decreased towards what it had been at intake (*T*40, *T*36). At this point therapy intervention was focused on social relatedness encouraging the family to arrange play dates for Erik and to monitor Erik's behavior for social appropriateness. These observations were then discussed in therapy with suggestions for better social effectiveness. Thus use of the RSCA to monitor progress in therapy helped to identify a core problem area for Erik that had not previously been identified and addressed (Fig. 3.4).

Erik learned to avoid situations that would provoke triggers to his anger such as participating in playground games with kids who bullied him because he liked the game. He chose to play games with kids who he liked even though the game was not as exciting. Erik learned to count to ten before acting on his anger, use self-talk, and leave the situation when he felt he was getting out of control. Erik's parents put him on a behavioral point system for which he lost points if he had a meltdown at home or at school. Over time the frequency of Erik's angry outbursts decreased as did his anger score on the BYI-II. On the RSCA, Erik's Emotional Reactivity Score decreased and his Sense of Mastery and Sense of Relatedness Scores increased.

Erik's RSCA Profile 3 months later (7.13.2011) (Fig. 3.5) illustrated significantly increased Sense of Mastery (*T*67) in the very high range; increased

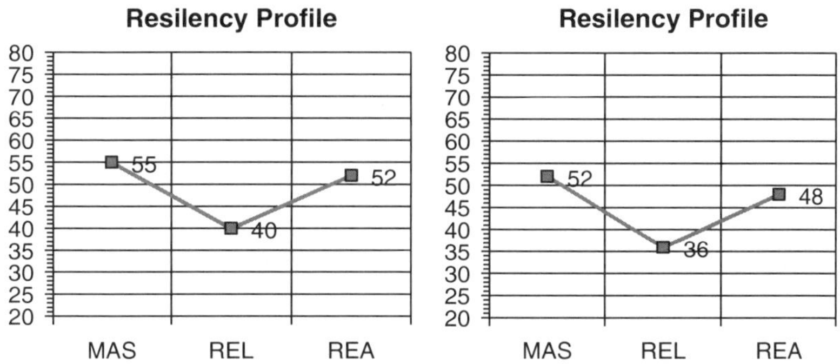

Fig. 3.4 RSCA profiles for Erik in March 2011 (3.17.11) and (3.31.11)

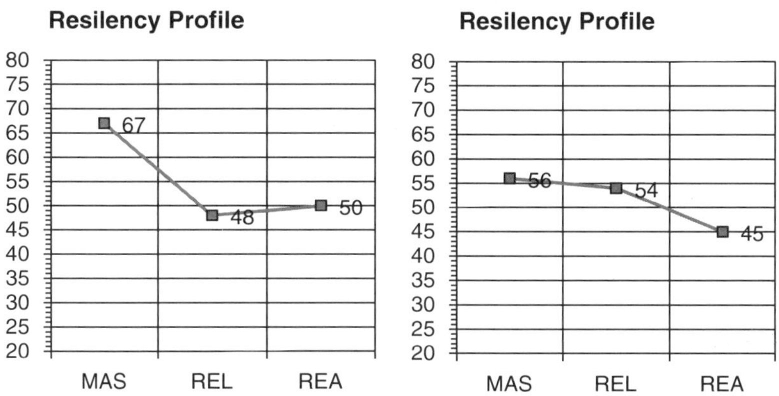

Fig. 3.5 RSCA profiles for Erik summer (7.13.11) and fall 2011 (10.06.11)

Sense of Relatedness (*T*48) in the average range, and a maintained Emotional Reactivity Score in the average range (*T*50). It is likely that Erik's Sense of Mastery was higher than previously because Erik was not in school, did not have homework, and was attending camp engaging in fun activities. Increased Sense of Relatedness may have been related to the structured social activities at camp where teams were structured and supervised by camp counselors as opposed to the unstructured socializing that had taken place at recess and lunch during the school year.

Erik's RSCA Profile 3 months later (10.06.2011) (Fig. 3.5) shows a Sense of Mastery Score decreased back to the above average range (*T*56) consistent with being back in school and faced with increased academic demands. Sense of Relatedness has increased slightly (*T*54) and Emotional Reactivity has decreased (*T*45) and is in the average range. This profile reflects a time when Erik had returned to the school that had been new to him the year before, and to peers, teachers who know him and an environment with which he was familiar. It should be noted that Erik's lowered Emotional Reactivity reflects his increased awareness and sense of control in this area, although he remained somewhat emotionally reactive (Fig. 3.5).

These positive changes allowed Erik's parents to focus on other behaviors such as Erik's tendency to bully his younger sister at home. Although the two siblings generally were good friends and played well together, Erik would occasionally lose control and bully his sister. Work began on helping Erik be aware of this behavior and his inability to control it. Erik was coached in how to diffuse his own anger by thinking of something funny.

In summary, Erik RSCA profile indicates a steady decrease in Emotional Reactivity across treatment consistent with the goals of treatment. In addition there was an increase in Sense of Mastery which may have been related to decreased Emotional Reactivity and a greater sense of control in this area. Erik's profile indicated the most vulnerability in Sense of Relatedness. Some gains were indicated after treatment focus shifted to enhancement of social skills. The example provided above illustrates that the experience of personal resilience is modifiable and not "carved in stone" as a trait interpretation of the construct would imply.

Summary

In summary this chapter presents the Resiliency Scales for Children and Adolescents as a tool for translating resiliency theory for application with children and adolescents ages 9–18.

Three global scales are designed to reflect three developmental systems that have been consistently identified as core aspects of personal resiliency, Sense of Mastery, Sense of Relatedness, and Emotional Reactivity. Research suggests that these three scales reflect the underlying constructs in a reliable and valid manner. In addition these three scales are linked with specific areas of intervention that may help to enhance personal resiliency through these three developmental systems. Outcome studies tracking changes in RSCA Global Scores over time may be used to assess the effectiveness of interventions. Two Index scores combining the three global scale scores may be used to assess perceived personal resources (the Resource Index) and the discrepancy between Emotional Reactivity and perceived personal resources (the Vulnerability Index). The RSCA Index scores, particularly the Vulnerability Index score may be used along with the RSCA Personal Resiliency Profile for preventive screening to select youth who might benefit from preventive intervention to enhance personal resiliency.

Unique characteristics of the RSCA are the following. The RSCA describes three core developmental systems underlying resiliency that are well documented in the literature and consistent with factor analytic studies (Prince-Embury, 2007). The RSCA was normed on a US representative sample systematically stratified by race/ethnicity and parent education level allowing *T* scores to be determined based on a representative normative sample that is represented in the US Census. Further analysis by Prince-Embury (2009) suggests that there are no systematic differences in RSCA scores across race/ethnicity that are not accounted for by differences in parent education level. The *T* score metric allows comparison across developmental system to identify areas of relative strength or vulnerability. Identification of three areas of personal resilience allows targeted interventions to enhance personal resiliency and/or identify those who may be more at risk in the face of adversity. In summary, the RSCA passes the test of sound theoretical and psychometric foundation as well as clinical and research utility.

References

Ainsworth, M. D. S. (1989). Attachments beyond infancy. *American Psychologist, 44*, 709–716.

Armsden, G. C., & Greenberg, M. T. (1987). The Inventory of Parent and Peer Attachment: Individual differences and their relationship to psychological well-being in adolescence. Journal of Youth and Adolescence, ***16***, 427–454.

Ayyash-Abdo, H., & Sanchez-Ruiz, M. J. (Unpublished manuscript). Resilience, hope, and personality among Lebanese adolescents.

Bandura, A. (1977). Self-efficacy: Toward a unifying theory of behavioral change. *Psychological Review, 84*, 191–215.

Bandura, A. (1993). Perceived self-efficacy in cognitive development and functioning. *Educational Psychologist, 28*(2), 117–148.

Barrera, M. J. (1986). Distinctions between social support concepts, measures and models. *American Journal of Community Psychology, 14*, 413–445.

Beck, A., Beck, J., Jolly, J., & Steer, R. (2005). *Beck Youth Inventories—Second Edition*. San Antonio, TX: Harcourt Assessment.

Block, J. H., & Block, J. (1980). The role of ego-control and ego-resilience in the organization of behavior. In W. A. Collins (Ed.), *Development of cognition, affect and social relations. The Minnesota Symposia on child psychology* (Vol. 13, pp. 39–101). Hillsdale, NJ: Lawrence Erlbaum.

Bolby, J. (1982). Attachment and loss a retrospect and prospect. *American Journal of Orthopsychiatry, 52*(4), 664–668.

Bolby, J. (1988). Developmental psychiatry comes of age. *American Journal of Psychiatry, 145*, 1–10.

Bowlby, J. (1969). *Attachment and loss: Vol. 1. Attachment. The international psycho-analytical library* (Vol. 79, pp. 1–401). London: The Hogarth Press and the Institute of Psycho-Analysis.

Bretherton, I., & Munholland, K. A. (1999). Internal working models in attachment: A construct revisited. In J. Cassidy & P. Shaver (Eds.), *Handbook of attachment: Theory, research and clinical application* (pp. 89–111). New York, NY: Guilford.

Brooks, R., & Goldstein, S. (2001). *Raising resilient children; fostering strength, hope and optimism in your child.* New York, NY: Contemporary Books.

Brooks, R., & Goldstein, S. (2008). The mindset of teachers capable of fostering resilience in students. *Canadian Journal of School Psychology, 23*, 114–126.

Cicchetti, D. V. (1994). Guidelines, criteria, and rules of thumb for evaluating normed and standardized assessment instruments in psychology. *Psychological Assessment, 6*, 284–290.

Cicchetti, D., Ganiban, J., & Barnett, D. (1991). Contributions from the study of high-risk populations to understanding the development of emotion regulation. In J. Garber & K. Dodge (Eds.), *The development of emotion regulation and dysregulation* (pp. 15–48). New York, NY: Cambridge University Press.

Cicchetti, D., & Tucker, D. (1994). Development and self-regulatory structures of the mind. *Development and Psychopathology, 6*(4), 533–549.

Cohen, S., & Wills, T. A. (1985). Stress, social support, and the buffering hypothesis. *Psychological Bulletin, 98*, 310–357.

Connors, C. K. (1997). *Connors-Wells Adolescent Symptoms Scale; Short Form (CASS)*. Toronto: Multi-Health Systems, Inc.

Cowen, E. L., Pryor-Brown, L., Hightower, A. D., & Lotyczewski, B. S. (1991). Age perspectives on the stressfulness of life events for 10–12 year old children. *School Psychology Quarterly, 6*, 240–250.

Cui, L., Teng, X., Li, X., & Oei, T. P. S. (2010). The factor structure and psychometric properties of the Resiliency Scale in Chinese undergraduates. *European Journal of Psychological Assessment, 26*(3), 162–171.

Doll, B., Zucker, S., & Brehm, K. (2004). *Resilient classrooms: Creating healthier environments for learning.* New York, NY: Guilford.

Dumont, M., & Provost, M. A. (1999). Resilience in adolescents: Protective role of social support, coping strategies, self-esteem, and social activities on experience of stress and depression. *Journal of Youth and Adolescence, 28*(3), 343–363.

Eisenberg, N., Champion, C., & Ma, Y. (2004). Emotion-related regulation: An emerging construct. *Merrill-Palmer Quarterly, 50*, 236–259.

Erikson, E. H. (1963). *Childhood and society* (2nd ed.). New York, NY: W.W. Norton & Company.

Hayes, W. L. (1994). Statistics (5th ed.). Ft. Worth, TX: Harcourt Brace.

Hogan, B. E., Linden, W. M., & Najarian, B. (2002). Social support interventions: Do they work? *Clinical Psychology Review, 22*, 381–440.

Jackson, Y., & Warren, J. (2000). Appraisal, social support and life events: Predicting outcome behavior in school-age children. *Child Development, 71*, 1441–1453.

Jordani, R. B. (2008). *Translation and validation of the Resilliency Scales for Children and Adolesents.* Dissertation, CAPES, Brazil.

Kaplan, H. B. (2005). Understanding the concept of resilience. In S. Goldstein & R. B. Brooks (Eds.), *Handbook of resilience in children* (pp. 223–237). New York, NY: Kluwer Academic/Plenum.

Kumar, G., Steer, R., & Gulab, N. (2010). Profiles of personal resiliency in child and adolescent inpatients. *Journal of Psychoeducational Assessment, 28*(4), 315–325.

Luthar, S. S. (2006). *Resiliency in low SES adolescents.* Unpublished study.

Luthar, S. S., Cicchetti, D. C., & Becker, B. (2000). The construct of resilience: A critical evaluation and guidelines for future work. *Child Development, 71*(3), 543–562.

Luthar, S. S., & Zelazo, L. B. (2003). Research on resilience: An integrative review. In S. S. Luthar (Ed.), *Resilience and vulnerability: Adaptation in the context of childhood adversities* (pp. 510–549). New York, NY: Cambridge University Press.

Masten, A. S. (1994). Resilience in individual development: Successful adaptation despite risk and adversity. In M. C. Wang & E. W. Corden (Eds.), *Educational resilience in inner city America; challenges and perspectives* (pp. 3–25). Hillsdale, N.J: Erlbaum.

Masten, A. S. (2001). Ordinary magic: Resilience processes in development. *American Psychologist, 56*, 227–238.

Masten, A. S., Burt, K. B., & Coatsworth, J. D. (2006). Competence and psychopathology in development. In D. Cicchetti & D. Cohen (Eds.), *Handbook of developmental psychopathology* (2nd ed., Vol. 3, pp. 696–738). New York, NY: Wiley.

Masten, A. S., & Coatsworth, J. D. (1998). The development of competence in favorable and unfavorable environments: Lessons from research on successful children. *American Psychologist, 53*, 205–220.

Masten, A. S., & Curtis, W. J. (2000). Integrating competence and psychopathology: Pathways toward a comprehensive science of adaptation in development [Special issue]. *Development & Psychopathology, 12*, 529–550.

Masten, A. S., & Obradovic, J. (2006). Competence and resilience in development. *Annals of the New York Academy of Science, 1094*, 13–27.

Masten, A. S., & Powell, J. L. (2003). A resilience framework for research, policy, and practice. In S. S. Luthar (Ed.), *Resilience and vulnerability: Adaptation in the context of childhood adversities* (pp. 1–25). New York, NY: Cambridge University Press.

Masten, A. S., Roisman, G. I., Long, J. D., Burt, K. B., Obradovic, J., Riley, J. R., et al. (2005). Developmental cascades: Linking academic achievement and externalizing and internalizing symptoms over 20 years. *Developmental Psychology, 41*, 733–746.

Mowder, M., Cummings, J., & McKinney, R. (2010). Resiliency Scales for children and adolescents: Profiles of juvenile offenders. *Journal of Psychoeducational Assessment, 28*(4), 326–337.

Piers, E. (2002). *Piers-Harris children's self-concept scale* (2nd ed.). Los Angeles, CA: Western Psychological Services.

Prince-Embury, S. (2006a). *Resiliency Scales for adolescents: Profiles of personal strengths*. San Antonio, TX: Harcourt Assessments, Inc.

Prince-Embury, S. (2006b). *Adolescent risk behavior inventory*. Unpublished study.

Prince-Embury, S. (2006c). *Negative life events inventory*. Unpublished study.

Prince-Embury, S. (2007). *Resiliency Scales for Children and Adolescents: Profiles of personal strengths*. San Antonio, TX: Harcourt Assessments, Inc.

Prince-Embury, S. (2008). Resiliency Scales for Children and Adolescents, psychological symptoms and clinical status of adolescents. *Canadian Journal of School Psychology, 23*, 41–56.

Prince-Embury, S. (2009). The Resiliency Scales for Children and Adolescents as related to parent education and race/ethnicity in children. *The Canadian Journal of School Psychology, 24*(2), 167–182.

Prince-Embury, S. (2010a). Psychometric properties of the Resiliency Scales for Children and Adolescents and use for youth with psychiatric disorders. *Journal of Psychoeducational Assessment, 28*(4), 291–303.

Prince-Embury, S. (2010b). Assessment for integrated screening and prevention using the Resiliency Scales for Children and Adolescents. In B. Doll, W. Pfohl, & J. Yoon (Eds.), *Handbook of youth prevention science*. New York, NY: Routledge.

Prince-Embury, S., & Courville, T. (2008a). Comparison of one, two and three factor models of personal resilience using the Resiliency Scales for Children and Adolescents. *Canadian Journal of School Psychology, 23*, 11–25.

Prince-Embury, S., & Courville, T. (2008b). Measurement invariance of the Resiliency Scales for Children and Adolescents with respect to sex and age cohorts. *Canadian Journal of School Psychology, 23*, 26–40.

Prince-Embury, S., & Steer, R. (2010). Profiles of personal resiliency for normative and clinical samples of children and adolescents using the Resiliency Scales for Children and Adolescents. *Journal of Psychological Assessment, 28*(4), 303–315.

Reivich, K., Gilham, J. E., Chaplin, T. M., & Seligman, M. E. P. (2005). From helplessness to optimism: The role of resilience in treating and preventing depression in youth. In S. Goldstein & R. B. Brooks (Eds.), *Handbook of resilience in children* (pp. 223–237). New York, NY: Kluwer Academic/Plenum.

Reynolds, W. (2004). *Reynolds bully victimization scale*. San Antonio, TX: Harcourt Assessment.

Rothbart, M. K., & Derryberry, D. (1981). Development of individual differences in temperament. In M. E. Lamb & A. L. Brown (Eds.), *Advances in developmental psychology* (Vol. 1, pp. 37–86). Hillsdale, NJ: Erlbaum.

Rutter, M. (1987). Psychosocial resilience and protective mechanisms. *American Journal of Orthopsychiatry, 57*, 316–331.

Rutter, M. (1993). Resilience: Some conceptual considerations. *Journal of Adolescent Health, 14*, 626–631.

Saklofske, D. H., & Nordstokke, D. (2011). The relationship of the RSCA with personality and Motivation measures in Canadian young adult samples. Society for Personality Assessment, March, Boston. T.

Sarason, B. R., Shearon, E. N., Pierce, G. R., & Sarason, I. G. (1987). Interrelationships of social support measures. Theoretical and practical implications. *Journal of Personality and Social Psychology, 52*, 813–832.

Schutte, N. S., Malouff, J. M., Hall, L. E., Haggerty, D. J., Cooper, J. T., Golden, C. J., et al. (1998). Development and validation of a measure of emotional intelligence. *Personality and Individual Differences, 25*, 167–177.

Seligman, M. E. P., Reivich, K., Jaycox, L., & Gillham, J. (1995). *The optimistic child*. New York, NY: Houghton Mifflin.

Siegel, D. J. (1999). *The developing mind: How relationships and the brain interact to shape who we are*. New York, NY: Guilford.

Sroufe, L. A., Carlson, E. A., Levy, A. K., & Egeland, B. (1999). Implications of attachment theory for developmental psychopathology. *Development and Psychopathology, 11*, 1–13.

Thompson, R. A. (1990). Emotion and self-regulation. In R. Dienstbier (Series Ed.) and R. A. Thompson (Vol. Ed.), *Nebraska symposium on motivation: Socioemotional development* (pp. 367–467). Lincoln: University of Nebraska Press.

Thompson, R. A. (2000). The legacy of early attachments. *Child Development, 71*(1), 145–152.

Thompson, R. A., Flood, M. F., & Goodvin, R. (2006). Social support and developmental psychopathology. In D. Cicchetti & D. J. Cohen (Eds.), *Developmental psychopathology: Risk, disorder, and adaptation* (2nd ed., Vol. 3, pp. 1–37). Hoboken, NJ: Wiley.

Tignor, B., & Prince-Embury, S. (2013). Resilience in Kenyan youth living in the slums and suburbs of Nairobi: An explanatory and descriptive study. In S. Prince-Embury & D.H. Saklofske (Eds.), *Resilience in Children, Adolescents, and Adults: Translating Research into Practice* (pp. 257–278). New York, Springer.

Van Wyk, H. (2011). *The relationship between vulnerability factors and life satisfaction in adolescents: A cross cultural study*. Unpublished thesis, University of the Free State, South Africa.

Werner, E. E., & Smith, R. S. (1982). *Vulnerable but invincible: A longitudinal study of resilient children and youth*. New York, NY: McGraw-Hill.

White, R. W. (1959). Motivation reconsidered: The concept of competence. *Psychological Review, 66*, 297–333.

Wyman, P. A., Cowen, E. L., Work, W. C., & Kerley, J. H. (1993). The role of children's future expectations in self-system functioning and adjustment to life stress: A prospective study of urban at-risk children (Special issue). *Development and Psychopathogy, 5*, 649–661.

The Devereux Suite: Assessing and Promoting Resilience in Children Ages 1 Month to 14 Years

4

Paul A. LeBuffe, Katherine M. Ross, Jennifer L. Fleming, and Jack A. Naglieri

For the past several decades, the concept of resilience has received increasing attention. From the early work of Emmy Werner, Norm Garmezy, Michael Rutter, and other pioneering resilience researchers, resilience has grown to become a topic of critical importance for a variety of child-serving professions, all with the goal of promoting children's resilience so they are better able to face life's many challenges. This growth in the importance of resilience can be explicitly seen by an examination of the professional literature over the last three decades. We conducted a search of the Social Sciences Citation Index to find the number of published articles which included the word "resilience" and its variants in the title or topic fields. As can be seen in Fig. 4.1, the results of these searches revealed a substantial increase from >20 citations in 1990 to over 1,200 citations in 2010.

One facet of resilience, social and emotional competence, has also gained prominence in recent years. Social and emotional competence has been defined as "the ability of children to successfully interact with other children and adults in a way that demonstrates an awareness of, and ability to manage, emotions in an age- and context-appropriate manner" (LeBuffe, Shapiro, & Naglieri, 2009, p. 5). These important competencies serve as protective factors, buffering children from the negative effects of risk and adversity and thereby supporting their resilience (Masten & Garmezy, 1985). The importance of promoting social and emotional competence as a way to build resilience is increasingly being recognized in practice, policy, and research.

In regard to practice, several fields have begun to incorporate standards related to resilience and social and emotional competencies. For example, in the recent revision of the National Association of School Psychologists (NASP) Model for Comprehensive and Integrated School Psychological Services (2010), one of the core competencies of school psychologists is the provision of "effective services to help children and youth succeed academically, socially, behaviorally and emotionally" (p. 1). Additionally, school psychologists are expected to "promote recognition of risk and protective factors" (p. 7) and "promote wellness and resilience" (p. 7) of all children. These practice standards reflect the value of recognizing and targeting these competencies that directly impact the well-being of children.

The importance of recognizing and promoting children's social and emotional competencies is also evident in recent policy changes. As of the

P.A. LeBuffe, M.A. (✉) • K.M. Ross, B.S.
J.L. Fleming, M.S.
Devereux Center for Resilient Children, Villanova, PA, USA
e-mail: plebuffe@Devereux.org; kross@Devereux.org; Jflemin2@Devereux.org

J.A. Naglieri, Ph.D.
Devereux Center for Resilient Children, Villanova, PA, USA

University of Virginia, Charlottesville, VA, USA
e-mail: jnaglieri@gmail.com

S. Prince-Embury and D.H. Saklofske (eds.), *Resilience in Children, Adolescents, and Adults: Translating Research into Practice*, The Springer Series on Human Exceptionality,
DOI 10.1007/978-1-4614-4939-3_4, © Springer Science+Business Media New York 2013

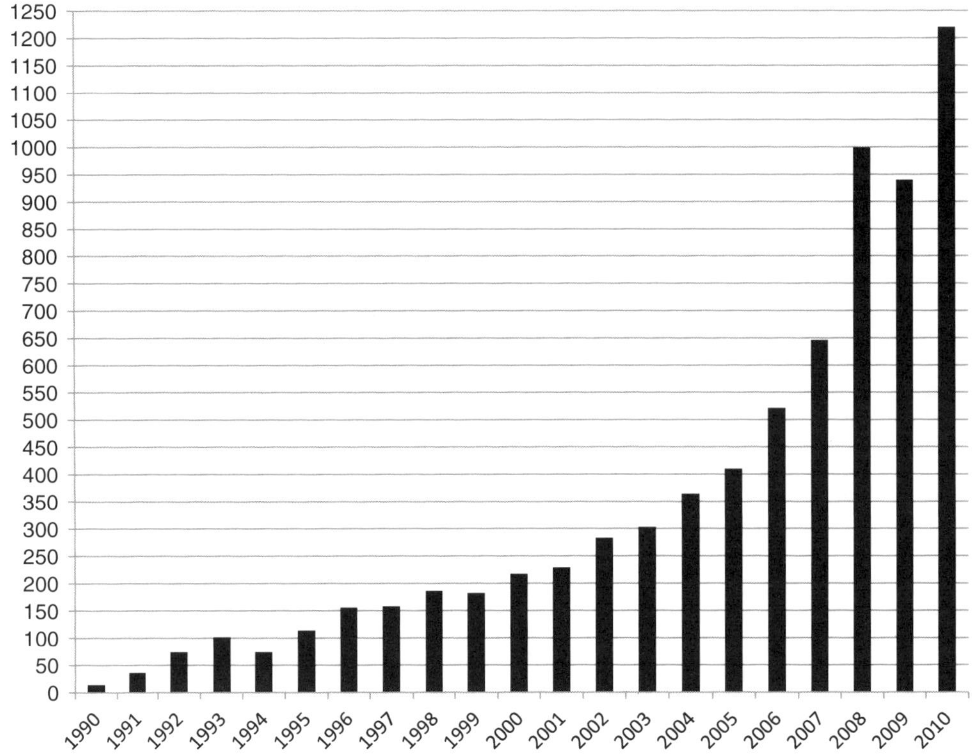

Fig. 4.1 Number of citations with "resilience" in the title or topic fields from 1990 to 2010

fall of 2011, eight states had adopted or were drafting explicit K-12 educational standards in the social and emotional domain. The remaining 42 states as well as six United States Territories had included some social and emotional learning (SEL) goals or benchmarks in their educational standards (CASEL, 2011). Similarly, all states had preschool educational standards related to SEL, with 48 of these states having comprehensive, free standing standards for SEL. In addition, the Academic, Social and Emotional Learning Act of 2011 was introduced to the 112th Congress. This proposed legislation is still under consideration as this chapter is being written, but if passed, will support the implementation of SEL programs in the schools, particularly through providing funds through the Elementary and Secondary Education Act (ESEA) to support training in SEL programs for principals and teachers. These standards suggest the recognition of the importance of promoting social and emotional skills within all children.

To meet these standards, a variety of evidence-based SEL programs are available for preschool and school-age children. Research supports the use of these programs and the benefits to children who experience well-implemented SEL programs. Durlak, Weissberg, Dymnicki, Taylor, and Schellinger (2011) conducted a meta-analysis of 213 school-based studies involving more than 270,000 students that investigated the outcomes of universal SEL programs. They found that students in well-implemented SEL programs showed positive outcomes compared to students in control groups in a wide range of domains. The SEL programs resulted in increased social and emotional skills; improved attitudes toward self, school, and others; decreased behavioral concerns; and, importantly, an average 11 % point gain in tests of academic achievement.

In addition to curricula designed to promote children's social and emotional competencies, assessments are also needed to provide professionals with assistance in planning interventions and evaluating outcomes. For SEL programs, in particular, strength-based assessments are particularly useful as they provide a framework for identifying and teaching these competencies. Epstein (2004) defined strength-based assessment as "the measurement of those emotional and behavioral skills, competencies, and characteristics that create a sense of personal accomplishment; contribute to satisfying relationships with family members, peers, and adults; enhance one's ability to deal with adversity and stress; and promote one's personal, social and academic development" (p. 4). An increasing number of strength-based assessments are available to professionals, such as the Devereux Suite of Assessments discussed in this chapter, the Behavioral and Emotional Rating Scale, Second Edition (BERS-2; Epstein, 2004), the Resiliency Scales for Children and Adolescents (RSCA; Prince-Embury, 2007), the Developmental Assets Profile (Search Institute, 2004), and the Social–Emotional Assets and Resilience Scales (SEARS; Merrell, 2011).

There are a variety of benefits to using strength-based assessment. Perhaps the most notable of these is that they can be readily used within a primary prevention or promotion model (LeBuffe & Shapiro, 2004). By using a strength-based approach, one can identify the absence of any necessary skills or competencies, and begin to implement strategies designed to target those skills before challenging behaviors or difficulties occur. In contrast, the use of a deficit-oriented approach would be implemented only after problem behaviors or pathologies would arise. Furthermore, a strength-based approach can be useful even after problem behaviors have occurred. This approach would allow professionals to gain a more comprehensive understanding of the child and provide opportunities to use more prosocial strategies to help children meet their needs.

With the increasing emphasis placed on resilience and SEL, the newly developed state and practice standards, and the availability of a variety of evidence-based SEL programs, it is essential that well-developed and psychometrically sound assessments are available to assess children's strengths and needs, guide planning, and evaluate outcomes. The Devereux Suite of Assessments was developed specifically to serve these needs.

The Devereux Suite of Assessments

The Devereux Center for Resilient Children's suite of assessments consists of four different behavior rating scales developed to measure within-child protective factors related to resilience. The four measures differ primarily in the age of the child being rated and encompass ages 1 month through 14 years (eighth grade). For all four forms, the child is rated by either a teacher or a parent. These two informant classes were chosen because they have the most contact with the child and are often viewed as the most important adults in the life of the child. The Devereux assessments are based on the risk and resilience framework, and the belief that building a child's protective factors will mitigate the impact of risk. The common set of overarching goals that drove the creation of Devereux assessments are discussed later in this chapter. These goals led to a number of similarities between the assessments that are reflected in their development, psychometric properties, and intended uses.

Each assessment in the Devereux Suite was standardized using a nationally representative sample and has a different set of norms for parent and teacher raters. Parents and teachers rate how often they have seen the child exhibit a specific set of behaviors within the last 4 weeks using a Likert Scale ranging from 0 (*Never*) to 4 (*Very Frequently*). Each assessment is available in both paper and online formats and in both English and Spanish. Results are reported using *T*-scores and percentile ranks for each specific protective factor as well as a total score. Suggested wording is provided to describe ranges of *T*-scores to aid in communicating the results to parents, teachers and, if appropriate, the child. The term, "Strength" is used for protective factor *T*-scores of 60 or above. In the national standardization samples, 16% of children received scores in the Strength range. *T*-Scores of 41–59 inclusive, which were

Early Childhood Scales				School Age Scales
DECA-I	DECA -T	DECA	DECA-P2	DESSA
Attachment/ Relationships	Attachment/ Relationships	Attachment	Attachment/ Relationships	Social-Awareness
				Relationship Skills
				Optimistic Thinking
Initiative	Initiative	Initiative	Initiative	Goal-Directed Behavior
				Personal Responsibility
				Decision Making
	Self-Regulation	Self - Control	Self-Regulation	Self-Awareness
				Self-Management

Fig. 4.2 Comparison of Devereux assessment scales across the age span

received by 68% of children in the standardization sample, are described as "Typical." For *T*-scores of 40 or below, which were received by 16% of the standardization sample, the term "Need" is recommended.

Low scores in the Need range on both the individual scale scores and the total score can be used to help identify children who are at-risk and in need of additional support in building social and emotional skills. The *T*-scores also allow administrators to compare specific protective factors within and across children and to chart progress across time. The ultimate purpose of the Devereux Suite of Assessments is to promote the resilience of children by enabling professionals to identify children who lack strong social and emotional competencies (i.e., within-child protective factors) so that preventive interventions can be delivered to support the development of those competencies before the child encounters significant or additional risk.

The Devereux Suite provides a developmental continuum of within-child protective factors that spans infancy through the eighth grade. Based on cross-sectional research with a total of more than 6,600 children, the Devereux Suite also helps elucidate the emergence of within-child protective factors. Figure 4.2 shows the developmental progression of protective factor scales from our early childhood assessments to our school age assessments. Each of these scales will be defined in the next section.

Each of the Devereux assessments has strong psychometrics. During development, the reliability of each form was evaluated and yielded results meeting or exceeding the guidelines outlined by Wasserman and Bracken (2003). Strong validity was also demonstrated through a series of studies for each assessment. With the development and revision of each assessment, the Devereux Center for Resilient Children aimed to provide additional interpretive tools, exceed previous expectations, and reflect the changing characteristics of our nation's children. Therefore, each assessment is presented below in the order of development by the Devereux Center for Resilient Children. Table 4.1 provides a descriptive summary of each assessment.

Devereux Early Childhood Assessment

The Devereux Early Childhood Assessment (DECA; LeBuffe & Naglieri, 1999) was the first assessment developed by the Devereux Center for Resilient Children. The DECA was standardized on a national sample of 2,017 children aged 2–5 years and was designed to be used by preschool program directors, teachers, preschool mental health providers, and early childhood special educators to evaluate protective factors related to resilience in children ages 2–5. We present the results of the reliability and validity studies in the DECA Technical Manual (LeBuffe & Naglieri, 1999).

The 37 DECA items are organized into two dimensions—protective factors and behavioral concerns. The protective factors included are

Table 4.1 Description of Devereux Suite

Rating scale	Year of publication	Number of items	Age range	Standardization sample size
Devereux Early Childhood Assessment-Infant (DECA-I)	2007	33	4 Weeks to 18 months	987
Devereux Early Childhood Assessment-Toddler (DECA-T)	2007	36	18 Months to 3 years	1,196
Devereux Early Childhood Assessment (DECA)	1999	37	2–5 Years	2,017
Devereux Early Childhood Assessment for Preschoolers, Second Edition (DECA-P2)	2012	38	3–5 Years	3,553
Devereux Student Strengths Assessment (DESSA)	2009	72	5–14 Years	2,494
Devereux Student Strengths Assessment-Mini (DESSA-mini)	2011	Four 8-item forms	5–14 Years	1,250

Initiative (11 items), Self-control (8 items), and Attachment (8 items). A screener for behavioral concerns (10 items) is included to help identify children with emerging problem behaviors. Items on the Initiative scale assess the child's use of independent thought and action to meet his or her needs. This is measured through items such as "start or organize play with other children" or "try or ask to try new things or activities." The Self-control scale includes items concerning the child's ability to experience a range of feelings and express them appropriately using words and actions. "Accept another choice when her/his first choice was unavailable" and "calm herself/himself down when upset" are two example items from the Self-control scale. Attachment items ascertain if the child has developed mutual, strong, and long-lasting relationships with other children and adults. The scale contains items such as "show affection for familiar adults" and "trust familiar adults and believe what they say." In addition, a Total Protective Factors Scale is provided. The behavioral concerns items measure a wide variety of problem behaviors seen in some young children. It should be noted that the DECA is the only tool in the Devereux Suite that includes behavioral concerns.

It is important to note that at the time of this writing the second edition of the DECA is in the final stages of development. The second edition has a larger standardization sample (3,553) and new norms. More information about this edition can be found in the manual that will be published along with the rating scale.

Devereux Early Childhood Assessment for Infants

Responding to the growing awareness of promotion, prevention, and early intervention in infants and toddlers, the Devereux Early Childhood Assessment for Infants and Toddlers (DECA-I/T; Powell, Mackrain, & LeBuffe, 2007) was created. The Devereux Early Childhood Assessment for Infants (DECA-I) was standardized on a national sample of 987 infants between 4 weeks and 18 months of age. Separate norms were created for several different month intervals, as age trends were present in the data (1 month up to 3 months, 3 months up to 6 months, 6 months up to 9 months, and 9 months up to 18 months). The results of the reliability and validity studies are presented in the Technical Manual (Powell et al., 2007).

The DECA-I has 33 items comprising two protective factor scales: Initiative (18 items) and Attachment/Relationships (15 items). The Attachment/Relationships scale assesses if a mutual, strong, lasting relationship has developed between the infant and a significant adult. The Initiative scale determines the infant's ability to use independent thought or actions to meet his or her needs.

Devereux Early Childhood Assessment for Toddlers

The Devereux Early Childhood Assessment for Toddlers (DECA-T; Powell et al., 2007) was developed simultaneously with the DECA-I, and therefore shares many of the same characteristics. The description of development and the standardization sample in addition to the results of the reliability and validity studies are presented in the same Technical Manual (Powell et al., 2007). The DECA-T was standardized on a national sample of 1,196 toddlers between 18 months and 3 years of age.

The Toddler form has 36 items comprising three protective factors scales: Attachment/Relationships (18 items), Initiative (11 items), and Self-regulation (7 items). The Self-regulation scale measures the toddler's ability to gain control of and manage emotions and sustain focus and attention.

Devereux Student Strengths Assessment

The Devereux Center for Resilient Children expanded into school-aged populations to address several issues: (1) to continue to serve our "DECA graduates," or children who had been benefiting from the DECA program and were now entering the school system, (2) to provide a tool for educators to address emerging state SEL standards, and (3) to recognize the importance of building protective factors through a child's life, beyond the preschool years.

The Devereux Student Strengths Assessment (DESSA; LeBuffe et al., 2009) is a rating scale designed to assess social–emotional competencies that serve as protective factors for children in kindergarten through the eighth grade. The DESSA was standardized on a national sample of 2,494 children in grades K through 8 by teachers and parents using both paper and pencil and online versions of the scale. Results of the reliability and validity studies are presented in the DESSA Manual (LeBuffe et al., 2009).

The DESSA is completed by parents, teachers, or staff of child-serving agencies, including after-school, social service, and mental health programs. The assessment is composed of 72 entirely strength-based items. We developed the DESSA to closely reflect the SEL core competencies that are articulated by the Collaborative for Social, Emotional, and Academic Learning (CASEL). These core competencies are also closely aligned with emerging state SEL standards. The DESSA is organized into eight conceptually derived scales that provide information about social–emotional competencies. They are: Self-awareness (7 items), Social-awareness (9 items), Self-management (11 items), Goal-Directed Behavior (10 items), Relationship Skills (10 items), Personal Responsibility (10 items), Decision Making (8 items), and Optimistic Thinking (7 items).

The combination of these scales is used to obtain a Social–Emotional Composite score. This composite score provides an overall indication of the strength of the child's social–emotional competence and the eight DESSA scales are used to create profiles for individuals as well as the entire classroom that describe the strengths and needs of the student and/or groups of students as compared to national norms. This information can also be used to compare ratings across raters, environments, and time to monitor progress and evaluate outcomes.

A brief universal screener and ongoing progress monitoring form called the DESSA-mini is also available. The DESSA-mini is available in four different, 8-item forms. It was developed using items from the DESSA and the same standardization sample, so it shares many of the same properties as the full DESSA. For more information, please refer to the DESSA-mini manual (Naglieri, LeBuffe, & Shapiro, 2011).

The Devereux Suite of Assessments as a Measure of Behaviors Related to Resilience

As previously mentioned, the Devereux Suite of Assessments was developed on the foundation of risk and resilience literature. Our assessments aim to measure within-child protective factors, which are thought to mitigate the impact of risk

Table 4.2 Results of the DESSA protective factor study

Risk	Competence	*n*	Mean	SD
High risk	Low competence	14	123.86	15
	Average/high competence	17	116.41	18
Average/low risk	Low competence	37	117.19	18
	Average/high competence	78	97.58	13

Note: On the Devereux Behavior Rating Scale—School Form, the mean is set to 100 and the standard deviation to 15. Higher scores indicate greater behavioral problems

in children's lives. Therefore, higher scale scores on the protective factor scales should be associated with decreasing the impact of risk. We investigated this hypothesis in a series of similar studies for each of the four assessments. The most recent of the studies is described in the DESSA manual (LeBuffe et al., 2009) and is summarized here. A sample of 149 parents and caregivers completed the DESSA as a measure of within-child protective factors, two risk questionnaires as a measure of Total Risk, and The Devereux Behavioral Rating Scale—School Form (DSF; Naglieri, LeBuffe, & Pfeiffer, 1993, 1994) as a measure of problem behaviors associated with mental health diagnoses. The two risk questionnaires were modified from the Major Life Events Checklist (Work, Cowen, Parker, & Wyman, 1990) and the Daily Hassles Checklist (Kanner, Coyne, Schaefer, & Lazarus, 1981) with permission from the authors. A two-way ANOVA was conducted and the results indicated that social and emotional competence, as measured by the DESSA, reduces negative outcomes for children with varying levels of risk (high risk and average/low risk). In other words, for both high risk and low risk children, higher scores on the DESSA were associated with less behavioral concerns. The results of this study are presented in Table 4.2. Main effects existed for the Risk ($F(1)=16.62, p<0.001, d=0.93$) and Competence ($F(1)=18.71, p<0.001, d=1.11$) variables. These results support the contention that the DESSA does indeed measure protective factors related to resilience. These findings have been replicated in four additional studies conducted during the development of the DECA, the DECA-I, the DECA-T, and the revised DECA.

Applications of the Devereux Suite of Assessments in Promoting Resilience

In developing the Devereux Suite of Assessments, we have been guided by three overarching goals: simplicity, excellence, and innovation to enhance professional practice. Assessments that achieve only one or two of these goals are unlikely to ultimately benefit children or other consumers, which is the ultimate goal of the assessment process (National Association for the Education of Young Children, 2003). If assessments are too complex, they are unlikely to be used by teachers and other professionals that already have too many demands on their time. If they lack psychometric excellence, error variance will have too much influence on assessment results leading to poor decisions regarding the child. Finally, as practice standards and the evidence base in the field evolve, assessments must provide new tools and interpretive techniques to maintain their utility. The challenge has always been balancing these three goals given that, in some cases, optimizing one characteristic may jeopardize another. For instance, in general, reliability is enhanced as the number of items is increased; however, this adds length to the assessment, which can impair simplicity. As the sections that follow indicate, we believe that we have found a satisfactory balance of these three desired criteria.

Simplicity

There are a number of considerations in ensuring the simplicity of an assessment. The most obvious of these is the reading level of the items and directions. In developing the Devereux Suite, we took a number of steps to ensure that the items would be comprehended by a wide variety of individuals, including those with only a basic level of English proficiency. First, we repeatedly checked the reading level during the development of the item pool. Typically we used the Flesch-Kincaid Grade Level method provided in the Microsoft Word program and strived for a sixth grade or less reading level. In addition, during initial pilot testing, we asked parents and teachers completing the assessment to indicate if they had trouble understanding or completing the item. Any item that was rated as hard to understand by 20% or more of the raters was dropped from the standardization form of the assessments. Finally, as the assessments are revised and renormed (e.g., the DECA), we conduct focus groups with teachers and parents to identify any problematic items. These and other approaches result in items and directions that are clear and easy to understand.

The format of the assessment itself also contributes to simplicity. In addition to a clean and crisp appearance, we strive to develop forms that are intuitive and easy to score. For instance, in the DECA materials, the order of the scales in the score summary boxes on the record form, the norms table, and the Individual Child Profile always follows the same order from left to right. Similarly, parent data is always presented first (either on the top or left side) in every table in the manual, the norms table, and the Individual Child Profile. Such consistency makes information easier to find and reduces error. Another key feature enhancing simplicity is the inclusion of the norms tables, whenever possible, in the actual record form. This eliminates the need to reference the manual when scoring and interpreting the results.

Perhaps the most important and most controversial means of enhancing simplicity is the elimination of multiple rating forms and keeping the number of norms tables to a minimum. For each assessment in the Devereux Suite, there is only one record form. This obviously eliminates the need to keep an inventory of different forms on hand. In order to have only one form, the items have to be appropriate for all raters. This requirement is met by careful item development and ensuring that each item describes a behavior that can be observed in both classroom and home settings. The use of only one form for all raters also has practical advantages as outlined below in the discussion of rater comparisons.

Multiple norms tables, which are often due to age-based norms, increase the possibility of error.[1] There is always a chance that the professional will inadvertently consult the wrong table, or as we have found, teachers and other professionals sometimes "guestimate" the child's birth date and age. If there are age-based norms tables, this can result in significant error. To eliminate the need for age-based norms, we examined age trends in both the pilot and standardization forms of the Devereux assessments and eliminated any items that showed age trends. Consequently, whereas some assessments have multiple norms tables based on age, all of the assessments in the Devereux Suite, with the exception of the DECA-Infant form, have just one norm table for parents and one for teachers. With infants, there were such strong age trends that we decided to present age-based norms.

Many assessments also present norms based on gender again adding to the number or complexity of the norms tables. In the Devereux Suite, we have chosen not to present norms based on gender. Although this does promote the goal of simplicity, our primary reason was value-driven. Separate norms by gender disguise the real differences in girls' and boys' social and emotional competence. We have consistently found that girls tend to exhibit slightly stronger social and emotional skills. Separate norms by gender would equate this higher raw score average for girls with the lower raw score average obtained by boys; both would receive a *T*-score of 50 and a percentile rank of 50. In the Devereux Suite, we decided to preserve this raw score difference by having

[1] For example, one commonly used assessment in school settings presents 39 different norms tables extending over more than 250 pages.

Table 4.3 Internal reliability (Alpha) coefficients for the Devereux Suite

Rating scale	Scale	Teacher raters
Devereux Early Childhood Assessment-Infant (DECA-I)	Total Protective Factors	0.93–0.94
Devereux Early Childhood Assessment-Toddler (DECA-T)	Total Protective Factors	0.95
Devereux Early Childhood Assessment (DECA)	Total Protective Factors	0.94
Devereux Student Strengths Assessment (DESSA)	Social Emotional Composite	0.99
Devereux Student Strengths Assessment-Mini (DESSA-mini)	Form 1–4	0.91–0.92

only one set of norms based on both genders. As a result, in general girls will receive a slightly higher raw and standard score than boys, which reflects a real difference in their social and emotional competence.

Psychometric Excellence

Our second goal in creating the Devereux Suite of Assessments was to meet or exceed professional standards, especially those presented in the Standards for Educational and Psychological Testing (AERA, APA, & NCME, 1999). These standards identify the appropriate standardization sample, reliability, and validity evidence needed to support behavioral assessments. We strive to amply describe how we met and tested psychometric excellence in each assessment's technical manual.

A large and representative standardization sample ensures quality norms. According to Wasserman and Bracken (2003), the main purpose of a standardization sample is to serve as an accurate representation of the population that the assessment is intended to measure. Therefore, we followed their suggestions when developing the Devereux Suite and ensured that the standardization samples were representative of the population of interest according to gender, race, ethnicity, region, and poverty status. Our latest standardization sample (as outlined in the upcoming DECA-P2 Technical Manual) is also representative of parental education. Additionally, which each assessment, we collected a larger standardization sample than previously obtained. As Table 4.1 indicates, each sample meets or exceeds 987 cases.

Good reliability is essential for all measurements used for research as well as in applied settings to ensure accuracy. Reliability is important to the practitioner because it reflects the amount of error in the measurement. Prior to publication, we evaluate every assessment with respect to internal reliability, test–retest reliability, and interrater reliability. Internal reliability (Alpha) coefficients are reported in Table 4.3 for our assessments. Test–retest reliability is obtained when an adult assesses the same child on two separate occasions and yields very similar results. Interrater reliability is obtained when two adults assess a child that they have a similar relationship with and their results are closely correlated. The Devereux Suite reports the results of these and additional studies in each technical manual.

Validity refers to the extent to which empirical evidence and theory supports the recommended uses and interpretations of scores derived from an assessment. For each of our assessments, we demonstrate content, criterion, and construct validity. Content validity is mostly established through careful literature reviews, collaboration with experts in the field, and surveying potential users of the assessment to ensure that the items on the assessment thoroughly sample the constructs they are intended to measure. Criterion validity is an assessments' ability to accurately identify children's membership in a particular group, or in the case of our assessments, accurately identify children who are "seriously emotionally disturbed." Evidence for criterion validity is demonstrated in each technical manual. We have also tested our Suite on construct validity. At the time of the original DECA publication, a similar tool was not available, so the construct validity evidence was limited to the risk and protective factor study previously described. However, the field of strength-based assessments related to resilience has evolved since 1999 and we have been able to demonstrate construct validity in our latest assessments by examining convergent validity with similar measures. For example, scores on the DESSA were correlated with scores on the Behavioral and Emotional Rating Scale-Second Edition (BERS-2; Epstein, 2004) and the Behavior Assessment System for Children-Second Edition (BASC-2; Reynolds & Kamphaus, 2004). Strong correlations between similar scales were obtained.

Innovation to Enhance Professional Practice

Our work in developing assessments of behaviors related to resilience began in the context of early care and education. As a result, we have been very influenced by the position statement of the National Association for the Education of Young Children on "Early Childhood Curriculum, Assessment and Program Evaluation," (NAEYC, 2003). These standards stress that assessments should be, "connected to specific beneficial purposes," (NAEYC, 2003, p. 1). That is, assessment should not solely be an estimate of a child's ability or performance in a given area, but should inform professional practice to benefit the child. The Devereux Suite provides specific tools and techniques to inform practice in three areas: assessing a child's social and emotional strengths and needs, guiding interventions and strategies to support the child's development, and evaluating outcomes.

Assessing Social and Emotional Strengths and Needs

In addition to scale scores which are found on all credible assessments, the Devereux Suite provides a rubric to assist professionals in better understanding the social and emotional competence of the child or children being assessed. The "rater comparison" technique allows the direct comparison of the results obtained from the ratings completed by two adults, typically a teacher and a parent. The goal in comparing the ratings of a child obtained from a parent and a teacher is to better understand the generality or situational specificity of the child's demonstration of social and emotional competencies. For instance, a child might show good self-regulation in a well-structured classroom environment, but not in a more chaotic home situation. Similarly a child who is a recent immigrant might show good initiative at home where he comprehends the language spoken by adults, but not demonstrate this competence in the less familiar and intelligible classroom.

The essential question to ask when comparing ratings obtained from two adults is, *does this difference in scores exceed what I expect by chance and represent a reliable difference in the perceptions of the child's behavior?* To help practitioners answer this important question, the Devereux Suite manuals provide a table of minimal differences required between the two raters in order to conclude that a reliable (i.e., statistically significant) difference exists. The values in the table are based on the standard error of the difference between the scores, calculated using the formula provided by Anastasi and Urbina (1997). For instance, a 10-point *T*-score difference is required for significance when comparing Initiative scale scores obtained from a parent and teacher rating on the DECA. Differences of >10 points can be accounted for by chance. It is important to note that these comparisons can be made for each scale, allowing the determination of agreement on a scale-by-scale basis. Therefore, one might note that the teacher and parent agree on their report of the child's Initiative and Self-regulation, but not Attachment.

In addition to providing a richer and more nuanced view of the child's behavior across settings and informants, the rater comparison technique is also designed to promote parent–professional collaboration. When results are reviewed with the parents, we recommend that the professional proceed in this order:

1. Begin by noting areas where both raters perceive strengths (if any). This sharing of

a positive view of the child's competencies establishes a positive tone for the meeting.

2. Then note areas of agreement that fall in the typical or need ranges. Noting a shared perception of an area of need can build empathy and lay the foundation for a joint strategy to support the child.
3. End by noting areas where the perceptions differ. The approach here should be to better understand why the child shows more competence in one setting than another so that strategies can be shared.

The desired outcomes of this process are a shared understanding of the child's social and emotional strengths and needs, better insight into what helps the child succeed or fail in different settings, and a shared commitment to implementing strategies based on a common understanding of the child and mutual respect between the adults.

Guiding Interventions and Strategies

One of the "specific, beneficial purposes" identified by NAEYC is, "identifying significant concerns that may require focused intervention for individual children" (2003, p. 1). Scale scores have a significant limitation in this respect—they do not provide specific enough information to guide targeted or focused intervention. Often constructs such as within-child protective factors contain subscales or clusters of conceptually related items. For instance, on the DECA Self-control scale, some items relate to anger management (e.g., handle frustration well, calm herself/himself down when upset, control her/his anger) while others concern interpersonal challenges (e.g., cooperate with others, share with other children, listen to or respect others). A child with a score in the need range on this scale might have difficulty with one or the other or both sets of items.

To provide the level of specificity necessary to guide individualized, specific, behaviorally grounded interventions, the Devereux Suite features item-level norms. That is, for each item, we identify a range of scores on that item that was obtained by the lowest 16% of children in the national standardization sample (this is equivalent to a *T*-score of 40 or below and represents a need), was obtained by the 68% of children in the middle of the distribution (i.e., a typical score at the item level), or the top 16% of children (i.e., a strength). We encourage the administrator to examine these item-level norms to determine the specific nature of the child's difficulties and also to identify the specific strengths that the child is exhibiting. We then suggest that these two kinds of items be incorporated into a "Strengths–Needs–Strategies" planning approach to support the child. For instance, on the DESSA, a child received a *T*-score of 32 on the Self-management scale. A review of the items indicated that the child was struggling with transitions. A review of his item-level strengths revealed that he excelled at "following rules," and also liked to "take on additional work or responsibilities." The teacher combined these two important pieces of information about the child in a strategy in which she invited the child to help create the transition rules and routines for the classroom and then teach them to his peers. This kind of targeted intervention requires a finer analysis of the ratings than that provided solely by scale scores.

With the emergence of SEL standards, there is an increasing need for teachers to address the social and emotional competencies of the class as a whole. The Devereux Classroom Profile[2] was developed to assist teachers in using their time and resources to greatest effect. The Classroom Profile is generated by the online administration, scoring and interpretation programs for all four assessments in the Devereux Suite. The Classroom Profile is a color-coded document and therefore is not reproduced as a figure in this chapter. A sample profile can be found however at www.CenterforResilientChildren.org. The Devereux Classroom Profile is essentially a matrix in which each child is a row and each within-child protective factor is a column. Each cell in this matrix then indicates the score a given child received on a specific protective factor. On the Devereux

[2]On the DECA-I and DECA-T, this form is referred to as the Devereux Group Profile.

Classroom Profile, a green-shaded cell indicates a strength, a blue-shaded cell a typical score, and a red-shaded cell a need. By examining the distribution of green, blue, and red cells in each column (i.e., for each protective factor), the administrator can quickly discern the relative strengths and needs of a group of children. One might note, for instance, that Attachment is the area with the greatest number of children with a strength and that Self-control is the protective factor with the greatest number of children with a need. This information can then be used to plan classroom-wide strategies to promote self-control or reinforce attachment. There are many other uses of the Classroom Profile. See www.CenterforResilientChildren.org for more information.

At a yet higher level, results from the Devereux assessments can inform school-wide efforts. For the past 4 years, we have had the privilege of partnering with the Anchorage, Alaska School District and Ms. Ann Bryson, Social and Emotional Learning Coach for Anchorage in field trials of the DESSA. This experience has been of great value to us at the Devereux Center for Resilient Children and has taught us much about how schools that are committed to promoting the resilience of their children can use assessments to guide those efforts. In the 2010–2011 School Year, two of the principals in Anchorage, Diane Hoffbauer at the Alaskan Native Cultural Charter School and Marcus Wilson at North Star Elementary examined DESSA results for their entire schools and noted that many of their children were showing areas of need on the Optimistic Thinking and Decision-Making scales. This insight has led them to focus their entire school community on the promotion of these two protective factors in the 2011–2012 school year. This is a good example of how assessments can, as NAEYC suggested, connect to specific, beneficial purposes.

Assessing Outcomes

The growing emphasis on evidence-based practice and accountability in education and human services has led to a demand for measurable outcomes that substantiate the efficacy of SEL programs and other interventions to promote resilience in children. The Devereux Suite was intentionally designed to help meet this demand. All of the Devereux assessments feature a pretest–posttest comparison technique that is both powerful and flexible in measuring outcomes. Similar to the rater comparison technique described above, the essential question with pretest–posttest comparisons is, *does the amount of change observed in the scale T-scores between pretest and posttest exceed what I would expect by chance?* To answer this important question we provide a table that, for a given pretest *T*-score, gives the range of expected variation in posttest *T*-scores based on both chance variation and regression to the mean. These ranges are based on the standard error of prediction (Atkinson, 1991). If the posttest *T*-score falls above this range, then the child has shown reliable improvement in that protective factor. If the posttest *T*-score falls within the range of expected variation, then no reliable change has occurred. If the posttest *T*-score is below the range, then the child has shown deterioration or worsening in the protective factor. These ranges are provided for each scale on the assessment so the professional can note improvement, no change, or worsening on each scale for a single child. This information can then be used to evaluate and modify interventions at the individual child level. If the child shows improvement in a given area, the interventions are having their desired effect. If no change or worsening is noted, the interventions are ineffective and need to be increased in intensity, frequency or duration, or changed altogether.

Once outcome data has been evaluated for each child, the results can be aggregated for a classroom. For example, using this approach a teacher might note that of all the children showing a need on the Attachment scale at pretest, 75% have shown improvement on the posttest. However, of children showing a need on the Self-control scale at pretest, only 25% showed reliable improvement. The promotion of Self-control could then become an area identified in the teacher's professional development plan or a focus of supervision. These data could even be aggregated at the school level leading a principal to identify areas where the teachers excel at promoting protective factors and areas where, as a group, they are having less success. This could lead to school-wide quality improvement efforts (as in the case of the schools in Anchorage discussed above) or to targeted professional development for the faculty.

This section has reviewed just some of the ways in which the Devereux Suite of Assessments can provide education and human service professionals with new tools and approaches to promoting the resilience of children. Assessments are not used to their full advantage when practitioners stop at recording a scale score. Rather, they can be used to better understand the child, plan more specific and targeted interventions to support the child, and evaluate our efforts so that we can continually improve outcomes and promote the resilience of all children.

Conclusion: A New and Valuable Approach to Promotion and Prevention

This chapter began with a brief review of the ways in which the concept of resilience has gained recognition and prominence in research, practice, and policy. The evidence base for the critical role of social and emotional competence and resilience in school and life success continues to expand at an exponential rate; more state departments of education are promulgating SEL standards, and leading professional organizations like the National Association of School Psychologists now expect their members to assess and promote social and emotional competence and resilience. The Devereux Suite of Assessments was developed to support and promote these positive trends.

Our experience over the past 15 years has also indicated that the shift to strength-based assessments can directly influence how teachers, counselors, psychologists, and front-line human service workers view children and also their role as a child-serving professional. Across educational, child welfare and behavioral health treatment settings, three themes have emerged.

Theme 1: A More Balanced View of the Child

One of the most profound changes among professionals is the recognition of a student's strengths, particularly when that student had been identified as seriously emotionally disturbed. For instance, one of the teachers in Anchorage commented, "*Being that my students are in a self-contained special education classroom, I was surprised that several of my students are 'typical' in more areas than I would have thought.*" Similarly, in a pilot study of the DESSA conducted at a private school in Pennsylvania serving children who had been identified as seriously emotionally disturbed, although the majority of the 25 students had Social and Emotional Composite scores in the Need range, only four students (16%) did not have at least one scale score in the Typical range (Dopp & LeBuffe, 2010). The use of well-developed strength-based assessments often makes evident the normative or superlative behaviors of children with special needs that sometimes get overlooked. In a survey of 75 teachers from Anchorage and an elementary school in the state of Washington (Ball & Hughes, 2009) 68% agreed that the DESSA gave them new and unique information about the students in their class. By making the positive behaviors of children obvious, strength-based assessments lead to a more balanced view of the child.

Theme 2: A Better Basis for Collaboration

At least since the publication of the Child and Adolescent Service System Program Principles (Stroul & Friedman, 1986), professionals in child-serving systems have been expected to collaborate with parents in decision-making and education/treatment planning regarding their child. By focusing on the promotion of child strengths, rather than solely on the reduction of problem behaviors, strength-based assessments can promote stronger collaboration with parents as seen in these comments by teachers in Anchorage, "*The DESSA would help give specific vocabulary for explaining strengths and weaknesses,*" "*The parallels and differences between the two surveys would be a jumping off point for discussion of student behaviors in class and at home,*" and "*The DESSA is a way we can be on the same team to build up a child.*"

The very act of recognizing a child's strengths in a meaningful way can have a large positive impact on parent–professional relationships. Park and Turnbull (2002) surveyed 68 family members regarding what they considered to be "quality indicators" for the professionals who worked with their special-needs children. The first theme to emerge from their qualitative analysis of the focus group results was, "Respect for Children," which included both treating children with dignity and being positive toward children. Park and Turnbull noted (p. 119) that "families wanted professionals to look at the positive side of their children. Many families expressed frustration when professionals focused only on what the child cannot do without considering the child's strengths and preferences." Clearly, assessments such as those in the Devereux Suite can help professionals meet this reasonable and important expectation of parents.

Theme 3: A Reason for Hope

The promotion of social and emotional competence and resilience is, at its core, an optimistic business. Beginning with the observations of children who, to use Emmy Werner's phrase, "defied the odds," to the more recent conclusion of Masten (2001) that resilience is "Ordinary Magic" that all children are capable of attaining if basic human resources and adaptational systems are protected, the study of resilience has always focused on promoting healthy human outcomes. Now that the field has good tools including the Devereux Suite of Assessments and Prince-Embury's Resilience Scale for Children and Adolescents, professionals can identify children at risk of negative developmental outcomes because their within-child protective factors are lacking or not as strong as we would expect. This gives us the opportunity to intervene and add or strengthen protective factors before risk factors overwhelm the child and jeopardize development, health, and happiness. Armed with good measures of behaviors related to resilience, we are in a better position to assure parents, children, and ourselves that, in the words of our colleague Dr. Tom Lottman, "Risk is not destiny."

References

Academic, Social, and Emotional Learning Act of 2011, H.R. 2437, 112th Cong. (2011). Retrieved from http://www.govtrack.us/congress/billtext.xpd?bill=h112-2437

American Educational Research Association, American Psychological Association, & National Council on Measurement in Education. (1999). *Standards for educational and psychological testing*. Washington, DC: Author.

Anastasi, A., & Urbina, S. (1997). *Psychological testing* (7th ed.). Upper Saddle River, NJ: Prentice Hall.

Atkinson, L. (1991). Three standard errors of measurement and the Wechsler memory scale-revised. *Psychological Assessment: A Journal of Consulting and Clinical Psychology, 3*, 136–138.

Ball, A., & Hughes, C. (2009). *Examining the contextual validity of the DESSA and DESSA-mini for use in primary and middle school settings*. Villanova, PA: Unpublished Research Report for the Devereux Center for Resilient Children.

Collaborative for Academic, Social, and Emotional Learning. (2011). *SEL in your state*. Retrieved from http://casel.org/research/sel-in-your-state/

Dopp, A., & LeBuffe, P. (2010). *A pilot study of the efficacy and acceptability of the Devereux Student Strengths Assessment in an approved private school*. Villanova, PA: Unpublished Research Report from the Devereux Center for Resilient Children.

Durlak, J. A., Weissberg, R. P., Dymnicki, A. B., Taylor, R. D., & Schellinger, K. B. (2011). The impact of enhancing students' social and emotional learning: A meta-analysis of school-based universal interventions. *Child Development, 82*, 405–432.

Epstein, M. H. (2004). *Behavioral and Emotional Rating Scale, Second Edition: Examiner's manual*. Austin, TX: PRO-ED, Inc.

Kanner, A. D., Coyne, J. C., Schaefer, C., & Lazarus, R. S. (1981). Comparison of two modes of stress measurement: Daily hassles and uplifts versus major life events. *Journal of Behavioral Medicine, 4*, 1–39.

LeBuffe, P. A., & Naglieri, J. A. (1999). *Devereux Early Childhood Assessment: User's guide and technical manual*. Lewisville, NC: Kaplan.

LeBuffe, P. A., & Shapiro, V. B. (2004). Lending "strength" to the assessment of preschool social–emotional health. *The California School Psychologist, 9*, 51–61.

LeBuffe, P. A., Shapiro, V. B., & Naglieri, J. A. (2009). *The Devereux Student Strengths Assessment (DESSA) manual*. Lewisville, NC: Kaplan.

Masten, A. S. (2001). Ordinary magic. *American Psychologist, 56*(3), 227–238.

Masten, A. S., & Garmezy, N. (1985). Risk, vulnerability and protective factors in developmental psychopathology. In B. B. Lahey & A. E. Kazdin (Eds.), *Advances in clinical child psychology* (Vol. 8, pp. 1–512). New York, NY: Plenum.

Merrell, K. W. (2011). *Social–Emotional Assets and Resilience Scales*. Lutz, FL: PAR Assessments.

Naglieri, J. A., LeBuffe, P. A., & Pfeiffer, S. I. (1993). *Devereux Behavior Rating Scale - School Form*. San Antonio, TX: The Psychological Corporation.

Naglieri, J. A., LeBuffe, P. A., & Shapiro, V. B. (2011). *The Devereux Student Strengths Assessment-Mini manual*. Lewisville, NC: Kaplan.

National Association for the Education of Young Children, & National Association of Early Childhood Specialists in State Departments of Education. (2003). *Early childhood curriculum, assessment, and program evaluation: Building an effective, accountable system in programs for children birth through age 8 (Joint Position Statement)*. Washington, DC: NAEYC.

National Association of School Psychologists. (2010). Model for comprehensive and integrated school psychological services. *School Psychology Review, 39*, 320–333.

Park, J., & Turnbull, A. P. (2002). Quality indicators of professionals who work with children with problem behavior. *Journal of Positive Behavior Interventions, 4*(2), 118–122.

Powell, G., Mackrain, M., & LeBuffe, P. (2007). *Devereux Early Childhood Assessment for Infants and Toddlers, technical manual*. Lewisville, NC: Kaplan.

Prince-Embury, S. (2007). *Resiliency Scales for Children and Adolescents: Profiles of Personal Strengths*. San Antonio, TX: Harcourt Assessments, Inc.

Reynolds, C. R., & Kamphaus, R. W. (2004). *Behavior Assessment System for Children-Second Edition: manual*. Circle Pines, MN: American Guidance Service.

Search Institute. (2004). *Developmental Assets Profile*. Minneapolis, MN: Author.

Stroul, B. A., & Friedman, R. M. (1986). *A system of care for seriously emotionally disturbed children and youth*. Washington, DC: CASSP Technical Assistance Center, Georgetown University Child Development Center.

Wasserman, J. D., & Bracken, B. A. (2003). Psychometric characteristics of assessment procedures. In I. Weiner, D. Freedheim, J. Schinka, & W. Velicer (Eds.), *Handbook of psychology* (pp. 43–66). New York, NY: Wiley.

Work, W. C., Cowen, E. L., Parker, G. R., & Wyman, P. A. (1990). Stress resilient children in an urban setting. *Journal of Prevention, 11*, 3–17.

Classroom Resilience: Practical Assessment for Intervention

5

Samuel Y. Song, Beth Doll, and Kelly Marth

Resilience research has proven to be helpful to those committed to improving academic and psychosocial outcomes for students within schools. Empirical descriptions of children who succeed despite growing up in very adverse living conditions have been used as an undergirding foundation to applied practice in schools (Doll & Cummings, 2008; Doll et al., 2009; Werner, 2006). However, a major challenge has been the translation of diverse resilience constructs and research (described in detail in Chap. 1) into practical assessments of resilience that are meaningful in schools. School practitioners require assessment strategies that capture the foundations of developmental resilience research, while also relating in important ways to the empirical precursors to school success and using procedures that are resource efficient and highly beneficial for educational planning.

Applied practice in schools includes two groups of mental health professionals: *community professionals* (e.g., psychiatrists who provide monthly medication consultations) who work primarily outside the school system but collaborate with schools in a consultative manner; and *school professionals* (e.g., school psychologists or school counselors) who are employees of the school system and are credentialed by state education departments. Applied practices to strengthen resilience in schools may look quite different depending on whether practitioners are community professionals or school professionals. Community professionals are often focused on assessing resilience "within the person" because much of the funding for community agencies is tied to third-party reimbursements that target a single student (Doll, 2010). School professionals on the other hand are more likely to assess resilience "within the context" as long as they can demonstrate that these strategies yield meaningful improvements in students' school success. School professionals must frequently negotiate complex factors within the school system to influence their districts' commitment to the promotion of resilience within an educational climate that emphasizes academic learning. Whereas community professionals typically reside within agencies that recognize social, emotional, and psychological wellness to be core to their missions.

Until recently, resilience-promoting assessment and intervention strategies have emphasized

S.Y. Song, Ph.D., N.C.S.P. (✉) • K. Marth
Counseling & School Psychology Department,
Seattle University, Loyola Hall 215, 901 12th Ave,
Box 222000, Seattle, WA 98122-1090, USA
e-mail: songs@seattleu.edu

B. Doll, Ph.D.
College of Education and Human Sciences,
University of Nebraska Lincoln, 238 Mabel Lee Hall,
Lincoln, NE 68588-0234, USA
e-mail: Bdoll2@unl.edu

S. Prince-Embury and D.H. Saklofske (eds.), *Resilience in Children, Adolescents, and Adults: Translating Research into Practice*, The Springer Series on Human Exceptionality,
DOI 10.1007/978-1-4614-4939-3_5, © Springer Science+Business Media New York 2013

"within the person" frameworks (Knitzer, 2005), which may be a significant reason why previous assessment tools have often been impractical for widespread use in the schools (Prince-Embury & Saklofske, 2011). This chapter will describe the early steps in an effort to bridge this research-to-school-practice gap by developing an assessment and school change strategy that is sensitive to the needs of school professionals.

The *ClassMaps Consultation (CMC)* framework (Doll et al., 2009; Doll, Zucker, & Brehm, 2004) is a pioneering effort to translate resilience research into applied practice in schools by teachers and school mental health professionals. First, characteristics of school contexts were identified that have been empirically associated with the social, emotional, and academic success of chronically underprivileged students. Then, the ClassMaps Survey (CMS) was developed and field tested, with subscales that assess each of the identified characteristics. Subsequently, the CMS is being used within a data-based problem-solving cycle to prompt classrooms and schools to strengthen their resilience-promoting characteristics. Within the CMC framework, allowance was always made for the possibility that additional resilience-promoting characteristics would be identified, and these could easily be integrated into the data-based problem-solving cycle. The Protective Peer Ecology Scale (PPEcoS; Song, 2004, 2006) is a prime example. The PPEcoS assesses an aspect of schools' peer culture that was not part of the original ClassMaps Framework but is nevertheless highly related to schools' promotion of developmental resilience. To enhance the scales' relevance to school practice, both the CMS and the PPEcoS assess resilience as a characteristic of the school context (rather than as a "within the person" construct) and both emphasize positive characteristics that promote resilience in preference to assessing the absence of pathology. In the remainder of this chapter, we will first describe the ClassMaps Framework, then describe the development and technical soundness of the CMS and the PPEcoS, and finally describe the place of these assessment tools within the larger task of promoting students' resilience in schools.

Resilience Framework

The ClassMaps Framework is based on developmental resilience research and an ecological framework and has the goal of being useful for school practitioners. Within this broad theoretical framework, an empirical approach was first employed to identify characteristics that were consistent with the framework. Multiple longitudinal studies have identified very similar family and community characteristics that predict school success in vulnerable children growing up with multiple adversities (Doll & Lyon, 1998; Werner, 2006). These characteristics include nurturing by adults, forming a close bond with at least one caretaker, finding friendships with peers, holding expectations of efficacy and competence, developing an internal locus of control or sense of self-determination, and expanding their capacity for self-control. Similarly in the educational literature, there is substantial consensus that three key features of schools and classrooms influence academic engagement in students: (a) relatedness in which teachers and classmates contribute to a caring and supportive social community; (b) perceived competence in which students expect to be successful in school and so behave in ways that predispose them to experience success; and (c) autonomy in which students act as executive directors of their own learning experiences (Fredricks, Blumenfeld, & Paris, 2004; Furrer & Skinner, 2003; National Research Council [NRC], 2004). Thus, high quality relationships and supports for students' developing autonomy and perceived competence are characteristics of success-promoting tiers of influence within students' ecosystems.

Resilience is conceptualized then as a set of environmental characteristics that make up the ecology of school classrooms, which can be assessed and enhanced through intervention strategies. Accordingly, these factors found in the empirical literature were then operationalized in the CMS to provide an assessment tool that could serve as a first step towards strengthening classroom learning ecologies and supporting students' academic engagement (Doll et al., 2009; Doll,

Zucker, et al., 2004). The CMS emphasizes three aspects of relatedness (students' relationships with their teachers, students' relationships with their classmates, and families' involvement in students' schooling), and three aspects supporting student autonomy (students' efficacy for their own academic success, students' self-determination for goals and decisions related to their schooling, and their self-control of their own goal-directed behaviors). The six ecological factors emphasized in the CMS have also been demonstrated in educational and psychological research to be critical to students' achievement in classrooms and influence student's motivational response to school (Bandura, 1997; Brophy, 2004; Deci & Ryan, 2000; Masten et al., 1999; Masten & Powell, 2003; NRC/IOM, 2004).

Relational Characteristics of Resilient Classrooms

Social relationships have long been recognized as essential building blocks of resilience and psychological wellness. Learning is essentially a social activity that emerges out of interpersonal interactions between and among adults and children. However, the relationships in classrooms are unique because they are necessarily constructed among a very few adult teachers and many students. Relationships among students are also unique because school settings almost always represent the earliest opportunity for children to interact with each other outside of the close monitoring of their families. Both adult–child and child–child relationships can be characterized by either positive (prosocial) or negative (conflictual) features, and it is increasingly apparent that these are isomorphic features. Conflict does not always signify the absence of caring, and prosocial interactions are not necessarily conflict free.

Teachers' Relationships with Students. A strikingly consistent finding of developmental resilience researchers has been that effective relationships with caring adults are critically important protective factors for children growing up in disadvantaged homes and communities (Werner, 2006). In schools, the most important adult relationships are those that students form with their teachers. Teachers are an enduring presence in the lives of children, represent the most familiar adult outside of their parents for many students, and act as important "secure bases" that allow children to explore and take risks intellectually, socially, and emotionally (Kesner, 2000; Pianta, 1999). Effective teacher–student relationships are caring, trusting, respectful, and fair. The support that students receive from their teachers contributes to their behavioral competence (Hamre & Pianta, 2005), academic progress (Murray & Malmgren, 2005), and social success (Pianta & Stuhlman, 2004). Particularly when they are struggling with family and community disadvantages, students who feel valued and respected by their teachers are more committed to learning and better able to cope with adversity (National Research Council/Institute of Medicine, 2004).

Like students' relationships with parents, students can be taught strategies to strengthen their relationships with teachers by sustaining interactions over time and demonstrating respect for teachers' expectations and requests (Consortium on the School-Based Promotion of Social Competence, 1994). Alternatively, teachers strengthen these relationships by being warm, caring, fair, and helpful and by modeling responsible behavior (Brophy, 2004; Wentzel, 2002). Effective teachers use humor and encouragement to empower students' independence and autonomy. The challenge for teachers is that these relationships are asymmetrical (adults retain more responsibility for and power over the relationship than students) and simultaneous (with teachers interacting with all students in a classroom at any single moment) (Consortium on the School-Based Promotion of Social Competence, 1994). Thus, teachers must master the very difficult art of interacting personally and effectively with large groups of individual students. The CMS assesses student perceptions of teacher–student relationships with the My Teacher subscale described in detail later.

Peer Relationships. Developmental resilience researchers have also demonstrated the significance of peer relationships in children's development (Werner, 2006). Peer relationships refer to students' interactions with their classmates in all forms such as friendships, acquaintances, and enemies. Friendships form when two students mutually prefer one another's company and provide important sources of support for one another such as companionship, assistance, comfort, and fun (Johnson, Johnson, Buckman, & Richards, 1998). Peer friendships have been significantly correlated with academic achievement (Pellegrini, 2005; Wentzel & Caldwell, 1997), as students who have friends at school are more engaged in academic and school activities (Pellegrini, 2005; Wentzel & Watkins, 2002). Therefore, the CMS's My Classmates subscale assesses the degree to which students' believe that their friendships at school are rewarding.

Peer conflict is a normative experience within peer relationships, as even friends may tease one another and have arguments that need to be problem solved. Indeed, one study found that most students reported that their classmates teased them (60%) or argued with them (67%; Doll, 2006). Still, when peer conflict is unresolved, this can lead to a decline in classroom student involvement (Ladd, Birch, & Buhs, 1999). Intense peer conflict has been shown to lead to academically disengagement and school dropout (Barclay & Doll, 2001). The Kids In This Class subscale of the CMS measures peer conflict perceived by students within classrooms.

While peer conflict is common among friends, bullying often occurs between non-friends and within peer groups. Bullying is when peer aggression becomes a pattern between more powerful students against weaker students who cannot make the bullying stop (Aluede, Adeleke, Omoike, & Afen-Akapida, 2008; Olweus, 1993). Bullying occurs among students at a regular rate of 10–20% (Nansel, Overpeck, & Pilla, 2001). The negative consequences of bullying are clear and include academic challenges, e.g., absenteeism, difficulty concentrating on learning, school drop out, and psychological challenges such as social skills deficits, higher rates of depression, and anxiety (Aluede et al., 2008; Paul & Cillessen, 2003). Peer bullying may be measured by the degree to which students worry about peers becoming aggressive towards them such as in the I Worry That subscale of the CMS.

Protective Peer Ecology. A recent extension of the peer relationships dimension of resilient classrooms focuses on how peers protect one another from bullying and provide social support for one another. This aspect of peer relationships has been argued to be the most influential context for bullying prevention (Song, 2006; Song, Doll, Swearer, Johnsen, & Siegel, under review; Song & Stoiber, 2008), and as such may be the best target for bullying prevention. Peers can effectively help correct the inherent power imbalance between bullies and victims and address school environments that encourage bullying (i.e., inaction of school personnel). For example, because peers are typically present during the majority of bullying interactions, they can detect even the covert occurrences of bullying and, therefore, intervene on bullying more effectively than adult school personnel (e.g., Craig & Pepler, 1997). Peers may also be preferred over adults when victims of bullying are deciding to whom to come for help. This aspect of peer relationships, protective peers, is measured by the PPEcoS (Song, 2006).

Home–School Relationships. A final resilience-promoting relationship occurs between home and school. Home–school relationships refer to all types of interactions between a student's family and the school contexts, e.g., direct in-person and indirect communication. A number of studies have shown the positive effects that come from a strong home–school relationship. For example, student outcomes have been demonstrated for higher rates of work completion (Epstein & Van Voorhis, 2001), higher grades and test scores (Fan, 2001; Hill et al., 2004), better attendance, fewer suspensions, and likelihood to complete school (Anguiano, 2004; Fan, 2001; Hill et al., 2004). Key school practices that encourage this relationship are implementing parent-centered practices that promote involvement, inviting parents to participate, and expecting parents to do so

(Hoover-Dempsey et al., 2005). The Talking With My Parents subscale from the CMS describes the home–school relationship from the students' perspective.

Autonomy-Promoting Characteristics of Resilient Classrooms

Academic Self-Efficacy. Developmental resilience research has supported that a student's confidence in succeeding on a task is a critically important protective factor for children growing up in disadvantaged homes and communities (Werner, 2006). Success in school is also strongly influenced by self-efficacy beliefs (Bandura, 1997; Pajares & Schunk, 2001; Schunk & Pajares, 2005). Self-efficacy is shaped in school classrooms by regular and prompt feedback on student work, direct and indirect experiences of success and failure, and encouragement from their teachers and peers (Brophy, 2004; Pastorelli et al., 2001). Students' academic efficacy is measured by The Believing In Me subscale of the CMS.

Self-Determination. The second autonomy-promoting resilience factor is self-determination, the ability to manage one's learning productively. Students who are self-determined can set productive goals for their learning, behave according to these goals, and allot the appropriate amount of effort to achieve them (Masten et al., 1999). Responsible learning, taking credit for achievements, developing reasonable plans to address academic failures, and intrinsic motivation to succeed also characterize self-determined students (Assor, Kaplan, & Roth, 2002; Masten, 2001). Self-determination may be promoted in classrooms that value skill competency using specific and attainable mastery goals instead of competitive performance goals (Pajares & Schunk, 2001). The CMS assesses students' self-determination with the Taking Charge subscale.

Behavioral Self-Control. Resilience in classrooms also includes behavioral self-control. Behavioral self-control incorporates autonomy in that students' learn to management themselves in terms of appropriate, rule-governed, and goal-directed actions (Bandura, 1997; Bear, 2005). Behavioral choices, expectations set for behavior, and the degree to which students meet their self-imposed expectations all influence behavioral self-control in students. Empirical work has substantiated the interaction between behavioral conduct and academic success (Hawkins et al., 2003; Osher, Bear, Sprague, & Doyle, 2010), academic underachievement (Lane, Pierson, & Givner, 2003), and students' grades (McDermott, Mordell, & Stoltzfus, 2001; Osher et al., 2010). Behavioral self-control is also linked to key relationship factors in classrooms such as weakened relationships with their teachers and peers. Many prominent evidence-based interventions have been designed to improve behavioral self-control in classrooms (Bear, 2005; Mitchem, Young, West, & Benyo, 2001; Osher et al., 2010). These management strategies fall into types that are more adult imposed or student centered (Bear, 2005). Strategies that are more likely to strengthen students' self-regulated discipline and control are student-centered approaches. Students' class wide behavioral control is assessed on the Following Class Rules subscale of the CMS.

Resilience Operationalized for Assessment

The ClassMaps Survey

Efforts to strengthen the resilience-promoting characteristics of classrooms depend on the availability of a technically sound and eminently practical measure of classroom resilience that can guide and evaluate classroom change efforts. With this ultimate purpose in mind, the CMS (Doll, Spies, Champion, et al., 2010; Doll, Spies, LeClair, Kurien, & Foley, 2010) has been developed through an ambitious program of research extending through the past 14 years. As a first step, a careful research review was conducted to identify the characteristics of classrooms that were strongly related to the success of students who learned there (Doll, Zucker, et al., 2004). Three relational characteristics (teacher–student relationships, peer relationships, home–school relationships) and three autonomy-promoting characteristics (academic efficacy, academic self-determination, and behavioral self-control) were identified through this research review. Next, student survey items were developed to describe each characteristic, resulting in a pilot survey with six subscales. Items were field tested across elementary and middle school students; quantitative data was used to describe the technical properties of the CMS while qualitative data was gathered to examine teachers and students' perceptions of the items' clarity, relevance, and acceptability. Results were used to refine the survey through three successive forms: the CMS 2004; CMS 2005; and CMS 2007. Refinements resulted in an eight-subscale CMS 2007 that closely matched the six classroom characteristics identified initially. The eight CMS 2007 subscales include: My Teacher (teacher–student relationships), My Classmates (peer friendships), Talking With My Parents (home–school relationships), Believing In Me (academic self-efficacy), Taking Charge (academic self-determination), Following Class Rules (behavioral self-control), Kids In This Class (peer conflict), and I Worry That (worries about peer aggression). The technical properties (reliability, factor structure, and validity) of the CMS 2007 were then examined in two comprehensive studies: one with elementary students (Doll, Spies, LeClair, et al., 2010) and the second with middle school science students (Doll, Spies, Champion, et al., 2010).

Item Development and Field Testing. The item development phase of the CMS research was intended to yield a survey with separate subscales for each of the six classroom characteristics. Ideally, each subscale could then be used independent of the others, depending upon the focus and content of classroom intervention efforts. Consequently, each subscale's internal consistency needed to be adequate to support its independent use. Between 6 and 8 items were written for each characteristic, resulting in a 40-item version of the survey. This pilot version was administered to 400 middle school students (Doll et al., 1999). Results showed that the pilot survey had six factors (as predicted) but the subscales' internal consistency was inadequate for the peer relationships subscale (0.56). Feedback from both students and teachers was used to refine the items' wording, format, and practical utility.

Next, with the assistance of elementary school teachers, the 40 items were simplified so that elementary students could easily understand them. Each item used a uniform 3-point Likert-type response format: "Yes," "Sometimes," or "No." The 40-item CMS 2004 was then administered in 82 classrooms in rural and urban Midwestern communities (Doll & Siemers, 2004; Doll, Song, & Siemers, 2004). Results showed that CMS 2004 had seven factors: two peer relationships factors (peer friendships and peer conflict) and one factor for each of the remaining five classroom characteristics. Most items loaded on their predicted factor. However, the internal consistency of both the Believing In Me and the Taking Charge subscales fell below 0.70 (0.64 and 0.55, respectively) and so was insufficient to support the use of these subscales as stand-alone measures.

Subscale Refinement. The CMS was further revised and strengthened over a 2-year span. The CMS 2005 version included rewritten items using a 4-point Likert-type scale: Never, Sometimes, Often, and Almost Always. Several items were dropped from the Following Class Rules subscale, because they contributed little to the subscale's internal consistency. Also, and at the request of a school partner, an additional peer relationships subscale describing students' worries about peer aggression was added (I Worry That). The CMS 2007 version separated the peer relationships subscale into two subscales: My Classmates (peer friendships) and Kids In This Class (peer conflict) because these had consistently factored into two parts across previous analyses. Additional revisions simplified the language and eliminated all double negatives from item wording, and the peer conflict items were rewritten as negative items (e.g., "Kids in this class argue a lot with each other").

Negative items on the Kids In This Class subscale and the I Worry That subscale were reverse scored so that higher scores still represented more positive perceptions of the classroom. Finally, items were refined to better represent empirical findings for the Believing In Me subscale and the Taking Charge subscale.

These revisions successfully raised the internal consistency reliability of the subscales from an average of 0.66 to an average of 0.74 (Doll & Spies, 2007). The dimensionality of the CMS 2007 demonstrated an eight-factor solution in which all items loaded on their predicted subscale. Subsequently, using a sample of 1,056 science students (Grades 5–8), a factor analysis of seven of the eight CMS 2007 subscales (absent the I Worry That subscale) supported a seven factor solution with coefficient alphas ranging from 0.80 to 0.91 (Doll, Champion, & Kurien, 2008).

Concurrent Validity of the CMS. As additional evidence of the CMS' technical soundness, several studies compared the CMS subscales with other well-established and theoretically similar measures. Using a high school sample, significant correlations ranging from 0.47 to 0.80 were found for parallel scales of CMS 2004 and the Yale School Development Program School Climate Survey (Paul, 2005). With an elementary sample, and as predicted, the Friendship Features Scale correlated significantly with the My Classmates subscale of the CMS 2005 ($r=0.81$) and did not correlate with the Kids in This Class subscale ($r=0.28$). In a middle school sample, all subscales of the CMS 2007 correlated with middle school students' positive ratings of the science instruction that they received in the class (Doll et al., 2008). Its utility as a measure of classroom learning environments was supported in two intervention studies that used the CMS to evaluate interventions to strengthen classroom resilience characteristics (Murphy, 2002; Nickolite & Doll, 2008). A third study used the CMS 2007 to examine differences in English Language learner students' perceptions of their classrooms (LeClair, Doll, Osborn, & Jones, 2009).

Construct Validity of the CMS. Most recently, two studies have examined the factor structure of the CMS 2007. Using a sample of 345 third through fifth grade students, the first study demonstrated that most CMS items (53 of the 55) loaded strongly onto their theoretically predicted subscale, the internal consistency of all subscales was strong (α equal to or greater than 0.75), and the subscale means were consistent across grade and gender (Doll, Spies, LeClair, et al., 2010). The second study, conducted with 1,019 fifth- through eighth-grade science students (Doll, Spies, Champion, et al., 2010), used a confirmatory factor analysis to reaffirm that the survey factored into the predicted subscales and demonstrate that subscales correlated as predicted with four additional scales. In the second study, internal consistency for the CMS subscales was somewhat stronger (α equal to or greater than 0.82).

The CM Survey was developed to provide a practical yet psychometrically sound assessment of the six characteristics of classroom resilience. Because resilience research using sociometrics has demonstrated that the aggregation of student judgments across all students in a class provides an appropriate description of classmates' social behaviors (Barclay, 1992; Gresham, 1986), it was expected that aggregated student judgments could also be useful to describe classroom resilience. The CMS is part of a larger intervention model in schools called ClassMaps Consultation (CMC), which requires quick and efficient administration methods of the surveys such as through simple computer technology, which also prints out data files immediately for data graphs or data reports. In practice, the student survey data had other benefits that were not anticipated. One of the most important benefits was that the surveys added a new tier of influence (peer ecology) to the intervention planning process, which most teachers had not accessed, due to the discussions with classroom students. These new insights into the peer ecology were often important keys to intervention, as students' perceptions of their own classroom were related in important ways to their behaviors in the same classrooms.

The Protective Peer Ecology Scale

Following a similar conceptual rationale for development as the CMS, the PPEcoS (Song, 2004, 2006) was developed more specifically to address school bullying by assessing a key resilience factor within the peer ecology. The original elementary school version of the PPEcoS (Song, 2004, 2006) was developed from a comprehensive review of developmental research, focus group interviews with school personnel and children, and expert review. It demonstrated strong psychometric properties in preliminary studies (Song, 2006; Song & Siegel, 2006a; Song, Siegel, & Doll, 2009; Song & Sogo, 2010). Peer protection measures perceptions of the peer context regarding classmates' protection from bullying. Ratings are obtained through students' responses on a 5-point scale (never to always) to the prompt, "If I'm being bullied, my peers would try to stop the bullying." All items loaded strongly on a single factor accounting for a cumulative total of 50.5% of the variance explained by the factor. Internal consistency using coefficient alpha was 0.86 indicating adequate reliability, and the subscales related both significantly and in the expected directions with known correlates (i.e., positive relations with positive peer relationship variables and negative relations with being bullied variables).

The middle school version of the PPEcoS (Song, 2005) was also developed to measure four critical variables of the protective peer ecology: peer protection, peer encouragement of bullying, peer protector, and peer encourager of bullying. The middle school version was developed through a series of focus group interviews consisting of relevant school personnel, i.e., school administrator, teachers, school counselors, and school psychologists. Peer protection and peer encouragement of bullying subscales measure perceptions of the peer context regarding classmates' protection from bullying and classmates' encouragement of bullying. Ratings are obtained through students' responses on a 5-point scale (never to always) to the prompt, "If I'm being bullied…" Peer protection from bullying is a subscale comprising eight items (e.g., my peers would try to stop the bullying) that measures students' perceptions that peers would intervene if they were bullied. The peer encouragement of bullying subscale is a 5-item subscale that includes items such as "my peers would laugh." The third subscale peer protector includes eight items designed to assess a student's inclination to protect others from bullying (e.g., I would try to make the others stop bullying) that students rate on a 5-point scale (never to always) in response to the prompt, "If I know that someone in my school is being bullied…" Finally, the peer encourager of bullying subscale is five items with the same prompt and format, but the items assess a student's inclination to encourage bullying in the peer context (e.g., I would laugh).

All four subscales of the first draft of the PPEcoS-Middle School Version had adequate dimensionality and reliability (Hamm et al., 2010; Song & Sogo, 2010). Preliminary analyses of the dimensionality of the scale have provided strong support for the four factors based on exploratory factor analysis using principal axis factoring (Hamm et al., 2010; Song & Sogo, 2010). Using a sample of 428 sixth through eighth graders from the Northeastern USA, all items loaded strongly on their respective factors (ranged between 0.50 and 0.90) and independently, explaining a total of 67.4% of the variance, coefficient alphas all strong indicating adequate reliability, and bivariate correlations were significant and in the expected direction with known correlates.

A second study using a rural middle school sample across multiple sites further supported the preliminary findings indicating strong psychometric properties for the PPEcoS (Hamm et al., 2010). Following a randomized control trial design, Native American and White students' ($N=165$) social, behavioral, and academic adjustment was assessed in intervention compared with control schools. More so than White students, Native American students evidenced particular gains in achievement and perceptions of the school social/affective context, which included the PPEcoS. In this study, the PPEcoS demonstrated comparable Cronbach's α across Native American ($\alpha=0.91$) and White ($\alpha=0.89$) participants, as well as by gender ($\alpha=0.87$ for female participants; $\alpha=0.91$ for male participants).

Next Steps

This chapter has provided an illustration of how developmental resilience research can be translated into survey assessments that describe the degree to which essential resilience-promoting characteristics are present within schools and classrooms. It described ClassMaps' resilient classroom framework of ClassMaps and two operationalizations of the framework: the ClassMaps Surveys and the PPEcoS. Results of both surveys can be aggregated across all students in a class or a school, providing a useful index of the degree to which these characteristics are present or absent. The resulting data can be a foundation for subsequent interventions using a simple data-based problem-solving cycle (Doll, Zucker, et al., 2004). Schools might change key routines and practices in response to the data, or they might engage teachers, parents, or students in problem-solving discussions to evaluate the accuracy of the data and suggest modifications that might be responsive to the data. For example, in response to data showing frequent playground fights over playground rules, one school created a common booklet of "school rules" for several popular recess games (e.g., tetherball, four-square, one-goal basketball), carefully explained the rules to all teachers and recess supervisors, and explicitly taught the rules during each class's physical education period. The frequency of playground fights fell as a result. When simple modifications of routines are not sufficient, schools might use data for ambitious data-based problem-solving meetings in the school and community (Osher & Kendziora, 2010). If problem-solving meetings are insufficient, evidence-based curricula might be implemented in response to identified weaknesses captured by data. The ultimate test of the utility of the ClassMaps Framework is its translation into school learning environments that contribute to the resilience of students who learn there.

Even though the ClassMaps Framework is essentially a population-based model that emphasizes interventions that strengthen school environments (Doll & Cummings, 2008), we are not arguing that the framework can be used instead of "within the person" practices. Indeed, even within the strongest classroom environments, there will be students who continue to struggle with autonomy or interpersonal relationships. These struggling students will benefit from individualized assessment and intervention to strengthen their personal coping skills. However, school-based efforts to build more and stronger natural supports for students social, emotional, and academic competence ought to limit the number of struggling students in any one school or classroom. The long-term goal of ClassMaps school resilience research is to identify the most useful blend of "within the person" and contextual strategies to maximize students' success given available community resources.

Translating resilience research to clinical practice is challenging, which is why the foundation laid for this chapter focused on a pioneering model of doing that well (Doll et al., 2009; Doll, Zucker, et al., 2004). Continued efforts in expanding and extending this model as well as adaptations of it are crucial for resilience research to continue to be helpful to all children despite the obstacles that face them daily.

References

Aluede, O., Adeleke, F., Omoike, D., & Afen-Akapida, J. (2008). A review of the extent, nature, characteristics and effects of bullying behaviour in schools. *Journal of Instructional Psychology, 35*, 151–158.

Anguiano, R. P. V. (2004). Families and schools: The effect of parental involvement on high school completion. *Journal of Family Issues, 25*, 61–85.

Assor, A., Kaplan, H., & Roth, G. (2002). Choice is good, but relevance is excellent: Autonomy-enhancing and suppressing teacher behaviours predicting students' engagement in schoolwork. *British Journal of Educational Psychology, 72*, 261–278.

Bandura, A. (1997). *Self-efficacy: The exercise of control*. New York, NY: W. H. Freeman.

Barclay, J. R. (1992). Sociometry, temperament and school psychology. In T. R. Kratochwill, S. Elliott, & M. Gettinger (Eds.), *Advances in school psychology* (Vol. 8, pp. 79–114). Hillsdale, NJ: Lawrence Erlbaum Associates.

Barclay, J. R., & Doll, B. (2001). Early prospective studies of the high school dropout. *School Psychology Quarterly, 16*, 357–369.

Bear, G. G. (2005). *Developing self-discipline and preventing and correcting misbehavior*. Boston, MA: Pearson Allyn and Bacon.

Brophy, J. (2004). *Motivating students to learn* (2nd ed.). Mahwah, NJ: Lawrence Erlbaum Associates.

Consortium on the School-Based Promotion of Social Competence. (1994). The school-based promotion of social competence: Theory, research, practice, and policy. In R. J. Haggerty, L. R. Sherrod, N. Germezy, & M. Rutter (Eds.), *Stress, risk, and resilience in children and adolescents* (pp. 268–316). New York, NY: Cambridge University Press.

Craig, W. M., & Pepler, D. J. (1997). Observations of bullying and victimization in the school yard. *Canadian Journal of School Psychology, 13*(2), 41–59.

Deci, E. L., & Ryan, R. M. (2000). The "What" and "Why" of goal pursuits: Human needs and the self-determination of behavior. *Psychological Inquiry, 11*, 227–268.

Doll, B. (2006, July). *Resilient classrooms: Places where all kids succeed*. An invited workshop at the 3rd Annual NASP Summer Conference: Critical skills and issues in school psychology, Chicago, IL.

Doll, B. (2010, August). *Noticing our success: School psychology's pivotal responsibility for scaling up effective youth mental health practices*. An invited address at the 2010 convention of the American Psychological Association, San Diego, CA.

Doll, B., Champion, A., & Kurien, S. (2008, February). *Social and psychological context for high quality classrooms*. A poster presented at the 2008 Annual Convention of the National Association of School Psychologists, New Orleans.

Doll, B., & Cummings, J. A. (2008). *Transforming school mental health services: Population-based approaches to promoting the competency and wellness of children*. Thousand Oaks, CA: Corwin.

Doll, B., Kurien, S., LeClair, C., Spies, R., Champion, A., & Osborn, A. (2009). The ClassMaps Survey: A framework for promoting positive classroom ecologies. In R. Gilman, S. Huebner, & M. Furlong (Eds.), *Handbook of positive psychology in the schools* (pp. 213–227). New York, NY: Routledge.

Doll, B., & Lyon, M. (1998). Risk and resilience: Implications for the practice of school psychology. *School Psychology Review, 27*, 348–363.

Doll, B., & Siemers, E. (2004, April). *Assessing instructional climates: The reliability and validity of ClassMaps*. A poster presented at the annual convention of the National Association of School Psychologists, Dallas, TX.

Doll, B., Song, S. Y., & Siemers, E. (2004). Classroom ecologies that support or discourage bullying. In S. M. Swearer & D. Espeleage (Eds.), *Bullying in the schools: A social and ecological perspective on intervention and prevention*. Mahwah, NJ: Lawrence Erlbaum.

Doll, B., & Spies, R. A. (2007, March). *The CMS*. A paper presented at the Annual Convention of the National Association of School Psychologists, New York.

Doll, B., Spies, R. A., Champion, A., Guerrero, C., Dooley, K., & Turner, A. (2010). The ClassMaps Survey: A measure of students' perceptions of classroom resilience. *Journal of Psychoeducational Assessment, 28*, 338–348.

Doll, B., Spies, R. A., LeClair, C., Kurien, S., & Foley, B. P. (2010). Student perceptions of classroom learning environments: Development of the ClassMaps Survey. *School Psychology Review, 39*, 203–218.

Doll, B., Zucker, S., & Brehm, K. (1999, April). Reliability and validity of ClassMaps. A poster presentation at the annual convention of the National Association of School Psychologists, Las Vegas, NV. [ERIC Document Reproduction Services No. ED 435 934].

Doll, B., Zucker, S., & Brehm, K. (2004). *Resilient classrooms: Creating healthy environments for learning*. New York, NY: Guilford Publications.

Epstein, J. L., & Van Voorhis, F. L. (2001). More than minutes: Teachers' roles in designing homework. *Educational Psychologist, 36*, 181–193.

Fan, X. (2001). Parental involvement and students' academic achievement: A growth modeling analysis. *Journal of Experimental Education, 70*, 27–61.

Fredricks, J. A., Blumenfeld, P. C., & Paris, A. H. (2004). School engagement: Potential of the concept, state of the evidence. *Review of Educational Research, 74*, 59–109.

Furrer, C., & Skinner, C. (2003). Sense of relatedness as a factor in children's academic engagement and performance. *Journal of Educational Psychology, 95*, 148–162.

Gresham, F. (1986). Conceptual issues in the assessment of social competence in children. In P. Strain, M. Guralnick, & H. Walker (Eds.), *Children's social behavior: Development, assessment and modification*. New York, NY: Academic.

Hamm, J., Farmer, T., Robertson, D., Dadisman, K., Murray, A., Meece, J., & Song, S. Y. (2010). Effects of a developmentally based intervention with teachers on Native-American and White adolescents' schooling adjustment. Journal of Experimental Education, *78*, 343–377.

Hamre, B., & Pianta, R. (2005). Can instructional and emotional support in the first-grade classroom make a difference for children at-risk for school failure? *Child Development, 76*, 949–967.

Hawkins, J. D., Smith, B. H., Hill, K. G., Kosterman, R. F. C., Catalano, F. C., & Abbott, R. D. (2003). Understanding and preventing crime and violence: Findings from the Seatle Social Development Project. In T. P. Thornberry & M. D. Krohn (Eds.), *Taking stock of delinquency: An overview of findings from contemporary longitudinal studies* (pp. 255–312). New York, NY: Kluwer Academic/Plenum.

Hill, N. E., Castellino, D. R., Lansford, J. E., Nowlin, P., Dodge, K. A., Bates, J. E., et al. (2004). Parent academic involvement as related to school behavior, achievement, and aspirations: Demographic variations across adolescence. *Child Development, 75*, 1491–1509.

Hoover-Dempsey, K. V., Walker, J. M. T., Sandler, H. M., Whetsel, D., Green, C. L., Wilkins, A., et al. (2005). Why do parents become involved? Research findings and implications. *The Elementary School Journal, 106*, 105–130.

Johnson, D. W., Johnson, R. T., Buckman, L. A., & Richards, P. S. (1998). The effect of prolonged implementation of cooperative learning on social support within the classroom. *The Journal of Psychology, 119*, 405–411.

Kesner, J. E. (2000). Teacher characteristics and the quality of child–teacher relationships. *Journal of School Psychology, 28*, 133–149.

Knitzer, J. (2005). Advocacy for children's mental health: A personal journey. *Journal of Clinical Child and Adolescent Psychology, 34*(4), 612–618.

Ladd, G. W., Birch, S. H., & Buhs, E. S. (1999). Children's social and scholastic lives in kindergarten: Related spheres of influence? *Child Development, 70*, 1373–1400.

Lane, K., Pierson, M. R., & Givner, C. C. (2003). Teacher expectations of student behavior: Which skills do elementary and secondary teachers deem necessary for success in the classroom?. Education & Treatment of Children, *26*(4), 413–430.

LeClair, C., Doll, B., Osborn, A., & Jones, K. (2009). English language learners' and non-English language learners' perceptions of the classroom environment. *Psychology in the Schools, 46*, 568–577.

Masten, A. S. (2001). Ordinary magic: Resilience processes in development. *American Psychologist, 56*, 227–238.

Masten, A. S., Hubbard, J. J., Gest, S. D., Tellegen, A., Garmezy, N., & Ramirez, M. (1999). Competence in the context of adversity: Pathways to resilience and maladaptation from childhood to late adolescence. *Development and Psychopathology, 11*, 143–169.

Masten, A. S., & Powell, J. L. (2003). A resilience framework for research, policy, and practice. In S. S. Luthar (Ed.), *Resilience and vulnerability: Adaptation in the context of childhood adversities* (pp. 1–25). New York, NY: Cambridge University Press.

McDermott, P. A., Mordell, M., & Stoltzfus, J. (2001). The organization of student performance in American schools: Discipline, motivation, verbal learning, and nonverbal learning. *Journal of Educational Psychology, 93*, 65–76.

Mitchem, K. J., Young, K. R., West, R. P., & Benyo, J. (2001). CWPASM: A Classwide Peer-Assisted Self-Management Program for general education classrooms. *Education and Treatment of Children, 24*, 111–141.

Murphy, P. (2002). *The effect of classroom meetings on the reduction of recess problems: A single case design*. Unpublished doctoral dissertation, University of Denver, Denver, CO.

Murray, C., & Malmgren, K. (2005). Implementing a teacher–student relationship program in a high-poverty urban school: Effects on social, emotional, and academic adjustment and lessons learned. *Journal of School Psychology, 43*, 137–152.

Nansel, T. R., Overpeck, M., & Pilla, R. S. (2001). Bullying behaviors among US youth: Prevalence and association with psychosocial adjustment. *Journal of the American Medical Association, 285*, 2094–2100.

National Research Council/Institute of Medicine. (2004). *Engaging schools: Fostering high school students' motivation to learn*. Washington, DC: The National Academies Press.

Nickolite, A., & Doll, B. (2008). Resilience applied in school: Strengthening classroom environments for learning. *Canadian Journal of School Psychology, 23*, 94–113.

Olweus, D. (1993). *Bullying at school*. Cambridge, MA: Blackwell Publishers.

Osher, D., Bear, G. G., Sprague, J. R., & Doyle, W. (2010). How can we improve school discipline? *Educational Researcher, 39*, 48–58.

Osher, D., & Kendziora, K. (2010). Building conditions for learning and healthy adolescent development: A strategic approach. In B. Doll, W. Pfohl, & J. Yoon (Eds.), *Handbook of youth prevention science* (pp. 121–140). New York, NY: Routledge.

Pajares, F., & Schunk, D. H. (2001). Self-beliefs and school success: Self-efficacy, self-concept, and school achievement. In R. J. Riding & S. G. Rayner (Eds.), *Self perception* (pp. 239–265). Westport, CT: Ablex Publishing.

Pastorelli, C., Caprara, G. V., Barbaranelli, C., Rola, J., Rozsa, S., & Bandura, A. (2001). *The structure of children's perceived self-efficacy: A cross-national study*. European Journal of Psychological Assessment, *17*, 87–97. doi:10.1027//1015-5759.17.2.87

Paul, K. (2005). *SchoolMaps: A reliability and validity study for a secondary education school climate instrument*. Unpublished doctoral dissertation, University of Nebraska, Lincoln.

Paul, J., & Cillessen, A. (2003). Dynamics of peer victimization in early adolescence: Results from a four-year longitudinal study. In M. J. Elias & J. E. Zins (Eds.), *Peer harassment, and victimization in the schools: The next generation of prevention* (pp. 25–43). New York, NY: US Haworth Press.

Pellegrini, A. D. (2005). Recess: Its role in education and development. Mahwah, NJ: Lawrence Erlbaum Associates, Publishers.

Pianta, R. C. (1999). *Enhancing relationships between children and teachers*. Washington, DC: American Psychological Association.

Pianta, R. C., & Stuhlman, M. W. (2004). Teacher–child relationships and children's success in the first years of school. *School Psychology Review, 33*, 444–458.

Prince-Embury, S., & Saklofske, D. (2011). Introductory chapter. In S. Prince-Embury & D. Saklofske (Eds.), *Translating resiliency theory for application with children and adolescents*. New York, NY: Springer.

Schunk, D. H., & Pajares, F. (2005). Competence perceptions and academic functioning. In A. J. Elliot & C. S. Dweck (Eds.), *Handbook of competence and motivation* (pp. 85–104). New York, NY: Guilford Publications, Inc.

Song, S. Y. (2004). Protective Peer Ecology Against Bullying Scale. Unpublished measure.

Song, S. Y. (2005). Protective Peer Ecology Against Bullying Scale: Middle School Version. Unpublished measure.

Song, S. Y. (2006). The role of protective peers and positive peer relationships in school bullying: How can peers help? (Doctoral dissertation, University of Nebraska-Lincoln). *Dissertation Abstracts International, 67*, 8A.

Song, S. Y., Doll, B., Swearer, S. M., Johnsen, L., & Siegel, N. (under review). How peer protection is related to school bullying: An examination of the protective peers hypothesis.

Song, S.Y., Siegel, N., Sogo, W. & Doll, B. (2009). The protective peer ecology and bullying prevention in low resource schools. Symposium presented at the 2009 Annual Convention of the National Association of School Psychologists, Boston, MA.

Song, S.Y. & Siegel, N. (2006a). Middle school bullying prevention: Processes in a protective peer ecology. Poster presented at the 2006 Annual Convention of the American Psychological Association, New Orleans, LA.

Song, S. Y., & Sogo, W. (2010). A hybrid framework for intervention development: Social justice for bullying in low resource schools. In B. Doll, W. Pfohl, & J. Yoon (Eds.), *Handbook of youth prevention science*. Mahwah, NJ: Lawrence Erlbaum Publishing.

Song, S. Y., & Stoiber, K. (2008). Children exposed to violence at school: Understanding bullying and evidence-based interventions [Special issue on children exposed to violence]. *Journal of Emotional Abuse, 8*(1/2), 235–253.

Wentzel, K. R. (2002). Are effective teachers like good parents? Teaching styles and student adjustment in early adolescence. *Child Development, 73*, 287–301.

Wentzel, K. R., & Caldwell, K. (1997). Friendships, peer acceptance, and group membership: Relations to academic achievement in middle school. *Child Development, 68*, 1198–1209.

Wentzel, K. R., & Watkins, D. E. (2002). Peer relationships and collaborative learning as contexts for academic enablers. *School Psychology Review, 31*, 366–377.

Werner, E. E. (2006). What can we learn about resilience from large-scale longitudinal studies? In S. Goldstein & R. B. Brooks (Eds.), *Handbook of resilience in children* (pp. 91–105). New York, NY: Springer.

6 Translating Resilience Theory for Application with Children and Adolescents By Parents, Teachers, and Mental Health Professionals

Sam Goldstein, Robert Brooks, and Melissa DeVries

He likes to do stuff if people are nice to him.

Comment by Noah's Mother.

This parent's observation about the type of environment her child would function and feel best in is a frequent comment made by parents of children struggling to meet the academic, social, emotional, and behavioral expectations of childhood in the twenty-first century. Mental health and educational professionals have increasingly become sensitized to the important role the behavior of adults and the environments in which children are placed serve in helping or hindering their growth and development. This area of practice and science has come to fall under the umbrella of resilience.

We begin this chapter with a brief overview of the research on resilience to set the important foundation that the ideas and strategies offered have a basis in science. We then provide an overview of the essential characteristics of a resilient mindset followed by discussions of the mindsets and practices of adults capable of nurturing resilience in children.

S. Goldstein, Ph.D. (✉) • M. DeVries, Ph.D.
Neurology, Learning and Behavior Center, 230 South 500 East, Suite 100, Salt Lake City, UT 84102, USA
e-mail: info@samgoldstein.com; mldevries@gmail.com

R. Brooks, Ph.D.
Harvard University, Assistant Clinical Professor of Psychology, Department of Psychiatry, Needham, MA 02492, USA
e-mail: contact@drrobertbrooks.com

The Study of Resilience

The study of resilience traces its roots back a scant 50 years. Early on, the field of study was not extensive and the number of researchers devoting their careers to the examination of this phenomenon was fairly small. The field, as Michael Rutter noted in 1987 reflected not so much a search for factual phenomena but "for the developmental and situational mechanisms involved in protective processes" (p. 2). The interest was and is not just on what factors insulate and protect, but how they went about exerting their influence. Resilience studies were reserved for high risk-populations with a particular focus on those youth demonstrating resilience or the ability to overcome the emotional, developmental, economic, and environmental challenges they faced growing up.

Research about resilience has expanded significantly and with greater urgency over the last 30 years. There are a number of reasons for this phenomenon. First, as the technological complexity of the late twentieth century increased, the number of youth facing adversity and the number of adversities they faced appeared to be increasing. More youth were and are at risk. Second, there has been an accelerated interest in not only understanding risk and protective factors and their operation, but in determining whether this information can be distilled into clinically relevant interventions (e.g., Fava & Tomba, 2009;

S. Prince-Embury and D.H. Saklofske (eds.), *Resilience in Children, Adolescents, and Adults: Translating Research into Practice*, The Springer Series on Human Exceptionality,
DOI 10.1007/978-1-4614-4939-3_6, © Springer Science+Business Media New York 2013

Wolchik, Schenck, & Sandler, 2009) that may not only increase positive outcome for those youth facing risk, but also can be applied to the population of children in general in an effort to create, as Brooks and Goldstein (2001) point out, a "resilient mindset" in all youth.

A definition of mindsets is essential. We have noted, "Mindsets are assumptions and expectations we have for ourselves and others that guide our behavior and our interactions." The concept of mindsets can be extended to include not only these self-perceptions but the ways in which we understand the behavior of others. For example, it is essential for adults to appreciate that the assumptions they hold for themselves and children, which are often unstated, have profound influence in determining effective parenting and teaching practices, the quality of relationships with children, and the positive or negative climate that is created in the home and classroom settings.

The importance of such a mindset goes hand in hand with the perception that no child is immune from pressure in our current, fast-paced, stress-filled environment, an environment we have created to prepare children to become functional adults. Even children fortunate to not face significant adversity or trauma, or to be burdened by intense stress or anxiety, experience the pressures around them and the expectations placed upon them. Thus, this field has increasingly focused on identifying those variables that predict resilience in the face of adversity and developing models for effective application (Rutter, 2006). The belief then is that every child capable of developing a resilient mindset will be able to deal more effectively with stress and pressure, to cope with everyday challenges, to bounce back from disappointments, adversity, and trauma, to develop clear and realistic goals, to solve problems, to relate comfortably with others, and to treat oneself and others with respect.

A number of longitudinal studies over the past few decades have set out to develop an understanding of these processes, in particular the complex interaction of protective and risk factors with the goal of developing a model to apply this knowledge in clinical practice (Donnellan, Conger, McAdams, & Neppl, 2009; Garmezy, Masten, & Tellegen, 1984; Luthar, 1991; Rutter, Cox, Tupling, Berger, & Yule, 1975; Rutter & Quinton, 1994; Werner & Smith, 1982, 1992, 2001). These studies have made major contributions in two ways. First, they have identified resources across children's lives that predicted successful adjustment for those exposed to adversity, and second, they began the process of clarifying models of how these protective factors promote adaptation (Wyman, Sandler, Wolchik, & Nelson, 2000).

Whether these processes can be applied to all youth in anticipation of facing adversity remains to be demonstrated (Ungar, 2008). Masten (2001) suggests that the best recent evidence demonstrates that in fact resilience processes are not only effective but can be applied. She points out the recovery to near normal functioning found in children adopted away from institutional settings, characterized by deprivation. The positive outcome for many Romania adoptees appears to reflect this process (Beckett et al., 2006; Kreppner et al., 2007; Masten, 2001). Aames (1997), as cited in Rutter and the English and Romania Adoptees Study Team (1998), documents a significant degree of developmental catch up cognitively and physically in many of these children.

The concept of resilience is fairly straightforward if one accepts the possibility of developing an understanding of the means by which children develop well emotionally, behaviorally, academically, and interpersonally either in the face of risk and adversity, or not. Such a model would offer valuable insight into those qualities that likely insulate and protect in the face of wide and varied types of adversities, including children experiencing medical problems (Brown & Harris, 1989), family risks (Beardslee, 1989; Beardslee & Podorefsky, 1988; Hammen, 1997; Worsham, Compas, & Ey, 1997), psychological problems (Hammen, 1997; Hauser, Allen, & Golden, 2006), divorce (Sandler, Tein, & West, 1994), loss of a parent (Lutzke, Ayers, Sandler, & Barr, 1999), as well as school problems (Skinner & Wellborn, 1994).

Competent, appropriate parenting, for example, that which provides a democratic or authoritative model, parental availability, monitoring, and support, are powerful protective factors reducing the risk of antisocial behavior (Dubow, Edwards, & Ippolito, 1997; Masten et al., 1999). In fact, it appears to be the case that youth functioning well in adulthood regardless of whether they faced adversity or not, may share many of the same characteristics in regards to stress hardiness, communication skills, problem solving, self-discipline, and connections to others. Though the earliest studies of resilience suggested the role of "exceptional characteristics" within the child that led to "invulnerability" (Garmezy & Nuechterlein, 1972), it may well be that resilience reflects very ordinary development processes to explain adaptation (Masten, 2001; Masten & Coatsworth, 1998). Though, as noted, a focus on symptoms and symptom relief, that is one assessing risk alone, may be satisfactory for identification of immediate needs and diagnoses within a psychopathology model, such data are necessary though not sufficient to improve future functioning. It has been well documented that not all children facing significant risk and adversity develop serious adolescent and adult psychiatric, lifestyle, and academic problems. Risk factors also do not appear to be specific to particular outcomes but relate to more broad developmental phenomena. It is likely, as noted, that there is a complex, multidimensional interaction between risk factors, biological functioning, environmental issues, and protective factors that combines to predict outcome (e.g., Kim-Cohen & Gold, 2009).

Within this framework, resilience can be defined as a child's achievement of positive developmental outcomes and avoidance of maladaptive outcomes under adverse conditions (Rutter, 2006; Wyman et al., 1999).

Essential Characteristics of a Resilient Mindset

Resilient children possess certain qualities and/or ways of viewing themselves and the world that are not readily apparent in youngsters who have not been successful in meeting challenges. The mindset (Brooks & Goldstein, 2001, 2011) that children have about themselves influences the behaviors and skills they develop. In turn, these behaviors and skills influence this mindset so that a dynamic process is constantly operating.

The mindset of resilient children contains a number of noteworthy characteristics that are associated with specific skills. These include the following:

- Feeling loved and accepted.
- Possessing realistic goals and expectations.
- Believing they have the ability to solve problems and make sound decisions.
- Viewing mistakes, setbacks, and obstacles as challenges to confront rather than as stressors to avoid.
- Relying on effective coping strategies that promote growth and are not self-defeating.
- Having an awareness and acceptance of their weaknesses and vulnerabilities, viewing these as areas for improvement rather than as unchangeable flaws.
- Recognizing and enjoying their strong points and talents.
- Possessing a self-concept filled with images of strength and competence.
- Feeling comfortable with others and possessing effective interpersonal skills with peers and adults alike.
- Being able to seek out assistance and nurturance in a comfortable, appropriate manner from adults who can provide the support they need.
- Displaying the capacity to define the aspects of their lives over which they have control and to focus their energy and attention on those rather than on factors over which they have little, or any, influence.

An understanding of the features of a resilient mindset can provide parents and other caregivers with guideposts for nurturing inner strength and optimism in their children. Adults adhering to these guideposts can employ effective practices in each interaction with children to reinforce a resilient mindset. While the outcome of a specific situation may be important, even more essential are the lessons learned from the process of dealing with each issue or problem. The knowledge gained supplies the nutrients from which the seeds of resiliency will flourish.

The following are key characteristics of the mindset of adults who are effective in nurturing resilience in children:

- Understanding of the lifelong impact adults have on children, including instilling a sense of hope and resilience.
- Belief that children's learning and their behavior has as much, if not more, to do with the influence of adults than what children might bring into the situation.
- Belief that all children yearn to be successful and that adults must ask how they can adapt their own behavior, expectations, and environments around them to meet children's needs.
- Recognition that if adults are to relate effectively to children, they must be empathic, always attempting to perceive the world through the eyes of the child.
- Understanding that discipline is a teaching process rather than a process of intimidation and humiliation.
- Realization that one of the greatest obstacles to learning is the fear of making mistakes and feeling embarrassed or humiliated.
- Subscription to a strength-based model, which includes identifying and reinforcing each child's "islands of competence."

Teachers and other educational professionals will also find the following characteristics to be important components of their mindset in the academic setting in order to nurture resilience in children:

- Belief that attending to the social–emotional needs of children is not an "extra-curriculum" that draws time away in school or at home from teaching or studying academic subjects.
- Appreciation that the relationships forged between children and their teachers, parents, and other adults are the foundation for successful learning and a safe and secure environment.
- Recognition that children will be more motivated to learn when they feel a sense of ownership for their own education.

Mindsets and Practices of Adults Capable of Nurturing Resilience in Children

Brooks and Goldstein (2001, 2003) proposed guideposts that form the scaffolding for reinforcing a resilient mindset and lifestyle in children and adolescents. These guideposts are relevant for all interactions clinicians, educators, parents, and other caregivers have with children whether coaching them in a sport, helping them with homework, engaging them in an art project, asking them to assume certain responsibilities, assisting them when they make mistakes, teaching them to share, or disciplining them. While the specific avenues and practices through which these guideposts can be applied will differ from one child and one situation to the next, the guideposts remain constant. In our discussion, we provide several examples to illustrate how these guideposts can be translated into specific strategies that can then be applied. While some examples place more emphasis on educators and others on parents, all caregivers can embody these guideposts and apply the strategies to their interactions with children on a daily basis.

Being Empathic

Empathy is a basic foundation of any relationship and is a major component of emotional intelligence (Goleman, 1995). Simply defined, empathy is the capacity of adults to place themselves inside the shoes of children and to see the world through their eyes. Empathy does not imply that adults agree with what children do, but rather they attempt to appreciate and validate their point of view. It is easier for children to develop empathy when they interact with adults who model empathy on a daily basis.

It is not unusual for adults to believe they are empathic, but the reality is that empathy is more fragile or elusive than many realize. It is easier to be empathic when children do what we ask them to do, meet our expectations, and are warm and loving. Being empathic is tested when we are upset, angry, or disappointed with children. When adults feel this way, many will say or do things that actually work against a child developing resilience.

To strengthen empathy, adults must keep in mind several key questions, questions that we frequently pose in our clinical practices and workshops. They include the following:

- "How would I feel if someone said or did to me what I just said or did to this child?"
- "When I say or do things with children, am I behaving in a way that will make them most responsive to listening to me?"
- "What words would I hope a child uses to describe me?"
- "Do I behave in ways that would prompt a child to describe me in the way I hope?"
- "How would a child actually describe me and how close is that to how I hope that child would describe me?"

As an example, when 10-year-old Michael insisted on completing a radio kit by himself but was unable to do so, his father, Mr. Burton, angrily retorted, "I told you it wouldn't work. You don't have enough patience to read the directions carefully." Mr. Burton's message worked against the development of a resilient mindset in his son since it contained an accusatory tone, a tone focusing on Michael's shortcomings rather than on his strengths. It did not offer assistance or hope.

Similarly, a teacher may attempt to motivate a student who is not performing adequately by exhorting the student to "try harder." While the teacher may be well intentioned, the comment is based on the assumption that the student is not willing to expend the time and energy necessary to succeed. Thus, such a remark is frequently experienced as accusatory and judgmental. When children feel accused, they are less prone to be cooperative. Consequently, the teacher's comment is not likely to lead to the desired results, which, in turn, may reinforce the teacher's belief that the student is unmotivated and not interested in "trying."

In contrast, an empathic teacher might wonder, "If I were struggling in my role as a teacher, would I want another teacher or my principal to say to me, 'If you just tried a little harder you wouldn't have this problem'?" When we have offered this question at workshops, many teachers laugh and say they would be very annoyed if they were accused of not trying. The question prompts them to reflect upon how their statements are interpreted by their children. There are several other exercises that can be introduced at workshops to reinforce empathy in teachers. Teachers can be requested at workshops to share with their colleagues their response to the following questions:

- "Of all of the memories you have as a student, what is one of your favorite ones, something that a teacher or school administrator said or did that boosted your motivation and self-dignity?"
- "Of all of the memories you have as a student, what is one of your worst ones, something that a teacher or school administrator said or did that lessened your motivation and self-dignity?"
- "As you reflect upon both your positive and negative memories of school, what did you learn from both and do you use these memories to guide what you are doing with your children today?"
- "What memories are my children taking from their interactions with me?"
- "Are they the memories I would like them to take?"
- "If not, what must I change so that the memories they will take will be in accord with the memories I hope they take?"

Parents or teachers can monitor their interactions with children, with emphasis placed on taking the child's perspective, examining what aspects of a situation are resilience builders and should be maintained as good practice, and identifying which aspects of the situation worked against that child developing a resilient mindset in order that those statements and behaviors be modified to reflect a more empathic approach.

Communicating Effectively and Listening Actively

Empathy is closely associated with the ways in which adults communicate with children. Communication is not simply how we speak with another person. Effective communication involves actively listening to children, understanding and validating what they are attempting to say, and responding in ways that avoid power struggles by not interrupting them, by not telling them how they should be feeling, by not derogating them, and by not using absolute words such as *always* and *never* in an overly critical, demeaning fashion (e.g., "You never help out"; "You always act disrespectful"). Resilient children demonstrate a capacity to communicate their feelings and thoughts effectively. Their parents, teachers, and other adults in their lives serve as important models in the process.

Parents, teachers, and clinicians may consider the following questions useful in fostering empathy through communication styles that reinforce a resilient mindset:

- "Do my messages convey and teach respect?"
- "Am I fostering realistic expectations in children?"
- "Am I helping children learn how to solve problems?"
- "Am I nurturing empathy and compassion?"
- "Am I promoting self-discipline and self-control?"
- "Am I setting limits and consequences in ways that permit children to learn from me rather than resent me?"
- "Am I truly listening to and validating what children are saying?"
- "Do children know that I value their opinion and input?"
- "Do children know how special they are to me?"
- "Am I assisting children to appreciate that mistakes and obstacles are part of the process of learning and growing?"
- "Am I comfortable in acknowledging my own mistakes and apologizing to children when indicated?"

If adults keep these questions in mind, they can communicate in ways that reinforce a resilient mindset.

Changing Negative Scripts

Well-meaning adults have been known to apply the same approach with children for weeks, months, or years even when the approach has proven ineffective. For instance, a set of parents reminded (nagged) their children for years to clean their rooms, but the children failed to comply. When asked why they used the same unsuccessful message for years, they responded, "We thought they would finally learn if we told them often enough."

Similar to the reasoning offered by these parents, many adults believe that children should be the ones to change, not them. Others believe if they change their approach, it is like "giving in to a child" and they are concerned that their children will take advantage of them. Adults with a resilient mindset of their own recognize that if something they have said or done for a reasonable amount of time does not work, then they must change their "script" if children are to change theirs. This position does not mean giving in to the child or failing to hold the child accountable. It suggests that adults must have the insight and courage to consider what they can do differently, lest they become entangled in useless, counterproductive power struggles. It also serves to teach children that there are alternative ways of solving problems and it helps them learn to be more flexible and accountable in handling difficult situations.

While many parents, educators, and others say they subscribe to these assumptions, their actions frequently belie their assertion. For example, it is not unusual to hear the following statements offered by adults at consultations we have conducted.

"This child is unmotivated to change. She just won't take responsibility for her behavior." Or, "We've been using this strategy for 5 months. He's still not responding. He's resistant and oppositional."

We believe in perseverance, but if the same approach has been employed for 5 months without any positive outcome, one can ask, "Who are the resistant ones here?"

The parents and teachers most often resistant to change are those who equate acquiescing to the child with failure on the part of the adult. For these adults, any new strategy will be tainted by feelings of resentment. However, as a perceptive teacher once pointed out, "Asking what is it that

I can do differently should not be interpreted as blaming ourselves but rather as a source of empowerment." She continued, "Isn't it better to focus on what we can do differently rather than continue to wait for someone else to change first? We may have to wait forever and continue to be frustrated and unhappy."

A helpful exercise to illustrate the power of personal control and the need to change "negative scripts" that exist in our lives is to think about one or two instances when the usual script was altered and to consider what resulted as a consequence of the new script. Many adults are able to describe very positive results. Unfortunately, others report less satisfactory results, often reinforcing the belief that they had gone out of their way for children, but the children did not reciprocate. When the outcome of a change in script is not positive, a problem-solving attitude should be introduced by asking, "With hindsight, is there anything you would do differently today to lessen the probability of an unfavorable result?" Better still, having one or two back-up scripts in mind should the first prove ineffective conveys the positive message that a strategy that initially sounds promising may not yield the results we wish; however, rather than feeling defeated, we should learn from the experience and be prepared with alternative actions. We must keep in mind that a new script may create the conditions that encourage children to change their behaviors.

Loving Children in Ways that Help Them to Feel Special and Appreciated

It is well established that a basic foundation of resilience is the presence of at least one adult (hopefully several) who believes in the worth and goodness of the child. The late psychologist Julius Segal referred to that person as a "charismatic adult," an adult from whom a child "gathers strength" (Segal, 1988). One must never underestimate the power of one person to redirect a child toward a more productive, successful, satisfying life. Parents, keeping in mind the notion of a charismatic adult, might ask each evening, "Are my children stronger people because of the things I said or did today or are they less strong?"

When parents are asked to recall a favorite occasion from their childhood when their parents served as a charismatic adult for them, one of the most common memories involves doing something pleasant and alone with the parent. The power of these "special times" is recalled by many adults. It is recommended that parents create these occasions in the lives of their children. Parents of young children might say, "When I read to you or play with you, it is so special that even if the phone rings I won't answer it." One young child said, "I know my parents love me. They let the answering machine answer calls when they are playing with me."

Time alone with each child does not preclude family activities that also create a sense of belonging and love. Sharing evening meals and holidays, playing games, attending a community event as a family, or taking a walk together are all opportunities to convey love and help children feel special in the eyes and hearts of their parents.

Just as parents can create an atmosphere in which children feel appreciated, teachers can also initiate strategies to convey the message that they genuinely care about each student. While most teachers appreciate that they will be influential in the lives of their children for years to come, many are not aware of the extent of their impact. When teachers recognize the power of their influence and identify and implement strategies to do so in positive ways, it can add meaning and purpose to their role, while lessening disillusionment and burnout (Brooks, 1991; Brooks & Goldstein, 2001; Goldstein & Brooks, 2007).

Schools have been spotlighted, for example, as environments in which self-esteem, hope, and resilience can be fortified, often with simple gestures from the teachers toward their students. A smile, a warm greeting, a note of encouragement, a few minutes taken to meet alone with a student, and an appreciation of and respect for different learning styles are but several of the activities that define a "charismatic teacher" (Brooks, 1991). These and other factors, which help children and adolescents to deal more effectively with stress, to overcome adversity, and to become resilient have received increased emphasis in the research literature in the past 20 years (Brooks, 1994; Brooks & Goldstein, 2001, 2003;

Doll, Jones, Osborn, Dooley, & Turner 2011; Goldstein & Brooks, 2005; Katz, 1997; Werner & Smith, 1992).

Teachers are often unaware that they are or have been "charismatic adults" in the life of a student. To emphasize this issue we ask teachers to consider if they have ever received unexpectedly, a note from a former student thanking them for the positive impact they had on the student's life. While many have been fortunate to be the recipient of such a note, others have not, although they are equally deserving of such feedback.

We frequently ask participants at our workshops if there are teachers who had a significant influence on their lives whom they have failed to acknowledge via a note or letter. It is not unusual for many teachers to voice regret they have not thanked several such "charismatic adults." Some have written notes to the latter following the workshop.

We use these exercises to suggest that while we may not receive formal confirmation that we have worn the garb of "charismatic adults," if we approach each day with the belief that today may be the day we say or do something that directs a child's life in a more positive path, we will be more optimistic about our role as parents or teachers, and our children will be the beneficiaries of more realistic, hopeful expectations.

Helping Children Experience Success By Identifying and Nurturing Their "Islands of Competence"

Resilient children do not deny their problems. Such denial runs counter to mastering challenges. However, in addition to acknowledging and confronting problems, resilient youngsters are able to identify and utilize their strengths. Unfortunately, many children who feel poorly about themselves and their abilities experience a diminished sense of hope. Adults sometimes report that the positive comments they offer their children fall on "deaf ears," resulting in parents becoming frustrated and reducing positive feedback.

It is important for adults to be aware that when children lack self-worth they are less receptive to accepting positive feedback. Adults should continue to offer this feedback, but must recognize that true self-esteem, hope, and resilience are based on children experiencing success in areas of their lives that they and significant others deem to be important. This requires adults to identify and reinforce a child's "islands of competence." Every child possesses these islands of competence or areas of strength and we must nurture these rather than overemphasize the child's weaknesses. When children discover their islands of competence, they are more willing to confront those areas that have been problematic for them.

Researchers and clinicians have emphasized the significance of recruiting selected areas of strength or "islands of competence" in building self-confidence, motivation, and resilience (Deci & Flaste, 1995; Katz, 1994; Rutter, 1984). Rutter (1984), in describing resilient individuals, observed, "Experiences of success in one arena of life led to enhanced self-esteem and a feeling of self-efficacy, enabling them to cope more successfully with the subsequent life challenges and adaptations" (p. 604). Katz (1994) noted, "Being able to showcase our talents, and to have them valued by important people in our lives, helps us to define our identities around that which we do best" (p. 10).

Recognizing and honoring a child's islands of competence can be difficult when such "islands" do not meet our expectations. Adults must learn to accept children for who they are and not what they envisioned or hoped they would be. Our acceptance of children for who they are is made more challenging by how different children are from birth because of their temperament. Chess and Thomas (1987), two of the pioneers in measuring temperamental differences in newborns, observed that some youngsters enter the world with so-called "easy" temperaments, others with cautious or "slow-to-warm-up" temperaments, while still others with "difficult" temperaments. Understanding of such individual differences can help adults foster resilience in children by setting the stage for each child's success.

Fortunately, in the past 20 years there have been an increasing number of publications to help parents and teachers appreciate, accept, and respond effectively to a child's temperament and learning style (Carey, 1997; Keogh, 2003; Kurcinka, 1991; Levine, 2002, 2003; Sachs, 2001). For example, acceptance does not imply that we excuse inappropriate, unacceptable behavior but rather that we understand this behavior and help to modify it in a manner that does not assault a child's self-esteem and sense of dignity. It means setting realistic expectations for children, careful not to set the bar too high or too low. If the bar is set too high, children will continually experience failure and are likely to feel they are a disappointment to the important adults in their lives. Setting the bar too low may rob children of experiences that test their abilities and their capacity to learn to manage setbacks. Very low expectations also convey the message, "We don't think you are capable."

Just as parents must accept temperamental differences in their children, it is also important for educators to appreciate that each child has different learning styles and strengths (Gardner, 1983; Levine, 2002; Mather & Goldstein, 2008). This requires that teachers familiarize themselves with such topics as multiple intelligences and learning styles and assist children in feeling competent by teaching them in ways in which they can learn best. Teachers and other adults should work under the assumption that all children wish to learn and to succeed and if they seem unmotivated or unengaged, they may believe they lack the ability to achieve in school or life.

We often hear teachers refer to children as lazy or unmotivated. As we have noted, once these accusatory labels are used and a negative mindset dominates, educators are more likely to respond to these children with annoyance. The mindset of an effective educator constantly echoes, "I believe that all children desire to learn. It they are disinterested and feel defeated, we must figure out how best to reach and teach them."

Subscribing to this view has a profound impact on the ways in which we respond to children, especially those who are struggling. When children lose faith in their ability to learn and when feelings of hopelessness pervade their psyche, they are vulnerable to engaging in counterproductive or self-defeating ways of coping. They may quit at tasks, clown around, pick on other children, or expend little time and effort in academic requirements. When a student feels that failure is a foregone conclusion, it is difficult to muster the energy to consider alternative ways of mastering learning demands.

Teachers who observe such counterproductive behaviors may easily reach the conclusion that the student is unmotivated or lazy, or not caring about school. As negative assumptions and mindsets dominate, teachers are less likely to consider more productive strategies for reaching the student. Instead, thoughts turn into punitive actions, e.g., what punishments would finally get through to the student. However, if educators subscribe to the belief that each student wishes to succeed, negative assumptions are less likely to prevail.

Educators are also more likely to maintain a sense of optimism, and a desire to assist those students who appear to be struggling, if they understand that focusing on a child's social/emotional development and well-being is not an extra curriculum that draws time away in school from teaching or studying academic subjects. It is unfortunate that a dichotomy has arisen in many educational quarters prompting some educators to perceive that nurturing a child's emotional and social health is mutually exclusive from the goal of teaching academic material. This dichotomy has been fueled, in part, by the emergence of high stakes testing and an emphasis on accountability. The following refrain is heard in many schools: "We barely have time to get through the assigned curriculum. We really don't have the time to focus on anything else."

There are numerous strategies that teachers can offer to assist children to feel more confident and competent, and to experience successes at school. At the beginning of the school year, teachers can meet with each student for a few minutes and ask, "What are you interested in? What do you like to do? What do you think you do well?" While some children will respond eagerly, others may simply say, "I don't know." In that case, teachers can respond, "That's okay, it often takes time to figure out what you're good at. I'll try to be of help."

A high school teacher noted that given all of the children attending his classes, he did not have the time to meet with each individually at the beginning of the year. Instead, he devised a questionnaire that he sent out to each student a week before school began. He told them that it was not mandatory that they complete the questionnaire, but if they did it would help him to be a more effective teacher. The questionnaire focused on a number of areas, several of which asked children to list what they perceived to be their strengths and weaknesses. In the 7 years in which he had sent out the questionnaire, not one student had failed to return it. This teacher found the information he obtained to be an invaluable resource in connecting with children.

Strengthening a student's feeling of well-being, self-esteem, and dignity should not be an afterthought. If anything, a student's sense of belonging, security, and self-confidence in the classroom provides the scaffolding that supports the foundation for enhanced learning, motivation, self-discipline, responsibility, and the ability to deal more effectively with obstacles and mistakes (Brooks, 1991, 2004).

Helping Children Realize that Mistakes Are Experiences from Which to Learn

While setting realistic expectations for children can help to reduce the amount of failure they experience, one of the most powerful approaches for reinforcing a feeling of competence in children is to lessen their fear of failure. There is a significant difference in the way in which resilient children view mistakes compared with youngsters who are not resilient. Resilient children tend to perceive mistakes as opportunities for learning. In contrast, children who are not very hopeful often experience mistakes as an indication that they are failures. In response to this pessimistic view, they are likely to flee from challenges, feeling inadequate and often blaming others for their problems. If parents are to raise resilient children, they must help them develop a healthy attitude about mistakes from an early age.

Adults can assist children to develop a more constructive attitude about mistakes and setbacks. This task can be facilitated if adults consider what their children's answers would be to the following questions:

- "When your parents or teacher make a mistake, when something doesn't go right, what do they do?"
- "When you make a mistake, what do your parents or teacher say or do to you?"

In terms of the first question, adults serve as significant models for handling mistakes. It is easier for children to learn to deal more effectively with mistakes if they see important adults in their lives doing so. However, if they observe adults blaming others or becoming very angry and frustrated when mistakes occur or offering excuses in order to avoid a task, children are more likely to develop a self-defeating attitude towards mistakes. In contrast, if children witness adults using mistakes as opportunities for learning, they are more likely to do the same.

The second question also deserves serious consideration. Many well-meaning adults become anxious and frustrated with children's mistakes. Given these feelings they may say or do things that contribute to children fearing rather than learning from setbacks. For instance, parental or teacher frustration may lead to such comments as: "Were you using your brains?" or "You never think before you act!" or "I told you it wouldn't work!" These and similar remarks serve to corrode a child's sense of dignity and self-esteem.

No one likes to make mistakes or fail, but adults can use children's mistakes as teachable moments. They can engage children in a discussion of what they can do differently next time to maximize chances for success. Using empathy, they can refrain from saying things that they would not want said to them (e.g., how many parents would find it helpful if their spouse said to them, "Were you using your brains?").

The fear of making mistakes and failing also permeates every classroom and if it is not actively addressed it remains an active force, compromising the joy and enthusiasm that should be part of the learning process. It is the proverbial elephant in the room and in this case, one that may be on a destructive rampage; yet it is not acknowledged.

Effective educators can begin to overcome the fear of failure by identifying this elephant in the room. The fear must be openly addressed with children. One technique for doing so is for teachers to ask their class at the beginning of the school year, "Who feels they are going to make a mistake and not understand something in class this year?" Before any of the children can respond, teachers can raise their hand as a way of initiating a discussion of how the fear of making mistakes affects learning.

It is often helpful for teachers to share some of their own anxieties and experiences about making mistakes when they were children. They can recall when they were called upon in class, when they made mistakes or when they failed a test. This openness often invites children to share some of their thoughts and feelings about making mistakes. Teachers can involve the class in problem solving by encouraging them to suggest what they can do as teachers and what the children can do as a class to minimize the fear of failure and appearing foolish. Issues of being called on and not knowing the answer can be discussed. Effective teachers recognize that when the fear of failure and humiliation are actively addressed in the classroom, children will be more motivated to take realistic risks and to learn.

If adults are to reinforce a resilient mindset in children, their words and actions must convey a belief that we can learn from mistakes. The fear of making mistakes and being humiliated is one of the most potent obstacles to learning, one that is incompatible with a resilient lifestyle.

Developing Responsibility, Compassion, and a Social Conscience By Providing Children with Opportunities to Contribute

Parents and teachers often ask what they can do to foster an attitude of responsibility, caring, and compassion in children. One of the most effective ways of nurturing responsibility is offering children opportunities to help others.

Parents and teachers would be well advised to say as often as possible to their children, "We need your help" rather than "Remember to do your chores." In addition, adults who involve their children in charitable endeavors, such as walks for hunger or AIDS or food drives, appreciate the value of such activities in fostering self-esteem and resilience. Responsibility and compassion are not promoted by "lectures" but rather by opportunities for children to assume a helping role and to become part of a "charitable family," a family that is engaged in acts of compassion and giving.

Opportunities can also be provided for children to help by contributing to the school milieu, which can foster a more positive attachment to school and increase motivation for learning (Brooks, 1991; Rutter, 1990; Werner, 1993). Examples include the following: older children with learning problems reading to younger children; a hyperactive child being asked to assume the position of "attendance monitor," which involves walking around the halls to take attendance of teachers while the latter are taking attendance of children; and the use of cooperative learning in which children of varying abilities work together as a team bringing their own unique strengths to different projects.

When children are enlisted in helping others and engaging in responsible behaviors, parents and teachers communicate trust in them and faith in their ability to handle a variety of tasks. In turn, involvement in these tasks reinforces several key characteristics of a resilient mindset including empathy, a sense of satisfaction in the positive impact of one's behaviors, a more confident outlook as islands of competence are displayed, and the use of problem-solving skills.

Teaching Children to Solve Problems and Make Decisions

Children with high self-esteem and resilience believe that they are masters of their fate and that they can define what they have control over. A vital ingredient of this feeling of control is the belief that when problems arise, they have the ability to make decisions and solve their problems.

Resilient children are able to articulate problems, consider different solutions, attempt what they judge to be the most appropriate solution, and learn from the outcome (Shure, 1996; Shure & Aberson, 2005).

If adults are to reinforce this problem-solving attitude in children, they must refrain from constantly telling children what to do. Instead it is more beneficial to encourage children to consider different possible solutions. To facilitate this process, for example, parents might wish to establish a "family meeting time" every week or every other week during which problems facing family members can be discussed and solutions considered.

As Shure (1996) has found in her research, even preschool children can be assisted to develop effective and realistic ways of making choices and solving problems. When children initiate their own plans of action with the guidance of parents, their sense of ownership and control is reinforced, as is their resilience.

Problems need not arise, however, in order for children to be invited to participate in decision making. Children can be encouraged to provide ongoing feedback and input on a regular basis, a process that serves to enhance empathy and promotes a sense of responsibility and ownership in children. When children feel their voice is being heard, they are more likely to work cooperatively with parents and teachers and more motivated to meet challenges.

Examples of this have been found in classrooms, for instance, where teachers request anonymous feedback from children. One high school teacher asked children to draw him, describe him, list what they liked about his teaching style and the class, and what they would recommend he change. Another teacher requested that children complete a one-page report card about him whenever he filled out report cards on them. He asked children to rate him on such dimensions as discipline style, response to student questions, teaching style, and fairness towards all children. The exercise actually increased achievement scores and cooperation; this was not surprising since the children felt respected.

Responsibility and ownership in children can also be reinforced by engaging children in a discussion about the benefits or drawbacks of educational practices that are typically seen as "givens," including such activities as tests, reports, and homework. In addition, educators can strengthen a feeling of student ownership by incorporating a variety of choices in the classroom, none of which diminishes a teacher's authority but rather empowers children to feel a sense of control over their own education.

At home, children can feel empowered by being allowed to participate in establishing household rules. Parents can utilize family meeting times, as discussed earlier, to reinforce children's choice and ownership in disciplinary practices by asking children to consider such questions as.

"What rules do you think we need at home for everyone to feel comfortable and cooperate with each other?"

"Even as your parent I may forget a rule. If I do, this is how I would like you to remind me. (Parents can then list one or two ways they would like to be reminded.) Now that I have mentioned how I would like to be reminded, how would you like me to remind you?" (When children inform parents how they would like to be reminded should they forget a rule, they are less likely to experience the reminder as a form of nagging and more likely to hear what the parent has to say. It is easier for children to consider ways of being reminded if parents first serve as models by offering how they would like to be reminded).

"What should the consequences be if we forget a rule?"

When children's input is welcomed on a regular basis, it gives them a sense of control and empowerment that has the capacity to shape their decision making processes in and outside of the home and school settings. It encourages a sense of ownership for rules and consequences, thereby promoting responsibility and self-discipline. The issue of self-discipline relates to the final point, namely, effective forms of discipline.

Disciplining in Ways that Promote Self-discipline and Self-worth

To be a disciplinarian is one of their most important roles that adults assume in nurturing resilience in children (Brooks & Goldstein, 2007a, 2007b). In this role adults must remember that the word *discipline* relates to the word *disciple* and thus is a teaching process. The ways in which children are disciplined can either reinforce or erode self-esteem, self-control, and resilience.

Two of the major goals of effective discipline are as follows: (a) to ensure a safe and secure environment in which children understand and can define rules, limits, and consequences, and (b) to reinforce self-discipline and self-control so that children incorporate these rules and apply them even when parents and other caregivers are not present. A lack of consistent, clear rules and consequences often contributes to chaos and to children feeling that adults do not care about them. On the other hand, if adults are harsh and arbitrary, if they resort to yelling and spanking, children are likely to learn resentment rather than self-discipline.

There are several key principles that adults can follow to employ discipline techniques that are positive and effective. Given the significant role that discipline plays in parenting and educational practices and in nurturing resilience, they are described in detail. Although many of the following examples focus on discipline practices of parents, the underlying principles can be adapted and applied by educators as well.

Practice Prevention. It is vital for adults to become proactive rather than reactive in their interactions with children, especially in regard to discipline. For example, discipline problems were minimized in one household when a young, hyperactive boy was permitted to get up from the dinner table when he could no longer remain seated. This approach proved far more effective than the previous one used by the parents, namely, to yell and punish him; when a punitive atmosphere was removed, this boy also learned greater self-control.

Work as a Parental Team. In homes with two parents, it is important that parents set aside time for themselves to examine the expectations they have for their children as well as the discipline they use. This dialogue can also occur between divorced parents. While parents cannot and should not be clones of each other, they should strive to arrive at common goals and disciplinary practices, which most likely will involve negotiation and compromise. This negotiation should take place in private and not in front of children.

Be Consistent, Not Rigid. The behavior of children sometimes renders consistency a Herculean task. Some children, based on past experience, believe that they can outlast their parents or teachers and that eventually adults will succumb to their whining, crying, or tantrums. If guidelines and consequences have been established for acceptable behavior, it is important that adults adhere to them. However, adults must remember that consistency is not synonymous with rigidity or inflexibility. A consistent approach to discipline invites thoughtful modification of rules and consequences such as when a child reaches adolescence and is permitted to stay out later on the weekend. When modifications are necessary, they should be discussed with children so that they understand the reasons for the changes and can offer input.

Select One's Battlegrounds Carefully. Adults can find themselves reminding and disciplining their children all day long. It is important for adults to ask what behaviors merit discipline and which are not really relevant in terms of nurturing responsibility and resilience. Obviously, behaviors concerning safety deserve immediate attention. Other behaviors will be based on the particular values and expectations in the home or classroom. If children are punished for countless behaviors, if adults are constantly telling them what to do in an arbitrary manner, then the positive effects of discipline will be lost.

Rely When Possible on Natural and Logical Consequences. Children must learn that there are consequences for their behavior. It is best if these consequences are not harsh or arbitrary and are based on discussions that parents have had with their children. Discipline rooted in natural and logical consequences can be very effective. *Natural* consequences are those that result from a child's actions without parents having to enforce them such as a child having a bicycle stolen because it was not placed in the garage. While *logical* consequences sometimes overlap with natural consequences, logical consequences involve some action taken on the part of parents in response to their child's behavior. Thus, if the child whose bicycle was stolen asked parents for money to purchase a new bicycle, a logical consequence would be for the parents to help the child figure out how to earn the money needed to pay for the new bicycle.

Positive Feedback and Encouragement Are Often the Most Powerful Forms of Discipline. Although most of the questions we are asked about discipline focus on negative consequences or punishment, it is important to appreciate the impact of positive feedback and encouragement as disciplinary approaches. Adults should "catch children doing things right" and let them know when they do. Children crave the attention of their parents and teachers. It makes more sense to provide this attention for positive rather than negative behaviors. Well-timed positive feedback and expressions of encouragement and love are more valuable to children's self-esteem and resilience than stars or stickers. When children feel loved and appreciated, when they receive encouragement and support, they are less likely to engage in negative behaviors.

A Final Word on Applying the Practices to Nurture Resilience in Our Children

At the end of one of our workshops, a teacher said, "I love your ideas, but I'm too stressed out to use them." Similar commentary has been offered by parents who report that they are often too busy trying to manage their family and work lives to try anything new. These remarks capture an important consideration.

Although the strategies we advocate do not take time away from teaching or parenting, but rather help to create environments that are less stressful and more conducive to building children's resilience, we can appreciate parents' and teachers' frustration that change requires additional time, a commodity that is not readily available. Some teachers, and parents alike are hesitant to leave their "comfort zone" even when this zone is filled with stress and pressure. They would rather continue with a known situation that is less than satisfying than engage in the task of entering a new, unexplored territory that holds promise but also uncertainty.

If adults are to be effective and if they are to apply many of the ideas described in this chapter, they must venture from their "comfort zone" by utilizing techniques for dealing with the stress and pressure that are inherent in their work. Each can discover his or her own ways for managing stress. For instance, some can rely on exercise, others on relaxation or meditation techniques, all of which can be very beneficial. In addition to these approaches there has been research conducted by Kobasa and her colleagues (Holt, Fine, & Tollefson, 1987; Kobasa, Maddi, & Kahn, 1982; Martinez, 1989) under the label of "stress hardiness" that examines the characteristics or mindset of individuals who experience less stress than others while working or parenting in the same environment.

This "stress hardy" mindset involves "3 C's" (the first letter of each of the words of the mindset begins with the letter "C"). The three components are interrelated and when we describe them at our workshops we encourage the audience to reflect upon how they might apply this information to lessen stress and burnout.

The first C represents "commitment." Stress hardy individuals do not lose sight of why they are doing what they are doing. They maintain a genuine passion or purpose for their efforts rather than feeling as if they are "being forced to" do something. If the latter pervades one's mindset, a sense of commitment and purpose is sacrificed, replaced by feelings of stress and burnout. As an antidote to burnout, parents and teachers are encouraged to recall what it is they like best about their role and why they made the decision to have, or work with, children in the first place. Discussions like this can help to reinvigorate their dreams and goals.

The second C is for "challenge." Adults who deal more effectively with stress have developed a mindset that views difficult situations as opportunities for learning and growth rather than as stress to avoid. For example, a principal of a school faced a challenging situation. Her school was located in a neighborhood that had changed in a few short years from a middle class population with much parent involvement to a neighborhood with a lower socioeconomic makeup and less parent involvement. There were several key factors that contributed to the decrease in parent involvement, including less flexibility for many parents to leave work in order to attend a school meeting or conference as well as many parents feeling unwelcome and anxious in school based upon their own histories as children in the school environment.

Instead of bemoaning this state of affairs and becoming increasingly upset and stressed, this particular principal and her staff realized that the education of their children would be greatly enhanced if parents became active participants in the educational process; consequently, they viewed the lack of involvement as a challenge to meet rather than as a stress to avoid. Among other strategies, they scheduled several staff meetings in the late afternoon and moved the site of the meetings from the school building to a popular community house a few blocks away. These changes encouraged a number of the parents to attend the meetings since the new time was more accommodating to their schedules and the new location helped them to feel more comfortable since it was held on their "turf."

We have found other examples of parents stepping up to challenges, that could otherwise be viewed as stressful, to increase their learning and growth, and ultimately benefit their child. For instance, parents of children with disabilities often prove to be amazing advocates not only for their own children but for all children with disabilities with the school setting. Some parents have gone above and beyond their duties as parents, becoming well versed in special education laws and disability rights, working with the school district to increase disability awareness and to assist other families in the process of accessing special education services.

In each of these situations, the relationship between parents and teachers was greatly enhanced by individuals rising to rather than running from a challenge, and the children were the beneficiaries.

The third C is "control" or what we call "personal control" since some individuals may mistakenly view the word control as a form of controlling others. Control, as used in stress hardiness theory, implies that individuals who successfully manage stress and pressure focus their time and energy on factors over which they have influence rather than attempting to change things that are beyond their sphere of control. Although many individuals believe they engage in activities over which they have influence or control, in fact, many do not. We worked with groups of parents and teachers who were feeling burned out. We reviewed the basic tenets of stress hardiness theory and asked if they focused their energies on factors within their domain of control. They replied in the affirmative.

We then asked them to list what would help their roles to be less stressful. Their answers, as one insightful participant quickly identified, included things over which they had little, if any, control. The group then found that focusing on what they could do differently to improve the environment was empowering and lessened stressful feelings. The mood of pessimism and burnout that had pervaded the room began to change.

Conclusions

The day-to-day interactions educators, mental health professionals, and most importantly parents have with children are influential in determining the quality of lives that children will lead (Sheridan, Eagle, & Dowd, 2005). Adults can serve as charismatic individuals to children. They can assume this role by understanding and fortifying in children the different characteristics of a resilient mindset, by believing in them, by conveying unconditional love, and by providing them with opportunities that reinforce their islands of competence and feelings of self-worth and dignity. Nurturing resilience is an immeasurable, lifelong gift we can offer children. It is part of our legacy to the next generation.

References

Beardslee, W. R., & Podorefsky, D. (1988). Resilient adolescents whose parents have serious affective and other psychiatric disorders: Importance of self-understanding and relationships. *American Journal of Psychiatry, 145*, 63–69.

Beardslee, W. R. (1989). The role of self-understanding in resilient individuals. *The American Journal of Orthopsychiatry, 59*, 266–278.

Beckett, C., Maughan, B., Rutter, M., Castle, J., Colvert, E., Groothues, C., et al. (2006). Do the effects of early severe deprivation on cognition persist into early adolescence? Findings from the English and Romanian Adoptees study. *Child Development, 77*, 696–711.

Brooks, R. (1991). *The self-esteem teacher.* Loveland, OH: Treehaus Communications.

Brooks, R. (1994). Children at risk: Fostering hope and resilience. *American Journal of Orthopsychiatry, 64*, 545–553.

Brooks, R. (1998). Parenting a child with learning disabilities: Strategies for fostering self-esteem, motivation, and resilience. In T. Citro (Ed.), *The experts speak: Parenting a child with learning disabilities* (pp. 25–45). Waltham, MA: Learning Disabilities Association of Massachusetts.

Brooks, R. (2005). The power of parenting. In S. Goldstein & R. Brooks (Eds.), *Handbook of resilience in children* (pp. 297–314). New York, NY: Kluwer Academic/Plenum.

Brooks, R., & Goldstein, S. (2001). *Raising resilient children: Fostering strength, hope, and optimism in your child.* New York, NY: McGraw-Hill.

Brooks, R., & Goldstein, S. (2003). *Nurturing resilience in our children. Answers to the most important parenting questions.* New York, NY: McGraw-Hill.

Brooks, R., & Goldstein, S. (2007a). *Raising a self-disciplined child.* New York, NY: McGraw-Hill.

Brooks, R., & Goldstein, S. (2007b). *Understanding and managing children's classroom behavior* (2nd ed.). New York, NY: Wiley.

Brooks, R., & Goldstein, S. (2011). Raising resilient children. In G. P. Koocher & A. M. LaGreca (Eds.), *The parents' guide to psychological first aid* (pp. 142–150). New York, NY: Oxford.

Brown, G. W., & Harris, T. O. (1989). *Life events and illness.* New York: Guilford Press.

Carey, W. B. (1997). *Understanding your child's temperament.* New York, NY: Macmillan.

Chess, S., & Thomas, A. (1987). *Know your child.* New York, NY: Basic Books.

Deci, E. L., & Flaste, R. (1995). *Why we do what we do: Understanding self-motivation.* New York: Guilford.

Doll, B., Zucker, S., & Brehm, K. (2004). *Resilient classrooms.* New York, NY: Guilford.

Doll, B., Jones, K., Osborn, A., Dooley, K., & Turner, A. (2011). The promise and the caution of resilience models for schools. *Psychology in the Schools, 48*, 651–659.

Donnellan, M. B., Coner, K. J., McAdams, K. K., & Neppl, T. K. (2009). Personal characteristics and resilience to economic hardship and its consequences: Conceptual issues and empirical illustrations. *Journal of Personality, 77*, 1645–1676.

Dubow, E. F., Edwards, S., & Ippolito, M. F. (1997). Life stressors, neighborhood disadvantage, and resources: A focus on inner-city children's adjustment. *Journal of Clinical Child Psychology, 26*, 130–144.

Fava, G. A., & Tomba, E. (2009). Increasing psychological well-being and resilience by psychotherapeutic methods. *Journal of Personality, 77*, I1903–I1934.

Gardner, H. (1983). *Frames of mind.* New York: Basic Books.

Garmezy, N., Masten, A. S., & Tellegen, A. (1984). The study of stress and competence in children: A building block for developmental psychopathology. *Child Development, 55*, 97–111.

Garmezy, N., & Nuechterlein, K. (1972). Invulnerable children: The fact and fiction of competence and disadvantage. *The American Journal of Orthopsychiatry, 42*, 328–329.

Goldstein, S., & Brooks, R. (Eds.). (2005). *Handbook of resilience in children.* New York, NY: Kluwer Academic/Plenum.

Goldstein, S., & Brooks, R. (2007). *Understanding and managing children's classroom behaviour.* New York, NY: Wiley.

Goleman, D. (1995). *Emotional intelligence.* New York, NY: Bantam Books.

Hammen, C. (1997). Children of depressed parents: The stress context. In S. A. Wolchik & I. N. Sandler (Eds.), *Handbook of children's coping: Linking theory and intervention* (pp. 131–159). New York, NY: Plenum Press.

Hauser, S., Allen, J., & Golden, E. (2006). *Out of the woods: Tales of resilient teens.* Cambridge, MA: Harvard University Press.

Hechtman, L. (1991). Resilience and vulnerability in long term outcome of attention deficit disorder. *Canadian Journal of Psychiatry, 36*, 415–421.

Holt, P., Fine, M. J., & Tollefson, N. (1987). Mediating stress: Survival of the hardy. *Psychology in the Schools, 24*, 51–58.

Katz, M. (1994, May). From challenged childhood to achieving adulthood: Studies in resilience. *Chadder*, 8–11.

Katz, M. (1997). *On playing a poor hand well*. New York: Norton.

Keogh, B. K. (2003). *Temperament in the classroom: Understanding individual differences*. Baltimore, MD: Brookes Publishing.

Kim-Cohen, J., & Gold, A. L. (2009). Measured gene–environment interactions and mechanisms promoting resilient development. *Current Directions in Psychological Science, 18*, 138–142.

Kobasa, S. C., Maddi, S. R., & Kahn, S. (1982). Hardiness and health: A prospective study. *Journal of Personality and Social Psychology, 42*, 168–177.

Kreppner, J. M., Rutter, M., Beckett, C., Castle, J., Colvert, E., Groothues, C., et al. (2007). Normality and impairment following profound early institutional deprivation: A longitudinal follow-up into early adolescence. *Developmental Psychology, 43*, 931–946.

Kurcinka, M. S. (1991). *Raising your spirited child*. New York, NY: HarperCollins.

Levine, M. D. (2001). *A mind at a time*. New York, NY: Simon & Schuster.

Levine, M. D. (2002). *A mind at a time*. New York: Simon & Schuster.

Levine, M. D. (2003). *The myth of laziness*. New York, NY: Simon & Schuster.

Luthar, S. S. (1991). Vulnerability and resilience: A study of high-risk adolescents. *Child Development, 62*, 600–616.

Lutzke, J. R., Ayers, T. S., Sandler, I. N., & Barr, A. (1999). Risks and interventions for the parentally bereaved child. In S. A. Wolchik & I. N. Sandler (Eds.), *Handbook of children's coping: Linking theory and intervention* (pp. 215–245). New York, NY: Plenum.

Martinez, J. G. (1989). Cooling off before burning out. *Academic Therapy, 24*(3), 271–284.

Masten, A.S. (2001). Ordinary magic: Resilience processes and development. *American Psychologist, 56*, 227–238.

Masten, A. S., Best, K. M., & Garmezy, N. (1990). Resilience and development: Contributions from the study of children who overcome adversity. *Development and Psychopathology, 2*, 425–444.

Masten, A. S., & Coatsworth, J. D. (1998). The development of competence in favorable and unfavorable environments: Lessons from research on successful children. *American Psychologist, 53*, 205–220.

Masten, A. S. (1999). Resilience comes of age: Reflections on the past and outlook for the next generation of research. In M. D. Glantz, J. Johnson, & L. Huffman (Eds.), *Resilience and development: Positive life adaptations* (pp. 282–296). New York, NY: Plenum.

Mather, N., & Goldstein, S. (2008). *Learning disabilities and challenging behavior: A guide for educators* (2nd ed.). Baltimore, MD: Brookes Publishers.

Reivich, K., & Shatte, A. (2002). *The resilience factor*. New York, NY: Broadway Books.

Rutter, M. (1985). Resilience in the face of adversity: Protective factors and resistance to psychiatric disorders. *British Journal of Psychiatry, 147*, 598–611.

Rutter, M. (1987). Psychosocial resilience and protective mechanisms. *American Journal of Development*. New York, NY: Irvington Publishers.

Rutter, M. (1990). Psychosocial resilience and protective mechanisms. In J. Rolf, A. S. Masten, D. Cicchetti, K. H. Nuechterlein, & S. Weintraub (Eds.), *Risk and protective factors in the development of psychopathology* (pp. 181–214). New York, NY: Cambridge University Press.

Rutter, M. (2006). Implications of resilience concepts for scientific understanding. *Annals of the New York Academy of Sciences, 1094*, 1–12.

Rutter, M., Cox, A., Tupling, C., Berger, M., & Yule, W. (1975). Attainment and adjustment in two geographical areas: I. The prevalence of psychiatric disorder. *The British Journal of Psychiatry, 126*, 493–509.

Rutter, M., & Quinton, D. (1984). Long-term follow-up of women institutionalized in childhood: Factors promoting good functioning in adult life. *British Journal of Developmental Psychology, 18*, 225–234.

Rutter, M., & The English and Romanian Adoptees (ERA) Study Team. (1998). Developmental catch-up and deficit, following adoption after severe global early privation. *Journal of Child Psychology and Psychiatry, 39*, 465–476.

Sachs, B. E. (2001). *The good enough child: How to have an imperfect family and be perfectly satisfied*. New York, NY: HarperCollins.

Sandler, I. N., Tein, J., & West, S. G. (1994). Coping, stress and psychological symptoms of children of divorce: A cross-sectional and longitudinal study. *Child Development, 65*, 1744–1763.

Segal, J. (1988). Teachers have enormous power in affecting a child's self-esteem. *The Brown University Child Behavior and Development Newsletter, 4*, 1–3.

Sheridan, S. M., Eagle, J. W., & Dowd, S. E. (2005). Families as contexts for children's adaptation. In S. Goldstein & R. Brooks (Eds.), *Handbook of resilience in children* (pp. 165–179). New York, NY: Kluwer Academic/Plenum.

Shure, M. B. (1996). *Raising a thinking child*. New York, NY: Pocket Books.

Shure, M. B., & Aberson, B. (2005). Enhancing the process of resilience through effective thinking. In S. Goldstein & R. Brooks (Eds.), *Handbook of resilience in children* (pp. 373–394). New York, NY: Kluwer Academic/Plenum.

Skinner, E. A., & Wellborn, J. G. (1994). Coping during childhood and adolescence: A motivational perspective. In D. R. Lerner & M. Perlmutter (Eds.), *Life-span development and behavior* (pp. 91–123). Hillsdale, NJ: Erlbaum.

Ungar, M. (2008). Resilience across cultures. *British Journal of Social Work, 38*, 218–235.

Werner, E. E., & Smith, R. S. (1992). *Overcoming the odds: High risk children from birth to adulthood*. Ithaca, NY: Cornell University Press.

Werner, E. (1993). Risk, resilience, and recovery: Perspectives from the Kauai Longitudinal Study. *Development and Psychopathology, 5*, 503–515.

Werner, E. E., & Smith, R. S. (1982). *Vulnerable but invincible: A study of resilient children*. New York, NY: McGraw Hill.

Werner, E. E., & Smith, R. S. (2001). *Journeys from childhood to mid-life: Risk, resilience and recovery*. Ithaca, NY: Cornell University Press.

Wolchik, S. A., Schenck, C. E., & Sandler, I. N. (2009). Promoting resilience in youth from divorced families: Lessons learned from experimental trials of the New Beginnings program. *Journal of Personality, 77*, 1833–1868.

Worsham, N. L., Compas, B. E., & Ey, S. (1997). Children's coping with parental illness. In S. A. Wolchik & I. N. Sandler (Eds.), *Handbook of children's coping: Linking theory and intervention* (pp. 195–215). New York, NY: Plenum.

Wyman, P. A., Cowen, E. L., Work, W. C., Hoyt-Meyers, L. A., Magnus, K. B., & Fagen, D. B. (1999). Caregiving and developmental factors differentiating young at-risk urban children showing resilient versus stress-affected outcomes: A replication and extension. *Child Development, 709*, 645–659.

7 Mental Health Promotion in the Schools: Supporting Resilience in Children and Youth

Barry Mallin, John R. Walker, and Benjamin Levin

Willie Sutton is famously known for answering a reporter, Mitch Ohnstad, who asked why he robbed banks by saying, *"because that's where the money is."* It is a good bet that if those working in the field of wellness promotion were asked, "Why do you focus your efforts on schools?" the answer would be "Because that's where the children are."

The many benefits of getting to children early, with a focus on promoting strengths and preventing problems, have been emphasized in theory and supported by evidence from the earliest days of community psychology (Cowan, 1975). Doll and Cummings (2008) describe the recent emergence of a shared vision for population-based services that amalgamates the insights of developmental research on children's healthy development and psychological disturbance with public health service delivery models. Many population-based practice models have emerged with theoretical unpinning ranging from generally behavioral approaches (Sanders, 1996), to positive psychology (Seligman, 1995), to ecological-systems theory (Bronfenbrenner, 1979). Models of mental health promotion (Jané-Lopis, Barry, Hosman, & Patel, 2005) focus on tailoring intervention to the settings in which people are living—such as the workplace, the school, and, the community. In this chapter, we support the proposition that school systems routinely and appropriately engage in mental health promotion strategies that support resilience in children and youth. We review the basic principles of prevention science as the larger context for a discussion of interventions that support resilience. To relate the principles of mental health promotion to educational practice, we describe a range of intervention approaches with evidence of effectiveness. While demonstrating that these programs fit well with the general philosophy and mandate of school systems, we also discuss the necessary considerations to support implementation and sustainability, incorporating considerations from the effective schools literature and the insights of those who have lead the implementation of successful programs.

B. Mallin, Ph.D. (✉)
Department of Psychology, Faculty of Arts, University of Manitoba, P519A Duff Roblin Bldg 190 Dysart Rd, Winnipeg, MB, Canada R3T 2N2
e-mail: mallin@ad.umanitoba.ca

J.R. Walker, Ph.D.
Department of Clinical Health Psychology, St. Boniface Hospital, University of Manitoba, M1-409 Avenue Taché Ave, Winnipeg, MB, Canada R2H 2A6
e-mail: jwalker@cc.umanitoba.ca

B. Levin, Ph.D.
Theory and Policy Studies, Ontario Institute for Studies in Education, University of Toronto, 252 Bloor Street West, Toronto, ON, Canada M5S 1V6
e-mail: ben.levin@utoronto.ca

Resilience and the Schools

In their review of the construct of resilience, Luthar, Cicchetti, and Becker (2000) provided a helpful definition of resilience: "Resilience refers

S. Prince-Embury and D.H. Saklofske (eds.), *Resilience in Children, Adolescents, and Adults: Translating Research into Practice*, The Springer Series on Human Exceptionality, DOI 10.1007/978-1-4614-4939-3_7, © Springer Science+Business Media New York 2013

to *a dynamic process encompassing positive adaptation within the context of significant adversity*. Implicit within this notion are two critical conditions: (1) exposure to significant threat or severe adversity, and (2) the achievement of positive adaptation despite major assaults on the developmental process…" (p. 543). In describing the evolution of research in the field, the authors noted that while initial research focused on the characteristics of the child, later research has suggested that an understanding of resilience requires study of a variety of factors including (a) characteristics of the child; (b) aspects of their families; and (c) characteristics of the wider social environment. Further, they note that research has moved from a focus on identifying *protective factors* to understanding *protective processes* (Luthar et al., 2000). Resilience has been studied in various circumstances including (a) positive outcomes in high-risk children; (b) sustained competence in children under stress; and (c) good recovery from trauma (Masten, Best, & Garmezy, 1990). Common positive outcomes which have been the focus of this research have been successful academic performance, positive relationships with peers, and positive relationships with adults (Luthar et al., 2000).

Masten (2001), in reviewing the literature on resilience argued that resilience, rather than being an unusual and exceptional phenomenon is the norm. "Resilience appears to be a common phenomenon arising from ordinary human adaptive processes. The great threats to human development are those that jeopardize the systems underlying these adaptive processes, including brain development and cognition, caregiver-child relationships, regulation of emotion and behavior, and the motivations for learning and engaging in the environment (p. 234)." She suggested that work on the promotion of health and mental health in children should focus not only on the reduction of risks and psychopathology but also incorporate the promotion of competence, especially in the developmental systems that support adaptive responding in the environment. She also noted that there are relatively few low-risk children with maladaptive outcomes and children with low risk and children identified as doing well in spite of high risk are often very similar in terms of competence and environmental supports. In other words, similar characteristics support positive outcomes in children at high and low risk. Sapienza, Julianna, and Masten (2011) identified the most widely reported correlates of resilience arising from research on children and youth:

- Positive relationships with caring adults.
- Effective care giving and parenting.
- Intelligence and problem-solving skills.
- Self-regulation skills.
- Perceived efficacy and control.
- Achievement motivation.
- Positive friends or romantic partners.
- Faith, hope, spirituality.
- Beliefs that life has meaning.
- Effective teachers and schools.

Although not explicitly mentioned until the last point in this list, clearly the school has a strong role to play in almost every one of these correlates of resilience.

Another important concept from the area of child development, *developmental cascades*, has influenced thinking on resilience and mental health promotion in the education system. Compelling longitudinal research in this area is described in two special issues of the journal *Development and Psychopathology* in 2010. Much of this work has focused on preschool and school-aged children. According to Masten and Cicchetti (2010): "Developmental cascades refer to the cumulative consequences for development of the many interactions and transactions occurring in developing systems that result in spreading effects across levels, among domains at the same level, and across different systems or generations. Theoretically these effects may be direct and unidirectional, direct and bidirectional, or indirect through various pathways, but the consequences are not transient: developmental cascades alter the course of development (p. 491)." Examples of developmental cascades are common, beginning with adaptive behavior early in childhood. The longitudinal research designs used in studying cascade effects evaluate whether these effects are present over and above effects of within-time covariation and stability over time in key variables.

Lewin-Bizan, Bowers, and Lerner (2010) describe a longitudinal study in which they focused on four assessments over 4 years (ages 11–14) assessing associations among contextual factors and youth development. They found that positive parenting (parental warmth and monitoring) was a major contextual asset predicting subsequent intentional self-regulation; intentional self-regulation predicted subsequent positive youth development (competence, confidence, character, connection, and caring); and positive youth development in turn predicted later youth contribution (positive views and actions related to helping in the community). Positive youth development was not related to later scores for youth problematic outcomes (delinquency, substance use, and depression).

Bornstein, Hahn, and Haynes (2010), in a longitudinal study of 117 families in the community, found that children with lower social competence at age 4 years exhibited more externalizing and internalizing behaviors at ages 10 and 14. Children who exhibited more internalizing behaviors at age 4 years exhibited more internalizing behaviors at age 10 and more externalizing behaviors at age 14. These relationships were present even when there were statistical controls for maternal education and the child's intellectual functioning. Burt and Roisman (2010) studied a large community sample across five time points from age 54 months through age 15 years. They found cross-domain effects from early externalizing problems through effects on both academic and social competence into later internalizing problems. Effects held across gender and were largely unaffected by inclusion of socioeconomic status, early caregiving, and early cognitive ability as covariates in the model. This observational study shows the very negative consequences of early externalizing problems. In considering cascading effects of a preventative intervention, Patterson, Forgatch, and DeGarmo (2010) presented results from their randomized controlled trial (RCT) of an intervention with families with children with antisocial behavior (excessive noncompliance, arguing, teasing, hitting, and temper tantrums) using the Parent Management Training—Oregon Model. This intervention teaches parents strategies to reduce coercion and increase positive parenting with their children and other family members. Children who received the intervention showed reduced rates of delinquency 4 years later and also reduced rates of depression (which may have been related to improved peer relations). Mothers who participated in the program also showed lower levels of depression and improved financial status 4 years later—clear cascade effects. While interventions to support resilience may be helpful at any point in development, these studies highlight the advantages of intervening early in the life span (e.g., Patterson et al., 2010).

Mental Health Promotion and the Schools

Despite a long-standing appreciation of the need to view the person in context, mental-health services typically focus on children, adolescents, and families seeking help with well-established problems. Public health and community psychology endorse a model that provides promotion, prevention, and early intervention services engaging the social structure that affects young people, including the school (Bronfenbrenner, 1992; Cowan, 1975). Consciously or not, schools play an important part in the development of all aspects of children's mental health including skills related to resilience. Starting in their very early years children spend a large proportion of their waking hours in school developing academic skills, life skills, and forming lifelong relationships. Because of this continuing contact with children and families and the opportunity to model and directly teach many proficiencies, schools are ideally placed for conscious, directed and rigorously evaluated activities to promote physical and mental health.

Mental health problems are common among youth even during the preschool years (Kessler, Berglund, Demler, Jin, & Walters, 2005). One in ten children experience severe impairments of functioning in the home, the school, or the community (New Freedom Commission on Mental Health, 2003). Unfortunately, in the USA and

Canada less than 20% of children in need receive required services (Kirby & Keon, 2006; Tolan & Dodge, 2005). Access to specialized educational and support services varies as a function of income (Howell, 2004), involvement with the social welfare or justice systems (Burns et al., 2004; Skowyra & Cocozza, 2006), ethnicity (Kataoka, Zhang, & Wells, 2002), and local government policies (Sturm, Ringel, & Andreyeva, 2003). In schools the effects of this lack of adequate supports can be seen in attention difficulties, highly problematic behavior, confrontational relationships, aggravated physical complaints, and lower academic achievement, all with potential adverse long-term social and physical consequences (Gunner, 2007; Tolan & Dodge, 2005).

The importance of addressing children's mental health needs is well documented (Adelman & Taylor, 1998). In accepting their mandate to provide an appropriate education to all children, schools routinely implement programs directed at concerns such as relationship enhancement, responsible decision making, conflict resolution, managing bullying, outreach to parents, and anxiety reduction. When well implemented these are clear examples of school friendly, empirically supported, mental health promotion strategies even if schools do not label the efforts as such. By supporting resilience, schools help children fare better at home, in school, and in the community (Horner, Sugai, Todd, & Lewis-Palmer, 2005; Fergus & Zimmerman, 2005; Greenberg, Domitrovich, & Bumbarger, 2000; Kirby & Keon, 2006; Masten & Powell, 2003; US Department of Health and Human Services, 1999; Wagner, 2005). In the USA this perspective is clearly evident in the intent of the *No Child Left Behind Act* and the *Individuals with Disabilities Education Act* as well as the objectives of the *President's New Freedom Commission on Mental Health* (2003).

Schools are not the only influence on the developmental trajectory of youth, but the editor they do play a central role and characteristics of the school itself influence outcomes. In a comparative study of 12 London schools, Rutter, Maughan, Mortimore, Ouston, and Smith (1979) found that high delinquency rates correlated highly with truancy, lowest achieving students, an emphasis on punitive consequences, and low evidence of adult praise or social support. Conversely higher levels of achievement in high risk children are evident in school environments that actively promote relationships within the school and the community, maintain high appropriate academic expectations, and prepare children to deal effectively with stress (Comer, Haynes, Joyner, & Ben-Avie, 1996; Cowen, 1994; Cowan, Cohn, Cowan, & Pearson, 1996). It is important that schools strive provide an environment conducive to the growth of social and academic proficiency over time (Short & Shapiro, 1993; Wehlage, Rutter, Smith, Lesko, & Fernandez, 1989).

Given that the school environment plays an important role in enhancing students' positive development through a range of developmental stages, many prevention theorists view schools as the ideal venue for efforts to mitigate risk and build competencies (Simeonson, 1994; Wolin & Wolin, 1997).

Prevention Science

In support of this view, there are many aspects of the conceptual basis and historical development of prevention science that makes it a useful and appropriate model for school-based mental health work. Prevention science is an interdisciplinary field that developed out of work in community psychology and public health to establish an integrated model for prevention-related research and the consequent development and implementation of evidence-based practices. There is longstanding support for putting prevention at the forefront of services provided to families and children (McClellan & Trupin, 1989). The Ottawa Charter for Health Promotion (World Health Organization and Canadian Public Health Association, 1986) placed prevention and early intervention at the center of public policy, a position since supported in other respected policy documents (e.g., National Health Service, 1999; National Institute of Mental Health, 1998).

The focus is not just on the prevention and reduction of individual diagnosable disorders. Prevention science also seeks to promote positive adjustment for the general population (Kellam, Koretz, & Mościcki, 1999; Kellam & Langevin, 2003). It is inclusive of health promotion (Kok, 1993) and a resilience orientation of establishing and supporting confirmed protective factors (Raphael, 1992). The field emphasizes comprehensive, community-wide approaches (Chamberlin, 1992) acknowledging the demonstrated effectiveness of early intervention (Webster-Stratton, Reid, & Hammond, 2004) and supports tailoring interventions to the degree of need.

The discipline is more than simply aspirational. Prevention scientists are firmly committed to using rigorous science-based methods to develop strategies that are effective and appropriately evaluated. Kellam and Langevin (2003) provide a useful framework for understanding the scientific basis, focus, ecology, and reliance on evidence of prevention science. The phases of prevention research incorporate and expand on traditional laboratory science incorporating considerations of dissemination and sustainability. We present an adapted version of the six themes that comprise their framework for understanding evidence in prevention science in Table 7.1.

Table 7.1 Understanding evidence in prevention science

A. Phases of prevention research have different requirements for evidence
The efficacy phase is measured through clinical research trials "well-controlled laboratory settings where the intervention is studied under highly standardized conditions, using such procedures as randomized assignment to experimental and control groups, strict adherence to treatment protocols, and tight control over sources of extraneous variance" (Merrell & Buchanan, 2006, p. 168).
The effectiveness phase investigates the ability of a new treatment to translate into everyday practices that tend not have the tight controls characteristic of efficacy research, or "such vaunted but unrealistic procedures as matching of samples, random assignment, and strict intervention fidelity" (Merrell & Buchanan, 2006, p. 168).
The sustainability phase considers what administrative and training structures are required to maintain an effective intervention.
The going-to-scale phase evaluates how the intervention works when applied broadly in the community at a scale that is feasible to have wide impact.
The sustainability system-wide phase evaluates what is required to sustain interventions when they are implemented system wide. In many cases system-wide implementation is required for effects that may be demonstrated at a population level.
B. Prevention strategies are directed to individuals, small social contexts and larger societal structures.
The research design and data collection in prevention (or promotion) research will depend on level of intervention. Common levels of intervention are the child, the family, the classroom, the school, the school district, or the community.
C. Prevention programs recognize a hierarchy of risk: the total population; a smaller subpopulation at increased risk; or a still smaller subpopulation at very high risk.
Many of the protective and risk factors correlated with resilience apply across the population. Subpopulations may be identified and targeted for additional support if there are lower levels of protective factors and higher levels of risk factors. In the school system common higher risk subpopulations (at the community level) are children living with limited economic resources, lower parental education, or more disadvantaged neighborhoods. At the individual level, children with lower levels of pre-academic and academic skills or those with problems such as limited social skills, aggression, or reduced attention span have been identified as having higher risk.
D. Economic analysis is a central requirement of prevention research.
Successful program implementers have developed business models and mechanisms of dissemination to support training and resourcing practitioners to deliver worthwhile programs. Lack of a cost benefit analysis can lead to effective programs not being disseminated at all or a surfeit of short term, low impact initiatives (Turner & Sanders, 2006; Wolfe, 2006).

(continued)

Table 7.1 (continued)

E. Collaboration is required.

Both implementers and educational theorists note that sustainability issues, such as treatment fidelity, require attention and commitment to the larger social environment and in particular the human capital (Levin & Riffel, 1998; Turner & Sanders, 2006). There must be wide-scale buy in by the key players in an organization for programs to be sustained (teachers, parents, administrators, and government authorities).

F. Acceptance of a multidimensional framework for understanding evidence is essential.

It is important to understand the multidimensional concept of evidence and why it is central to the practice of prevention science. The common view of science presents it as entirely based on a narrow implementation of the basic scientific problem-solving model: observation, hypothesis generation, data collection, analysis, recommendation generation, intervention implementation, and further data collection (The Canadian Cochrane Network, 2003). Typically this model is implemented in the classic experimental process of the randomized controlled trial (RCT). Contemporary models of evidence in science recognize a hierarchy of research evidence as opposed to adherence to a single methodology or research design. Evidence hierarchies typically place meta-analyses and true experiments (RCTs) at the highest level with expert opinion on the lowest level. However one conceives the hierarchy, given the absence or inappropriateness of evidence at the highest level, decisions should be based on evidence at the next lower level (Hamilton, 2005) rather than relying excessively on untested opinion, however derived. Prevention science and educational researchers acknowledge that there are many procedures that yield trustworthy evidence (Berliner, 2002) including research using single-case designs and exploratory qualitative approaches including structured content analysis and naturalistic observations. It is important to appreciate that a greater range of considerations applies to the use of interventions. In practice non-empirical factors such as beliefs, familiarity, and comfort level matter. Evidence-based clinical practice (EBCP) guidelines are based on "the integration of best research evidence with clinical expertise and patient values" (Sackett, Straus, Richardson, Rosenberg, & Haynes, 2000, p. 1).

In support of the value of an evidence-based focus, school psychology defines data-based decision making and accountability as fundamental to its activities (NASP, 2009). The Task Force on Evidence-Based Interventions in School Psychology encourages the profession to "extend knowledge of evaluation criteria for evidence-based interventions" by collaborating with other professionals to ensure that interventions demonstrate effectiveness in the educational setting (Kratochwill & Shernoff, 2003, p. 390).

The Convergence of Educational Theory and Practice with Preventions Science Concepts

Aspects of a prevention approach are apparent in a wide range of current universal and targeted school practices. The evidence of a significant shift in school systems from a pathology oriented identification and treatment model to one that broadly defines mental health to encompass the promotion of social and emotional development and learning (Adelman, 1995; Adelman & Taylor, 1994) is most evident in the adoption of the *response to intervention (RtI)* approach (Fuchs, Mock, Morgan, & Young, 2003). *RtI* is a widely practiced model developed to provide services appropriate to the needs of all students. Common to properly implemented *RtI* approaches is a holistic ecological orientation beginning with the broader population and proceeding to the individual and entirely consistent with the prevention science focus on *individuals, small social contexts, and larger societal structures.*

RtI was designed with early identification and intervention in mind to avoid the *wait to fail* pitfall of the earlier *refer, test, place* model. It utilizes screening measures to identify students at risk in hopes of preventing persistent and severe difficulties. It also relies on data from progress monitoring, including benchmark assessment and curriculum-based measurement, as the basis of data-based decision making. This emphasis on the value of measurement reflects another hallmark of prevention science.

The RtI approach is based on the tiered provision of services starting with universal services that proceed to more intense interventions applied to a smaller number of at risk students. Models of RtI vary in specifics such as the number of tiers of service intensity envisioned and the labels attached (Fuchs et al., 2003; Marston, Muyskens, Lau, &

Canter, 2003; Tilly, 2006; Vaughn & Chard, 2006), but the tiered approach to interventions is equivalent to that used in prevention science (National Research Council and the Institute of Medicine, 2009).

As a relatively new approach, RtI is still subject to examination. Its insistence on scientifically validated interventions speaks to considerations of both *efficacy* and *effectiveness*. The funding structure in the USA that ties federal funding to demonstrated results speaks to the concept of *efficiency* and the need for economic evidence.

In the clinical realm, a compatible theoretical orientation is evident in the guiding document *School psychology: A blueprint for training and practice III* (Ysseldyke et al., 2006). These guidelines include a domain of competency titled Enhancing the Development of Wellness, Social Skills, Mental Health, and Life Competencies and explicitly state: "a prevention focus exists throughout the document" (p. 38). Ideally, this explicit support for a public health orientation will help school psychologists shape school systems to focus more on promotion approaches that encompass the entire school population rather than primarily on individual identified students (Strein, Hoagwood, & Cohn, 2003).

Examples of Programs to Support Resilience

There now are many mental health promotion programs that have been widely applied in the schools. These programs differ in the degree to which they:

- Are integrated with the usual functioning of the schools or are add on programs.
- Involve regular school staff or require additional staff.
- Are universal (for all students), selected (focused on students, schools, or families at higher risk), or indicated (focused on children who show evidence of having problems currently).
- Have evidence of efficacy, effectiveness, sustainability, going to scale, and sustainability system-wide.
- Have costs associated with training, implementation, and sustaining.
- Have evidence concerning longer-term costs and benefits.

Reviews such as that by Inman, van Bakergem, LaRosa, and Garr (2011), the special issue *Using Prevention Science to Address the Mental Health Issues in Schools* (Stormont, Reinke, & Herman, 2010) and many online resources have aggregated information focused on children and youth. Table 7.2 describes useful web portals that describe evidence-based programs and practices. In the following sections we provide examples of programs that are applied on a school-wide basis, at the classroom level, as indicated programs for children with particular risk factors, and as part of school efforts to support parents in their important role.

Programs Implemented on a School-Wide Basis

School-wide Positive Behavioral Interventions and Supports (SWPBIS): (http://www.pbis.org/default.aspx) This approach is probably the most comprehensive, aiming to influence the environment in the whole school. The program applies a behaviorally based systems approach to enhance the capacity of schools, families, and communities and promote effective student behaviors (Sugai, Sprague, Horner, & Walker, 2000). It is not a specific model but rather a framework or approach comprised of intervention practices and organizational systems for establishing the social culture, learning and teaching environment. The approach includes individual behavior supports needed to achieve academic and social success for all students, not just students with disabilities. It employs a tiered model of increasingly intense supports. Primary prevention strategies are for all students (Sugai & Horner, 2002) focusing on ecological aspects of the school, such as using effective teaching practices and curricula or explicit teaching of acceptable behavior (Lewis, Sugai, & Colvin, 1998; Martella & Nelson, 2003). Secondary prevention strategies target

Table 7.2 Evidence-based practices web resources

Center for the study and prevention of violence	
Blueprints for violence prevention	http://www.colorado.edu/cspv/blueprints
The Blueprints mission is to identify violence and drug prevention programs that meet a high scientific standard of effectiveness. Three criteria are given greater weight: evidence of deterrent effect with a strong research design, sustained effect, and multiple site replication. Blueprints *model* programs must meet all three of these criteria, while *promising* programs must meet only the first criterion	
The Office of Juvenile Justice and Delinquency	
Prevention Model Programs Guide	http://www.ojjdp.gov/mpg/
Designed to assist practitioners and communities in implementing evidence-based prevention and intervention programs. It describes over 200 evidence-based programs that address a range of issues, including substance abuse, mental health, and education. The evidence ratings are based on the evaluation literature summarizing four dimensions: • The conceptual framework of the program • Program fidelity • The evaluation design • Evidence demonstrating the prevention or reduction of problem behavior; the reduction of risk factors related to problem behavior; or the enhancement of protective factors related to problem behavior	
Effectiveness dimensions and the overall scores are used to classify programs into three categories to provide the user with a summary knowledge base of the supporting research.	
The Social Work Policy Institute	
Evidence-based practice	http://www.socialworkpolicy.org/research/evidence-based-practice-2.html
Two sections are presented: • The Evidence-Based Practice Resources section provides tools that can be used to identify EBPs, online resources that can inform the EBP process and a list of publications for further information • The Partnership examples section highlights some existing partnerships created between researchers and practitioners that further EBP	
What works Wisconsin	
Evidence-based Program Registries	http://whatworks.uwex.edu/Pages/2evidenceregistries.html
Lists evidence-based programs that have met specific criteria for effectiveness. The registries cover a range of areas including substance abuse and violence prevention as well as the promotion of positive outcomes such as school success and emotional and social competence. Generally, registries are used to find programs for implementation. However, registries may also be used to learn about evidence-based programs that serve as models as organizations modify their own programs.	

students who continue at risk for academic failure or behavior problems but are not in need of individual support (Nelson, Benner, Reid, Epstein, & Currin, 2002). Interventions most often are in small groups and include social skills training, empirically supported academic instruction or behavioral supports. Tertiary prevention programs focus on students who display persistent patterns of disciplinary problems (Nelson et al., 2002) and are strength-based. They could include use of full functional behavioral assessment and development of a behavior intervention plan. Simple measures such as office disciplinary referrals (Tidwell, Flannery, & Lewis-Palmer, 2003; Walker, Cheney, Stage, & Blum, 2005) are used to identify students and track progress.

SWPBS systems change strategies have been demonstrated to be empirically effective and efficient. Evidence from RCTs have been supportive (Bradshaw, Koth, Bevans, Ialongo, & Leaf, 2008; Horner et al., 2005). Adopted in excess of 9,000 schools in the USA, the US Department of Education has worked to scale-up the approach and maintain fidelity. A blueprint and self-assessment toolkit is available for SWPBIS implementers (Sugai et al., 2010).

Programs Implemented at the Classroom Level

The Good Behavior Game (GBG): A description of the GBG was first published by Barrish, Saunders, and Wolf (1969). Since this time the approach has been studied in a wide range of classroom situations and there has been an impressive accumulation of evidence on its effectiveness (Tingstrom, Sterling-Turner, & Wilczynski, 2006). While the program focuses on the early school years, it has also been successfully adapted to high school settings (Kleinman & Saigh, 2011). In a typical application, a classroom is divided into two (or more) teams. Lead by the teacher, members of the class work out expectations for positive behavior in the classroom. Each team receives marks on the chalk board for disruptive behavior while the teacher is teaching a particular class segment. The team with the fewest marks or both teams if they have a low level of disruptive behavior, win the game. Winning teams receive special privileges such as a special activity (often academically focused), early recess, lining up first for lunch, or special recognition of some kind. The emphasis is on ease of administration by the teacher during regular classroom activities and activity rewards that are easily available in the classroom. An advantage is that the program does not focus on a specific child with problematic behavior but rather focuses on encouraging cooperative and on task behavior in the classroom as a whole. This whole class approach is easier for a teacher to consistently deliver. There has been some concern about the focus on disruptive behavior, rather than positive behavior and the approach appears to work just as well when there is an emphasis on appropriate classroom behaviors rather than disruptive behavior (Tanol, Johnson, McComas, & Cote, 2010). The approach has been studied in a number of large-scale RCTs and the impact on behavior in the classroom is large (Kellam, Rebok, Ialongo, & Mayer, 1994; van Lier, Muthén, van der Sar, & Crijnen, 2004). What is especially promising about the approach is the long-term impact. A group based at the at the Prevention Research Center of Johns Hopkins School of Public Health studied this approach in schools in disadvantaged areas of Baltimore, Maryland (Kellam et al., 1994). They found that first-grade boys who were initially rated at or above the median on aggression, and who participated in the game throughout first and second grades, had lower levels of aggression in fourth, fifth, and sixth grades. Participants in these studies were followed as young adults and showed reduced drug and alcohol abuse/dependence disorders, regular smoking, and antisocial personality disorder (Kellam et al., 2008). A more recent RCT (Witvliet, van Lier, Cuijpers, & Koot, 2009) found that the GBG both reduced disruptive classroom behavior and improved peer acceptance. Reductions in externalizing behavior appeared to be partly mediated by the improvements in peer acceptance.

Recently Embry (2002) has updated the materials and procedures in a version called Pax-GBG (http://www.paxis.org/content/goodbehavior.aspx) to make it easier for teachers to implement and to broaden the focus of the game. This version adds additional elements to encourage positive interactions among students and individual emotion regulation. Kits, which include an implementation DVD, are available for use by teachers or schools.

The Fourth R: Skills for Youth Relationships (http://www.youthrelationships.org/about_fourth_r.html). Fourth R is taught as part of the regular curriculum. It is an inclusive strategy, based on a universal model of health promotion for all youth, focusing on effective methods to encourage youth participation and healthy choices (Burt, 2002; Farrow & Saewyc, 2002). Its goals can be mapped directly onto the core competencies identified by the Collaborative for Academic, Social, and Emotional Learning (CASEL, 2006): self-awareness (i.e., recognizing your emotions and values along with your strengths and limitations), social awareness (i.e., demonstrating empathy and understanding for others), self-management (i.e., goal-directed management of emotions and behaviors), relationship skills (i.e., establishing positive relationships, teaming, effective management of conflict), and responsible decision making (i.e., making principled, productive choices about personal and social behavior) (Christenson, Whitehouse, & VenGetson, 2007).

The program is taught in the classroom, using a thematic approach to reduce risk behaviors including violence/bullying, unsafe sexual behavior, and substance use. It was designed to address adolescent dating violence and related risk behaviors by teaching, in an integrated manner, evidence-based strategies such as negotiation, delay, and refusal skills, and exercises to define and rehearse responsibilities associated with healthy relationships. Examples of peer and dating conflicts faced by teens are provided, as are role-play instructions to increase interpersonal and problem-solving skills. Qualified teachers are trained in a 21-lesson curriculum comprised of three units containing seven 75-min classes each: (1) personal safety and injury prevention, (2) healthy growth and sexuality, and (3) substance use and abuse. An underlying theme of healthy, nonviolent relationship skills throughout the units increases generalization. Detailed lesson plans, video resources, role-play exercises, rubrics, and handouts develop skills to deal with pressures and nonviolent conflict resolution using graduated practice with peers. Slightly different exercises and activities are used for boys and girls to maximize relevance and minimize defensiveness on the part of participants. Efficacy studies have been supportive (Wolfe, Crooks, Chiodo, Hughes, & Jaffe, 2005). The program is funded by a private endowment, by a partnership with a national business consortium, and by sales of materials. It undertakes continuing development and evaluation and has a version modified to meet the requirements of aboriginal peoples.

Indicated Programs for Children with Particular Risk Factors

Incredible Years Child and Teacher Intervention (http://www.incredibleyears.com). The Incredible Years program was developed initially for clinic-referred children and families in the 3–7 year age range with difficulties with oppositional behavior and conduct problems (Webster-Stratton, Reid, & Stoolmiller, 2008). The clinic-based program has been extensively evaluated and found to be effective in reducing problem behavior, increasing social competence, and encouraging the use of more effective parenting techniques (Webster-Stratton & Herman, 2010). This treatment model was adapted for use by teachers as a preschool and early school-years preventive model with a focus on schools in economically disadvantaged communities. The program focuses on (a) supporting teacher classroom management skills and maintenance of a positive classroom environment, (b) encouraging teacher–parent involvement, and (c) developing child school readiness (social competence, emotional self-regulation, and absence of behavior problems). The child-focused component of the program (Dina Dinosaur Social Skills and Problem Solving Curriculum) involves 30 classroom lessons per year with brief teaching sessions (using DVD models) followed by skill practice sessions. Areas covered in the lessons include: (1) classroom rules, (2) empathy and emotion, (3) problem solving, (4) anger control, (5) friendship skills, (6) communication skills, and (7) school skills. Between 30 and 40 min are spent on these activities twice a week. In the RCT these sessions were co-lead by a member of the research staff to insure that all classes received a full dose of the activities. Observers who were blind to whether the class was in the control or intervention group visited the classrooms at the beginning and the end of the school year. These observations indicated that intervention teachers used more positive classroom management strategies and their students showed more social competence and emotional self-regulation and fewer conduct problems. Intervention teachers reported more involvement with parents than control teachers. Satisfaction with the program was very high regardless of grade level. This program has also been evaluated with positive results in the context of mental health consultation to preschool teachers in a Head Start program (Raver et al., 2009). The developers of this program indicate that more research is needed to evaluate whether the program can produce similar results with lower levels of teacher support and less direct monitoring of children and teachers. Webster-Stratton and Herman (2010) have developed a model and strategies for implementing this program in community and school settings with high fidelity. While the programs were developed initially with a focus on families living in economically disadvantaged communities, they are also suitable for universal use. The Incredible Years program has developed extensive resources for schools and workshops for teachers and other professionals. There has been some evaluation of the cost effectiveness of the various components of the program (parent, child, teacher) used individually or in combination (Foster, Olchowski, & Webster-Stratton, 2007).

Programs to Support Parents

The Family and Schools Together Program (FAST) (http://familiesandschools.org). FAST was designed based on family stress and prevention theory with a view to strengthening resiliency for at-risk children and at improving family functioning in collaboration with schools. It is in every sense what Christenson and Sheridan (2001) have defined as partnering with a "*student-focused philosophy* wherein educators and families cooperate, coordinate, and collaborate to enhance learning opportunities, educational progress and school success for students in four domains: academic, social, emotional, and behavioral" (p. 37).

FAST is a multisession group for families of elementary school children. To meet the needs of additional target populations, related curricula have been developed including: Baby FAST, Pre-K FAST, Kids FAST, Middle School FAST, and Teen FAST. FAST has been used in urban and rural settings in over 600 schools with diverse of ethnic backgrounds and socioeconomic status in 38 states (Kratochwill, McDonald, Levin, Bear-Tibbetts, & Demaray, 2004). It has been described as a blend of "family therapy principles, delinquency and substance abuse prevention strategies, psychiatric techniques, family systems theory, and group dynamics" (Sass, 1999, p. 2). FAST includes a well-developed evaluation protocol focused on measuring change toward the FAST program goals (McDonald et al., 1997). Results clearly demonstrate significant improvement both at home and at school (Coote, 2000).

The Kids FAST program is a voluntary program that that involves the whole family along with school and community members. Families elect to participate after being nominated by schools or through open enrolment. Ten weekly evening sessions of approximately 2½ h typically are held in a school. The program requires facilitation by a trained team and follow-up evaluation. Activities include "age appropriate lessons with music, to feeling charades, to creating a family flag, to dinners on and off site, to fun family play. A central component includes structured and unstructured playtime which include the parents and children" (Crozier, Rokutani, Russett, Godwin, & Banks, 2010, p. 210). Program cycles conclude with graduation ceremonies. For graduate families, FASTWORKS, is a structured, parent-led program meeting monthly in the school or community for 2 years or more with the goals of building an ongoing parent support network empowering parents to strengthen their families, to be their child's advocate, and to become leaders in the community and school. FAST has a well-developed business model based on fees for program-provided training and ongoing licensing. These support dissemination, further development and the required quality assurance through evaluation.

Triple—P (Positive Parenting Program) (http://www1.triplep.net/). Triple P is a multi-level, parenting and family support system developed at the University of Queensland in Brisbane, Australia. While not specifically school focused, the system is intended to be integrated with community organizations including schools. Triple P is an outstanding example of the implementation of every aspect of the prevention science model at a population level. It provides parents access to the program through mass media campaigns as well as by training service providers in schools, health centers, and child welfare systems. Triple P's efficacy and effectiveness have been extensively examined in the literature (e.g., Sanders, 1999, 2001; Sanders, Markie-Dadds, Tully, &

Bor, 2000; Sanders, Turner, & Markie-Dadds, 2002). The system is the only parenting support approach which has developed evidence for its effects at the population level through major studies in Australia (Sanders et al., 2008) and the USA (Prinz, Sanders, Shapiro, Whitaker, & Lutzker, 2009). Triple P is based firmly on social learning principles that highlight the transactional nature of parent–child interactions (e.g., Patterson, 1982). It incorporates behavior change techniques supported in child and family behavior therapy research (Sanders, 1996) and is grounded in public health research (e.g., Becker et al., 1992). Triple P planfully addresses the self-regulation of parental skill and the ecological context of parenting using a five level, tiered continuum of interventions of increasing strength directed to a variety of consumers.

Building on successful efficacy and effectiveness trials the dissemination, continuing evaluation, and quality control components have been designed to support practitioner growth and engage their work environments. (Backer, Liberman, & Kuehnel, 1986; Henggeler, Melton, Brondino, Scherer, & Hanley, 1997). The program retains tight control of practitioner training by having program accredited staff provide standardized professional training programs for all levels of Triple P intervention. It has a well-developed business model based on fees for training and materials that supports dissemination, further development, and evaluation.

Evidence-Based Kernels Approach

While Embry has been associated with revising and disseminating the GBG approach to classroom management (described above), he also has advocated for an approach which differs from many of the sophisticated programs described above. Embry (2004, 2008, 2011) argues that it is a challenge to implement and maintain highly structured programs with requirements for extensive staff training in complex environments. As an alternative, he suggests that researchers identify fundamental approaches used in promoting changes in behavior. He calls these units *evidence-based kernels*. In developing approaches to support healthy behavior in children (and across the age span), leaders can promote the use of kernels appropriate to the particular situation. Embry defines an evidence-based kernel as follows:

> An evidence-based kernel is an indivisible procedure empirically shown to produce reliable effects on behavior, including psychological processes. The unit is indivisible in the sense that it would be ineffective upon elimination of any of its components. Examples of kernels include timeout, written praise notes, self-monitoring, framing relations among stimuli to affect the value of a given stimulus, and increasing Omega-3 fatty acids in the diet in order to influence behavior. A kernel may increase the frequency of a behavior or it may make a behavior less likely. It can have its impact by altering antecedent or consequent events in the psychological environment of the person or it can affect behavior by directly manipulating a physiological function. Kernels, by definition, target a single behavior, whereas programs typically target multiple behaviors (Embry, 2011, p. 9).

Embry defines *behavioral vaccines* as the "repeated use of kernel or a simple recipe of kernels that prevent or reduce morbidity or mortality or improve wellbeing. Hand washing or buckling a seatbelt are clear health examples of behavioral vaccines" (Embry, 2011). Rather than requiring extensive training, kernels and behavioral vaccines may be easier to disseminate to organizations and the public at low cost because they:

- *Focus on small units of behavior change* that may be adopted by the consumers (parents, teachers, schools, children) or organizations (classrooms, schools, states) via simple verbal explanations, demonstrations, or symbolic modeling with less demanding requirements for training than more elaborate programs.
- Often *produce rapid behavior change* that supports the continued use of the approach.
- May be *evaluated in simple ABAB designs* which demonstrate the effectiveness of the approach. [ABAB designs involve the development of baseline assessment (A), then implementation of the procedure until a change is clearly demonstrated in the target behaviors (B), then removal of the procedure (A) to evaluate the effect on the target behaviors, and

then return to implementation of the procedure in the longer term (B)].

These approaches have informed a number of successful large-scale public health campaigns including interventions to reduce the sale of tobacco to young people, reduce tobacco use in young people, and increase positive social interactions and reduce violence in the schools (Embry, 2011). Embry argues that practitioners must make interventions like these attractive to consumers, widely marketed, and easily available at low cost in line with a public health model. These approaches are also suitable for use in routine health care consultations with health-care and educational service providers.

Challenges to Implementation of Evidence-Based Approaches

As described above, there are a number of well-evaluated interventions that support protective factors and reduce risk factors related to resilience in school-aged children. In every area of human services, however, there is concern about how to encourage the uptake and sustained use of approaches supported by research (e.g., Kratochwill & Shernoff, 2004). Leaders in the field have recognized that developing and evaluating effective approaches will not be enough to insure that they are adopted and sustained (Turner & Sanders, 2006). Background information in support of implementation is available in the literature on leadership development, knowledge translation, school improvement and effectiveness, policy development, public health, community psychology, and systems theory. Currently, there is a strong recognition of the need for systemic or large-scale approaches that integrate factors external and internal to schools that are known to make a difference in the provision of effective and sustainable educational program (Adelman & Taylor, 2004). There are many challenges to improving schools across an entire education system. International rankings such as the UN Human Development Index (hdr.undp.org/en/statistics), the Competitiveness Index of the World Economic Forum (http://www.weforum.org/en/initiatives/gcp/index.htm), or the Organisation for Economic Co-operation and Development's (OECD) Programme for International Student Assessment (PISA, http://www.oecd.pisa.org) have increased motivation by governments to focus on the quality of education systems at a national level. Globally, attention is beginning to shift to whole system reform because some countries are doing noticeably better through the use of effective educational strategies. A growing interest in benchmarking not just outcomes but also policies and strategies for whole populations has led to a surge of interest in how to improve education outcomes across a nation or a political subunit such as a state.

The research on large-scale improvement of the education system is growing but still not large with few careful studies of what is required. There are national or international correlation studies that attempt to link better outcomes with various factors. PISA, as one example, has been highly influential internationally (e.g., Schleicher, 2009), while various smaller studies have used similar correlational techniques at national levels (e.g., Creemers & Kyriakides 2008). However, understanding the correlates of strong performance, while vital, does not necessarily tell us how to get more of those factors and thus improve performance. Recently, more has been written about large-scale change. Fullan (2005, 2006, 2007, 2009, 2010) has been a key writer in this field and a number of others have contributed to a growing literature. Barber (2007, 2009) has provided an insider's account of what was required to move an entire national education system in England and discussed the broader lessons from this experience. Hopkins (2008) has described the English strategy in more conceptual terms. Recent papers describe educational change approaches focused on literacy used in the USA, (Fullan, 2009), Canada (Levin, 2008a, Fullan, 2009), Australia (Elmore, 2007), and Finland (Fullan, 2009). Summaries can be found in influential papers by Barber and Mourshed (2007) and Whelan (2009). A new report by the Kinsey Corporation (Mourshed, Chijioke, & Barber, 2010) is particularly focused on improvement in national systems across countries with different characteristics.

Four main challenges have been identified in producing changes in the education system: (1) the educational challenge of changing very large numbers of schools and classrooms on a sustained basis, (2) the bureaucratic challenge of improving the connections among different areas of social policy in pursuit of better outcomes for students, (3) the learning challenge of organizing complex systems to do this work while continually modifying the approach in light of new evidence and system feedback, and (4) the political challenge of galvanizing the effort required to support these other changes.

The educational challenge: The early view that policy measures or incentive structures will produce system change has given way to a clear understanding that policy is nothing without effective implementation (Levin, 2008b; McLaughlin, 1987; McLaughlin & Mitra, 2001) largely because education is a multifaceted social process. Efforts at large-scale educational change, therefore, necessarily involve careful consideration of the views, beliefs, and habits of many thousands of people—the children as well as the adults who work with them. Such efforts are shaped fundamentally not only by geography, history, local institutional structures and cultures, language, and custom but also by the way these affect individuals or small groups. This means that some things need to be done at scale across an entire system. Yet, strict top-down approaches based on mindless compliance cannot succeed in a field where people's desire is so central. People must be engaged in the work, and this means there must also be some degree of flexibility for participants. Balancing the appropriate degree of direction and flexibility is very challenging. Too much direction is demotivating to people, but too little direction means that good practices do not spread and ineffective practices can continue indefinitely.

The bureaucratic challenge: Performance in schools is powerfully shaped by social forces beyond the school, and in particular socioeconomic status (Raffo et al., 2009; Rothstein, 2004). Improving education outcomes therefore requires attention to related social policies. Early childhood factors, especially those related to resilience, need to be taken seriously (Fullan, 2009). Better results are possible if government departments and community organizations could work more closely together and bureaucratic organizational boundaries could be overcome to produce "joined up thinking." But creating effective working relationships across boundaries is challenging. Organizations will inevitably have different mandates, different legislative provisions, different stakeholder groups, and different professional cultures, all of which make it harder to collaborate effectively. There may be more potential for effective collaboration at local levels where it is possible to build the personal relationships required to sustain collaborative work.

The learning challenge: Most public policy systems are not designed with good feedback or learning loops (Wilson, 1989). Much of the emphasis in government goes to design and announcement, following which everyone tends to move on to the next pressing issue. An education strategy that involves real change across many elements of a large and complex system also requires a learning strategy so that there can be constant adjustment of plans and programs in light of emerging information on implementation and results. The main elements required for effective learning are reasonably straightforward—timely, high-quality information on the state of the system and processes to analyze that information and adjust plans accordingly (Gawande, 2007). Because systems typically organize information around administrative or operational needs rather than around results or even key processes it often is difficult to access high-quality information even on basic student progress indicators. Information only matters if it is used and data have to be interpreted, always a political process (Garmston & Wellman, 1999). It is especially important to focus discussion of data and evaluation on what to do next, rather than who is right or wrong.

The political challenge: Almost everything in government and politics works against political leaders defining a small number of key priorities and then staying focused on those priorities.

To think that doing the right thing in politics is a matter of the will of politicians is fundamentally to misunderstand the nature of the political process. Politicians are, by design, in the business of getting and staying elected, a condition necessary to advance any policy goal. This means they cannot get too far ahead of, or too far behind their citizens, must be keenly aware of the state of public opinion and equally aware that public opinion often is a slippery thing. People can and do change their focus and their ideas. Large, quick swings in attention can result from totally unexpected events—a natural disaster, a political scandal, or the departure of a key person. Moreover, public concern about an issue implies neither any depth of knowledge nor any consistency in ideas. People can and do have strong views on issues based on ignorance and their ideas can be quite contradictory; people can simultaneously be in favor of more spending and lower taxes. Politicians cannot ignore these moods or swings, and cannot chastise voters for their lack of knowledge or consistency. Political timelines are relatively short while the most important policy challenges are long term.

Fundamental Elements in Large-Scale Change

While these challenges to system change in education are important, some guidance can be derived by mapping them to the following seven fundamental elements in large-scale educational change proposed by Levin and Fullan (2008):

1. A small number of ambitious yet achievable goals, publicly stated.
2. A positive stance with a focus on motivation.
3. Multilevel engagement with strong leadership and a "guiding coalition."
4. Emphasis on capacity building with a focus on results.
5. Keeping a focus on key strategies while also managing other interests and issues.
6. Effective use of resources.
7. Constant and growing transparency including public and stakeholder communication and feedback.

For example, the special education system remains the primary response system for schools to individual student challenges, so an effort to support resilience would have to consider how these ideas relate to or should affect special education policy, funding, and practice. As another instance, classroom teachers are the primary connection of schools to students, so any improvement in schooling at a system level must consider how to expand the skills and understandings of tens of thousands of teachers. Adding a few pilot projects or special programs will simply not have the desired effect. At the same time, this is a field full of new program ideas, many of which are advocated on the basis of one person's beliefs or purported success in one or two places with a small number of students. The system as a whole requires a much stronger and more rigorous research and development effort, in which new program ideas are carefully tested and then expanded when (and only when) there is convincing evidence from multiple sources of their effectiveness. Education currently lacks this rigorous approach to innovation. And all of this has to be done in a way that takes account of the very strong advocacy groups that exist around children's issues.

These insights from successful large-scale educational reforms can be linked directly to considerations of mental health promotion and supporting resilience in the schools. Adelman & Taylor (2007), speaking of the need for the USA to develop an integrated perspective to avoid fragmentation and marginalization, state "Given that systemic change is of central importance in efforts to improve schools and schooling, we suggest policy decision makers must recognize and support a growing research and training agenda to advance understanding and capability for designing, implementing, and sustaining prototypes and taking them to scale (p. 71)."

Similarly, in Canada, Leadbeater (2010) describes the infrastructures to support the evaluation and dissemination of promotion, prevention, and intervention programs as immature. This is especially true for long-term projects as evidenced by issues with health research funding that is short term and renewable; a lack of either appropriate financial or academic merit incentives; the plethora of roles the researcher must assume for dissemination [e.g., advocate, marketer, trainer, quality assurance manager and continued evaluator of the program (p. 223)]; a lack of interdisciplinary structure and long-term team building; and fragmentation both in government and in service delivery. She argues for stable, integrated community and government infrastructures to support implementation.

From their international perspective Turner and Sanders (2006) offer additional considerations including the need to cultivate a more entrepreneurial focus and the development of a proper business case to benefit developers and allow proper training and resourcing of practitioners to deliver worthwhile programs. They also recommend identifying an "internal advocate" (what Steve Jobs called "an evangelist" at Apple computers) to enhance the interpersonal factors that further support the new program (Backer et al., 1986).

Table 7.3 describes web resources that provide helpful advice for the practitioner interested in implementing mental health promotion approaches. An excellent resource related to this topic is the chapter *Best practices in accessing the systems change literature* (Ervin & Schaughency, 2008) which provides "sample resources and references pertaining to literature

Table 7.3 Web resources concerning program implementation

The Collaborative for Academic, Social, and Emotional Learning (CASEL)	
Rubric for school-wide implementation of social and emotional learning	http://casel.org/wp-content/uploads/2011/04/Rubric.pdf
A detailed implementation rubric comprised of ten steps over three phases, along with a set of ongoing sustainability factors. It is discussed in detail in *Transforming School Mental Health Services* (Doll & Cummings, 2008) along with insights from other chapter authors.	
The Substance Abuse and Mental Health Services Administration (SAMHSA)	
EBP Implementation Resource Kits for Mental Health	http://mentalhealth.samhsa.gov/cmhs/communitysupport/toolkits/about.asp
Six resource kits to encourage the use of evidence-based practices as part of SAMHSA's and its Center for Mental Health Services (CMHS) science-to-services strategy.	
National Implementation Research Network (NIRN)	
Improving the Science of Implementation	http://www.fpg.unc.edu/~nirn/reviews/review-detail.cfm?reviewID=16
The site provides an extensive annotated list of reviews of collections of programs, curricula, guidelines, and tools to support effective implementation, research, and practice. One comprehensive publication is D. L. Fixsen, et al., (2005). *Implementation Research: A Synthesis of the Literature*, FPG Child Development Institute, University of North Carolina at Chapel Hill. http://www.fpg.unc.edu/~nirn/resources/publications/Monograph/index.cfm	
Communities and Schools Promoting Health	
A Gateway to information on comprehensive school health (CSH) and health promoting schools (HPS).	http://www.safehealthyschools.org/mental_health/mental_health_1.htm
This gateway website provides access to many resources in school health promotion. Extensive background information, explanation of the essential elements of the comprehensive school health approach are provided as well as tools such as lesson plans, webquests, sample policies, evaluation tools, and practical advice.	
Center for Mental Health in Schools at UCLA	
Information resource	http://smhp.psych.ucla.edu/
Guides to Policy and Program Development/Practice. The categories covered are guidebooks, guidance notes, practice notes, policy notes, tools and other resources addressing: (1) Barriers to Learning and Teaching: contains examples of policy formulations, prototypes of guidelines and standards, and a prototype for a school district proposal including planning tools for initial and ongoing planning. (2) Mental Health in Schools: includes a broad view of mental health in schools and of the value of embedding mental health into a comprehensive classroom and school-wide system to ensure all students have an equal opportunity to succeed at school. *NOTE*: The link provided takes you to the home page. From there click on Practitioner Toolbox, Resources & Networks and then on Guidebooks.	

from broader fields, theories of change past efforts and the change agent's role in the process"(p. 855).

Conclusion

Levin & Riffel (1998) point out that while change is complex and attempts at rationality are subject to limitations of human capacity and action an optimistic perspective comes from choosing to focus on the ability of people when motivated and supported to find ways of being in the world that are more conducive to "creating and sustaining the kind of schools, and the kind of society, that most of us want." (p. 125). The strategy proposed by Levin and Fullan (2008), while far from proven, remains a reasonable guiding proposition for those interested in large-scale improvement in student outcomes as is the model curriculum proposed by Reinke, Herman, Stormont, Brooks, and Darney (2010). However, like any major shift in focus, change will take some time. There is specific need for research related to schools on resilience and protective factors; the sustainability of outcomes of school-based interventions for emotional and behavioral problems and how school districts scale-up evidence-based prevention programs (Adelman & Taylor, 2004). Meeting the challenge of implementing mental health promotion strategies, starting at the preschool level and continuing through the school years, holds the promise of producing major improvements in the resilience of the population. Continuing to light the way with the twin torches of prevention science and informed implementation strategies will help us stumble less along the way.

References

Adelman, H. S. (1995). Education reform: Broadening the focus. *Psychological Science, 6*(1), 61–62.

Adelman, H. S., & Taylor, L. (1994). *On understanding intervention in psychology and education*. Westport: Praeger Publishers/Greenwood Publishing Group.

Adelman, H. S., & Taylor, L. (1998). Reframing mental health in schools and expanding school reform. *Educational Psychologist, 33*, 135–152.

Adelman, H.S., & Taylor, L. (2004). Mental health in schools: A shared agenda. Report on Emotional & Behavioral Disorder in Youth, 4(3). Retrieved July 2012 from http://smhp.psych.ucla.edu/publications/48%20Mental%20Health%20in%20Schools.pdf.

Adelman, H. S., & Taylor, L. (2007). Systemic change for school improvement. *Journal of Educational and Psychological Consultation, 17*, 55–77.

Backer, T. E., Liberman, R. P., & Kuehnel, T. G. (1986). Dissemination and adoption of innovative psychosocial interventions. *Journal of Consulting and Clinical Psychology, 54*(1), 111–118.

Barber, M. (2007). *Three paradigms of public-sector reform*. London: McKinsey.

Barber, M. (2009). Education, equity, and the economy. In M. Fullan (Ed.), *The challenge of change: Start school improvement now!* (2nd ed., pp. 207–222). Thousand Oaks, CA: Corwin Press.

Barber, M., & Mourshed, M. (2007). *How the world's best performing school systems come out on top*. London: McKinsey.

Barrish, H. H., Saunders, M., & Wolf, M. M. (1969). Good behavior game: Effects of individual contingencies for group consequences on disruptive behavior in a classroom. *Journal of Applied Behavior Analysis, 2*(2), 119–124.

Becker, D. M., Hill, D. R., Jackson, J. S., Levine, D. M., Sillman, F. A., & Weiss, S. M. (1992). *Health behavior research in minority populations: Access, design and implementation*. Washington, DC: US Department of Health and Human Services.

Berliner, D. C. (2002). Comment: Educational research: The hardest science of all. *Educational Researcher, 31*(8), 18–20.

Bornstein, M. H., Hahn, C., & Haynes, O. M. (2010). Social competence, externalizing, and internalizing behavioral adjustment from early childhood through early adolescence: Developmental cascades. *Development and Psychopathology, 22*(4), 717–735.

Bradshaw, C. P., Koth, C. W., Bevans, K. B., Ialongo, N., & Leaf, P. J. (2008). The impact of school-wide positive behavioral interventions and supports (PBIS) on the organizational health of elementary schools. *School Psychology Quarterly, 23*(4), 462–473.

Bronfenbrenner, U. (1979). Contexts of child rearing: Problems and prospects. *American Psychologist, 34*(10), 844–850.

Bronfenbrenner, U. (1992). Ecological systems theory. In R. Vasta (Ed.), *Six theories of child development: Revised formulations and current issues* (pp. 187–249). London: Jessica Kingsley Publishers.

Burns, B. J., Phillips, S. D., Wagner, H. R., Barth, R. P., Kolko, D. J., Campbell, Y., et al. (2004). Mental health need and access to mental health services by youths involved with child welfare: A national survey. *Journal of the American Academy of Child and Adolescent Psychiatry, 43*(8), 960–970.

Burt, M. R. (2002). Reasons to invest in adolescents. *Journal of Adolescent Health, 31*(6 Suppl 1), 136–152.

Burt, K. B., & Roisman, G. I. (2010). Competence and psychopathology: Cascade effects in the NICHD study of early child care and youth development. *Development and Psychopathology, 22*(3), 557–567.

Canadian Cochrane Network. (2003). *A primer on evidence-based clinical practice*. Retrieved July 2012, from http://www.cochrane.uottawa.ca/pdf/presentations/EBCPPrimer_July_2012.pdf.

CASEL Practice Rubric for Schoolwide SEL implementation. (2006). Retrieved July 2012, from http://casel.org/wp-content/uploads/2011/04/Rubric.pdf.

Chamberlin, R. W. (1992). Preventing low birth weight, child abuse, and school failure: The need for comprehensive, community-wide approaches. *Pediatrics in Review, 13*, 64–71.

Christenson, S. L., & Sheridan, S. M. (2001). *Schools and families: Creating essential connections for learning*. New York: Guilford Press.

Christenson, S. L., Whitehouse, E. L., & VenGetson, G. R. (2007). Partnering with families to enhance students' mental health. In B. Doll & J. A. Cummings (Eds.), *Transforming school mental health services: Population-based approaches to promoting the competency and wellness of student services* (pp. 69–101). Thousand Oaks, CA: Corwin Press.

Comer, J. P., Haynes, N. M., Joyner, E. T., & Ben-Avie, M. (1996). *Rallying the whole village: The comer process for reforming education*. New York: Teachers College Press.

Coote, S. (2000). *Families and schools together (FAST)*. Paper presented at the conference: Reducing criminality: Partnerships and best practices, Perth, Australia.

Cowan, P. A. (1975). *Community psychology: The emperor without clothes*. Washington, DC: American Psychological Association.

Cowen, E. L. (1994). The enhancement of psychological wellness: Challenges and opportunities. *American Journal of Community Psychology, 22*(2), 149–179.

Cowan, P. A., Cohn, D. A., Cowan, C. P., & Pearson, J. L. (1996). Parents' attachment histories and children's externalizing and internalizing behaviors: Exploring family systems models of linkage. *Journal of Consulting and Clinical Psychology, 64*, 53–63.

Creemers, B. P. M., & Kyriakides, L. (2008). *The dynamics of educational effectiveness: A contribution to policy, practice, and theory in contemporary schools*. New York: Routledge.

Crozier, M., Rokutani, L., Russett, J. L., Godwin, E., & Banks, G. E. (2010). A multisite program evaluation of families and schools together (FAST): Continued evidence of a successful multifamily community-based prevention program. *School Community Journal, 20*, 187–207.

Doll, B., & Cummings, J. A. (2008). *Transforming school mental health services: Population-based approaches to promoting the competency and wellness of children*. Thousand Oaks, CA: Corwin Press.

Elmore, R. F. (2007). Local school districts and instructional improvement. In W. D. Hawley & D. L. Rollie (Eds.), *The keys to effective schools: Education reform as continuous improvement* (pp. 189–200). Thousand Oaks, CA: Corwin Press.

Embry, D. D. (2002). The good behavior game: A best practice candidate as a universal behavioral vaccine. *Clinical Child and Family Psychology Review, 5*(4), 273–297.

Embry, D. D. (2004). Community-based prevention using simple, low-cost, evidence-based kernels and behavioral vaccines. *Journal of Community Psychology, 32*(5), 575–591.

Embry, D. D. (2011). Behavioral vaccines and evidence-based kernels: Nonpharmaceutical approaches for the prevention of mental, emotional, and behavioral disorders. *Psychiatric Clinics of North America, 34*(1), 1–34.

Ervin, R., & Schaughency, E. (2008). Best practices in accessing the systems change literature. In A. Thomas & J. Grimes (Eds.), *Best practices in school psychology V*. Bethesda, MD: National Association of School Psychologists.

Farrow, J. H., & Saewyc, E. (2002). Work group III: Identifying effective strategies and interventions for improving adolescent health at the individual level. *Journal of Adolescent Health, 31*(Suppl. 6), 226–229.

Fergus, S., & Zimmerman, M. A. (2005). Adolescent resilience: A framework for understanding healthy development in the face of risk. *Annual Review of Public Health, 26*, 399–419.

Fixsen D. L. (2005). *Implementation research: A synthesis of the literature*. FMHI Publication #231 Ed. Tampa, FL : The National Implementation Research Network, University of South Florida.

Foster, E. M., Olchowski, A. E., & Webster-Stratton, C. H. (2007). Is stacking intervention components cost-effective? An analysis of the Incredible Years program. *Journal of the American Academy of Child and Adolescent Psychiatry, 46*, 1414–1424.

Fuchs, D., Mock, D., Morgan, P. L., & Young, C. L. (2003). Responsiveness-to-intervention: Definitions, evidence, and implications for the learning disabilities construct. *Learning Disabilities Research and Practice, 18*, 157–171.

Fullan, M. (2005). *Leadership and sustainability: System thinkers in action*. Thousand Oaks, CA: Corwin Press.

Fullan, M. (2006). *Turnaround leadership*. San Francisco, CA: Jossey-Bass.

Fullan, M. (2007). Achieving large-scale reform. *Learning and Teaching for the Twenty-first Century, 2*, 137–144.

Fullan, M. (Ed.). (2009). *The challenge of change: Start school improvement now!* (2nd ed.). Thousand Oaks, CA: Corwin Press.

Fullan, M. (2010). *Motion leadership: The skinny on becoming change savvy*. Thousand Oaks, CA: Corwin Press.

Garmston, R. J., & Wellman, B. M. (1999). *The adaptive school: A sourcebook for developing collaborative groups*. Norwood, MA: Christopher-Gordon Publishers.

Gawande, A. (2007). *Better: A surgeon's notes on performance*. New York: Metropolitan Books.

Greenberg, M. T., Domitrovich, C., & Bumbarger, B. (2000). *Preventing mental health disorders in school-age children: A review of the effectiveness of prevention programs*. University Park, PA: Prevention Research Center for the Promotion of Human Development, College of Health and Human Development, Pennsylvania State University.

Gunner, M. R. (2007). Stress effects on the developing brain. In D. Romer & E. F. Walker (Eds.), *Adolescent psychopathology and the developing brain: Integrating brain and prevention science* (pp. 127–147). New York: Oxford University Press.

Hamilton, J. (2005). The answerable question and a hierarchy of evidence. *Journal of the American Academy of Child and Adolescent Psychiatry, 44*(6), 596–600.

Henggeler, S. W., Melton, G. B., Brondino, M. J., Scherer, D. G., & Hanley, J. H. (1997). Multisystemic therapy with violent and chronic juvenile offenders and their families: The role of treatment fidelity in successful dissemination. *Journal of Consulting and Clinical Psychology, 65*(5), 821–833.

Hopkins, R. (2008). *The transition handbook: From oil dependency to local resilience*. White River Junction, VT: Chealsea Green Publishing Co.

Horner, R. H., Sugai, G., Todd, A. W. & Lewis-Palmer, T. (2005). School-wide positive behavior support. In L. Bambara & L. Kern (Eds.), *Individualized supports for students with problem behaviors: Designing positive behavior support plans* (pp. 359–390). New York: Guilford Press.

Howell, C. L. (2004). Resilience in adult women students in higher education: Implications for academic achievement and persistence. ProQuest Information & Learning. *Dissertation Abstracts International Section A: Humanities and Social Sciences, 65*.

Inman, D. D., van Bakergem, K. M., LaRosa, A. C., & Garr, D. R. (2011). Evidence-based health promotion programs for schools and communities. *American Journal of Preventive Medicine, 40*(2), 207–219.

Jané-Lopis, E., & Anderson, P. (2005). *Mental health promotion and mental disorder prevention: A policy for Europe*. Nijmegen: Radboud University.

Jané-Lopis, E., Barry, M. M., Hosman, C., & Patel, V. (2005). Mental health promotion works: a review. *Promotion and Education, 61,* 67(Suppl. 2), 9–25.

Kataoka, S. H., Zhang, L., & Wells, K. B. (2002). Unmet need for mental health care among U.S. children: Variation by ethnicity and insurance status. *The American Journal of Psychiatry, 159*(9), 1548–1555.

Kellam, S. G., Brown, C. H., Poduska, J. M., Ialongo, N. S., Wang, W., Toyinbo, P., et al. (2008). Effects of a universal classroom behavior management program in first and second grades on young adult behavioral, psychiatric, and social outcomes. *Drug and Alcohol Dependence, 95*(Suppl. 1), S5–S28.

Kellam, S. G., Koretz, D., & Mościcki, E. K. (1999). Core elements of developmental epidemiologically based prevention research. *American Journal of Community Psychology, 27*(4), 463–482.

Kellam, S. G., & Langevin, D. J. (2003). A framework for understanding "evidence" in prevention research and programs. *Prevention Science, 4*(3), 137–153.

Kellam, S. G., Rebok, G. W., Ialongo, N., & Mayer, L. S. (1994). The course and malleability of aggressive behavior from early first grade into middle school: Results of a developmental epidemiologically-based preventive trial. *Journal of Child Psychology and Psychiatry, 35*, 259–281.

Kessler, R. C., Berglund, P., Demler, O., Jin, R., & Walters, E. E. (2005). Lifetime prevalence and age-of-onset distributions of DSM-IV disorders in the National Comorbidity Survey Replication. *Archives of General Psychiatry, 62*, 593–602.

Kirby, M. J., & Keon, W. J. (2006). *Out of the shadows at last: Transforming mental health, mental illness, and addiction services in Canada*. Ottawa: The Standing Senate Committee on Social Affairs, Science and Technology.

Kleinman, K. E., & Saigh, P. A. (2011). The effects of the good behavior game on the conduct of regular education New York city high school students. *Behavior Modification, 35*(1), 95–105.

Kok, G. (1993). Why are so many health promotion programs ineffective? *Health Promotion Journal of Australia, 3*(2), 12–17.

Kratochwill, T. R., McDonald, L., Levin, J. R., Bear-Tibbetts, H. Y., & Demaray, M. K. (2004). Families and schools together: An experimental analysis of a parent-mediated multi-family group program for American Indian children. *Journal of School Psychology, 42*(5), 359–383.

Kratochwill, T. R., & Shernoff, E. S. (2003). Evidence-based practice: Promoting evidence-based interventions in school psychology. *School Psychology Quarterly, 18*, 389–408.

Kratochwill, T. R., & Shernoff, E. S. (2004). Evidence-based practice: Promoting evidence-based interventions in school psychology. *School Psychology Review, 33*(1), 34–48.

Leadbeater, B. (2010). The fickle fates of push and pull in the dissemination of mental health programs for children. *Canadian Psychology, 51*(4), 221–230.

Levin, B. (2008a). *How to change 5000 schools*. Cambridge, MA: Harvard Education Press.

Levin, B. (2008b) *Thinking about knowledge mobilization*. Vancouver: Canadian Council on Learning and the Social Sciences and Humanities Research Council of Canada. Retrieved July 2012, from http://www.oise.utoronto.ca/rspe/Conference_Presentations_Publications/index.html.

Levin, B., & Fullan, M. (2008). Learning about systems renewal. *Educational Management Administration and Leadership, 36*(2), 289–303.

Levin, B., & Riffel, J. A. (1998). Conceptualising school change. *Cambridge Journal of Education, 28*(1), 113–127.

Lewin-Bizan, S., Bowers, E. P., & Lerner, R. M. (2010). One good thing leads to another: Cascades of positive

youth development among American adolescents. *Development and Psychopathology, 22*(4), 759–770.
Lewis, T. J., Sugai, G., & Colvin, G. (1998). Reducing problem behavior through a school-wide system of effective behavioral support: Investigation of a school-wide social skills training program and contextual interventions. *School Psychology Review, 27*, 446–459.
Luthar, S. S., Cicchetti, D., & Becker, B. (2000). The construct of resilience: A critical evaluation and guidelines for future work. *Child Development, 71*(3), 543–562.
Marston, D., Muyskens, P., Lau, M., & Canter, A. (2003). Problem-solving model for decision making with high-incidence disabilities: The Minneapolis experience. *Learning Disabilities Research and Practice, 18*(3), 187–200.
Martella, R. C., & Nelson, J. R. (2003). Managing classroom behaviour. *Journal of Direct Instruction, 3*(2), 139–165.
Masten, A. S. (2001). Ordinary magic: Resilience processes in development. *American Psychologist, 56*(3), 227–238.
Masten, A. S., Best, K. M., & Garmezy, N. (1990). Resilience and development: Contributions from the study of children who overcome adversity. *Development and Psychopathology, 2*, 425–444.
Masten, A. S., & Cicchetti, D. (2010). Developmental cascades. *Development and Psychopathology, 22*(3), 491–495.
Masten, A. S., & Powell, J. L. (2003). A resilience framework for research, policy, and practice. In S. S. Luthar (Ed.), *Resilience and vulnerability: Adaptation in the context of childhood adversities* (pp. 1–25). New York: Cambridge University Press.
McClellan, J., & Trupin, E. (1989). Prevention of psychiatric disorders in children. *Hospital and Community Psychiatry, 40*(6), 630–636.
McDonald, L., Billingham, S., Conrad, T., Morgan, A., Nina, O., & Payton, E. (1997). Families and schools together (FAST): Integrating community development with clinical strategies. *Families in Society, 78*(2), 140–155.
McLaughlin, M. W. (1987). Learning from experience: Lessons from policy implementation. *Educational Evaluation and Policy Analysis, 9*(2), 171–178.
McLaughlin, M. W., & Mitra, D. (2001). Theory-based change and change-based theory: Going deeper, going broader. *Journal of Educational Change, 2*(4), 301–323.
Merrell, K. W., & Buchanan, R. (2006). Intervention selection in school-based practice: Using public health models to enhance systems capacity of schools. *School Psychology Review, 35*, 167–180.
Mourshed, M., Chijioke, C., & Barber, M. (2010). *How the world's best performing school systems keep getting better*. London: McKinsey.
National Association of School Psychologists. (2009). *Appropriate academic supports to meet the needs of all students*. Bethesda, MD: National Association of School Psychologists.
National Health Service. (1999). *National service framework for mental health: Modern standards and service models*. London: The Stationery Office.
National Institute of Mental Health (1998). *Mental illness in America: The National Institute of Mental Health agenda*. Retrieved July 2012, from http://www.nimh.com.
National Research Council and the Institute of Medicine. (2009). *Preventing mental, emotional, and behavioral disorders among young people: Progress and possibilities*. Washington, DC: National Academies Press.
Nelson, J. R., Benner, G. J., Reid, R. C., Epstein, M. H., & Currin, D. (2002). The convergent validity of office discipline referrals with the CBCL-TRF. *Journal of Emotional and Behavioral Disorders, 10*, 181–188.
Patterson, G. R. (1982). *Coercive family process*. Eugene, OR: Castalia.
Patterson, G. R., Forgatch, M. S., & DeGarmo, D. (2010). Cascading effects following intervention. *Development and Psychopathology, 22*(4), 949–970.
Prinz, R. J., Sanders, M. R., Shapiro, C. J., Whitaker, D. J., & Lutzker, J. R. (2009). Population-based prevention of child maltreatment: The U.S. Triple P System Population Trial. *Prevention Science, 10*(1), 1–12.
Raffo, C., Dyson, A., Gunter, H., Hall, D., Jones, L., & Kalambouka, A. (2009). Education and poverty: Mapping the terrain and making the links to educational policy. *International Journal of Inclusive Education, 13*(4), 341–358.
Raphael, B. (1992). *Prevention in the mental health field*. Report presented at the 114th session of the National health and Medical Research Council, Canberra, Australia.
Raver, C., Jones, S., Li-Grining, C., Zhai, F., Metzger, M., & Solomon, B. (2009). Targeting children's behavior problems in preschool classrooms: A cluster-randomized controlled trial. *Journal of Consulting and Clinical Psychology, 77*, 302–316.
Reinke, W. M., Herman, K. C., Stormont, M., Brooks, C., & Darney, D. (2010). Training the next generation of school professionals to be prevention scientists: The Missouri Prevention Center Model. *Psychology in the Schools, 47*(1), 101–110.
Rothstein, R. (2004). *Class and schools: Using social, economic, and educational reform to close the black-white achievement gap*. Washington, DC: Economic Policy Institute.
Rutter, M., Maughan, B., Mortimore, P., Ouston, J., & Smith, A. (1979). *15000 Hours: Secondary schools and their effects on children*. Cambridge, MA: Harvard University Press.
Sackett, D. L., Straus, S. E., Richardson, W. S., Rosenberg, W., & Haynes, R. B. (2000). *Evidence-based medicine: How to practice and teach EBM* (2nd ed.). Edinburgh: Churchill Livingstone.
Sanders, M. R. (1996). New directions in behavioral family intervention with children. In T. H. Ollendick & R. J. Prinz (Eds.), *Advances in clinical child psychology* (pp. 283–330). New York: Plenum Press.

Sanders, M. R. (1999). Triple P-positive parenting program: Towards an empirically validated multilevel parenting and family support strategy for the prevention of behavior and emotional problems in children. *Clinical Child and Family Psychology Review, 2*(2), 71–90.

Sanders, M. R. (2001). Helping families change: From clinical interventions to population-based strategies. In A. Booth, A. C. Crouter, & M. Clements (Eds.), *Couples in conflict national symposium, November 1999, Pennsylvania State University* (pp. 185–219). Mahwah, NJ: Lawrence Erlbaum Associates.

Sanders, M. R., Markie-Dadds, C., Tully, L. A., & Bor, W. (2000). The Triple P-positive parenting program: A comparison of enhanced, standard, and self-directed behavioral family intervention for parents of children with early onset conduct problems. *Journal of Consulting and Clinical Psychology, 68*(4), 624–640.

Sanders, M. R., Ralph, A., Sofronoff, K., Gardiner, P., Thompson, R., Dwyer, S., et al. (2008). Every Family: A population approach to reducing behavioral and emotional problems in children making the transition to school. *Journal of Primary Prevention, 29*(3), 197–222.

Sanders, M. R., Turner, K. M. T., & Markie-Dadds, C. (2002). The development and dissemination of the Triple P-positive parenting program: A multilevel, evidence-based system of parenting and family support. *Prevention Science, 3*(3), 173–189.

Sapienza, J. K., Julianna, K., & Masten, A. S. (2011). Understanding and promoting resilience in children and youth. *Current Opinion in Psychiatry, 24*(4), 267–273.

Sass, J. (1999). *Comprehensive evaluation report for the Canadian replication of the Families and Schools Together (FAST) program*. Paper presented at the Annual Meeting of the American Evaluation Association, Orlando.

Schleicher, A. (2009). International comparisons of student learning outcomes. In A. Hargreaves, A. Lieberman, M. Fullan, & D. Hopkins (Eds.), *Second international handbook of educational change* (pp. 485–504). Dordrecht, The Netherlands: Springer.

Seligman, M. E. P. (1995). The effectiveness of psychotherapy: The consumer reports study. *American Psychologist, 50*(12), 965–974.

Short, R. J., & Shapiro, S. K. (1993). Conduct disorders: A framework for understanding and intervention in schools and communities. *School Psychology Review, 22*(3), 362–375.

Simeonson, R. J. (1994). *Risk, resilience and prevention: Promoting the well-being of all children*. Baltimore, MD: P. H. Brookes.

Skowyra, K., & Cocozza, J. J. (2006). A blueprint for change: Improving the system response to youth with mental health needs involved with the juvenile justice system. *Research and program brief*. Retrieved July 2012, from http://www.ncmhjj.com/Blueprint/pdfs/ProgramBrief_06_06.pdf.

Stormont, M., Reinke, W. M., & Herman, K. C. (2010). Introduction to the special issue: Using prevention science to address mental health issues in schools. *Psychology in the Schools, 47*(1), 1–4.

Strein, W., Hoagwood, K., & Cohn, A. (2003). School psychology: A public health perspective: I. Prevention, populations, and, systems change. *Journal of School Psychology, 41*(1), 23–38.

Sturm, R., Ringel, J. S., & Andreyeva, T. (2003). Geographic disparities in children's mental health care. *Pediatrics, 112*(4), e308–e315.

Sugai, G., & Horner, R. (2002). The evolution of discipline practices: School-wide positive behavior supports. *Child and Family Behavior Therapy, 24*(1–2), 23–50.

Sugai, G., Horner, R. H., Algozzine, R., Barrett, S., Lewis, T., Anderson, C., et al. (2010). *School-wide positive behavior support: Implementers' blueprint and self-assessment*. Eugene, OR: University of Oregon.

Sugai, G., Sprague, J. R., Horner, R. H., & Walker, H. M. (2000). Preventing school violence: The use of office discipline referrals to assess and monitor school-wide discipline interventions. *Journal of Emotional and Behavioral Disorders, 8*, 94–101.

Tanol, G., Johnson, L., McComas, J., & Cote, E. (2010). Responding to rule violations or rule following: A comparison of two versions of the Good Behavior Game with kindergarten students. *Journal of School Psychology, 48*(5), 337–355.

The President's New Freedom Commission on Mental Health. (2003). *Achieving the promise: Transforming mental health care in America. Final report* (DHHS Publication No. SMA 03-3832). Washington, DC: U.S. Government Printing Office.

Tidwell, A., Flannery, K. B., & Lewis-Palmer, T. (2003). A description of elementary classroom discipline referral patterns. *Preventing School Failure, 48*(1), 18–26.

Tilly, W. D. (2006). Response to an intervention: An overview: What is it? Why do it? Is it worth it? *The Special Edge, 19*(2), 1–10.

Tingstrom, D. H., Sterling-Turner, H. E., & Wilczynski, S. M. (2006). The good behavior game: 1969–2002. *Behavior Modification, 30*(2), 225–253.

Tolan, P. H., & Dodge, K. A. (2005). Children's mental health as a primary care and concern: A system for comprehensive support and service. *American Psychologist, 60*(6), 601–614.

Turner, K. M. T., & Sanders, M. R. (2006). Dissemination of evidence-based parenting and family support strategies: Learning from the Triple P–positive parenting program system approach. *Aggression and Violent Behavior, 11*(2), 176–193.

US Department of Health and Human Services. (1999). Children and mental health. In Mental health: A report of the Surgeon General. Rockville, MD: U.S. Department of Health and Human Services, Substance Abuse and Mental Health Services Administration, Center for Mental Health Services, National Institutes of Health, National Institute of Mental Health.

van Lier, P. A., Muthén, B. O., van der Sar, R. M., & Crijnen, A. A. (2004). Preventing disruptive behavior in elementary schoolchildren: Impact of a universal classroom-based intervention. *Journal of Consulting and Clinical Psychology, 72*(3), 467–478.

Vaughn, S., & Chard, D. (2006). Three-tier intervention research studies: Descriptions of two related projects. *Perspectives, 32*(1), 29–34.

Wagner, M., Newman, L., Cameto, R., & Levine, P. (2005). Changes over time in the early postschool outcomes of youth with disabilities: A report of findings from the National Longitudinal Transition Study (NLTS) and the National LongitudinalTransition Study-2 (NLTS2). Menlo Park, CA: SRI International.

Walker, B., Cheney, D., Stage, S., & Blum, C. (2005). Schoolwide screening and positive behavior supports: Identifying and supporting students at risk for school failure. *Journal of Positive Behavior Interventions, 7*, 194–204.

Webster-Stratton, C., & Herman, K. (2010). Disseminating Incredible Years series early-intervention programs: Integrating and sustaining services between school and home. *Psychology in the Schools, 47*, 36–54.

Webster-Stratton, C., Reid, M. J., & Hammond, M. (2004). Treating children with early-onset conduct problems: Intervention outcomes for parent, child, and teacher training. *Journal of Clinical Child and Adolescent Psychology, 33*(1), 105–124.

Webster-Stratton, C., Reid, M. J., & Stoolmiller, M. (2008). Preventing conduct problems and improving school readiness: evaluation of the Incredible Years Teacher and Child Training Programs in high-risk schools. *Journal of Child Psychology and Psychiatry, 49*, 471–488.

Wehlage, G. G., Rutter, R. A., Smith, G. A., Lesko, N., & Fernandez, R. R. (1989). *Reducing the risk*. New York: Falmer Press.

Whelan, F. (2009). *Lessons learned: How good policies produce better schools*. London: Fenton Whelan.

Wilson, J. (1989). *Bureaucracy*. New York: Basic Books.

Witvliet, M., van Lier, P. A., Cuijpers, P., & Koot, H. M. (2009). Testing links between childhood positive peer relations and externalizing outcomes through a randomized controlled intervention study. *Journal of Consulting and Clinical Psychology, 77*(5), 905–915.

Wolfe, B. E. (2006). Employing empirically supported treatments: A research-informed clinical practitioner perspective. *Clinical Psychology: Science and Practice, 13*, 171–178.

Wolfe, D. A., Crooks, C., Chiodo, D., Hughes, R., & Jaffe, P. (2005). *Impact of a comprehensive school-based prevention program: Changes in adolescents' knowledge, attitudes and behaviour about violence, sexual behaviour and substance use*. Unpublished manuscript, available by contacting the Author.

Wolin, S., & Wolin, S. J. (1997). Shifting paradigms: Taking a paradoxical approach. *Resiliency in Action, 2*, 23–28.

World Health Organization. (1986). Ottawa Charter for Health Promotion, presented at the First International Conference on Health Promotion, Ottawa. Retrieved July 2012, from http://www.who.int/hpr/NPH/docs/ottawa_charter_hp.pdf.

Ysseldyke, J., Burns, M., Dawson, P., Kelley, B., Morrison, D., Ortiz, S., et al. (2006). *School psychology: A blueprint for training and practice III*. Bethesda, MD: National Association of School Psychologists.

Resilience in Childhood Disorders

8

Emma A. Climie, Sarah M. Mastoras, Adam W. McCrimmon, and Vicki. L. Schwean

Resilience is most commonly characterized as a dynamic process encompassing good or positive outcome in an individual despite experiences of serious or significant adversity or trauma (Luthar, Cicchetti, & Becker, 2000). Resilience as a theoretical concept implies that two specific constructs be present. First, the presence of adversity or risk associated with life circumstances known to interfere with adjustment (Luthar & Cicchetti, 2000; Masten, 2001). Common indicators of risk include low socioeconomic status (SES), chronic exposure to violence or aggression, and traumatic life events such as a divorce (Luthar & Cicchetti, 2000). The second construct, the achievement of positive adaptation despite the presence of adversity, is typically measured via observable behaviors such as social competence, academic success, and secure attachment with caregivers as well as an absence of psychopathology (Luthar & Cicchetti, 2000). Individuals are considered to be resilient when they face significant adversity to development yet display positive outcomes (Masten & Coatsworth, 1998; Olsson, Bond, Burns, Vella-Brodrick, & Sawyer, 2003).

Spurred by efforts to prevent the development of psychopathology, research on childhood resilience emerged in the 1970s with researchers exploring the phenomenon of children who seemed to achieve positive outcomes in the context of significant adversity (e.g., Anthony & Koupernik, 1974; Garmezy, 1971, 1974; Rutter, 1979). Such efforts were directed towards illuminating those qualities of resilient children that could be enhanced in others so as to minimize the impact of negative life events through the development of targeted interventions and public policy (Masten, 2001). Several decades of research have ensued, involving description of resilient populations, understanding the process of change and development of resilience models, and the development of interventions to enhance resilience (Masten, 2007, 2011). Modern models of resilience typically depict the construct as involving an interaction where risk is moderated by organic, environmental attributes, and/or risk-activated variables (Masten, 2001). As such, both risk factors that lead to poor outcome and protective factors that moderate or ameliorate the effects of risk are identified.

Although many resilience models have been developed in reference to diverse threats and risks to development, the attention of the developers of the models has been on defining variable-focused versus person-focused approaches (Masten, 2001, 2002). Variable-focused models examine characteristics of individuals, environments, and

E.A. Climie, Ph.D. • S.M. Mastoras
• A.W. McCrimmon, Ph.D.
Education Tower – University of Calgary,
2500 University Drive NW, Calgary,
AB T2N 1N4, Canada
e-mail: eaclimie@ucalgary.ca; s.mastoras@ucalgary.ca; a.mccrimmon@ucalgary.ca

V.L. Schwean, Ph.D. (✉)
Faculty of Education, The University of Western Ontario,
London, ON, Canada
e-mail: vschwean@uwo.ca

S. Prince-Embury and D.H. Saklofske (eds.), *Resilience in Children, Adolescents, and Adults: Translating Research into Practice*, The Springer Series on Human Exceptionality,
DOI 10.1007/978-1-4614-4939-3_8, © Springer Science+Business Media New York 2013

experiences to better understand which aspects of these variables (e.g., protective factors) account for positive outcome despite adversity. Within this realm, effort has been specifically directed towards the identification of particular assets that compensate for and offset risk (Garmezy, Masten, & Tellegen, 1984; Masten, Garmezy, Tellegen, Pellegrini, Larkin et al., 1988) and developing interventions to mediate risk and enhance resilience (Conger, Conger, & Elder, 1997; Conger, Conger, Elder, Lorenz, Simons et al., 1992; Forgatch & DeGarmo, 1999; McLoyd, 1998). In contrast, person-focused models examine differences between resilient and non-resilient individuals to determine what naturally occurring aspects are important in this differentiation. Research in this realm has tended to investigate groups of individuals from the same adverse environment who demonstrate either adaptive or maladaptive outcomes (e.g., Cowen, Wyman, Work, & Parker, 1990; Masten, Hubbard, Gest, Tellegen, Garmezy et al., 1999; Wyman, Cowen, Work, Hoyt-Meyers, Magnus et al., 1999).

Resilience and Psychopathology

Although the focus of resiliency research has been to identify and enhance qualities or aspects of individuals who are able to thrive despite adversity, the majority of such efforts have involved typically developing individuals experiencing adversity from the environment such as low SES, exposure to violence, war and trauma, etc. In contrast, a paucity of research has examined resilience in children with psychological disorders, a circumstance that naturally introduces aspects of adversity and risk. Research across numerous clinical populations has demonstrated a high degree of heterogeneity in outcome indicators such as symptom severity, duration or course of disorder, degree of impairment or associated challenges, achievement in core domains of functioning, and development of comorbid psychological disorders (American Psychiatric Association, 2000; Curry, Silva, Rohde, Ginsburg, Kratochvil et al., 2011; Hinshaw & Lee, 2003). This heterogeneity provides a strong indication that some aspect of resiliency is at play in these populations. Moreover, researchers have shown that symptoms of internalizing disorders such as anxiety or depression can be reduced or moderated by the use of effective problem-solving strategies and positive peer relationships (Reivich, Gillham, Chaplin, & Seligman, 2005), highlighting the likelihood of identifying key protective factors that may shape outcomes among such individuals.

Given that psychopathology introduces risk and adversity to development through clinical symptomology and associated functional impairment, it is apparent that research investigating aspects of resilient individuals with psychopathology, including protective factors that can enhance such individuals' ability to thrive, is of paramount importance. This importance is even more apparent when considering the fact that resilience is largely unstudied in clinical populations. Paralleling the strengths-based movement in psychology, a resilience perspective would serve to shift the focus away from the disorder and its deficits towards the individual experiences, achievements, and personal and environmental strengths that can support these individuals. In effect, such a perspective would facilitate the "moving from a perspective of 'what is wrong' to 'what can make it right?'" (Modesto-Lowe, Yelunina, & Hanjan, 2011, p. 519). Indeed, particularly for those disorders believed to be predominantly lifelong, such as Attention-Deficit/Hyperactivity Disorder (ADHD), learning disabilities, or autism spectrum disorders, a resilience perspective promotes an acceptance of the disorder and moves beyond mere understanding of psychopathology. Instead, a strengths-based perspective allows us to learn from those who have coped well to promote effective management of the disorder and the establishment of positive qualities and environments that can support both short- and long-term well-being.

At this stage of research, much is known about the deficits, types of impairment, and poor outcomes associated with many childhood disorders. With this knowledge as the foundation, we believe that the field of child psychopathology is now in a position to apply these understandings to the related study of resilience and thriving.

Discerning the impact and interplay between risk and protective factors in predicting outcomes can not only expand knowledge of the risk processes and trajectories of clinical disorders (Luthar et al., 2000) but can also have significant practical implications. For example, assessment of resilience factors can serve to identify those children most at risk and can help in designing individualized and strengths-based interventions focused on nurturing positive qualities rather than simply eliminating deficits. Moreover, the positive nature of the resilience perspective can "carry a much more appealing message to parents, school staff, communities, and children themselves" (Masten, Herbers, Cutuli, & Lafavor, 2008, p. 80), one which may be particularly important given the frustrations and isolation often faced by the families and those working with children with psychological disorders (Ditrano & Silverstein, 2006).

Thus, there is a strong rationale for integrating the resilience perspective into the conceptualization and study of children with clinical disorders. In the remainder of this chapter, we will explore the key factors that warrant consideration within the field of resilience (e.g., choosing appropriate outcome variables, understanding how we examine resilience in a specific population) and discuss how these factors would apply to a clinical population. We will use children with ADHD as a case study to highlight our rationale.

Establishing a Framework for the Study of Resilience Among Clinical Populations

Luthar et al., (2000) have emphasized the need for studies of resilience to be grounded in sound theoretical frameworks, with "explicit conceptual consideration of how interrelations among the matrix of constructs examined may be affected by the nature of the specific adversity condition under study" (p. 553). We would contend that this initial conceptualization is particularly crucial when studying resilience among clinical populations, as effectively shifting the study of children with psychological disorders towards a resilience paradigm must necessarily involve the integration of models of child development, resilience and thriving, and developmental psychopathology with what is known about the specific disorder. Many lessons can be taken from the tremendous progress and conceptual challenges observed in the study of resilience over the past decades. Some of the primary considerations that warrant discussion in addressing these concerns and applying modern resilience paradigms to clinical populations are explored below, followed by a case study illustrating how these considerations would apply to the study of resilience in children with ADHD.

Integrating Ecological Systems and Developmental Perspectives

The study of resilience has shifted from an initial exploration of "invulnerable" children to one in which resilience is understood as a multidimensional and dynamic construct influenced by qualities both intrinsic to the child and within the broader environment, as well as by the nature of the risks encountered (Masten, 2001). Modern perspectives on resilience incorporate prominent aspects of ecological systems theory and related models (e.g., Bronfenbrenner, 1977; Cicchetti & Lynch, 1993), in which the child's development is understood to be affected by the interaction of variables at multiple levels of influence, including various microsystems (e.g., home, school) as well as broader meso- and exosystems. Indeed, researchers in the field of resilience have identified variables across three broad levels of influence that appear to be central to understanding resilience: (1) personality and other features within the child; (2) variables within the family; and (3) external support systems within the broader community (cf. Luthar et al., 2000).

A similar perspective emphasizing multiple levels of influence also pervades much of the literature in developmental psychopathology, where risk factors across various sources of influence have been studied that may increase risk or exacerbate the presentation of child disorders (Masten, 2006). This shared perspective should promote and support the integration of such models and should be retained as a basis of any study of resilience among clinical populations. Importantly, the transactional perspective of typical and atypical development not only implies that variables at multiple levels of influence should be considered in predicting outcomes but also points to the importance of exploring interactions between these variables (e.g., cumulative or buffering effects; Masten, 2006). The fundamental notions of developmental continuity and discontinuity must also be integrated into any conceptual framework, with consideration of the fact that resilience factors at play during one stage of development may not have the same function at other stages (Rutter, 1993), and the short- and long-term effects of a given factor may differ in important ways. Indeed, studies have occasionally identified variables that appear to be protective at one age but are later found to be risk factors in longitudinal work (e.g., Mikami & Hinshaw, 2006). Moreover, developmental perspectives may point to particular "turning points" wherein individuals are especially susceptible to the influence of particular risk or protective factors or face choices that can significantly alter the course of their development (Kim-Cohen, 2007; Rutter, 1987).

Defining Resilience: Choosing Outcome Variables

Defining resilience within any population is intrinsically related to the types of outcomes that are considered and evaluated. Within the study of resilience from environmental adversity, there has not been a consistent definition of resilience, with variations in the types of variables chosen as outcomes (e.g., competence in life domains, absence of psychopathology, external versus intrinsic indicators of well-being), the degree of performance required to be deemed resilient (i.e., good versus acceptable), and even whether resilience entails adaptation across one or multiple domains of functioning (Luthar et al., 2000; Masten, 2001). Similar issues will be encountered in applying resilience models to the study of clinical populations, and thus the selection of outcome variables requires careful deliberation. In particular, these decisions should be guided by current knowledge of the nature and prominent features of the adversity condition being studied, with priority given to those outcome domains most strongly associated with the condition (i.e., where individuals may be most at-risk for poor outcomes; Luthar et al., 2000). Thus, while many approaches used in prior resilience work can be adapted to fit with clinical populations, specific outcome decisions should correspond with what is known about the typical trajectories and challenges associated with the disorder of interest.

The oft-used criteria of an absence of psychopathology in studies of resilience to environmental adversity can be adapted in several ways to apply to individuals with preexisting psychopathology. The absence of frequently comorbid conditions may be a relevant outcome measure, primarily in cases where the disorder of interest is believed to act as a risk factor for the comorbid disorder. Thus, the absence of oppositional defiant disorder (ODD) or conduct disorder (CD) might be a meaningful outcome in a study of ADHD. Additionally, knowledge of typical progressions of the disorder itself can inform outcome decisions, as remission might be a more appropriate outcome in some disorders (e.g., depression, ODD) but less so in other disorders believed to be lifelong (e.g., ADHD, Mental Retardation).

Symptom severity might also be considered as a measure of resilience, though in many cases it may be more meaningful to use this as a covariate. Alternatively, a measured reduction in symptom severity might be a more valuable indicator, corresponding to Masten's (2001) description of resilience as including the potential recovery after a traumatic event. However, it should be noted that an absence of negative outcomes may not be sufficient to describe resilient individuals, as it has been argued that evaluating positive outcomes is an integral aspect of establishing resilient functioning (Masten et al., 2008). In particular, the achievement of competence in developmentally appropriate tasks (e.g., Masten & Coatsworth, 1998) may serve as a valuable indicator of those who have learned to cope successfully with their disorder. In this case, knowledge of both typical development and disorder-specific trajectories can be crucial in informing the aspects of competence to evaluate, what may be taken as "success" within that domain, and the ways in which such outcomes are measured. For instance, findings that children with ADHD often provide elevated ratings of their own functioning (often referred to as positive illusory bias; Owens, Goldfine, Evangelista, Hoza, & Kaizer, 2007) may influence whether or how well-being or competence is measured as a meaningful outcome within this population. In all cases, it is essential that outcomes and the operational definition of resilience taken are clearly delineated to ensure that generalizations and applications to practice are appropriate and supported (Luthar et al., 2000).

Defining Resilience: "Resilient Compared to Whom?"

Perhaps the most basic approach to studying resilience among clinical populations would be to evaluate them on measures of known resilience factors. More specifically, it would be important to examine their abilities on factors that have been established for other at-risk populations using standardized measures (e.g., *Resiliency Scales for Children and Adolescents* (RSCA); Prince-Embury, 2007), thereby looking for areas of strength within this population relative to normative samples.

Certainly, such an approach may be valuable when working individually with a child and may serve as the foundation for studying resilience at the group level by establishing baselines of functioning for the group. Moreover, identifying areas of normative strength or resilience among clinical populations would be highly valuable in its own right. Conversely, given the known challenges in life domains associated with many child disorders (as reflected in the requisite criteria of functional impairment in mental health diagnoses), this approach also has the potential to provide an overly negative portrayal of the population that adds little to our understanding of resilience. For instance, this methodology was recently utilized in a small-scale study of young adults with Asperger's syndrome (AS). Overall, individuals in this population were found to experience significant risk factors in conjunction with few protective factors to serve as a buffer (Montgomery, Schwean, Burt, Dyke, Thorne et al., 2008).

Importantly, this method does not mean that such protective factors are not relevant, and it cannot be assumed that the same level of a particular protective factor is required for individuals facing differing types of adversity. Indeed, it is possible that a normative weakness in a protective factor may in fact be a relative strength within the clinical population, and thus may still serve an important function. A similar point can also be made in regard to the measurement of outcomes. Specifically, whereas in some cases resilience might be aptly defined as functioning at a level comparable to typically developing children, in other cases a more appropriate indicator of resilience might be functioning at the higher end of what is seen within the clinical group, even if this represents functioning below age-appropriate norms.

This point speaks to a key aspect of resilience research within clinical populations: the importance of focusing on within-group analysis rather than comparisons to a typical population. Such comparisons allow for an exploration of the heterogeneity within clinical populations, including both how particular strengths may have been supported within individuals and the effect they may have on outcomes. An example of this approach can be found in recent work exploring the resilience profiles of clinical populations using the RSCA (Kumar, Steer, & Gulab, 2010; Prince-Embury & Steer, 2010). Specifically, the authors identified four resilience profiles within their clinical population indicative of average resiliency, low resource vulnerability, high vulnerability, and very high vulnerability, with no one profile representative of the overall clinical group. This finding highlights the diversity of qualities within clinical populations, which may provide insight into the divergent trajectories observed within these groups. This or similar forms of subgroup profiling may be a valuable tool in exploring the mechanisms through which some children with disorders achieve greater well-being and success.

Ultimately, both between- and within-group analysis may prove useful in the study of resilience in clinical populations. Within-group comparisons allow for a greater understanding of what distinguishes those individuals with better or worse outcomes within the population and the mechanisms through which those resilient individuals achieve their success. However, including non-disordered individuals can allow for an examination of pathways that may be unique or particularly influential within the clinical population and the ways in which protective factors may interact with the disorder to shape outcomes over time. In fact, it has been argued that it is the interaction between a potential protective factor and the specific risk (in this case, the presence of a clinical disorder) that is most valuable to our understanding of resilience (Rutter, 1987).

Choosing Variables for Study

Identifying key protective factors is an important component of investigating resilience within any population. In existing resilience literature, a core set of resilience factors have been identified that appear to have a positive influence regardless of the particular risk factors faced, including intelligence, self-esteem, SES, and parenting practices (Masten, 2001), as well as self-regulation, perceived efficacy, and spirituality (Masten et al., 2008). Other factors have been identified that may play particularly important functions in the face of particular risk factors, such as high supervision parenting within the context of high-risk neighborhoods (cf. Rutter, 1987). An important place to begin in exploring resilience among clinical populations may be to explore the influence of factors known to promote resilience in other at-risk populations, particularly given that many forms of environmental adversity that have been the focus of resilience research (e.g., poverty, parental conflict, abuse) may also be more likely within clinical populations. Although it is likely that the core protective factors previously identified will play a similar role within clinical populations, the type and degree of influence cannot be assumed. Specifically, given distinct risks and trajectories within and between clinical groups, it is possible that a particular factor may be more or less influential for distinct populations, or might even have a converse effect within a particular group. For instance, despite the prominence of self-esteem in discussions of resilient qualities, it is unclear at this stage what role the aforementioned positive illusory bias plays in the well-being of children with ADHD. Although this elevated self-concept has been proposed as potentially serving a self-protective function (Owens et al., 2009), it is also possible that it prohibits learning from experiences and adjusting future behaviors, thereby increasing longer-term risks (McQuade & Hoza, 2008). Thus, without specific exploration of the development and functions of self-esteem among children with ADHD, literature from other populations cannot be soundly generalized to this group.

In addition to the importance of exploring these core resilience factors, studies in resilience can also be informed by the specific deficits and/or risks faced by the clinical population in question, as there may be unique protective factors for distinct populations or factors that may be more influential in a given clinical population than for other groups. In some cases, knowledge of typical development may inform this approach, as understanding the processes and factors that contribute to the development of a skill or resource in typical populations may provide insight into how such factors may be promoted within the at-risk group.

Relatedly, coping mechanisms or strategies, in this case those corresponding to the types of deficits or challenges inherent in the disorder, may be another avenue of exploration (Rutter, 2007).

Exploring Pathways and Mechanisms of Action

Finally, perhaps the most important and fruitful aspect of applying resilience frameworks to the study of childhood disorders is the need to move beyond identifying protective factors (i.e., those factors that seem to predict more positive outcomes) to exploring specific mechanisms of action (Luthar et al., 2000; Rutter, 2007); that is, how, when, and why a given factor is protective in the face of a specific risk. Masten (2001) has reviewed a number of pathways to consider in understanding the role of protective factors, including main versus interaction effects as well as risk-activated protective factors. In addition, Rutter (1987) has outlined several mechanisms through which protective factors may invoke their influence, including "reduction of risk impact; reduction of negative chain reactions; establishment and maintenance of self-esteem and self-efficacy; and opening of opportunities" (p. 325). He argues that it is through understanding *how* protective factors come to be present and *how* they exert their effect that resilience research can be most useful in informing intervention.

This approach to understanding resilience requires research designs and theory-driven hypotheses that explore specific relationships between risk and protective factors and outcomes, including both mediating and moderating models of influence (Masten, 2001). Current understandings around the specific symptoms and associated challenges faced by members of the clinical group can guide the formation and evaluation of hypothesized pathways addressing specific experiences often faced by members of the group. For instance, a protective factor may be important for all individuals within a clinical population (e.g., if it has a direct influence on outcomes or moderates the impact of core aspects of the disorder on associated challenges) or it may only be important for those individuals displaying particular symptoms or experiencing particular associated challenges (e.g., those with the disorder who experience academic impairment). For this reason, mapping out the pathways from core symptoms to outcomes that has been established in the psychopathology literature can serve as a strong foundation for exploring particular avenues of resilience. In addition to enhancing our understanding of the mechanisms of resilience, this approach can have particular value in establishing individualized intervention plans based on the particular strengths and needs of a child. For instance, the intervention plans for a child experiencing significant peer rejection versus a child experiencing difficult parent–child relationships may take different forms, focused on nurturing the resilience factors most influential in compensating for the particular challenges faced by each child. Moreover, understanding the mechanism of action of a protective factor that is less malleable may inform hypotheses of other protective factors that could be cultivated to play a similar role.

Given these many considerations, we propose that the study of resilience among populations of psychopathology must begin with the establishment of a conceptual framework that integrates current knowledge and theory in each field and can serve to guide specific hypotheses that will be most relevant and useful in moving research forward and supporting child-focused interventions. An illustrative example using ADHD is provided below to demonstrate how each of the considerations above can inform the formulation of a framework of resilience and psychopathology and the value this can bring to informing research and, ultimately, front-line practice.

Case Example: Applying a Resilience Paradigm to the Conceptualization of ADHD

ADHD is a developmental disorder of behavioral inhibition hindering self-regulation, organization of behavior, and goal-directed thought and action (Schwean & McCrimmon, 2008). ADHD is characterized by pervasive inattention and/or hyperactivity-impulsivity that results in significant functional impairment across settings. Current estimates of the prevalence of this disorder are between 3 and 7% of school-aged children (American Psychiatric Association, 2000), making it one of the most commonly diagnosed disorders in children (Centers for Disease Control, 2005). Moreover, ADHD has been found to persist through adolescence and adulthood for at least 70% of individuals with the disorder (Barkley, 2006).

ADHD has been the focus of an abundance of research attention which has served to establish a strong theoretical and evidence base for understanding the disorder. For instance, considerable research exploring the underlying neurocognitive basis and resulting behavioral characteristics of the disorder has led to the prominent and well-supported model of behavioral disinhibition and executive function (Barkley, 1997, 2006). Significant efforts have also been devoted to documenting the risk trajectories and poor outcomes associated with ADHD, highlighting significant social difficulties (e.g., Hoza, Mrug, Gerdes, Hinshaw, Bukowski et al., 2005; Sibley, Evans, & Serpell, 2010; Stormont, 2001), poor academic functioning (e.g., DuPaul & Stoner, 2003; Hoza, Pelham, Waschbusch, Kipp, & Owens, 2001), increased family dysfunction (e.g., Deault, 2010; Johnston & Mash, 2001), and high rates of comorbid internalizing and externalizing disorders (e.g., Carlson & Meyer, 2009; Newcorn, Halperin, & Miller, 2009; Tannock, 2009). Another prominent research emphasis has explored the effects of treatment, including pharmaceutical as well as psychosocial interventions (e.g., Daly, Creed, Xanthopolos, & Brown, 2007; MTA Cooperative Group, 2004a, 2004b; Pliszka, 2007). Although this work has demonstrated evidence of reduced symptom severity with medication and/or combined medical-psychosocial interventions, results have been less encouraging in regard to both the effects on associated challenges and the long-term maintenance of improvements.

Taken together, research to date can be described as predominantly deficit-based and paints a grim portrait of the experiences and progression associated with ADHD. However, a focused look beyond the overwhelming evidence of deficits reveals significant heterogeneity in the experiences and outcomes of individuals with ADHD, with a subset of this group experiencing success in at least some domains of functioning and a smaller number experiencing success across all major domains (Biederman, Mick, & Faraone, 1998; Lee, Lahey, Owens, & Hinshaw, 2008; Owens, Hinshaw, Lee, & Lahey, 2009). Although the current understanding of risk factors and pathways within the ADHD population can shed some light on this heterogeneity, this approach represents only half the picture. An exploration of the role and functions of resilience mechanisms is necessary to complement and enrich this understanding and provide a more complete picture of ADHD trajectories. Research in this direction has been significantly more limited to date, though holds promise for the value of a resilience perspective in enhancing our understanding of ADHD. For instance, researchers have begun to identify areas of potential strength within the ADHD population, highlighting that these children are often intelligent (Katusic, Voigt, Colligan, Weaver, Homan et al., 2011), have supportive families (Coles, Pelham, & Gnagy, 2010), and are equally creative as their non-ADHD peers (Healey & Rucklidge, 2005). Moreover, several studies have begun to identify possible factors that may exert a positive influence on the outcomes of children with ADHD, including self-reflective processes, positive relationships with others, and positive academic self-concept (e.g., Chen & Taylor, 2006; Litner & Mann-Feder, 2009; Mikami & Hinshaw, 2003, 2006; Modesto-Lowe et al., 2011).

Ultimately, as a largely hereditary disorder with a lifelong course (Barkley, 2006), a perspective that moves away from preventing or "curing" ADHD to one focused on coping successfully with it is particularly relevant for this population. Moreover, given the significant risks conferred by ADHD, an understanding of ways in which these individuals can be supported is highly relevant for clinical and educational practice. However, as noted above, a more deliberate reflection of how resilience can be more effectively integrated with ADHD models and literature bases would be highly valuable in guiding and integrating this direction of research.

Considerations in Integrating the Resilience Perspective with the Study of ADHD

Integrating Ecological Systems and Developmental Perspectives

Literature to date on ADHD fits well with ecological systems perspectives, with increasing evidence of the role of environment in contributing to the severity, course, and associated outcomes of the disorder over development (Barkley, 2006). Risk factors found to contribute to negative trajectories provide a strong foundation for applying resilience paradigms that explore the roles of potential protective factors within this population. In addition to efforts to identify potential factors across child, family, and community contexts (e.g., Modesto-Lowe et al., 2011), fully incorporating a transactional perspective to explore resilience would require further exploration of the interdependence and interactions between these factors (e.g., does resilience change if the child has poor peer relationships but positive family relationships?). In fact, the recognition of bidirectional child–family influences within ADHD populations (e.g., Deault, 2010) provides a strong demonstration of such interactions and a promising starting place for resilience-based study. Developmental considerations are also central to understanding ADHD. Current understandings such as changes in the manifestation of symptoms over development (Hart, Lahey, Loeber, Applegate, & Frick, 1995), effects of early negative experiences on later outcomes (e.g., peer rejection on later depression/anxiety; Mikami & Hinshaw, 2006), and unique challenges that arise at different stages of development (e.g., driving or relationships in adulthood; Barkley, 2006) can inform approaches to resilience research and potential priorities for study.

Defining Resilience: Choosing Outcome Variables

As noted above, establishing the outcomes that will be used to identify resilient functioning should correspond closely to the risks and trajectories associated with the population of interest. In the case of ADHD, the strong evidence of impairment across virtually all domains of functioning suggests that each of these domains would be important to evaluate, including developmentally appropriate and salient measures of social, academic (or occupational), emotional, and behavioral functioning. This analysis may include both measures of positive functioning or competence as well as consideration of comorbid disorders given the extremely high rates of comorbidity for this group. However, this approach does not imply that resilience should require positive adaptation across all areas (Luthar et al., 2000). Indeed, given the risks conferred by ADHD, examining children who have strengths within distinct areas may provide an opportunity to learn more about the factors impacting these areas of resilience. Moreover, this approach more closely incorporates a strengths-based perspective, in which we celebrate and learn from the strengths that all children have, despite the challenges they may experience in other areas.

The extensive literature on ADHD can also serve to illustrate another important consideration in selecting outcomes, namely, how particular outcomes might be measured to be most meaningful for the condition of interest. For instance, the issue of the positive illusory bias described above suggests a need to tread carefully in using self-esteem and related aspects of self-concept as a measure of emotional well-being, as it is unclear how well this reflects true well-being or predicts longer-term adjustment. Another domain relevant to the ADHD population, behavioral competence, illustrates the importance of establishing clear and informed operational definitions of positive adaptation. Behavioral competence has been identified as a meaningful measure of functioning among school-age children and may involve both rule-abiding behavior as well as a lack of aggression or delinquency (Masten & Coatsworth, 1998). Behavioral competence would also be a salient outcome domain within the ADHD population given the high associations of ADHD with aggression and conduct problems (Newcorn et al., 2009). However, given that ADHD by definition involves certain developmentally inappropriate behaviors (American Psychiatric Association, 2000), a meaningful measure of behavioral competence within this population would have to be clearly defined and carefully measured to avoid confounding core behaviors of the disorder with associated challenges in aggression and delinquency.

Defining Resilience: "Resilient Compared to Whom?"

In examining resilience in an ADHD population, it is important to understand domains in which these children have relative weaknesses to establish a frame of reference appropriate for the group. This knowledge can inform how protective factors should be conceptualized and explored in a meaningful way for the group. As noted above, it may be important to examine factors both *between* children with and without ADHD as well as looking at influential factors *within* a group of children with ADHD.

Examining differences between children with and without ADHD may provide valuable information regarding the differential effects of variables on these groups. Specifically, what may be of benefit for typically developing children may be of added benefit for children with ADHD or a factor may only be influential for one of these populations. For example, in exploring protective factors that might moderate the effect of peer rejection on internalizing and externalizing outcomes, Mikami and Hinshaw (2003) found that goal-directed solitary play and popularity with adults were more influential for children with ADHD than non-ADHD peer-rejected children. In another example, Hinshaw, Zupan, Simmel, Nigg and Melnick (1997) found that authoritative parenting beliefs made a positive independent contribution to social functioning for children with ADHD but had less impact for children without ADHD. Importantly, knowing when and for whom a factor is more or less influential can guide hypotheses around the role and function of that factor.

In areas of known deficits (e.g., social skills, working memory), it may be especially important to compare abilities *within* the group of children with ADHD as opposed to comparing their performance to that of typically developing children. For example, one variable that may be an important protective factor for children is social support (e.g., Cohen & Wills, 1985; Demaray & Malecki, 2002). Some children with ADHD may have a greater amount of social support relative to others within this group in the form of strong parent and/or community support networks. Conversely, some of these children would have a lesser amount of social support as compared to others within the ADHD population. In this situation, it would be important to compare these groups to determine how social support may influence other variables (e.g., social skills, academic achievement, or depression) rather than compare their scores to children without ADHD.

Choosing Variables

When applying a resilience framework to a clinical population, it is important to consider what specific factors may play a role in affecting outcomes. Both protective and risk factors will play an influential role in children with ADHD and can contribute to understanding resilience trajectories. A person-centered approach wherein groups are compared based on functioning in outcome domains provides one means of identifying factors that may distinguish resilient children. However, current knowledge of risk factors also provides some direction for variable-focused studies.

As noted above, much is already known about the risk factors contributing to poor outcomes among children with ADHD, and this knowledge can inform the identification of potential protective factors. For instance, whereas harsh parenting practices are known to increase risk for subsequent CD development, positive parenting practices may reduce this risk (Modesto-Lowe et al., 2011). This understanding can in turn guide further hypotheses, such as potential factors or practices that may promote positive parenting within these families (e.g., parent social support, parent training). Findings from other populations may also be highly relevant to understanding the ADHD group. For instance, exploring factors that promote academic motivation and persistence among children with learning disabilities, or that compensate for poor parent–child interactions among children from unstable homes, would provide insight into key protective factors that may be relevant to this population. Ultimately, given the extent of knowledge regarding ADHD trajectories, selecting variables for study may be most informed by understanding and exploring risk and resilience pathways, as described further below.

Exploring Pathways and Mechanisms of Action

Exploring the specific functions of protective factors and their mechanism of action in influencing outcomes is a critical element of resilience efforts. Within the study of ADHD, the extensive work around risk factors and pathways provides a rich literature base from which to generate hypotheses around protective pathways and mechanisms. Mapping out pathways from the underlying cognitive deficits to behaviors, associated challenges, and outcomes can provide an initial avenue for identifying resilience mechanisms within this group. For instance, the various pathways through which ADHD core deficits and symptoms can lead to academic difficulties and reduced academic motivation (DuPaul & Stoner, 2003) suggest a number of avenues for exploring compensatory or protective processes that may minimize this link.

Similarly, hypotheses can be guided by current understandings of how associated challenges can lead to later poor outcomes (e.g., peer rejection to depression/anxiety), as well as the unique interactions between ADHD and associated challenges that may further propagate trajectories. For instance, Mikami and Hinshaw (2003) have proposed that the effects of peer rejection may be particularly detrimental for children with ADHD because of the increased likelihood of concurrent parent–child conflict. The effect of elevated self-concepts of social functioning might also moderate the effects of peer rejection for these children in some way. The experiences and challenges faced by those with ADHD are likely to vary based on the specific risk and protective factors faced throughout their development. As such, understanding the specific function and mechanisms behind protective factors and their interactions would be important in informing the forms of support most valuable for a given child, ways of nurturing particularly protective factors, and how to most effectively elicit existing strengths within the child, their family, and community to support their well-being.

Resilience Model of ADHD

These considerations can be integrated to formulate a conceptualization of how resilience can apply and be approached in research within the population of interest. Using this approach, a conceptual model was developed by some of the authors (Mastoras, Climie, Schwean, & Saklofske, 2010) that provides guidance to the formulation of hypotheses and planning of specific work in this area. This model is depicted in Fig. 8.1.

As can be seen, this model incorporates the primary domains of outcomes relevant to the ADHD population as described above. Both core deficits and associated challenges of the disorder have been incorporated within an ecological framework, though they have been separated to demonstrate the important distinction between those factors core to the disorder and experienced by all individuals versus those associated risks experienced by some but not all members. Broad protective and risk factors that have been identified among other populations have also been depicted to acknowledge their potential role. This framework also points to several potential pathways through which protective factors might function, including: (1) broad and direct influences on outcomes (global supportive factors), pathways that influence the severity and/or impact of core deficits on associated challenges or outcomes (protective factors), and pathways that compensate or buffer the impact of associated risks and negative experiences on overall outcome domains (compensatory factors). As well, links between outcome domains have been included as a key factor. Together, this model allows for more specific hypotheses regarding the function and mechanism of action of particular resilience variables, as well as the interaction between protective and risk factors over time.

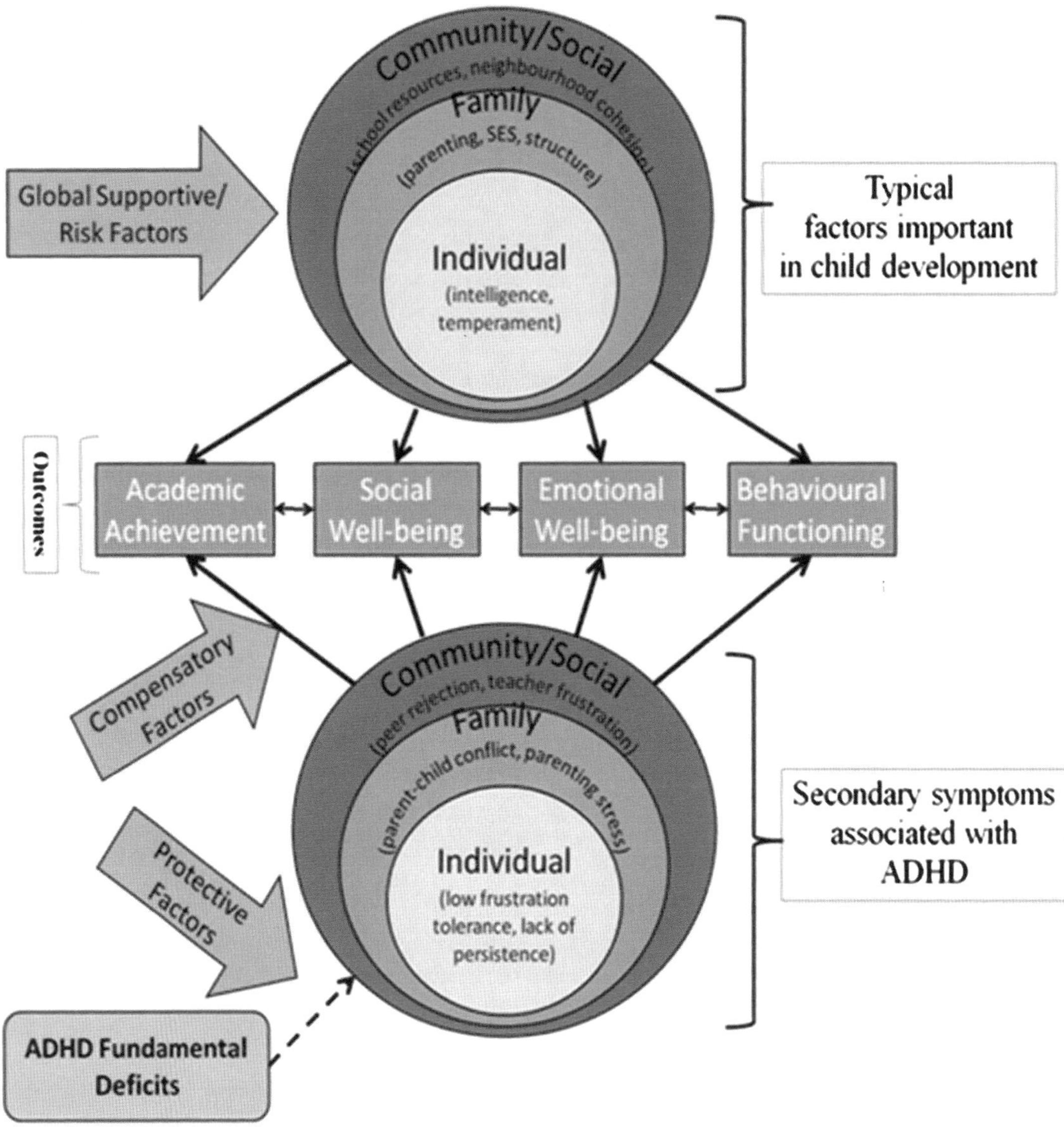

Fig. 8.1 A conceptual model of resilience in children with ADHD (Mastoras et al., 2010)

Key Factors in Extending a Resilience Approach to childhood disorders

Drawing from transactional models of child development, we have argued that biological risk factors (e.g., risks associated with lifelong difficulty in function and related to diagnosed medical disorders, as well as risks related to a history of prenatal, perinatal, neonatal, early developmental events or medical conditions which may affect the central nervous system) interact synergistically with environmental and psychosocial risk and protective factors to shape developmental outcomes in children.

Breakthroughs in neuroscience have increasingly demonstrated that a number of childhood conditions are "brain-based" and by their very nature predispose children to biological vulnerability (Swain et al., 2007; Piven & O'Leary, 1997). For example, there is compelling evidence that autism is related to a dysfunction of complex brain systems involving the frontal lobe and functionally related cortical and subcortical structures (Mash & Barkley, 2003). Although environmental risk factors may be contributory to heterogeneity amongst children presenting with autism as a function of factors such as IQ, language functioning, and early intervention, the prognosis is generally poor. In other conditions, the causal mechanisms are multifaceted and transactional and involve the complex interaction of biological and environmental factors (e.g., conduct disorders, anxiety, most depressions; and various areas of childhood exceptionality). Research suggests that these conditions may be more responsive to environmental interventions.

In this chapter, we have elucidated a model for the study of resiliency in ADHD. We believe that model has applicability to other areas of childhood disorders, as well as areas of exceptionality (e.g., learning disabilities, hearing impairments, physical and health disabilities, mental retardation) where children have already been exposed to a biological risk factor. As we have noted earlier in this chapter, application of the model, however, will require that attention be given to the following principles:

1. A comprehensive understanding of the condition under study to ensure that attention is appropriately drawn to those areas of the model that have greatest relevance to risks and protective factors related to the disorder. Under consideration should be potential etiologies, symptoms, and characteristics that define the condition, epidemiological findings, developmental course, associated and comorbid conditions, associated problems, as well as the general and specific literature that corroborates the importance of a relatively small set of global factors associated with developmental resilience (Masten, 1999).
2. Definitional issues have been raised earlier in this paper. One might argue that although defining resiliency as the ability to meet cultural age expectations is appropriate for those children who have not been exposed to a biological risk factor, that same definition is problematic for those youngsters who have experienced those risks during the pre- or perinatal periods. The biological risk is often significant enough that it eclipses a child's potential to meet the major expectations for children of that age and situation. In these cases, resilient behavior may better be determined by comparisons with age-mates experiencing the same or similar condition rather than typical peers.
3. The potentiation of inter-related risk factors (i.e., the cumulative impact of risk is exponential rather than linear) for poor outcomes on multiple indicators of development calls for sophisticated research designs and analysis (see Masten, 2001). Mash and Barkley (1996) argue that "rather than a direct causal pathway leading to a particular outcome, resilience involves ongoing interactions between a series of protective and/or vulnerability factors within the child and his/her surroundings and particular risk factors" (p. 19). Moreover, drawing from Rutter (1987), they contend that protective or vulnerability factors need to be conceptualized as processes rather than as absolutes since the same event or condition (e.g., early out-of-home placement) can operate as protective or vulnerability factors as a function of the overall context in which it occurs. These authors note that the multitude of interdependent and reciprocal influences, mechanisms, and processes involved in the etiology and course of childhood disorders clearly suggest a need for more complex theories (e.g., chaos theory), research designs, and data-analytic strategies.
4. The issue of comorbidity also assumes primacy in resiliency studies of childhood psychology and exceptionality. As noted by Haggerty, Sherrod, Garmezy and Rutter (1996), it is misleading to examine those factors that are associated with one condition alone, as these same factors may be concurrently related to a wider range of other manifestations of distress and disorder. Further, they

argue that a risk factor may contribute to the development of one disorder which, in time, contributes to the development of another. Thus, sources of risk and protection must be considered carefully in light of the co-occurrence of other conditions and problems.

5. We have established that environmental risks can be powerful moderators of development in infancy and childhood. Research has shown that process environmental features (i.e., those that are experienced more directly by the child) are highly predictive of subsequent outcomes in infancy and early childhood while status features, which are distal and broader and involve more indirectly experienced environmental events, are more predictive at school-age or later (Aylward, 1990, 1992, 1996). Thus, the application of resilience models to the study of childhood disorders must clearly attend to the nature of the environmental risk and developmental considerations (Bendersky & Lewis, 1994).
6. A related issue concerns the issue of timing in determining the potency of biological risk factors and the developmental risk they pose. In general, those risks that occur earliest are associated with the most serious developmental outcomes. Further, those children with an inherent biological vulnerability are more likely to be harmed by an adverse environment, and some environmental adversities, especially those that are long-standing or repeated, seem likely to induce a mental disorder in all but the most competent of children (Kopp & Kaler, 1989).

Intervention and Prevention

Findings indicating that certain children are resilient or invulnerable to stress have had a significant impact on the intervention and prevention literature and practice (Masten, 2001). A diversity of factors that have been linked to developmental resilience include early temperament; personal qualities such as self-esteem, ego-control, problem-solving skills, social competence, and autonomy; family stability; caring and secure parent–child relationships; attachment to at least one family member who engages in proactive, healthy behaviors; and, parental efficacy and reasoned disciplinary practices, amongst others. It is findings such as these that underscore the necessity of focusing not only on risk but also on those conditions that protect vulnerable children from dysfunction and lead to successful adaptations despite adversity (Cicchetti & Garmezy, 1993; Garmezy, 1985). According to Barkley & Mash (2001),

> research on resilience phenomena has changed the nature of the frameworks, goals, assessments, strategies, and evaluations in fields of prevention and treatment…. Goals now incorporate the promotion of competence as well as the prevention or amelioration of symptoms and problems. Strategies include the enhancement of assets as well as the reduction of risk or stressors, and the facilitation of protective processes as well as the treatment of illness or reduction of harmful processes. Assessments include assets and potential resources as well as problems and risks, competence as well as symptoms and disorder. These changes together reflect a major transformation in the conceptualization of prevention and intervention" (p.234).

Risk, protection, and resiliency are the central concepts in a risk and resilience model. Risk factors represent "any influences that increase the probability of onset, digression to a more serious state, or maintenance of a problem condition" (Kirby & Fraser, 1997, p. 11). Protective factors act to modify risk, either by directly reducing a disorder or dysfunction or by moderating the relationship among risk factors and problems or disorders, often called "buffering" effects (Fraser, Richman, & Galinsky, 1999). Promotive factors, on the other hand, exert positive effects regardless of risk exposure (Jenson & Fraser, 2006). Finally, resilience can be understood as the successful impact of protective factors on ameliorating or reducing risk factor outcomes and is usually defined as "the ability to function competently despite living or having lived in adversity" (Schofield & Beek 2005, p. 1283).

A key component of assessment from a resilience perspective is the concept of child competence and its systematic measurement. Although traditional child assessments have focused on the measurement of deficits and risks, the field is slowly undergoing a paradigm shift toward incorporating strengths-based practice to "discover and embellish, explore and exploit children's strengths and resources in the service of assisting them to achieve their goals" (Saleebey, 2006, p. 1). In particular, the literature now incorporates competence, strengths, assets, and abilities in the assessments of children to provide a more complete and accurate picture than those that focus on risks alone (Gilgun, Klein, & Pranis, 2000). Strength-based assessments are also crucial to demonstrating positive outcomes as a result of prevention and intervention strategies designed to offset deleterious outcomes particularly for vulnerable children.

However, there are obvious challenges related to the measurement of childhood strengths; most notably, the relative absence of assessment instruments focusing on constructs such as developmental strengths, resiliency, protective factors, assets, and competencies. Moreover, how to define these constructs for measurement purposes is highly problematic given that they are not simply dependent on the resources of the child but realize themselves through complex and dynamic interactions with the environment. A lack of consensus about how resiliency or competence should be defined and measured is also an issue. Thus, as Masten and Powell (2003) contend, the notion of multi-source, multi-modal assessment tied to issues such as "multiple developmentally appropriate domains of competence," the developmental process of a child, critical environmental or decision-making points, comorbidity, and other factors identified above are essential to establishing a reliable and valid assessment.

Interventions

A critical distinction that must be made when considering intervention concerns what is meant by the terms resilience and resiliency. Luthar et al. (2000) argue that the term resilience is most closely related to a "dynamic process" through interaction between the person and their environment at various levels. As such, in choosing the term resilience and the meaning ascribed to it, Luthar et al. contend the appropriate emphasis is given to the aspects of this construct which are most amenable to change; that is, decreasing risk factors and increasing protective factors to enhance the resilience. In contrast, resiliency represents the construct as a trait or characteristic which is not as amenable to intervention or change as it rests within the individual.

In alignment with Luthar et al.'s conceptualization of resilience, Masten (1994) has identified four strategies for fostering individual resilience and strengthening adaptive outcomes in children.

1. Reducing vulnerability and risk. Through the reduction of targeted risk factors, this approach attempts to circumvent high-risk situations before the individual encounters their effects (Fraser & Galinsky, 1997).
2. Reducing stressors. Potentiation effects can be reduced through interventions that lessen the effect of individual stressors or disrupt their accumulation.
3. Increasing available resources to mitigate the effect of risk.
4. Mobilizing protective processes that buffer the effects of risk factors, prevent the onset of a particular risk factor, or break the effects of potentiation. According to Smokowski (1998), "mapping such protective processes for intervention targets may be the single most important contribution resilience research makes to program development" (p. 340). He cautions that the strategies outlined by Masten are in no way mutually exclusive; rather, multifaceted prevention and intervention programs regularly integrate several of these objectives.

Luthar and Cicchetti (2000) provide further elaboration on applying the resilience perspective toward interventions. Key recommendations include: (a) interventions must have a strong base in theory; (b) interventions must have a strong basis in theory and research on the particular group being targeted; (c) efforts should be directed not only toward the reduction of negative outcomes or maladjustment among targeted groups but also toward the promotion of dimensions of positive adaption or competence; (d) interventions must be designed not only to reduce negative influences but also to capitalize on specific resources within particular populations; (e) interventions should target salient vulnerability and protective processes that operate across multiple levels of influence; (f) interventions must have a strong developmental focus; (g) the contextual relevance of the overall intervention aims, as well as of the specific intervention strategies, must be ensured; (h) intervention efforts should aim at fostering services that eventually can become self-sustaining; (i) data from intervention groups should be compared with those of appropriate comparison groups; and (j) there must be careful documentation and evaluation. The reader is strongly encouraged to consult this article for more detailed information regarding the application of resilience frameworks to intervention and social policy.

References

American Psychiatric Association. (2000). *Diagnostic and statistical manual of mental disorders (text revision)* (4th ed.). Washington, DC: American Psychiatric Association.

Anthony, E. J., & Koupernik, C. (Eds.). (1974). *The child in his family: Children at psychiatric risk*. New York: Wiley.

Aylward, G. P. (1990). Environmental influences and the developmental outcome of children at risk. *Infants and Young Children, 2*, 1–9.

Aylward, G. P. (1992). The relationship between environmental risk and developmental outcome. *Journal of Developmental and Behavioral Pediatrics, 13*, 222–229.

Aylward, G. P. (1996). Environmental risk, intervention and developmental outcome. *Ambulatory Child Health, 2*, 161–170.

Barkley, R. A. (1997). Behavioral inhibition, sustained attention, and executive functions: Constructing a unifying theory of ADHD. *Psychological Bulletin, 121*(1), 65–94.

Barkley, R. A. (2006). *Attention-deficit hyperactivity disorder: A handbook for diagnosis and treatment* (3rd ed.). New York: Guilford Press.

Bendersky, M., & Lewis, M. (1994). Environmental risk, biological risk, and developmental outcome. *Developmental Psychology, 30*(4), 484–494. doi:10.1037/0012-1649.30.4.484.

Biederman, J., Mick, E., & Faraone, S. V. (1998). Normalized functioning in youths with persistent attention deficit hyperactivity disorder. *The Journal of Pediatrics, 133*, 544–551. doi:10.1016/S0022-3476(98)70065-4 DOI:dx.doi.org.

Bronfenbrenner, U. (1977). Toward an experimental ecology of human development. *American Psychologist, 32*, 513–531.

Carlson, G., & Meyer, S. (2009). ADHD with mood disorders. In T. Brown (Ed.), *ADHD comorbidities: Handbook for ADHD complications in children and adults* (pp. 97–128). Arlington, VA: American Psychiatric Publishing.

Centers for Disease Control (CDC). (2005). Mental health in the United States: Prevalence of diagnosis and medication treatment for attention-deficit/hyperactivity disorder – United States, 2003. *Morbidity and Mortality Weekly Report, 54*, 842–847.

Chen, W., & Taylor, E. (2006). Resilience and self-control impairment. In S. Goldstein & R. Brooks (Eds.), *Handbook of resilience in children* (pp. 257–278). New York: Springer.

Cicchetti, D., & Lynch, M. (1993). Toward an ecological/transactional model of community violence and child maltreatment: Consequences for children's development. *Psychiatry, 56*, 96–118.

Cicchetti, D., & Garmezy, N. (1993). Prospects and promises in the study of resilience. *Development and Psychopathology, 5*(4), 497–502. doi:10.1017/S0954579400006118.

Cohen, S., & Wills, T. A. (1985). Stress, social support, and the buffering hypothesis. *Psychological Bulletin, 98*, 310–357.

Coles, E. K., Pelham, W. E., & Gnagy, E. M. (2010). Parental attributions for success in managing the behavior of children with ADHD. *Journal of Attention Disorders, 14*(2), 138–146.

Conger, R. D., Conger, K. J., & Elder, G. H. (1997). Family economic hardship and adolescent academic performance: Mediating and moderating processes. In G. Duncan & J. Brooks-Gunn (Eds.), *Consequences of growing up poor* (pp. 288–310). New York: Russell Sage.

Conger, R. D., Conger, K. J., Elder, G. H., Lorenz, F. O., Simons, R. I., & Whitbeck, L. B. (1992). A family process model of economic hardship and adjustment of early adolescent boys. *Child Development, 63*, 526–541.

Cowen, E. L., Wyman, P. A., Work, W. C., & Parker, G. R. (1990). The Rochester child resilience project: Overview and summary of first year findings. *Development and Psychopathology, 2*, 193–212.

Curry, J., Silva, S., Rohde, P., Ginsburg, G., Kratochvil, C., Simons, A., et al. (2011). Recovery and recurrence following treatment for adolescent major depression. *Archives of General Psychiatry, 68*, 263–270.

Daly, B. P., Creed, T., Xanthopolous, M., & Brown, R. T. (2007). Psychosocial treatments for children with attention deficit/hyperactivity disorder. *Neuropsychology Review, 17*(1), 73–89. doi:10.1007/s11065-006-9018-2.

Deault, L. C. (2010). A systematic review of parenting in relation to the development of comorbidities and functional impairments in children with attention-deficit/hyperactivity disorder (ADHD). *Child Psychiatry and Human Development, 41*, 168–192.

Demaray, C. M. K., & Malecki, K. (2002). The relationship between perceived social support and maladjustment for students at risk. *Psychology in the Schools, 39*(3), 305–316. doi:10.1002/pits.10018.

Ditrano, C. J., & Silverstein, L. B. (2006). Listening to parents' voices: Participatory action research in the schools. *Professional Psychology" Research and Practice, 37*(4), 359–366. doi:10.1037/0735-7028.37.4.359.

DuPaul, G. J., & Stoner, G. (2003). *ADHD in the schools: Assessment and intervention strategies* (2nd ed.). New York: Guilford Press.

Forgatch, M. S., & DeGarmo, D. S. (1999). Parenting through change: An effective prevention program for single mothers. *Journal of Consulting and Clinical Psychology, 67*, 711–724.

Fraser, M. W., & Galinsky, M. J. (1997). Toward a resiliency based model of practice. In M. W. Fraser (Ed.), *Risk and resilience* (pp. 265–275). Washington, DC: NASW Press.

Fraser, M. W., Richman, J. M., & Galinsky, M. J. (1999). Risk protection and resilience: Towards a conceptual framework for social work practice. *Social Work Research, 23*(3), 131–143.

Garmezy, N. (1971). Vulnerability research and the issue of primary prevention. *The American Journal of Orthopsychiatry, 41*, 101–116.

Garmezy, N. (1974). The study of competence in children at risk for severe psychopathology. In E. J. Anthony & C. Koupernik (Eds.), *The child and his Family* (Children at psychiatric risk, Vol. 3, pp. 77–97). New York: Wiley.

Garmezy, N. (1985). Stress-resistant children: The search for protective factors. In J. E. Stevenson (Ed.), Recent research in developmental psychopathology (*Journal of Child Psychology and Psychiatry Book suppl. No. 4*, pp. 213–233). Oxford, England: Pergamon Press.)

Garmezy, N., Masten, A. S., & Tellegen, A. (1984). The study of stress and competence in children: A building block for developmental psychopathology. *Child Development, 55*, 97–111.

Gilgun, J. F., Klein, C., & Pranis, K. (2000). The significance of resources in models of risk. *Journal of Interpersonal Violence, 15*(6), 631–650.

Haggerty, J., Sherrod, L., Garmezy, N., & Rutter, M. (1996). *Stress, risk and resilience in children and adolescents*. New York: Cambridge University Press.

Hart, E. L., Lahey, B. B., Loeber, R., Applegate, B., & Frick, P. J. (1995). Developmental change in attention-deficit hyperactivity disorder in boys: A four-year longitudinal study. *Journal of Abnormal Child Psychology, 23*, 729–749. doi:10.1007/BF01447474.

Healey, D., & Rucklidge, J. J. (2005). An exploration into the creative abilities of children with ADHD. *Journal of Attention Disorders, 8*(3), 88–95.

Hinshaw, S. P., & Lee, S. S. (2003). Conduct and oppositional defiant disorders. In E. J. Mash & R. A. Barkley (Eds.), *Child psychopathology* (2nd ed.). New York: Guilford Press.

Hinshaw, S. P., Zupan, B. A., Simmel, C., Nigg, J. T., & Melnick, S. (1997). Peer status in boys with and without attention-deficit hyperactivity disorder: Predictions from overt and covert antisocial behavior, social isolation, and authoritative parenting beliefs. *Child Development, 68*, 880–896.

Hoza, B., Mrug, S., Gerdes, A. C., Hinshaw, S. P., Bukowski, H. C., Gold, J. A., Kraemer, H., Pelham, W., Jr., Wigal, T., & Arnold, L. E. (2005). What aspects of peer relationships are impaired in children with attention-deficit/hyperactivity disorder? *Journal of Consulting and Clinical Psychology, 73*, 411–423.

Hoza, B., Pelham, W. E., Waschbusch, D. A., Kipp, H., & Owens, J. S. (2001). Academic task persistence of normally achieving ADHD and control boys: Performance, self-evaluations, and attributions. *Journal of Consulting and Clinical Psychology, 60*, 271–283.

Jenson, J. M., & Fraser, M. W. (2006). A risk and resilience framework for child, youth, and family policy. In J. M. Jenson & M. W. Fraser (Eds.), *Social policy for children & families: A risk and resilience perspective* (pp. 1–18). Thousand Oaks, CA: Sage Publications.

Johnston, C., & Mash, E. J. (2001). Families of children with attention-deficit/hyperactivity disorder: Review and recommendations for future research. *Clinical Child and Family Psychology Review, 4*, 183–207.

Katusic, M. Z., Voigt, R. G., Colligan, R. C., Weaver, A. L., Homan, K. J., & Barbaresi, W. J. (2011). Attention-deficit hyperactivity disorder in children with high intelligence quotient: Results from a population-based study. *Journal of Developmental and Behavioural Pediatrics, 32*(2), 103–109.

Kim-Cohen, J. (2007). Resilience and developmental psychopathology. *Child and Adolescent Psychiatric Clinics of North America, 16*, 271–283.

Kirby, L. D., & Fraser, M. W. (1997). Risk and resilience in childhood. In M. W. Fraser (Ed.), *Risk and resiliency in childhood: An ecological perspective* (pp. 10–33). Washington, DC: National Association of Social Workers.

Kopp, C. B., & Kaler, S. R. (1989). Risk in infancy: Origins and implications. *American Psychologist, 44*(2), 224–230.

Kumar, G., Steer, R. A., & Gulab, N. A. (2010). Profiles of personal resiliency in child and adolescent psychiatric inpations. *Journal of Psychoeducational Assessment, 28*, 315–325.

Lee, S. S., Lahey, B. B., Owens, E. B., & Hinshaw, S. P. (2008). Few preschool boys and girls with ADHD are well-adjusted during adolescence. *Journal of Abnormal Child Psychology, 36*, 373–383. doi:10.1007/s10802-007-9184-6.

Litner, B., & Mann-Feder, V. (2009). Fostering resilience in youth with ADHD. *Relational Child and Youth Care Practice, 22*(3), 35–39.

Luthar, S. S., & Cicchetti, D. (2000). The construct of resilience implications for intervention and social policy. *Development and Psychopathology, 12*, 857–885.

Luthar, S. S., Cicchetti, D., & Becker, B. (2000a). The construct of resilience: A critical evaluation and guidelines for future work. *Child Development, 71*, 543–562. doi:10.1111/1467-8624.00164.

Luthar, S. S., Cicchetti, D., Becker, B., Von-Eye, A., Schuster, C., Roosa, M. W., et al. (2000b). The construct of resilience: A critical evaluation and guidelines for future work. *Child Development, 71*(3), 543–575.

Mash, E.J., & Barkley, R.A. (Eds.) (2003). Child psychopathology (2nd Edition). New York: Guildford Publications.

Masten, A. S. (1994). Resilience in individual development: Successful adaptation despite risk and adversity. In M. Wang & E. Gordon (Eds.), *Risk and resilience in inner city America: Challenges and prospects* (pp. 3–25). Hillsdale, NJ: Erlbaum.

Masten, A. S. (1999). The promise and perils of resilience research as a guide to preventive interventions. In M. D. Glantz & J. L. Johnson (Eds.), *Resilience and development: Positive life adaptations* (pp. 251–257). New York: Plenum Press.

Masten, A. S. (2001). Ordinary magic: Resilience processes in development. *American Psychologist, 56*, 227–238. doi:10.1037/0003-066X.56.3.227.

Masten, A. S. (2002). Resilience in development. In C. R. Snyder & S. J. Lopez (Eds.), *Oxford handbook of positive psychology* (pp. 117–132). New York: Oxford University Press.

Masten, A. S. (2006). Developmental psychopathology: Pathways to the future. *International Journal of Behavioral Development, 30*, 47–54.

Masten, A. S. (2007). Resilience in developing systems: Progress and promise and the fourth wave arises. *Development and Psychopathology, 19*, 921–930.

Masten, A. S. (2011). Resilience in children threatened by extreme adversity: Frameworks for research, practice, and translational synergy. *Development and Psychopathology, 23*, 493–506.

Masten, A. S., & Coatsworth, J. D. (1998). The development of competence in favourable and unfavourable environments. *American Psychologist, 53*, 205–220. doi:10.1037/0003-066X.53.2.205.

Masten, A. S., Garmezy, N., Tellegen, A., Pellegrini, D. S., Larkin, K., & Larsen, A. (1988). Competence and stress in school children: The moderating effects of individual and family qualities. *Journal of Child Psychology and Psychiatry, 29*, 745–764.

Masten, A. S., Herbers, J. E., Cutuli, J. J., & Lafavor, T. L. (2008). Promoting competence and resilience in the school context. *Professional School Counseling, 12*(2), 76–84.

Masten, A. S., Hubbard, J. J., Gest, S. D., Tellegen, A., Garmezy, N., & Ramirez, M. (1999). Competence in the context of adversity: Pathways to resilience and maladaptation from childhood to late adolescence. *Development and Psychopathology, 11*, 143–169.

Masten, A. S., & Powell, J. L. (2003). A resilience framework for research, policy, and practice. In S. S. Luthar (Ed.), *Resilience and vulnerability: Adaptation in the context of childhood adversities* (pp. 1–25). Cambridge: Cambridge University Press.

Mastoras, S.M., Climie, E.A., Schwean, V.L., & Saklofske, D.H. (2010). *A conceptual model of socioemotional resilience in children with ADHD*. Poster presented at Canadian Psychological Association Annual Conference, Winnipeg, MB.

McLoyd, V. C. (1998). Socioeconomic disadvantage and child development. *American Psychologist, 53*, 185–204.

McQuade, J. D., & Hoza, B. (2008). Peer problems in Attention Deficit Hyperactivity Disorder: Current status and future directions. Developmental Disabilities Research Reviews, 14(4), 320–324. doi:10.1002/ddrr.35

Mikami, A. Y., & Hinshaw, S. P. (2003). Buffers of peer rejection among girls with and without ADHD: The role of popularity with adults and goal-directed solitary play. *Journal of Abnormal Child Psychology, 31*, 381–397.

Mikami, A. Y., & Hinshaw, S. P. (2006). Resilient adolescent adjustment among girls: Buffers of childhood peer rejection and attention-deficit/hyperactivity disorder. *Journal of Abnormal Child Psychology, 34*, 825–839.

Modesto-Lowe, V., Yelunina, L., & Hanjan, K. (2011). Attention-deficit/hyperactivity disorder: A shift towards resilience? *Clinical Pediatrics, 50*(6), 518–524.

Montgomery, J. M., Schwean, V. L., Burt, J. G., Dyke, D. I., Thorne, K. J., Hindes, Y. L., et al. (2008). Emotional intelligence and resiliency in young adults with Asperger's disorder. *Canadian Journal of School Psychology, 23*, 70–93.

MTA Cooperative Group. (2004a). National Institute of Mental Health Multimodal Treatment Study of ADHD. Follow-up: 24-month outcomes of treatment strategies for attention-deficit/hyperactivity disorder. *Pediatrics, 113*, 754–761.

MTA Cooperative Group. (2004b). National Institute of Mental Health Multimodeal Treatment Study of ADHD. Follow-up: Changes in effectiveness and growth after the end of treatment. *Pediatrics, 113*, 762–769.

Newcorn, J., Halperin, J., & Miller, C. (2009). ADHD with oppositionality and aggression. In T. Brown (Ed.), *ADHD comorbidities: Handbook for ADHD complications in children and adults* (pp. 157–172). Arlington, VA: American Psychiatric Publishing.

Olsson, C. A., Bond, L., Burns, J. M., Vella-Brodrick, D. A., & Sawyer, S. M. (2003). Adolescent resilience: A concept analysis. *Journal of Adolescence, 26*, 1–11.

Owens, E. B., Hinshaw, S. P., Lee, S. S., & Lahey, B. B. (2009). Few girls with childhood attention-deficit/hyperactivity disorder show positive adjustment during adolescence. *Journal of Clinical Child and Adolescent Psychology, 38*, 132–143. doi:10.1080/15374410802575313.

Owens, J. S., Goldfine, M. E., Evangelista, N. M., Hoza, B., & Kaiser, N. M. (2007). A critical review of self-perceptions and the positive illusory bias in children with ADHD. *Clinical Child and Family Psychology Review, 10*(4), 335–351. doi:10.1007/s10567-007-0027-3.

Piven, J., & O'Leary, D. (1997). Neuroimaging in autism. *Child and Adolescent Clinics of North America, 6*, 305–323.

Prince-Embury, S. (2007). *Resiliency scales for children and adolescents: Profiles of personal strengths*. San Antonio, TX: Harcourt Assessments.

Pliszka, S. R. (2007). Pharmacologic treatment of attention-deficit/hyperactivity disorder: efficacy, safety and mechanisms of action. *Neuropsychology Review, 17*(1), 67–72. doi:10.1007/s11065-006-9017-3.

Prince-Embury, S., & Steer, R. A. (2010). Profiles of personal resiliency for normative and clinical samples of youth assessed by the Resiliency Scales for Children and Adolescents. *Journal of Psychoeducational Assessment, 28*, 303–314.

Reivich, K., Gillham, J. E., Chaplin, T. M., & Seligman, M. E. P. (2005). From helplessness to optimism: The role of resilience in treating and preventing depression in young adults. In S. Goldstein & R. B. Brooks (Eds.), *Handbook of resilience in children* (pp. 203–222). New York: Plenum.

Rutter, M. (1979). Protective factors in children's responses to stress and disadvantage. In M. W. Kent & J. E. Rolf (Eds.), *Primary prevention of psychopathology: Social competence in children* (Vol. 3, pp. 49–74). Hanover, NH: University Press of New England.

Rutter, M. (1987). Psychosocial resilience and protective mechanisms. *The American Journal of Orthopsychiatry, 57*, 316–331.

Rutter, M. (1993). Resilience: Some conceptual considerations. *Journal of Adolescent Health, 14*, 626–631.

Rutter, M. (2007). Resilience, competence, and coping. *Child Abuse & Neglect, 31*, 205–209.

Saleebey, D. (2006). *The strengths perspective in social work practice* (4th ed.). Boston, MA: Allyn and Bacon.

Schofield, G., & Beek, M. (2005). Risk and resilience in long-term foster care. *British Journal of Social Work, 35*(8), 1283–1301.

Schwean, V., & McCrimmon, A. (2008). Attention-deficit/hyperactivity disorder: Using the WISC-IV to inform intervention planning. In A. Prifitera, D. Saklofske, & L. Weiss (Eds.), *WISC-IV: Clinical assessment and intervention*. Burlington, MA: Elsevier Academic Press.

Sibley, M. H., Evans, S. W., & Serpell, Z. N. (2010). Social cognition and interpersonal impairment in young adolescents with ADHD. *Journal of Psychopathology and Behavioral Assessment, 32*, 193–202.

Smokowski, P. R. (1998). Prevention and intervention strategies for promoting resilience in disadvantaged children. *The Social Service Review, 72*, 337–364.

Stormont, M. (2001). Social outcomes of children with AD/HD: Contributing factors and implications for practice. *Psychology in the Schools, 38*, 521–531.

Swain, J. E., Scahill, L., Lombroso, P. J., King, R. A., & Leckman, J. F. (2007). Tourette syndrome and tic disorders: A decade of progress. *Journal of the American Academy of Child and Adolescent Psychiatry, 46*(8), 947–968.

Tannock, R. (2009). ADHD with anxiety disorders. In T. Brown (Ed.), *ADHD comorbidities: Handbook for ADHD complications in children and adults* (pp. 131–152). Arlington, VA: American Psychiatric Publishing.

Wyman, P. A., Cowen, E. L., Work, W. C., Hoyt-Meyers, L., Magnus, K. B., & Fagen, D. B. (1999). Caregiving and developmental factors differentiating young at-risk urban children showing resilient versus stress-affected outcomes: A replication and extension. *Child Development, 70*, 645–659.

Part III

Resilience, Youth and Adults

9 The Ego-Resiliency Scale by Block and Kremen (1996) and Trait Ego-Resiliency

Sandra Prince-Embury

It is the opinion of this editor that a volume on translating resilience theory for application should include mention of the work of Jack Block, author of the Ego-Resiliency Scale (Block, 1989; Block & Kremen, 1996) and an originator of the construct of ego-resiliency. Dr. Block was unavailable to write a chapter himself as he passed away in 2010 just as this volume was being organized. Jacob "Jack" Block (April 28, 1924–January 13, 2010) was a well-known psychology professor at UC Berkeley. His main areas of research were personality theory, personality development, research methodology, personality assessment, longitudinal research, and cognition. He often collaborated with his wife and colleague Jeanne Block.

Block's most renowned body of work, undertaken primarily with his wife, was a longitudinal study on a cohort of more than 100 San Francisco Bay Area toddlers, who were studied regularly for nearly 30 years. The Blocks focused on the psychological makeup and history of the participants, tracking how their background influenced their later choices and the outcomes of their lives. This study, published in the book *Lives through Time* (Block & Block, 1971), was noteworthy not only for its contributions to the understanding of stability and change in personality but also for its inventive methodological approach.

Block's inclusion in this volume is warranted because he brought attention to the construct of "ego-resiliency" (Block, 1965; Block & Block, 1980), operationalized this construct as the "ego-resiliency scale" (Block, 1989) and generated an abundance of research relating to attributes associated with this construct. Ego-resiliency was conceptualized by Block as an aspect of personality which in turn served as a "structure for managing emotion," (Block, 2002). In his book *Personality as an Affect Processing System* (2002), Block presents his model of personality as an adaptive system for taking in and organizing information and maintaining nondisruptive levels of anxiety while responding to inner and outer demands. His proposed system consists of perceptual and control mechanisms operating in delicate balance.

Ego-control (EC) and ego-resiliency (ER) comprised the central mechanisms for understanding Block's model of an adaptive personality system (Block, 1950, 1951, 2002; Block & Block, 1980). Ego-Control refers to an adaptive system of impulse inhibition/expression, and ego-resiliency refers to an adaptive system for modifying one's level of control in response to situational demands. As a personality theorist, Block employed these mechanisms to explain relatively enduring traits of individuals.

Jack Block and associates developed self-report scales for both ego-control and ego-resiliency. Items were drawn from the Minnesota

S. Prince-Embury, Ph.D. (✉)
Resiliency Institute of Allenhurst, LLC,
625 North Edgemere Drive, West Allenhurst,
NJ 07711, USA
e-mail: Sandraprince-embury@earthlink.net

S. Prince-Embury and D.H. Saklofske (eds.), *Resilience in Children, Adolescents, and Adults: Translating Research into Practice*, The Springer Series on Human Exceptionality,
DOI 10.1007/978-1-4614-4939-3_9, © Springer Science+Business Media New York 2013

Multiphasic Personality Inventory (MMPI; Hathaway & McKinley, 1951) and the CPI (Gough, 1956), were written by Jack Block, or came from other sources that are at this time untraceable [see Block and Kremen (1996)]. The ego-resiliency scale (ER89) was developed to assess trait variation in psychological resilience. Originally, Block and Kremen (1996) administered the ER scale to research participants in the Block and Block Longitudinal Study of Cognitive and Ego Development (Block & Block, 1980). Participants at ages 18 and again at age 23 were asked to indicate the degree to which they agreed with 14 statements (e.g., "I quickly get over and recover from being startled," "I enjoy dealing with new and unusual situations") on a scale from 1 (*does not apply at all*) to 4 (*applies very strongly*). The coefficient of reliability for this sample was 0.76, providing adequate support that the scale measured one main factor. Across the 5 years between assessments, the test–retest reliabilities were 0.67 and 0.51 (adjusted for attenuation), for females and males, respectively.

Block's conceptualization of ego-resiliency differs from more recent conceptualizations of "resilience" as avoidance of negative outcomes in the face of adversity. Block's construct refers to a "personality trait" as opposed to the more "interactive and dynamic process" which is prevalent in current literature. In addition, Block's construct is based on the conceptualization of "ego," The ego was hypothesized by Freud as an organized part of the personality structure that includes defensive, perceptual, intellectual-cognitive, and executive functions. Conscious awareness was presumed to reside in the ego, although not all of the operations of the ego are conscious. Freud used the word ego to mean a set of psychic functions such as judgment, tolerance, reality testing, control, planning, defense, synthesis of information, intellectual functioning, and memory. Block suggested that ego functioning could be likened to "executive functioning" (Block, 2002, p. 29). Similarly, the term "ego-resiliency" might be likened to the concept of "emotion regulation" a concept prevalent in recent literature.

Ego-Control

According to Block the dimension of ego-control varies from overcontrol to under-control (Block, 2002; Block & Block, 1980). Overcontrolled individuals are described as relatively inhibited in action and affect-expressiveness to the point of at times being excessively constrained. Overcontrolled individuals were viewed as characteristically containing impulse and affect across situations, even when doing so may not be necessary. On the other hand, under-controlled individuals were viewed as characteristically expressing impulse and affect across situations, even when doing so may be inappropriate. Under-controlled individuals characteristically express affect and impulses relatively immediately and directly even when doing so may be socially or personally inappropriate. They are relatively unable to delay gratification, have fluctuating emotions, and are spontaneous, easily distracted, and relatively unbound by social customs (Block, 2002; Funder & Block, 1989). The consequences of overcontrol or under-control may be adaptive or maladaptive depending on circumstances. Overcontrol may facilitate disciplined and directed behavior, which can be advantageous in some situations. In other contexts, where spontaneity is desirable, overcontrol is likely to be limiting. In such situations, under-control can facilitate the expression of warmth, friendliness, and spontaneity, which are likely to be advantageous in promoting intimacy and the enjoyment of life. However, under-control can be maladaptive when it leads to erratic, unorganized, or dangerous behavior.

Block's conceptualization of ego-control contrasts fundamentally with that of other theorists who considered higher levels of control to be advantageous and adaptive under all conditions. This difference in theoretical interpretation may arise because these other investigators conceptualize EC as a variable that ranges from appropriate control to under-control, and therefore failed to theorize about or to measure the range between appropriate control and overcontrol.

Ego-Resiliency

According to the Blocks' theorizing, ego-resiliency is the ability to adapt one's level of control temporarily up or down as circumstances dictate (Block, 2002; Block & Block, 1980). Highly ego-resilient individuals were described as characteristically able to modify their level of control, either up or down, as may be appropriate or necessary according to the situational context. Individuals with a low level of ego-resiliency were described as more restricted to the same level of impulse containment or expression regardless of situational context. It is presumed that as a result of this adaptive flexibility, individuals with a high level of ego-resiliency are more likely to experience positive effect, and have higher levels of self-confidence and better psychological adjustment than individuals with a low level of ego-resiliency (Block & Kremen, 1996). It is presumed that when confronted by stressful circumstances, individuals with a low level of ego-resiliency may act in a stiff and perseverative manner or chaotically and diffusely, and in either case, the resulting behavior is likely to be maladaptive (Block & Kremen, 1996). Block's theoretical conceptualization of ego-resiliency is closely related to conceptions of good psychological functioning and appropriate and adaptive behavior across social contexts (Block & Block, 1980; Klohnen, 1996).

Block's definition of resiliency assumes a higher-order personality structure, a set of internalized, generalizing, and discriminating relations that encompass the range of circumstances that an individual will encounter. Block's Ego-Resiliency Scale includes behaviors related to the inferred personality traits above and beyond the specific mechanism of "ego-resiliency." Those who are not trait theorists might find little use for the scale in this regard. On the other hand, Block was critical of the modern, empirically based definition of resilience as survival in the face of adversity. He argued that it was not helpful to combine protective influences such as parental and societal support along with intrinsic characteristics of the individual in defining resilience (Block, 2002, p. 23).

In spite of the differences between Block's conceptualization of ego-resiliency and more prevalent definitions relating to surviving adversity, the ER has been shown to have high construct validity with respect to the latter. Higher scores on the ER have been found to predict the experience of fewer depressive symptoms after the terrorist attacks on 11th September (Fredrickson, et al., 2003), faster affective and physiological recovery from threat (Tugade & Fredrickson, 2004; Waugh, et al., 2008) and more successful adaptation to daily stressors (Ong et al., 2006). The ER scale was employed by Tugade and Fredrickson (2004), who found that positive emotionality and appraisal of threat moderate the relationship between resilience and the duration of cardiovascular reactivity following the induction of a negative emotion.

Fredrickson et al. (2003) using Block & Kreman's Ego-Resiliency Scale, replicating prior research, found that trait resilience was associated with a range of psychological benefits, both in day-to-day life and in coping with crises. First, people scoring high on trait resilience share a set of affect-related traits—low neuroticism coupled with high extraversion and high openness—that predispose them toward positive affectivity. Second, trait resilience—which itself can be considered a psychological resource—is associated with a host of other psychological resources, including life satisfaction, optimism, and tranquility. Third, people scoring higher on trait resilience were more likely to find positive meaning within the problems they faced as a result of the September 11 attacks. Fourth, people scoring higher on trait resilience endured fewer depressive symptoms following the September 11 attacks (Fredrickson et al., 2003). And, finally, those scoring high on trait resilience experienced more positive emotions: They were in better moods when tested and reported that since the attacks, they had experienced positive emotions more frequently (and negative emotions somewhat less frequently) than did their less-resilient peers. Examining the interrelations among these various correlates of resilience, Fredrickson et al. (2003) found that people's experiences of positive emotions after the

September 11 attacks could fully account for the relation between preexisting trait resilience and the later development of depressive symptoms. The implication here is that resilience is in some way related to an individual's ability to generate positive emotion.

In conclusion, Block's construct of ego-resiliency suggests trait like generalizability across circumstances and stability across time. Furthermore he defines ego-resiliency as central to normative, adaptive psychological functioning.

References

Block, J. (1950). An experimental investigation of the construct of ego-control. Unpublished Doctoral Dissertation, Stanford University, Stanford, CA.

Block, J. H. (1951). An experimental study of a topological representation of ego-structure. Unpublished Doctoral Dissertation, Stanford University, Stanford, CA.

Block, J. (1965). *The challenge of response sets: Unconfounding measuring, acquiescence and social desirability in the MMPI*. New York: Irvington.

Block, J. (1989). A revised Ego-Resiliency scale. Unpublished instrument. Department of Psychology, University of California, Berkeley.

Block, J. (2002). *Personality as an affect-processing system*. Mahwah, NJ: Erlbaum.

Block, J. H., & Block, J. (1971). *Lives through time*. Berkeley, CA: Bancroft.

Block, J. H., & Block, J. (1980). The role of ego-control and ego-resiliency in the organization of behavior. In W. A. Collins (Ed.), *Development of cognition, affect, and social relations: The Minnesota symposia on child psychology* (Vol. 13). Hillsdale, NJ: Erlbaum.

Block, J., & Kremen, A. M. (1996). IQ and ego-resiliency: Conceptual and empirical connections and separateness. *Journal of Personality and Social Psychology, 70*, 349–361.

Fredrickson, B., Tugade, M., Waugh, C. E., & Larkin, G. R. (2003). What good are positive emotions in crises? A prospective study of resilience and emotions following the terrorist attacks on the United States on September 11th, 2001. *Journal of Personality and Social Psychology, 84*(2), 365–376.

Funder, D. C., & Block, J. (1989). The role of ego-control, ego-resiliency, and IQ in delay of gratification in adolescence. *Journal of Personality and Social Psychology, 57*, 1041–1050.

Gough, H. G. (1956). *California Psychological Inventory administrator's guide*. Palo Alto, CA: Consulting Psychologists Press.

Hathaway, R. S., & McKinley, J. V. (1951). *Manual for the Minnesota Multiple Personality Inventory*. New York: Psychological.

Klohnen, E. C. (1996). Conceptual analysis and measurement of the construct of ego-resiliency. *Journal of Personality and Social Psychology, 70*, 1067–1079.

Ong, A. D., Bergeman, C. S., Bisconti, T. L., & Wallace, K. A. (2006). Psychological resilience, positive emotions, and successful adaptation to stress in later life. *Journal of Personality and Social Psychology, 91*(4), 730–749.

Tugade, M. M., & Fredrickson, B. L. (2004). Resilient individuals use positive emotions to bounce back from negative emotional experiences. *Journal of Personality and Social Psychology, 86*, 320–333.

Waugh, C. E., Fredrickson, B. L., & Taylor, S. F. (2008). Adapting to life"s slings and arrows: Individual differences in resilience when recovering from an anticipated threat. *Journal of Research in Personality, 42*, 1031–1046.

Perceived Self-Efficacy and its Relationship to Resilience

10

Ralf Schwarzer and Lisa Marie Warner

Conceptual Issues

The construct of perceived self-efficacy is the belief that one can perform novel or difficult tasks and attain desired outcomes, as spelled out in the Social Cognitive Theory (Bandura, 1997). This "can do"-cognition reflects a sense of control over one's environment and an optimistic belief of being able to alter challenging environmental demands by means of one's own behavior. Hence, it represents a self-confident view of one's capability to deal with certain stressors in life.

Self-efficacy makes a difference in how people feel, think, and act. Individuals with high levels of perceived self-efficacy trust their own abilities in the face of adversity, tend to conceptualize problems as challenges rather than as threats or uncontrollable situations, experience less negative emotional arousal in demanding tasks, think in self-enhancing ways, motivate themselves, and show perseverance when confronted with difficult situations (Bandura, 1997; Luszczynska, Gutiérrez-Doña, & Schwarzer, 2005).

In contrast, persons with low perceived self-efficacy tend to experience self-doubt and anxiety when they encounter environmental demands. They perceive demanding tasks to be threatening, avoid difficult situations, tend to cope less functionally with stressors, and are more likely to think in self-debilitating ways because they tend to take more responsibility for their failure than for their success. Also, they are more vulnerable to stress and depression (Bandura, 1997). This may result in a self-manifesting mechanism: Because persons high in self-efficacy tend to set themselves more ambitious goals and show more effort and persistence when facing difficulties, they develop more opportunities for experiencing mastery (Bandura, 1995). Mastery experience, in turn, increases self-efficacy beliefs. This reciprocal relationship between self-efficacy and behavior makes the maintenance or even increase in self-efficacy beliefs in highly self-efficacious individuals more likely. On the other hand, low self-efficacious persons tend to experience failure more often, as they invest less effort and give up more easily when they encounter difficulties. Combined with a self-debilitating attribution style, low self-efficacious individuals therefore tend to be more affected by failures (Jerusalem & Schwarzer, 1992). As Bandura (1995) stated "Disbelief in one's capabilities creates its own behavioral validation" (p. 4).

Self-Efficacy and Resilience

Self-efficacy not only affects human lives in highly stressful situations but also helps one to develop motivation and envision challenging

R. Schwarzer, Ph.D. (✉) • L.M. Warner, Ph.D.
Freie Universität Berlin Psychology,
Habelschwerdter Allee 45, Berlin, 14195, Germany
e-mail: ralf.schwarzer@fu-berlin.de;
lisa.warner@fu-berlin.de

S. Prince-Embury and D.H. Saklofske (eds.), *Resilience in Children, Adolescents, and Adults: Translating Research into Practice*, The Springer Series on Human Exceptionality,
DOI 10.1007/978-1-4614-4939-3_10, © Springer Science+Business Media New York 2013

goals in life. Thus, it influences private and professional decision-making throughout the course of one's life (Betz & Klein, 1996; Markman, Balkin, & Baron, 2002). Resilience, on the other hand, is mainly defined by coping adaptively with traumatic stressors. Hence, it is closely linked to the occurrence of demanding situations that one has to overcome. Resilient persons bend without breaking, and they quickly rebound from adversity, which reflects the "ordinary magic" of human adaptive systems (Masten, 2001). The concept of resilience is a multifaceted construct that also comprises several other personal resources, such as self-esteem, optimism, coping strategies, or good social relations (Condly, 2006). Resilience is usually understood as the ability to resist or bounce back from adversity (Bonanno, Brewin, Kaniasty, & La Greca, 2010; Tedeschi & Calhoun, 1995). Thus, resilience refers to rapidly returning to baseline functioning after exposure to trauma. Hence, one cannot be resilient if there is no stressor. However, self-efficacy can be present if the stressor has not yet happened or will not occur at all, such as when an individual thinks about and plans her or his future without having any specific challenges to fear (Berry & West, 1993). Therefore, high self-efficacy beliefs can have a positive impact on motivational processes even if specific stressors are absent. Being self-efficacious may, however, also be helpful to show resilience in the face of adversity. By activating affective, motivational, and behavioral mechanisms in taxing situations, self-efficacy beliefs can promote resilience. Self-efficacy therefore has sometimes been conceptualized as one component of resilience and posttraumatic growth (Rutter, 1987; Tedeschi & Calhoun, 1995; Werner, 1982).

The opposite is posttraumatic stress disorder (PTSD) that is negatively related to self-efficacy. As Luszczynska, Benight, and Cieslak (2009) write "Cross-sectional studies suggest medium to large effects of self-efficacy on general distress, severity and frequency of PTSD symptoms (weighted r values range from –0.36 to –77), whereas longitudinal studies indicate large effects on general distress and PTSD symptom severity (weighted r values range: –0.55 to –0.62)" (p. 51). Empirically, general self-efficacy correlates moderately to highly with other components of resilience (Hinz, Schumacher, Albani, Schmid, & Brähler, 2006). Resilience is hence empirically closely related to self-efficacy. However, theoretically it can be distinguished from self-efficacy beliefs because self-efficacy may be present even in the absence of stressors, as self-efficacy beliefs drive persons to strive proactively for goals and mold their own future (Diehl, Semegon, & Schwarzer, 2006).

Other Concepts Distinct from Self-Efficacy Beliefs

Self-efficacy beliefs are of a *prospective* and *operative* nature. Perceived self-efficacy can be characterized as competence-based, prospective, and action-related, as opposed to similar constructs that share only part of this portrayal (Bandura, 1997; Schwarzer, Boehmer, Luszczynska, Mohamed, & Knoll, 2005).

Self-efficacy beliefs are not mere *ability*, as an individual might be convinced that he or she is incapable to achieve certain outcomes, even though others would judge this person to be able of succeeding. For example, there are persons who think that certain actions are not within their scope, and thus they never try, even though they might not perform as badly as they think, for example, when high-school dropouts prevent themselves from attaining higher education, even though they would be capable of it. On the other hand, persons might also believe that they possess everything that is necessary to finish a marathon, even though their current fitness level makes it less than likely that an actual effort would be successful. However, in this example we would rather speak of positive illusions or unrealistic optimism than self-efficacy beliefs.

Self-efficacy is not *optimism*, as optimism is the belief that the future will be positive by any means. Optimism includes all kinds of causes, external and internal, and even chance. Self-efficacy, however, is the belief in being able to control and shape one's personal future and attain desired outcomes due to one's own actions and decisions (Bandura, 1997). Even though the empirical association between general self-efficacy and dispositional optimism is around $r=0.60$, optimism is theoretically the broader construct under which optimistic self-beliefs, such as self-efficacy, can be subsumed (Schwarzer, 1994). To continue with the marathon example, a highly or even unrealistically optimistic person might believe to be able to run a marathon without training, whereas a self-efficacious person would consider the necessity and his or her ability to train hard, for example in saying "I am confident that I can train hard enough to be able to finish a marathon race."

Moreover, self-efficacy is not the same as the expectation of certain outcomes, as *outcome expectancies* refer to the perception of the possible consequences of one's own acts (e.g., the acknowledgement by peers after having finished a marathon), whereas perceived self-efficacy pertains to personal *control* over one's own acts to achieve future outcomes (Bandura, 1992; Maddux, 1995).

The constructs of self-efficacy and *self-concept* are distinguishable, as individuals' self-concepts are higher-order constructs that not only contain the belief in being able to accomplish goals with one's own action, but they contain also diverse attributes and attitudes towards oneself. This includes an ideal self and the disparity of actual and ideal self, which makes the self-concept a more complex construct than self-efficacy. One of those components might be "I am a marathon runner," or "I am a couch potato," which can be highly salient for a person. However, another person might define his or her self-worth not through participating in sports or not, but for example by being a volunteer or a manager, or having a sense of humor. Comparative analyses found self-efficacy to be a better predictor of behavior than an individual's self-concept (Pajares & Kranzler, 1995). The reason is that self-efficacy is not only competence-based but is also operative (behavioral) and prospective.

Further, self-efficacy is not equivalent to the concept of *locus of control*, as locus of control refers to personal as well as environmental causes for an outcome. The construct of locus of control includes *external* causes for an outcome, such as luck, or task difficulty. In addition, it incorporates *internal* locus of control, such as ability or effort, which is closely related to self-efficacy beliefs. Having an internal locus of control, however, is not equivalent to being self-efficacious, as persons who believe that the cause of a certain outcome is inherent within themselves do not necessarily believe that they can change this internal factor (Condly, 2006). An example for internal and external locus of control would be "Finishing a marathon depends on the runner's training status (internal)/the race conditions (external)."

Self-efficacy is not *self-esteem*, as self-efficacy refers to an individual's evaluation of personal capabilities, whereas self-esteem reflects the person's overall judgment about him- or herself, including self-worth. Hence, self-esteem has an emotional connotation, such as "I have good characteristics," or "I am proud of myself for being so active in sports."

Autonomy is a fundamental and universal psychological need that may be defined primarily as the *experience of choice* and the ability to pursue activities that are intrinsically motivated (Deci & Ryan, 2008). To stay with our example, an item to assess autonomy might read "It is my free decision whether I want to train for and run a marathon 1 day." Usually studies find high correlations between trait autonomy and self-efficacy in specific domains (Vieira & Grantham, 2011). However, when autonomy is tested in relation to general self-efficacy, the two constructs appear to have discriminant validity (Warner et al., 2011).

Perceived behavioral control is conceptually very close to self-efficacy. Both concepts refer to individuals' beliefs in being able to attain certain outcomes. The difference between them is hard to understand, but the item phrasing is typically a bit different, as perceived behavioral control items mostly incorporate a statement about the *easiness* or *difficulty*, such as "*It is easy/difficult* for me to…," whereas self-efficacy items rather incorporate the "can-do"-component. Hence, they most likely start with an expression such as "I am sure that *I can do*…" A typical perceived behavioral control item would therefore be "It is *easy/difficult* for me to finish a marathon race." Even though some researchers see the two constructs as being the same (e.g., Fishbein & Cappella, 2006), others prefer to distinguish them (e.g., Ajzen, 2002).

General Self-Efficacy

According to Bandura (1997), self-efficacy beliefs can be classified into three dimensions: (a) level, (b) strength, and (c) generality. The *level* dimension refers to the difficulty of the tasks. For easy tasks with no barriers and difficulties, every person should have a similarly high level of self-efficacy. Varying demands and task difficulty, however, require varying levels of self-efficacy. The dimension of *strength* refers to how robust the self-efficacy beliefs are. Beliefs that are low in strength are easily diminished by failures to attain the desired outcome by means of own efforts. *Generality* of self-efficacy beliefs is low if an individual believes to be capable only in distinct situations and for very few behaviors. Self-efficacy has long been understood as being task- or domain-specific. Individuals were assumed to have more or less firm self-beliefs in different tasks or particular domains and specific situations, such as being able to succeed in a math test or being good at school in general. Bandura prefers this task and domain-specific approach to measure self-efficacy, as this reflects his initial conceptualization of the construct (Bandura, 1997). Along this line, specifically assessed self-efficacy beliefs were also found to predict specific outcomes best (Bandura, 1997; Schwarzer & Jerusalem, 1995a). Nonetheless, some researchers argue that it is of great interest to detect regularities and consistent patterns in human behaviors over a broad range of situations (Ajzen, 1988). For example, domain-specific measure of perceived self-efficacy may be useful to investigate coping with spider phobia or math problems. In contrast, if trait anxiety, depression, or similar global constructs are to be predicted, general constructs seem to be more adequate to serve as predictors.

Furthermore, both theoretical consideration and empirical research suggest that experiencing failure and success in various domains of life can generalize to a global perception of an individual's ability to deal with "life in general" (Wallston, Wallston, Smith, & Dobbins, 1987). Therefore, some researchers conceptualize self-efficacy as a more general construct (Harter, 1978; Schwarzer & Jerusalem, 1995a; Shelton, 1990; Sherer et al., 1982). The construct of general self-efficacy is assumed to consist of a global confidence in one's coping ability across a wide range of demanding or novel situations. Some studies found that using general measures of self-efficacy beliefs results in reduced predictive power of self-efficacy beliefs for certain outcomes (Earley & Lituchy, 1991; Pajares & Miller, 1995). Assessing global measures of self-efficacy, however, is very useful in some contexts, for example if multiple health behaviors (Luszczynska, Gibbons, Piko, & Teközel, 2004), multiple chronic diseases (Warner et al., 2011), various parenting tasks (Coleman & Karraker, 1998), or adolescents' adaptability to traumatizing experiences (Cheever & Hardin, 1999) are the target of research. An example for the use of general self-efficacy is a study on East Germans who migrated to the West when the Berlin wall came down: Over a 2-year observation period, initial general self-efficacy turned out to be the best single predictor of overall adjustment, as assessed by a number of outcomes, such as employment status, social integration, physical health, and subjective well-being (Schwarzer, Hahn, & Schröder, 1994; Schwarzer & Jerusalem, 1995b). In that case, the unique research context did not allow a closer examination of a variety of domain-specific coping outcomes with corresponding specific measures of self-efficacy, although this would have been desirable. General self-efficacy was hence defined as a stable sense to master a stressful or challenging situation, relevant for all kinds of behavioral domains (Schwarzer & Jerusalem, 1995a). It is further typically understood as encompassing all self-efficacy beliefs that people build up by experience over their entire life history (Watt & Martin, 1994).

Measurement of General Self-Efficacy

Scale Construction

The General Self-Efficacy scale was developed by Jerusalem and Schwarzer in 1978 in its original 20-item version, and it was first applied from 1979 to 1981 in a panel study with thousands of high-school students. This created the psychometric basis for the ten-item version (Jerusalem & Schwarzer, 1986; Schwarzer & Jerusalem, 1995a, 1999). The scale aims to assess a broad and stable sense of personal competence to deal effectively with a variety of stressful situations. Based on the German and English versions of the scale, bilingual native speakers translated and adapted the ten-item version to their respective languages (Scholz, Doña, Sud, & Schwarzer, 2002). The adaptations followed the "group consensus model" with several bilingual translators participating. The procedure included back translations and group discussions (Luszczynska et al., 2005). The items are answered via self-rating on a four-point scale. The responses are summed up to yield the final composite score, with a range from 10 to 40. The scale is designed for the adult population, including adolescents at least 12 years old.

Reliability

In samples from 25 nations, Cronbach's alphas ranged from 0.75 to 0.91, with a mean of 0.86 (Scholz et al., 2002). Exploratory as well as confirmatory factor analysis repeatedly confirmed the unidimensionality (Hinz et al., 2006; Leganger, Kraft, & Roysamb, 2000; Scherbaum, Cohen-Charash, & Kern, 2006; Scholz et al., 2002; Schwarzer, Bäßler, Kwiatek, Schröder, & Zhang, 1997). Test–retest reliability ranged between 0.47 and 0.75 in previous studies (Schwarzer, Mueller, & Greenglass, 1999). Item response analyses also showed that the scale discriminates well between individuals with high and low self-efficacy (Scherbaum et al., 2006).

Validity

The General Self-Efficacy Scale proved valid in terms of convergent and discriminant validity. For example, it correlated positively with self-esteem, dispositional optimism, favorable emotions, and work satisfaction (Luszczynska et al., 2005). Negative associations were found with depression, anxiety, stress, burnout, health complaints, anxiety, and physical symptoms (Hinz et al., 2006; Luszczynska et al., 2005; Schwarzer et al., 1999). Some studies find men to report higher levels of general self-efficacy than women (Hinz et al., 2006; Leganger et al., 2000; Schwarzer et al., 1999), and there is some empirical evidence that general self-efficacy beliefs slowly decrease with age (Hinz et al., 2006).

Norms

In most studies, the sum score lay around 29, with a standard deviation of 4. In addition, norms (*T* scores) were developed, based on a representative sample of 2,019 Germans between the age of 16 and 95 (Hinz et al., 2006).

Applicability

The General Self-Efficacy Scale could be used as an enhancement for measures of domain-specific self-efficacy beliefs. In addition to assessing general self-efficacy, further domain-specific assessments of self-efficacy should be appropriately tailored to the research questions (Samoocha, Bruinvels, Elbers, Anema, & van der Beek, 2010).

Dissemination

The General Self-Efficacy Scale is available free of charge in 33 languages on the internet at http://userpage.fu-berlin.de/~health/selfscal.htm. Raw data from 18,000 participants of different nations are available at http://userpage.fu-berlin.de/~health/world_24nations_25nov2006.sav. Recently, a five-item short form for survey studies has also been developed (Warner et al., 2011).

Research on General Self-Efficacy and How it Relates to Resilience in Children, Adolescents, and Adults

According to theory and research, self-efficacy makes a difference in how people think, feel, and act (Bandura, 1997). It has become a key variable in clinical, educational, social, developmental, health, and personality psychology (Bandura, 1997; Maddux, 1995; Schwarzer, 1992). In the following, some examples are given to illustrate how a general sense of efficacy helps children, adolescents, and adults overcome stressful situations without suffering long-lasting harm—hence, how a general sense of self-efficacy helps people to be resilient.

Children

Few studies have tested general self-efficacy in children below the age of 12 because they do not fall into the application range of the scale. The few studies that nevertheless focused on general self-efficacy in children found that schoolchildren (12–14 years of age), who reported higher general self-efficacy also reported lower depressive symptoms and dysfunctional thoughts (Pössel, Baldus, Horn, Groen, & Hautzinger, 2005) and more physical as well as emotional well-being (Kvarme, Haraldstad, Helseth, Sørum, & Natvig, 2009). First interventions to promote a general sense of self-efficacy were successful among schoolgirls, however not among schoolboys (Kvarme et al., 2010).

Adolescents

General Self-Efficacy and the Impact of Traumatization

Cheever and Hardin (1999) interviewed 1,427 freshmen and sophomores from three South Carolina high schools to find out whether during the previous year they were exposed to violent traumatizing experiences, such as physical assault, rape, or being held up with a weapon, or to nonviolent traumatic experiences, such as repeating a school grade, changing to a new school, or experiencing a natural disaster. The researchers found that higher levels of general self-efficacy were accompanied by lower self-reported health problems in this population.

General Self-Efficacy and Socioeconomic Status

Chinese college students who had a low socioeconomic status benefited from being high in general self-efficacy in terms of life satisfaction and subjective well-being (Tong & Song, 2004). In a sample of underprivileged rural African-American college students, general self-efficacy also related to future orientation, a construct that helps to explain the further development of youth (Kerpelman & Mosher, 2004).

General Self-Efficacy and Mental Health

Female high-school students with low levels of general self-efficacy were found to be at higher risk for developing eating disorders (Bennett, Spoth, & Borgen, 1991). An intervention to increase general self-efficacy also appeared to reduce students' depressive symptoms within the next 3 months (Pössel et al., 2005). Among Norwegian adolescents, general self-efficacy also correlated with life satisfaction and positive affect (Leganger et al., 2000).

General Self-Efficacy and Academic Performance

Students with high levels of general self-efficacy reported that they could self-regulate their attention better, work harder, monitor their efforts, and get better grades in school (Luszczynska et al., 2005; Luszczynska, Scholz, & Schwarzer, 2005; Usher & Pajares, 2008). Self-efficacious students also had lower levels of procrastination (Tuckman, 1991) and less state anxiety (Endler, Speer, Johnson, & Flett, 2001) and trait anxiety (Schneider et al., 2009). Self-efficacy beliefs also showed a generalization due to a cognitive–behavioral coping skills training to reduce test-anxiety in college students (Smith, 1989). The training helped reduce trait and state test anxiety, leading to higher academic performance in the training group compared to a waiting-list control group. It also enhanced specific self-efficacy beliefs towards test-anxiety management and academic performance. The training group further reported increases in a trait measure of general self-efficacy (Smith, 1989). Along with others studies, the latter study provides evidence that general self-efficacy beliefs are amenable to interventions in students (Dunlap, 2005; Smith, 1989).

Adults

General Self-Efficacy and Somatic Symptoms

Cancer patients reported fewer depressive symptoms and fatigue and better emotional, social, and cognitive functioning when they had a high level of self-efficacy (Luszczynska et al., 2005). Lower levels of depression were also found in patients with cardiovascular disease and arthritis. And those with gastrointestinal diseases reported lower levels of anxiety when they scored high on the General Self-Efficacy Scale (Barlow, Williams, & Wright, 1996; Luszczynska et al., 2005). In addition, ill persons had more positive illness representations when they were highly self-efficacious (Lau-Walker, 2006). Older low-functioning adults were found to have a lower increase in disabilities when they reported higher general self-efficacy earlier on (Kempen, Sonderen, & Ormel, 1999). In patients with musculoskeletal pain, general self-efficacy buffered the effect of pain on quality of life (Taylor, Dean, & Siegert, 2006).

General Self-Efficacy and Coping with Chronic Disease

Among cases of gastrointestinal disease, general self-efficacy was related to a less frequent use of passive coping strategies and to a more frequent use of active coping with pain (Luszczynska et al., 2005). Among patients with cancer, those who were high in general self-efficacy reported more frequently active coping, planning, positive reframing, humor, fighting spirit, and information seeking (Luszczynska et al., 2005). Those, who were low in general self-efficacy, however, reported use of maladaptive coping strategies, such as self-blame or behavioral disengagement more frequently (Luszczynska et al., 2005). Similarly, self-efficacious patients with rheumatoid arthritis used active pain coping strategies more often, whereas patients with lower self-efficacy were more likely to use passive coping strategies, which predicted poorer health outcomes after a 6-month period (Brown & Nicassio, 1987).

General Self-Efficacy and Mental Symptoms

Persons with psychological impairments had less state and trait anxiety, depression, negative affectivity, stress, and worries when they were high in general self-efficacy (Rimm & Jerusalem, 1999). For example, in patients with schizophrenia, general self-efficacy related to lower levels of depressive symptoms and maladaptive coping and higher quality of life (Vauth, Kleim, Wirtz, & Corrigan, 2007).

General Self-Efficacy and Health Behaviors

General self-efficacy predicts problematic drinking in clinical drinkers (Oei, Hasking, & Phillips, 2007) and also other health behaviors, such as smoking, physical activity, and a healthy diet (Luszczynska et al., 2005). In addition, women who were low in general self-efficacy were found to be at risk for developing eating disorders, such as binge eating or bulimia (Bardone, Perez, Abramson, & Joiner, 2003). Scoring high on general self-efficacy also was beneficial for physical health in patients with arthritis, multiple sclerosis, and diabetes (Fournier, de Ridder, & Bensing, 2002).

Health behaviors can be altered by self-efficacy interventions. For example, encouraging adults to believe that they have control about genetic testing led to increases in specific self-efficacy beliefs, which affected general self-efficacy beliefs as well (Hendy, Lyons, & Breakwell, 2006). Increasing self-efficacy for physical activity also resulted in more exercise (Ashford, Edmunds, & French, 2010). A higher sense of general self-efficacy even enhanced the likelihood that adults with physical disabilities engaged in health-promoting behaviors (Stuifbergen & Becker, 1994). Interventionists in this field should, however, keep in mind that we can have too much of a good thing: There is only little evidence as yet, but Haaga and Stewart (1992) report that participants with high efficacy did not recover very well from smoking lapses compared to those with moderate efficacy. Perceived self-efficacy hence has to be realistic to generate health motivation and should be optimistic, while at the same time not exceeding a certain limit, as unrealistic optimism leads to disappointment or harm.

General Self-Efficacy in Work Settings

Having high levels of general self-efficacy may also protect against stress at work. Studies that investigated workers in the information technology business as well as Chinese, German, and Syrian teachers found that they were all less likely to report symptoms of job burnout when they were high in general self-efficacy (Salanova, Peiró, & Schaufeli, 2002; Schwarzer & Hallum, 2008; Tang, Au, Schwarzer, & Schmitz, 2001). Workers in Costa Rica and Germany also reported higher job satisfaction when they were high in general self-efficacy (Luszczynska et al., 2005).

Self-efficacious patients with traumatic brain injury adjusted better to returning to work and had higher quality of life (Tsaousides et al., 2009). Similarly, general self-efficacy consistently predicted return to work in persons who had been on long-term sick leave (Brouwer, Reneman, Bültmann, van der Klink, & Groothoff, 2010). Helping low self-efficacious individuals to boost their belief in competence also increases the likelihood of reentering the job market (Eden & Aviram, 1993).

Furthermore, persons high in general self-efficacy were found to be more inclined to open up a new business than those low in self-efficacy (Markman et al., 2002).

Implications for Research and Practice

The positive effects of general self-efficacy beliefs on coping with various stressors and on proactive preparation for potential stressors make the construct of self-efficacy valuable for research on resilience. For children, much research on resilience has been conducted but little on general self-efficacy. This construct has been applied more intensively to adults, as the General Self-Efficacy Scale was not designed for populations younger than 12 years. Even though there are domain-specific self-efficacy scales for children, such as the Social Self-Efficacy Scale (the degree to which a child believes he or she could perform social tasks), or measures that combine different areas, such as school, family, and peer self-efficacy (Bradley & Corwyn, 2004; Ollendick & Schmidt, 1987), the development of a general self-efficacy scale for children could facilitate future research in this area.

In practice, the construct of perceived self-efficacy is very useful, as it is amenable to interventions. Also, it is clear which factors have to be considered in self-efficacy interventions to make them work. According to Bandura (1997), self-efficacy is generated by four sources: mastery experience, vicarious experience, verbal persuasion, and somatic and affective states.

Mastery experiences are postulated as being "the most effective source of efficacy information because they provide the most authentic evidence of whether one can master whatever it takes to succeed" (Bandura, 1997, p. 80). Building on operant conditioning, Bandura (1997) assumes that previous success fosters self-efficacy beliefs, as it represents desired outcomes and thereby enhances the likelihood of a certain behavior. On the other hand, failure undermines self-efficacy beliefs because it represents undesired outcomes (Bandura, 1997). However, one's subjective attributions of what caused success or failure can alter this paradigm: Failure, if attributed to low effort or insurmountable barriers to achievement, can actually enhance self-efficacy. Likewise, success, if attributed to chance or help from others, can diminish self-efficacy (Leganger et al., 2000). Self-efficacy for a particular behavior therefore not only predicts future behavior, but it is also influenced by one's interpretations of past behavior (Orsega-Smith, Payne, Mowen, Ho, & Godbey, 2007).

Vicarious experience, such as seeing others perform a behavior and observing the consequences of their actions, is also assumed to increase peoples' beliefs in their own capability to master similar tasks with comparable results (Bandura, 1997). Vicarious experience is a powerful source of self-efficacy beliefs because it provides the observer with strategies and techniques needed to attain desired goals or to overcome certain stressors (Wise & Trunnell, 2001).

Verbal or social persuasion is another source of self-efficacy belief according to the Social Cognitive Theory (Bandura, 1997). Persuasion is seen as someone else expressing faith in the capabilities of an individual (Bandura, 1997).

Perceptions of *somatic* and *affective states* are assumed to constitute self-efficacy beliefs as well. In general, people tend to read physiological signs, such as arousal or tension, as a sign of being unprepared for a task or of poor performance (Wood & Bandura, 1989). Hence, people are more likely to feel competent if they do not experience aversive arousal (Conger & Kanungo, 1988). According to Bandura, moderate levels of arousal are most adaptive when people face difficult tasks, as too low and too high arousal may impede performance (Bandura, 1997).

Most interventions that seek to promote self-efficacy beliefs prompt some of these sources with regard to task- or domain-specific self-efficacy beliefs (Ashford et al., 2010; Usher & Pajares, 2008). However, it is unrealistic to prepare children, adolescents, and even adults for the various traumatizing experiences they may have to deal with in life. A realistic option to make people more resilient is to promote a general sense of self-efficacy, which may help prepare for highly stressful and novel situations. It would also allow them to use adaptive coping strategies and endure such situations without suffering too much harm. Hence, boosting a general sense of self-efficacy is of special importance to render individuals resilient in the face of severe life stressors.

References

Ajzen, I. (1988). *Attitudes, personality and behaviour*. Milton Keynes: England Open University Press.

Ajzen, I. (2002). Perceived behavioral control, self-efficacy, locus of control, and the theory of planned behavior. *Journal of Applied Social Psychology, 32*(4), 665–683.

Ashford, S., Edmunds, J., & French, D. P. (2010). What is the best way to change self-efficacy to promote lifestyle and recreational physical activity? A systematic review with meta-analysis. *British Journal of Health Psychology, 15*(2), 265–288.

Bandura, A. (1992). Self-efficacy mechanism in psychobiologic functioning. In R. Schwarzer (Ed.), *Self-efficacy: Thought control of action* (pp. 355–394). Washington, DC: Hemisphere.

Bandura, A. (1995). Exercise of personal and collective efficacy in changing societies. In A. Bandura (Ed.), *Self-efficacy in changing societies* (pp. 1–45). New York: Cambridge University Press.

Bandura, A. (1997). *Self-efficacy: The exercise of control*. New York: Freeman.

Bardone, A. M., Perez, M., Abramson, L. Y., & Joiner, T. E. (2003). Self-competence and self-liking in the prediction of change in bulimic symptoms. *International Journal of Eating Disorders, 34*(3), 361–369.

Barlow, J. H., Williams, B., & Wright, C. (1996). The general self-efficacy scale in people with arthritis. *Arthritis Care and Research, 9*(3), 189–196.

Bennett, N. A. M., Spoth, R. L., & Borgen, F. H. (1991). Bulimic symptoms in high school females: Prevalence and relationship with multiple measures of psychological health. *Journal of Community Psychology, 19*(1), 13–28.

Berry, J. M., & West, R. L. (1993). Cognitive self-efficacy in relation to personal mastery and goal setting across the life span. *International Journal of Behavioral Development, 16*(2), 351–379.

Betz, N. E., & Klein, K. L. (1996). Relationships among measures of career self-efficacy, general self-efficacy, and global self-esteem. *Journal of Career Assessment, 4*(3), 285–298.

Bonanno, G. A., Brewin, C. R., Kaniasty, K., & La Greca, A. M. (2010). Weighing the costs of disaster: Consequences, risks, and resilience in individuals, families, and communities. *Psychological Science in the Public Interest, 11*, 1–49.

Bradley, R. H., & Corwyn, R. F. (2004). Life satisfaction among European American, African American, Chinese American, Mexican American, and Dominican American adolescents. *International Journal of Behavioral Development, 28*(5), 385–400.

Brouwer, S., Reneman, M. F., Bültmann, U., van der Klink, J. J. L., & Groothoff, J. W. (2010). A prospective study of return to work across health conditions: Perceived work attitude, self-efficacy and perceived social support. *Journal of Occupational Rehabilitation, 20*(1), 104–112.

Brown, G. K., & Nicassio, P. M. (1987). Development of a questionnaire for the assessment of active and passive coping strategies in chronic pain patients. *Pain, 31*(1), 53–64.

Cheever, K. H., & Hardin, S. B. (1999). Effects of traumatic events, social support, and self-efficacy on adolescents' self-health assessments. *Western Journal of Nursing Research, 21*(5), 673–684.

Coleman, P. K., & Karraker, K. H. (1998). Self-efficacy and parenting quality: Findings and future applications. *Developmental Review, 18*(1), 47–85.

Condly, S. J. (2006). Resilience in children: A review of literature with implications for education. *Urban Education, 41*(3), 211–236.
Conger, J. A., & Kanungo, R. N. (1988). The empowerment process: Integrating theory and practice. *Academy of Management Review, 13*(3), 471.
Deci, E. L., & Ryan, R. M. (2008). Hedonia, eudaimonia, and well-being: An introduction. *Journal of Happiness Studies, 9*(1), 1–11.
Diehl, M., Semegon, A. B., & Schwarzer, R. (2006). Assessing attention control in goal pursuit: A component of dispositional self-regulation. *Journal of Personality Assessment, 86*(3), 306–317.
Dunlap, J. C. (2005). Problem-based learning and self-efficacy: How a capstone course prepares students for a profession. *Educational Technology Research and Development, 53*(1), 65–85.
Earley, P. C., & Lituchy, T. R. (1991). Delineating goal and efficacy effects: A test of three models. *Journal of Applied Psychology, 76*(1), 81–98.
Eden, D., & Aviram, A. (1993). Self-efficacy training to speed reemployment: Helping people to help themselves. *The Journal of Applied Psychology, 78*(3), 352–360.
Endler, N. S., Speer, R. L., Johnson, J. M., & Flett, G. L. (2001). General self-efficacy and control in relation to anxiety and cognitive performance. *Current Psychology, 20*(1), 36–52.
Fishbein, M., & Cappella, J. N. (2006). The role of theory in developing effective health communications. *Journal of Communication, 56*(Suppl 1), S1–S17.
Fournier, M., de Ridder, D., & Bensing, J. (2002). Optimism and adaptation to chronic disease: The role of optimism in relation to self-care options of type 1 diabetes mellitus, rheumatoid arthritis and multiple sclerosis. *British Journal of Health Psychology, 7*(4), 409–432.
Haaga, D. A., & Stewart, B. L. (1992). Self-efficacy for recovery from a lapse after smoking cessation. *Journal of Consulting and Clinical Psychology, 60*(1), 24–28.
Harter, S. (1978). Effectance motivation reconsidered: Toward a developmental model. *Human Development, 21*(1), 34–64.
Hendy, J., Lyons, E., & Breakwell, G. M. (2006). Genetic testing and the relationship between specific and general self-efficacy. *British Journal of Health Psychology, 11*(Pt 2), 221–233.
Hinz, A., Schumacher, J., Albani, C., Schmid, G., & Brähler, E. (2006). Bevölkerungsrepräsentative Normierung der Skala zur Allgemeinen Selbstwirksamkeitserwartung [Population-representative norm for the general self-efficacy scale]. *Diagnostica, 52*(1), 26–32.
Jerusalem, M., & Schwarzer, R. (1986). Selbstwirksamkeit [Self-efficacy]. In R. Schwarzer (Ed.), *Skalen zur Befindlichkeit und Persönlichkeit [Scales to assess well-being and personality]* (pp. 15–28). Berlin: Institut für Psychologie, Freie Universität.
Jerusalem, M., & Schwarzer, R. (1992). Self-efficacy as a resource factor in stress appraisal processes. In R. Schwarzer (Ed.), *Self-efficacy: Thought control of action* (pp. 195–213). Washington, DC: Hemisphere.
Kempen, G. I. J. M., Sonderen, E. V., & Ormel, J. (1999). The impact of psychological attributes on changes in disability among low-functioning older persons. *The Journals of Gerontology Series B: Psychological Sciences and Social Sciences, 54B*(1), P23–P29.
Kerpelman, J. L., & Mosher, L. S. (2004). Rural African American adolescents' future orientation: The importance of self-efficacy, control and responsibility, and identity development. *Identity: An International Journal of Theory and Research, 4*(2), 187–208.
Kvarme, L. G., Haraldstad, K., Helseth, S., Sørum, R., & Natvig, G. K. (2009). Associations between general self-efficacy and health-related quality of life among 12-13-year-old school children: A cross-sectional survey. *Health and Quality of Life Outcomes, 7*, 85.
Kvarme, L. G., Helseth, S., Sørum, R., Luth-Hansen, V., Haugland, S., & Natvig, G. K. (2010). The effect of a solution-focused approach to improve self-efficacy in socially withdrawn school children: A non-randomized controlled trial. *International Journal of Nursing Studies, 47*(11), 1389–1396.
Lau-Walker, M. (2006). Predicting self-efficacy using illness perception components: A patient survey. *British Journal of Health Psychology, 11*(4), 643–661.
Leganger, A., Kraft, P., & Roysamb, E. (2000). Perceived self-efficacy in health behaviour research: Conceptualisation, measurement and correlates. *Psychology and Health, 15*(1), 51.
Luszczynska, A., Benight, C. C., & Cieslak, R. (2009). Self-efficacy and health-related outcomes of collective trauma: A systematic review. *European Psychologist, 14*, 51–62. doi:10.1027/1016-9040.14.1.51.
Luszczynska, A., Gibbons, F. X., Piko, B., & Teközel, M. (2004). Self-regulatory cognitions, social comparison, perceived peers' behaviors as predictors of nutrition and physical activity: A comparison among adolescents in Hungary, Poland, Turkey, and USA. *Psychology and Health, 19*(5), 577–593.
Luszczynska, A., Gutiérrez-Doña, B., & Schwarzer, R. (2005). General self-efficacy in various domains of human functioning: Evidence from five countries. *International Journal of Psychology, 40*(2), 80–89.
Luszczynska, A., Scholz, U., & Schwarzer, R. (2005). The general self-efficacy scale: Multicultural validation studies. *Journal of Psychology, 139*(5), 439–457.
Maddux, J. E. (1995). *Self-efficacy, adaptation, and adjustment: Theory, research, and application*. New York: Plenum.
Markman, G. D., Balkin, D. B., & Baron, R. A. (2002). Inventors and new venture formation: The effects of general self-efficacy and regretful thinking. *Entrepreneurship Theory and Practice, 27*(2), 149–165.
Masten, A. S. (2001). Ordinary magic: Resilience processes in development. *American Psychologist, 56*, 227–238. doi:10.1097/01.PSY.0000073873.74829.23.
Oei, T. P. S., Hasking, P., & Phillips, L. (2007). A comparison of general self-efficacy and drinking refusal self-efficacy in predicting drinking behavior. *The American Journal of Drug and Alcohol Abuse, 33*(6), 833–841.

Ollendick, T. H., & Schmidt, C. R. (1987). Social learning constructs in the prediction of peer interaction. *Journal of Clinical Child Psychology, 16*(1), 80–87.

Orsega-Smith, E. M., Payne, L. L., Mowen, A. J., Ho, C.-H., & Godbey, G. C. (2007). The role of social support and self-efficacy in shaping the leisure time physical activity of older adults. *Journal of Leisure Research, 39*(4), 705–727.

Pajares, F., & Kranzler, J. (1995). Self-efficacy beliefs and general mental ability in mathematical problem-solving. *Contemporary Educational Psychology, 20*(4), 426–443.

Pajares, F., & Miller, M. D. (1995). Mathematics self-efficacy and mathematics performances: The need for specificity of assessment. *Journal of Counseling Psychology, 42*(2), 190–198.

Pössel, P., Baldus, C., Horn, A. B., Groen, G., & Hautzinger, M. (2005). Influence of general self-efficacy on the effects of a school-based universal primary prevention program of depressive symptoms in adolescents: A randomized and controlled follow-up study. *Journal of Child Psychology and Psychiatry, 46*(9), 982–994.

Rimm, H., & Jerusalem, M. (1999). Adaptation and validation of an Estonian version of the general self-efficacy scale (ESES). *Anxiety, Stress, and Coping, 12*(3), 329–345.

Rutter, M. (1987). Psychosocial resilience and protective mechanisms. *The American Journal of Orthopsychiatry, 57*(3), 316–331.

Salanova, M., Peiró, J., & Schaufeli, W. B. (2002). Self-efficacy specificity and burnout among information technology workers: An extension of the job demand-control model. *European Journal of Work and Organizational Psychology, 11*(1), 1–25.

Samoocha, D., Bruinvels, D. J., Elbers, N. A., Anema, J. R., & van der Beek, A. J. (2010). Effectiveness of web-based interventions on patient empowerment: A systematic review and meta-analysis. *Journal of Medical Internet Research, 12*(2), e23.

Scherbaum, C. A., Cohen-Charash, Y., & Kern, M. J. (2006). Measuring general self-efficacy: A comparison of three measures using item response theory. *Educational and Psychological Measurement, 66*(6), 1047–1063.

Schneider, S., Houweling, J. E. G., Gommlich-Schneider, S., Klein, C., Nündel, B., & Wolke, D. (2009). Effect of maternal panic disorder on mother-child interaction and relation to child anxiety and child self-efficacy. *Archives of Women's Mental Health, 12*(4), 251–259.

Scholz, U., Doña, B. G., Sud, S., & Schwarzer, R. (2002). Is general self-efficacy a universal construct? Psychometric findings from 25 countries. *European Journal of Psychological Assessment, 18*(3), 242–251.

Schwarzer, R. (1992). *Self-efficacy: Thought control of action*. Washington DC: Hemisphere Publishing Corporation.

Schwarzer, R. (1994). Optimism, vulnerability, and self-beliefs as health-related cognitions: A systematic overview. *Psychology and Health, 9*(3), 161–180.

Schwarzer, R., Bäßler, J., Kwiatek, P., Schröder, K., & Zhang, J. X. (1997). The assessment of optimistic self-beliefs: Comparison of the German, Spanish, and Chinese versions of the general self-efficacy scale. *Applied Psychology: An International Review, 46*(1), 69–88.

Schwarzer, R., Boehmer, S., Luszczynska, A., Mohamed, N. E., & Knoll, N. (2005). Dispositional self-efficacy as a personal resource factor in coping after surgery. *Personality and Individual Differences, 39*(4), 807–818.

Schwarzer, R., Hahn, A., & Schröder, H. (1994). Social integration and social support in a life crisis: Effects of macrosocial change in East Germany. *American Journal of Community Psychology, 22*(5), 685–706.

Schwarzer, R., & Hallum, S. (2008). Perceived teacher self-efficacy as a predictor of job stress and burnout. *Applied Psychology: An International Review, 57*(Suppl 1), 152–171.

Schwarzer, R., & Jerusalem, M. (1995a). General self-efficacy scale: A user's portfolio. Causal and control beliefs. In J. Weinman, S. Wright, & M. Johnston (Eds.), *Measures in health psychology* (pp. 35–37). Windsor: NFER-Nelson.

Schwarzer, R., & Jerusalem, M. (1995b). Optimistic self beliefs as a resource factor in coping with stress. In S. E. Hobfoll & M. W. de Vries (Eds.), *Extreme stress and communities: Impact and intervention* (pp. 159–177). Dordrecht: Kluwer.

Schwarzer, R., & Jerusalem, M. (1999). *Skalen zur Erfassung von Lehrer- und Schülermerkmalen [Scales to assess attributes teachers and students]*. Berlin: Freie Universität Berlin.

Schwarzer, R., Mueller, J., & Greenglass, E. (1999). Assessment of perceived general self-efficacy on the internet: Data collection in cyberspace. *Anxiety, Stress, and Coping, 12*(2), 145–161.

Shelton, S. H. (1990). Developing the construct of general self-efficacy. *Psychological Reports, 66*, 987–994.

Sherer, M., Maddux, J. E., Mercandante, B., Prentice-Dunn, S., Jacobs, B., & Rogers, R. W. (1982). The self-efficacy scale: Construction and validation. *Psychological Reports, 51*, 663–671.

Smith, R. E. (1989). Effects of coping skills training on general self-efficacy and locus of control. *Journal of Personality and Social Psychology, 56*(2), 228–233.

Stuifbergen, A. K., & Becker, H. A. (1994). Predictors of health-promoting lifestyles in persons with disabilities. *Research in Nursing and Health, 17*(1), 3–13.

Tang, C. S.-K., Au, W.-T., Schwarzer, R., & Schmitz, G. (2001). Mental health outcomes of job stress among Chinese teachers: Role of stress resource factors and burnout. *Journal of Organizational Behavior, 22*(8), 887–901.

Taylor, W. J., Dean, S. G., & Siegert, R. J. (2006). Differential association of general and health self-efficacy with disability, health-related quality of life and psychological distress from musculoskeletal pain in a cross-sectional general adult population survey. *Pain, 125*(3), 225–232.

Tedeschi, R. G., & Calhoun, L. G. (1995). *Trauma & transformation: Growing in the aftermath of suffering*. Thousand Oaks, CA: Sage.

Tong, Y., & Song, S. (2004). A study on general self-efficacy and subjective well-being of low SES college students in a Chinese university. *College Student Journal, 38*(4), 637–642.

Tsaousides, T., Warshowsky, A., Ashman, T. A., Cantor, J. B., Spielman, L., & Gordon, W. A. (2009). The relationship between employment-related self-efficacy and quality of life following traumatic brain injury. *Rehabilitation Psychology, 54*(3), 299–305.

Tuckman, B. W. (1991). The development and concurrent validity of the procrastination scale. *Educational and Psychological Measurement, 51*(2), 473–480.

Usher, E. L., & Pajares, F. (2008). Sources of self-efficacy in school: Critical review of the literature and future directions. *Review of Educational Research, 78*(4), 751–796.

Vauth, R., Kleim, B., Wirtz, M., & Corrigan, P. W. (2007). Self-efficacy and empowerment as outcomes of self-stigmatizing and coping in schizophrenia. *Psychiatry Research, 150*(1), 71–80.

Vieira, E. T., Jr., & Grantham, S. (2011). University students setting goals in the context of autonomy, self-efficacy and important goal-related task engagement. *Educational Psychology, 31*(2), 141–156.

Wallston, K. A., Wallston, B. S., Smith, S., & Dobbins, C. J. (1987). Perceived efficacy and health. *Current Psychological Research and Reviews, 6*(1), 5–25.

Warner, L. M., Ziegelmann, J. P., Schüz, B., Wurm, S., Tesch-Römer, C., & Schwarzer, R. (2011). Maintaining autonomy despite multimorbidity: Self-efficacy and the two faces of social support. *European Journal of Aging, 8*(1), 3–12.

Watt, S. E., & Martin, P. R. (1994). Effect of general self-efficacy expectancies on performance attributions. *Psychological Reports, 75*(2), 951–961.

Werner, E. (1982). *Vulnerable but invincible: A longitudinal study of resilient children and youth*. New York: McGraw-Hill.

Wise, J. B., & Trunnell, E. P. (2001). The influence of sources of self-efficacy upon efficacy strength. *Journal of Sport and Exercise Psychology, 23*(4), 268–280.

Wood, R., & Bandura, A. (1989). Social cognitive theory of organizational management. *Academy of Management Review, 14*(3), 361–384.

Development and Use of the Resilience Scale (RS) with Middle-Aged and Older Adults

11

Gail Wagnild

Introduction

Until the late 1980s, the study of resilience was relatively new with most research focusing on children (Rutter, 1985, 1987; Werner, 1984, 1990). Much of "health" related research used models grounded in pathology, which emphasized identifying and diagnosing problems and developing approaches to cure or treat problems. In the last 20 years, a more positive approach to health has been taken, with a greater emphasis on recognizing capabilities and building on a foundation of strength. Because "resilience" connotes the ability to cope effectively and adapt successfully when faced with adversity, it became a useful, popular, and perhaps novel way of viewing adaptation to stress. It was from this paradigm shift that the Resilience Scale™ (RS) was developed.

The Resilience Scale was created in 1987 and initial psychometric analysis was conducted in two early studies in 1989 and 1990. Since then, it has been used worldwide and translated into at least 36 languages. *In the last 4 years alone, there have been more than 5,000 requests to use the RS for a variety of purposes including research, employment assistance programs, clinical assessment, education, and continuing education conferences and workshops. The RS has been used with a variety of populations including youth, young and middle-aged adults, and elders.

In this chapter, a review of the development and early psychometric analysis of the RS is presented followed by resilience research with specific adult populations. Although the RS has been used extensively in youth and young adults, the focus of this chapter will be on middle-aged and older adults. This is followed by a brief overview of how the RS can be used as an assessment tool in clinical settings.

G. Wagnild, R.N., Ph.D. (✉)
The Resilience Center, Billings, MT, USA
e-mail: gwagnild@resiliencecenter.com

**Albanian, Arabic, Bahasa Indonesian, Bosnian, Chinese, Creole, Czech, Danish, Dutch, Finnish, French, German, Hebrew, Icelandic, Italian, Japanese, Lithuanian, Malay, Norwegian, Polish, Portuguese (Brazil and Portugal), Russian, Sinhalese, Slovakian, Slovenian, Spanish (South America/Mexico), Spanish (Spain), Sri Lankan, Swedish, Tamil, Thai, Turkish, Urdu, and Zulu*

S. Prince-Embury and D.H. Saklofske (eds.), *Resilience in Children, Adolescents, and Adults: Translating Research into Practice*, The Springer Series on Human Exceptionality,
DOI 10.1007/978-1-4614-4939-3_11, © Springer Science+Business Media New York 2013

History and Background of the Resilience Scale

What Does the Resilience Scale Measure?

Until the mid-1980s, the term "healthy aging" was often seen as a contradiction in terms in that many viewed growing older as a time of the "Dreaded Ds:" depression, dependence, dementia, disability, and disease. Even so, many elders were aging successfully; meaning they maintained their independence, optimism in the face of loss, were fully engaged in life, and continued to face life's challenges with courage and enthusiasm. In short, they were living vital lives.

The question many were asking was "How can we promote healthy and vital aging in the midst of losses associated with growing older including functional, sensory, and cognitive decline, lifestyle changes, and death of friends and family?" Clearly some people were dealing with adversity and living life to the fullest despite loss, while others were giving up in despair. For instance, Montross et al. (2006) reported that the majority of study participants viewed themselves as aging well despite having chronic physical illnesses and some disability.

As we shifted our focus from viewing aging as a time of inevitable decline to one full of possibilities, we began to look at characteristics of elders that promoted healthy aging. In the latter part of the twentieth century, we began to see the term "resilience" used to describe elders living strong and healthy lives (Colerick, 1985). Since then, numerous writers have proposed that resilience may very well be an essential key to healthy aging (Harris, 2008; Resnick, 2010; Rowe & Kahn, 2000).

An early qualitative study by Wagnild and Young (1990) sought to understand why some older women adjusted successfully to adversity, while others became defeated. Interviews were conducted with 24 well-adapted women with a mean age of 78 who exhibited a high level of morale and were fully engaged in their lives despite having experienced a recent and major loss (e.g., loss of a spouse, health, or employment). Five essential characteristics underlying their successful adaptation were identified constituting the core construct of resilience. These characteristics were further defined with a comprehensive review of the literature on coping and adaptation.

The five characteristics were Purpose, Equanimity, Self-Reliance, Perseverance, and Existential Aloneness. These are now considered the "resilience core" and strengthening the core will enable a person to exhibit a very healthy resilience response to adversity (Wagnild, 2009). Much like a fitness coach will encourage athletes to strengthen their physical core, the resilience core can be strengthened and practiced, too. The stronger the core, the healthier one's response to adversity and setbacks. Each of the five core characteristics is defined as follows.

Purpose

To have a purposeful life is to have a life full of meaning and direction. It may be the most important characteristic of resilience because it provides the foundation for the other four characteristics. Life without purpose is futile and aimless. Purpose provides the driving force in life. People with purposeful lives have learned to derive meaning from their experiences, however initially devastating these experiences may be. Major adversities can be transformed into opportunities for personal growth and life satisfaction.

Equanimity

To live life with equanimity is to have a sense of balance and harmony. Resilient people have learned to avoid extreme responses to stress and adversity and "sit loose in the saddle." Resilient people understand that life is full of joys and sorrows, neither all good nor all bad, and they are open to many possibilities. This is one of the reasons resilient people are viewed as optimistic, because even when the situation looks doubtful, they are probably on the lookout for opportunities. They have also learned to draw on their own and others' experiences and wisdom and to use this to guide their responses. Equanimity also manifests itself in humor. Resilient individuals can laugh at themselves and their circumstances.

Self-Reliance

To be self-reliant is to believe in yourself. Self-reliant people have a clear understanding of their capabilities and limitations. It comes from experience and leads to confidence in one's abilities. Throughout a lifetime, individuals encounter challenges that are met successfully. At other times, people fail. Self-reliant individuals have learned from these experiences and developed many problem-solving skills. Furthermore, they use, adapt, strengthen, and refine these skills throughout a lifetime. This increases self-reliance.

Perseverance

Perseverance is the determination to keep going despite difficulties, discouragement, and disappointment. Repeated failure or rejection can be formidable roadblocks and can prevent us from moving forward and achieving our goals. Resilient individuals tend to finish what they begin. Bouncing back, one of the hallmark features of resilience, takes perseverance in getting back up when knocked down.

Existential Aloneness

People with existential aloneness understand that their life path is unique and that while some experiences can be shared, others must be faced alone. Resilient people are aware that there is continuity of oneself through the many stages and changes one experiences throughout a lifetime. Aloneness can be a wellspring for creativity, comfort, and self-acceptance. Existential aloneness confers a feeling of freedom and a celebration of uniqueness.

Development of the Resilience Scale

The above core characteristics of resilience served as the conceptual foundation for the Resilience Scale (RS). Initially, a 50-item scale was developed and pretested in 1988 using verbatim statements from qualitative interviews to capture the essence of resilience as described and explained by interview respondents. The scale was reviewed by two psychometricians and two nurse researchers prior to further testing and minor changes were made in the wording of items. After initial analysis, the scale was reduced to 25 items. The 25-item RS was the first and earliest published instrument designed to measure resilience directly (Wagnild & Young, 1993). There are five items per core characteristic totaling 25 items.

Initial Psychometric Testing of the RS

The initial psychometric testing of the RS was completed with a large sample of middle-aged and older adults residing in a Pacific Northwest community (Wagnild & Young, 1993). 1,500 surveys were randomly mailed and 810 responded (54% response rate). In addition to the RS, sociodemographic questions and measures of adaptation (i.e., life satisfaction, morale, and depression) were asked as well as a self-report of health status.

Surveys with missing data were eliminated resulting in 782 completed surveys available for analysis. The final sample ranged in age from 53 to 95 years with a mean age of 71.1 years (SD=6.5). The majority was female (62.3%) and most were married (61.2%). Most were retired (79.9%) and lived with a spouse (59.4%). Almost half (47.0%) reported very good to excellent health with about 15% reporting fair to poor health. All but 14 of the participants were of European-American descent and thus ethnicity was not analyzed separately.

The internal consistency of the RS was excellent (alpha coefficient=0.91). Scores ranged from 25 to 175 points. Scores greater than 144 indicated moderately high to high resilience, scores between 121 and 144 indicated moderately low to moderate levels of resilience, and scores of 120 and below indicated low resilience (see Table 11.1).

An exploratory principal components factor analysis suggested a two-factor solution with 17 items in Factor I that suggested self-reliance, independence, determination, invincibility, mastery, resourcefulness, and perseverance. This factor was labeled Personal Competence. The eight

Table 11.1 Interpretation of RS scores

Scale	Scoring				
RS	Very low	Moderately low	Moderate	Moderately high	Very high
	25–120	121–130	131–144	145–160	161–175

Table 11.2 Correlations between the RS and depression, morale, life satisfaction, and health status

Scales	Beck Depression Inventory	Philadelphia Geriatric Center Morale Scale	Life Satisfaction Index-A	Self-reported health status
RS	−0.41	0.32	0.37	−0.30

items constituting Factor II represented adaptability, balance, flexibility, and a balanced perspective of life. They reflected acceptance and a sense of peace despite adversity. This factor was labeled Acceptance of Self and Life. The two factors (personal competence and acceptance of self and life) were double-loaded on both factors, however, limiting support for this analysis. Subsequent studies have not consistently supported the above two factors. There is growing support for a one-dimensional scale with one underlying factor.

Concurrent validity was assessed by correlating the RS score with measures of depression using the Beck Depression Inventory (Beck & Beck, 1972), life satisfaction using the Life Satisfaction Index A (Neugarten, Havighurst, & Tobin, 1961), morale using the Philadelphia Geriatric Center Morale Scale (Lawton, 1975), and self-reported health status. The RS was significantly correlated to these measures (see Table 11.1).

Resnick and Inguito (2011) studied the psychometric properties and clinical applicability of the RS in two samples of elders, each participant reporting at least three comorbidities (residents of a continuing care retirement community and women with post hip fracture). While the alpha coefficient was adequate in each sample (0.91 and 0.83), the researchers identified a poor fit of several items in the scale and recommended additional items to differentiate those who are very resilient as most individuals scored high in resilience in their study. Higher resilience was associated with fewer negative and more positive outcome expectations, stronger self-efficacy expectations, and more time exercising in one sample but not the other. The RS results are frequently negatively skewed and items are currently being considered that will differentiate those scoring in the high range of resilience (Table 11.2).

Interpreting the RS

All items are scaled in a positive direction so that a higher score reflects greater resilience. No scores are reversed or otherwise modified prior to calculating scores. RS scores range from 25 to 175.

Response choices for the RS use a seven-point Likert scale to rate the individual evaluation of the item. The respondent's choices range from one (strongly disagree) to seven (strongly agree). The RS uses total scores rather than scores for each of the five characteristics. A higher total score indicates higher resilience.

In most studies, resilience is not related to gender or education. Resilience does appear to increase with age. In a large sample of 1,061 adults who completed the online RS (www.resiliencescale.com) (mean age = 36 years), the average RS score was 135.5 (19.68) and the alpha coefficient was 0.93. As age increased, the RS scores increased as presented in Table 11.3.

Overview of Research with Middle-Aged and Older Adults Using the RS

Several studies in the 1990s supported reliability and validity data for the RS. Populations studied in these earlier studies included undergraduate

Table 11.3 Average scores by age ($n = 1.061$)

Age	18–29	30–39	40–49	50–59	≥60
RS score	133	135	137	140	143

and graduate students, first-time mothers, and residents in public housing (Wagnild, 2009; Wagnild & Young, 1993). The alpha coefficient has been consistently acceptable and moderately high (0.73–0.95). Validity of the RS has also been consistently supported with hypothesized and statistically significant associations with morale, self-esteem, life satisfaction, depression, and perceived stress.

Support for the reliability and validity of the RS continued with studies of middle-aged and older adults. Resilience was correlated with positive aspects of successful aging including stress management and better health (Wagnild, 2000), and health-promoting behaviors (Wagnild, 2000; Wagnild & Branam, 2011). Leppert, Gunzelmann, Schumacher, Strauss, and Brähler (2005) studied 599 older adults in Germany whose average age was about 70. The average RS score was 132.6 (22.17) with an alpha coefficient of 0.94. Those elders who reported lower subjective body complaints reported higher resilience. Resilience was a significant predictive variable for physical well-being. Strauss et al. (2007) studied the influence of resilience on fatigue in cancer patients undergoing radiation therapy. Resilience, using the RS, strongly predicted the patients' fatigue at the beginning of radiation therapy. The authors concluded that resilience is a psychological predictor of quality of life and coping in cancer patients. They added that resilience does not appear to have influence on treatment related fatigue during radiation therapy, however.

Resilience has been associated with forgiveness (Broyles, 2005), morale (March, 2004; Wagnild & Young, 1993), purpose in life, sense of coherence, self-transcendence (Nygren et al., 2005), and self-efficacy (Caltabiano & Caltabiano, 2006). Resilience has also been inversely associated with depression (Wagnild, 2009; Wagnild & Young, 1993), perceived stress (March, 2004), and anxiety (Humphreys, 2003).

Wagnild and Young (1989) studied 39 female caregivers of spouses with Alzheimer's disease and found relationships between resilience and caregiver burden (−0.18, $p<0.01$), self-reported health status (−0.25, $p<0.01$), and morale (0.54, $p<0.01$). March (2004) studied 83 middle-aged and older adults in Australia (mean age of 72 years) and reported correlations between resilience and morale, stress, and number of stressful events ($r=0.71$, −0.43, and −0.40, respectively, all $p<0.01$). Broyles (2005) reported a relationship between resilience and forgiveness ($r=0.34$, $p<0.01$) among 497 older adults residing in a planned community whose average age was 65.4. The mean RS score was 143.0 (16.3).

Torma (2010) explored factors associated with increased risk of disability in 224 older adults (mean age of 62.1) with fibromyalgia in addition to factors that protected or enhanced physical function and promoted health. Greater resilience was significantly correlated with low pain ratings ($r=-0.21$, $p<0.005$), high levels of physical function ($r=0.32$, $p<0.001$), and low fibromyalgia impact ($r=-0.40$, $p<0.01$).

Selected Studies Using the RS Among Middle-Aged and Older Adults

Recent studies using the RS are reviewed in this section in order to present relationships between the RS and study variables associated with healthy aging. These study findings offer further support for the reliability and validity of the RS in a variety of study populations.

The RS is often used to investigate the relationship of resilience to other psychosocial variables. For instance, Lee, Brown, Mitchell, and Schiraldi (2008) explored the association between resilience and self-esteem, optimism, religiousness, cultural interdependency, and belief in higher education in a population of 200 elderly Korean women and 170 daughters. These women had experienced adversity including psychological and physical losses of war and difficulties associated with relocation. Self-esteem,

Table 11.4 Sample description and correlates of resilience

	Mothers	Daughters
Sample size	200	170
Alpha coefficient	0.94	0.94
Mean RS (SD)	128.1 (27.9)	123.8 (26.6)
Bivariate correlations		
Self-esteem	0.69**	0.62**
Optimism	0.47**	0.53**
Religiousness	0.22**	0.07
Belief in education	0.07	0.27**
Cultural interdependency	0.31**	0.16

**$p<0.01$ (two-tailed)

Table 11.5 Sample description and RS summary

	Sweden	Thailand
Sample size	422	200
Age group		
60–69	172	81
70–79	156	96
≥80	94	23
Alpha coefficient	0.94	0.92
Test–retest reliability	0.78	0.83
RS mean (SD)	144 (20.9)	146 (18.1)

optimism, religiousness, and cultural interdependency were significantly correlated with resilience among the elderly mothers. Length of time in the USA, age entering the USA, physical and psychological war-related adversities, current relocation difficulties, self-esteem, optimism, cultural interdependency, and belief in education were all significantly associated with daughters' resilience. In linear regression, self-esteem and optimism were important predictors of resilience (see Table 11.4).

Choowattanapakorn, Aléx, Lundman, Norberg, and Nygren (2010) compared the level of resilience of adults 60 years and older in Sweden and Thailand. They found that the resilience scores were almost the same between these two groups of elders. Swedes who described themselves as unhealthy had lower resilience scores (133.0) though this was not true for the Thai sample. Single Thai elders had significantly higher resilience scores than either Swedes or married, divorced/separated, and widowed Thai individuals (see Table 11.5).

Table 11.6 Correlations between the RS and psychosocial measures

Sense of coherence	0.35
Purpose in life	0.53
Self-transcendence	0.49
Mental health	0.37

**$p<0.01$

Table 11.7 Sample description and psychosocial correlates of RS

Sample size	59
Mean age	52
Alpha coefficient	0.95
Dizziness-specific anxiety	−0.46

In an earlier study of the oldest old in Sweden, Nygren et al. (2005) reported correlations of psychosocial measures with the RS as follow (Table 11.6).

Tschan et al. (2011) conducted a 1-year follow-up study that identified neurootological patients at risk for developing secondary somatoform dizziness and vertigo (SVD). Patients with higher scores on resilience, sense of coherence, and satisfaction with life were less likely to acquire secondary SVD over a year's time. Patients with normal recovery at year one had significantly higher scores on the RS (Table 11.7).

Martins et al. (2011) investigated whether positive self-perceived oral health is associated with resilience in a sample of 496 community-dwelling adults aged 64 and older. Each participant received a brief oral examination to assess number of teeth. High resilience in addition to income and no changes in diet due to dental problems were associated with positive self-perceived oral health. The authors hypothesized that resilient older persons with poor oral status would be more likely to perceive their oral health as good than less resilient older persons. People with high resilience were 18% more likely to rate their oral health as good, independent of other variables (Table 11.8).

Table 11.8 Sample description and RS results

Sample size	496
Mean age	70.6
Percent completely edentate	53.2%
Alpha coefficient	0.78
Mean RS (SD)	141.1 (13.3)

Table 11.9 Sample description and RS results

Sample size	277
Mean age	75
Alpha coefficient	0.94
Mean RS (SD)	148.0 (19.0)
Correlations	
Physical health status	0.23*
Mental health status	0.42*

*$p \leq .005$

Wells (2010) studied resilience in older adults living in rural, suburban, and urban areas to determine if resilience levels varied as a result of location. In multiple regression analysis, the strongest predictor of resilience was higher perceived mental health status. No sociodemographic factors except income were found to correlate with resilience. Higher income was associated with lower resilience levels. The author suggested that this unusual finding may be related to the economic downturn in 2008 and loss of investments in the high income group. Strong social networks, good physical, and mental health were protective factors for resilience (Table 11.9).

Wagnild & Branam (2011) interviewed 20 older women who lived in frontier communities and asked them about their health-promoting behaviors, self-reported health status, and resilience. Scores on the RS were significantly related to health and health behaviors. They concluded that even though these women were isolated from services and frequently isolated from face-to-face interaction, they were able to live a healthy old age (Table 11.10).

Wagnild (2009) surveyed a random selection of middle-aged and older adults from a Pacific Northwest readership of a senior publication. A total of 770 respondents completed the RS and the Health Promoting Lifestyle Profile (Walker, Sechrist, & Pender, 1987). The sample was further divided into those scoring low on resilience (<125) and high (>160). The results are presented in Table 11.11.

Table 11.10 Sample description and RS results

Sample size	20
Mean age	75.7
Alpha coefficient	0.94
Mean RS (SD)	147.1 (18.3)
Correlations	
Physical health status	0.59*
Health-promoting lifestyle	0.50*

*$p < 0.01$

Putting the Resilience Scale to Work

Most assessment instruments for middle-aged and older adults focus on problems such as loss, fear, anxiety, depression, confusion, and so forth. This is because most people seek help for problems they are experiencing. In conventional assessments, however, clients rarely have the opportunity to talk about their own goals or focus on their strengths and positive aspects of their lives. This information, seldom elicited, is unavailable to the caregiver, family, or other providers, and personal awareness may be lost as well (Kivnick & Stoffel, 2005).

Assessing resilience is done so that individual resilience can be strengthened; an important goal for aging adults (Harris, 2008). There are two parts to the resilience-based assessment.

Part 1: The Resilience Scale

The RS is useful for screening persons for resilience levels and identifying those at greater risk for low resilience. The scale is simple and direct and offers an overall assessment of psychological resilience. Individual items within the scale also identify specific areas within resilience that offer ideas for further introspection and exploration. Items such as "My life has purpose," or "I can

Table 11.11 Sample description and comparison between low and high resilience on healthy lifestyle behaviors using *t*-test

	Low resilience	High resilience	Total sample
Sample size	110	238	770
Mean age	72.8	71.8	71.9
Mean RS (SD)	107.2 (19.3)	167.3 (4.8)	147.0 (21.4)
T-test (2-tailed)	Mean score	Mean score	*T* Significance*
Health rating	2.9	3.8	−8.7
Depression	1.8	2.0	−6.5
Lifestyle total	118.0	158.0	−16.9
Self-actualization	33.0	47.6	−22.1
Health responsibility	23.3	30.0	−9.9
Nutrition	17.3	20.7	−8.9
Interpersonal support	17.8	24.5	−14.9
Stress management	16.1	21.9	−5.8

*$p<0.01$

usually find something to laugh about," can serve as springboards for further self-assessment.

Analysis and feedback for scores can be readily accessed at www.resiliencescale.com.

Part 2: Open-Ended Questions

Using the underlying five core characteristics of the Resilience Scale, open-ended questions can be asked for a more in-depth understanding of resilience. These questions help individuals begin to realize what is important and gives hope and meaning to life.

Examples of questions for each core area are included below.

Purpose

Living a life of significance may be the single most important outcome that older adults hope to achieve. The following questions help people explore their own life and identify what they do that gives meaning.

What in your life gives you the most meaning?

Why do you get up every morning?

Do you have a philosophy or religious beliefs that guide you in your life?

Perseverance

Answering the questions below will provide insight into an individual's ability to keep moving forward and do not give up despite setbacks and adversity.

When you have experienced difficulties in your life, what have you done to get through them?

Do you finish what you begin?

Are you a quitter?

Equanimity

The questions below are designed to elicit information related to perspective and outlook on life. Individuals who have a balanced view of life are more resilient.

How do you handle disappointments in your life?

Do you see the glass as half full or half empty when faced with failures?

Do you worry about and dwell on the negative "What ifs" when facing a challenge?

Self-Reliance

Individuals who can learn to depend on their own capabilities and competencies experience self-confidence and greater self-esteem.

What do you do well? Can you depend on yourself?

How do others who know you well say you respond to difficult situations? Are you resourceful?

Existential Aloneness

Questions on this core characteristic encourage individuals to understand what sets them apart and recognize how they are unique. People who are able to accept their personal life path recognize "continuity of self through changing times" (Wagnild & Young, 1990, p. 254).

Are you willing to go it alone even if it is not a popular choice?

What sets you apart from everyone else?

Do you accept who you have become?

Summary

The RS is an established instrument used to assess an individual's resilience, defined as the resilience core described above. Internal consistency of the RS is acceptable with alpha coefficients usually between 0.85 and 0.94. The RS score consistently differentiates between low and high resilience, and less consistently between moderately high and high resilience. Use of one total score reflects one underlying factor although there has been weak support for a two-factor or more solution in factor analyzes.

The RS is consistently and inversely related to measures of poor adaptation to adversity and stress including depression, anxiety, perceived stress, and positively related to measures of successful aging including morale, life satisfaction, optimism, self-esteem. The RS is usually related to behaviors associated with healthy aging such as health-promoting behaviors, self-care, and chronic disease management.

Overall the RS is a useful tool for screening individuals at risk for poor adaptation to adversity and unhealthy aging. It can be used to identify individual strengths and help individuals recognize their personal resilience and areas where they are already strong. There is a growing interest in factors that enhance healthy aging and research findings using the RS suggest that individual resilience may indeed be one of these factors.

References

Beck, A. T., & Beck, R. W. (1972). Screening depressed patients in family practice: A rapid technique. *Psychological Reports, 52*, 81–85.

Broyles, L. C. (2005). *Resilience: Its relationships to forgiveness in older adults*. Unpublished doctoral dissertation, University of Tennessee, Knoxville.

Caltabiano, M. L., & Caltabiano, N. J. (2006). *Resilience and health outcomes in the elderly*. Paper presented at the 39th national conference of the Australian Association of Gerontology, Sydney, New South Wales.

Choowattanapakorn, T., Aléx, L., Lundman, B., Norberg, A., & Nygren, B. (2010). Resilience among women and men aged 60 years and over in Sweden and in Thailand. *Nursing Health Science, 12*, 329–335.

Colerick, E. J. (1985). Stamina in later life. *Social Science and Medicine, 21*, 997–1006.

Harris, P. B. (2008). Another wrinkle in the debate about successful aging: The undervalued concept of resilience and the lived experience of dementia. *International Journal of Aging & Human Development, 67*, 43–61.

Humphreys, J. (2003). Research in sheltered battered women. *Issues in Mental Health Nursing, 24*, 137–152.

King, S. D. (2009). *Midlife and older gay men and their use of physical and mental health services: Exploring the effects of health enablers, health need, psychosocial stress and individual health coping*. Dissertation, Ohio State University, Graduate Program in Social Work. http://etd.ohiolink.edu/view.cgi?acc_num=osu1257437705. Retrieved October 14, 2011.

Kivnick, H. Q., & Stoffel, S. A. (2005). Vital involvement practice: Strengths as more than tools for solving problems. *Journal of Gerontological Social Work, 46*, 85–116.

Lawton, M. P. (1975). The Philadelphia Geriatric Center Morale Scale: A revision. *Journal of Gerontology, 30*, 85–89.

Lee, H. S., Brown, S. L., Mitchell, M. M., & Schiraldi, G. R. (2008). Correlates of resilience in the face of adversity for Korean women immigrating to the US. *Journal of Immigrant and Minority Health, 10*, 415–422.

Leppert, K., Gunzelmann, T., Schumacher, J., Strauss, B., & Brähler, E. (2005). Resilience as a protective personality characteristic in the elderly. *Psychotherapie, Psychosomatik, Medizinischle Psychologier, 55*, 365–369.

March, M. (2004). *Well being of older Australians: The interplay of life adversity and resilience in late life development*. Unpublished doctoral dissertation, Charles Sturt University, Australia.

Martins, A. B., dos Santos, C. M., Hilgert, J. B., de Marchi, R. J., Hugo, F. N., & Padilha, D. M. P. (2011). Resilience and self-perceived oral health: A hierarchical approach. *Journal of the American Geriatrics Society, 59*, 725–731.

Montross, L. P., Depp, C., Daly, J., Reichstadt, J., Golshan, S., Moore, D., et al. (2006). Correlates of self-rated successful aging among community-dwelling older adults. *The American Journal of Geriatric Psychiatry, 14*, 43–51.

Neugarten, B., Havighurst, R., & Tobin, S. (1961). The measure of life satisfaction. *Journal of Gerontology, 16*, 134–143.

Nygren, B., Aléx, L., Jonsén, E., Gustafson, Y., Norberg, A., & Lundman, B. (2005). Sense of coherence, purpose in life and self-transcendence in relation to perceived physical and mental health among the oldest old. *Aging and Mental Health, 9*, 354–362.

Resnick, B. (2010). Successful aging. Rooted in resilience. *Advance for NPs & PAs, 1*, 31–32. 34–35, 47.

Resnick, B., & Inguito, P. L. (2011). The Resilience Scale: Psychometric properties and clinical applicability in older adults. *Archives of Psychiatric Nursing, 25*, 11–20.

Rowe, J. W., & Kahn, R. L. (2000). Successful aging and disease prevention. *Advances in Renal Replacement Therapy, 7*, 70–77.

Rutter, M. (1985). Resilience in the face of adversity. *The British Journal of Psychiatry, 147*, 598–611.

Rutter, M. (1987). Psychosocial resilience and protective mechanisms. *The American Journal of Orthopsychiatry, 57*, 316–331.

Strauss, B., Brix, C., Fischer, S., Leppert, K., Füller, J., Roehrig, B., et al. (2007). The influence of resilience on fatigue in cancer patients undergoing radiation therapy (RT). *Journal of Cancer Research and Clinical Oncology, 133*, 511–518.

Torma, L. M. (2010). *Fibromyalgia pain and physical function: The influence of resilience*. Unpublished doctoral dissertation, Oregon Health & Science University, Portland.

Tschan, R., Best, C., Beutel, M. E., Knebel, A., Wiltink, J., Dieterich, M., et al. (2011). Patients' psychological well-being and resilient coping protect from secondary somatoform vertigo and dizziness (SVD) 1 year after vestibular disease. *Journal of Neurology, 258*, 104–112.

Wagnild, G. (1991). *Resilience among elderly residents of public housing*. Unpublished raw data.

Wagnild, G. (2000). *Resilience and health-promoting behaviors among community-dwelling adults*. Unpublished raw data.

Wagnild, G. (2009). *The Resilience Scale user's guide for the US English version of the Resilience Scale and the 14-item Resilience Scale (RS-14)*. Worden, MT: The Resilience Center.

Wagnild, G., & Branam, V. (2011). *Elderly frontier women: Role models for healthy aging*. Submitted for publication.

Wagnild, G., & Young, H. M. (1989). Resilience among caregivers. Unpublished raw data.

Wagnild, G., & Young, H. M. (1990). Resilience among older women. *Image – the Journal of Nursing Scholarship, 22*, 252–255.

Wagnild, G., & Young, H. M. (1993). Development and psychometric evaluation of the Resilience Scale. *Journal of Nursing Measurement, 1*, 165–177.

Walker, S. N., Sechrist, K. R., & Pender, N. J. (1987). The health-promoting lifestyle profile: Development and psychometric characteristics. *Nursing Research, 36*, 76–81.

Wells, M. (2010). Resilience in older adults living in rural, suburban, and urban areas. http://www.rno.org/journal/index.php/online-journal/article/viewFile/239/284. Retrieved December 10, 2011.

Werner, E. E. (1984). Resilient children. *Young Children, 40*, 68–72.

Werner, E. E. (1990). Resilient offspring of alcoholics: A longitudinal study from birth to age 18. *Journal of Studies on Alcohol, 47*, 34–40.

The Connor–Davidson Resilience Scale

12

Sandra Prince-Embury

One frequently used assessment of resilience in adults is the Connor–Davidson Resilience Scale (CD-RISC) (Connor & Davidson, 2003). The CD-RISC is unique in that it was developed specifically for the purpose of assessing treatment effects of pharmacotherapy and other modalities and has shown sensitivity in detecting symptom changes associated with drug treatment. In the words of the authors (Connor & Davidson, 2003) their interest in resilience as a factor in the treatment of anxiety, depression and stress reaction "arose in part from a finding that fluoxetine produced greater therapeutic benefit on stress coping than placebo in PTSD (Connor et al., 1999). Change documented by the CD-RISC included initial symptom alleviation and subsequent changes in patient well-being.

The original CD-RISC is an instrument that consists of 25 self-rated items (Connor & Davidson, 2003). Each item is rated on a five point frequency response ranging from 0 (not at all true) to 4 (true nearly all of the time). The total score range is between 0 and 100. Higher scores correspond to greater resilience. The rating is based on how the subject has felt over the past month. The CD-RISC currently exists in a 25 item version as well as 10 and 2 item versions.

Approved translations of the CD-RISC currently exist in the following languages: Afrikaans, Bahasa Indonesian (2 and 10 item versions only), Chinese (Taiwan and Peoples Republic), Dutch, Farsi, Finnish, French (France, Belgium), German, Hindi, Italian, Japanese, Kiswahili, Korean, Norwegian, Portuguese (Europe, Brazil), Quechua, Russian, Serbian, Spanish (Europe, Caribbean, South America), Turkish, Urdu. An approved Arabic version of the CD-RISC2 also exists.

According to the authors, the CD-RISC builds upon the work of previous research on hardiness, action orientation, self-efficacy, confidence, adaptability, patience, and endurance in the face of adversity, as well as on the characteristics of historical figures who embody the concept of resilience. The authors report that in reviewing the account of Sir Edward Shackleton's heroic expedition in the Antarctic in 1912 (Alexander, 1998), they noted that the expedition's leader possessed many personal characteristics compatible with resilience and that this may perhaps have contributed to the successful survival of each member of the expedition in the face of overwhelming odds.

These observations prompted the authors to undertake the development of a short self-rated resilience measure. The content of the scale was drawn from a number of sources including Kobasa's work on the construct of hardiness

S. Prince-Embury, Ph.D. (✉)
Resiliency Institute of Allenhurst, LLC,
625 North Edgemere Drive, West Allenhurst,
NJ 07711, USA
e-mail: sandraprince-embury@earthlink.net

S. Prince-Embury and D.H. Saklofske (eds.), *Resilience in Children, Adolescents, and Adults: Translating Research into Practice*, The Springer Series on Human Exceptionality,
DOI 10.1007/978-1-4614-4939-3_12, © Springer Science+Business Media New York 2013

(Kobasa, 1979). These items reflect control, commitment, and change viewed as challenge. Items were also drawn from the work of Rutter (1985). These items reflected the development of a strategy with a clear goal or aim, being action orientated, having a strong self-esteem/confidence, manifesting adaptability when coping with change, having social problem solving skills, showing humor in the face of stress, strengthening effect of stress, taking on responsibilities for dealing with stress, having secure/stable affection bonds, and previous experiences of success and achievement. From Lyons (1991), items assessing patience and the ability to endure stress or pain were included. Lastly, from Shackleton's experiences, it was noted that the role of faith and a belief in benevolent intervention ("good luck") were likely important factors in the survival of the expedition, suggesting a spiritual component to resilience," (Connor & Davidson, 2003).

The original samples in which the CD-RISC were tested included a general nonclinical group of 577 and four additional clinical groups; primary care outpatients ($n=139$); psychiatric outpatients in private practice ($n=43$); subjects in a study of generalized anxiety disorder ($n=25$); and subjects in two clinical trials of PTSD ($n=22$), (Connor & Davidson, 2003). Analysis of the 25 item version yielded strong psychometric properties (Connor & Davidson, 2003). The internal consistency of the CD-RISC for the original nonclinical group was good with a Cronbach's alpha coefficient of 0.89. Test-retest reliability for a small clinical sample was good with an intra-class coefficient of 0.87. Convergent validity was expressed for the CD-RISC by positive correlations with the Kobasa hardiness measure in psychiatric outpatients ($n=30$; Pearson $r=0.83$, $p<0.0001$) and negative correlations with the Perceived Stress Scale (PSS-10), ($n=24$; Pearson $r=-0.76$, $p<0.001$). The authors concluded, based on their initial studies (Connor & Davidson, 2003), that the CD-RISC exhibited validity relative to other measures of stress and hardiness, and reflected different levels of resilience in populations that were thought to be differentiated by their degree of resilience as well as other significant ways (e.g., general population vs. patients with anxiety disorders).

Based on these findings, Connor and Davidson (2003) suggested that the CD-RISC had demonstrated good internal consistency and test-retest reliability in both community and clinical samples. When compared to other measures, the scale exhibited validity relative to stress and hardiness and reflected different levels of resilience in differentiated populations. The general population mean was established as a total score of 80. Lower mean scores are observed in various treatment-seeking populations: primary care, 72; psychiatric outpatients, 68; generalized anxiety disorder, 62; major depression, 58; and PTSD, 50. Clinical improvement was found associated with up to a 25% increase in resilience, depending on the level of global improvement. Improvements in CD-RISC score were noted in proportion to overall clinical global improvement. The greatest increase was noted in subjects with the highest global improvement; CD-RISC scores decreased or remained unchanged in individuals with minimal or no global improvement. According to its developers, the CD-RISC findings helped to demonstrated that resilience is quantifiable, modifiable, and can improve with pharmacologic and psychotherapeutic interventions.

Additional construct validity was reported by Campbell-Sills, Cohan, and Stein (2006) who found that resilience was negatively associated with neuroticism, and positively related to extraversion and conscientiousness. In addition, CD-RISC scores manifested statistically significant and salient relationships with three of the five factor model personality constructs. Correlations of resilience with neuroticism, extraversion, conscientiousness, openness, and agreeableness were (–) 0.65, 0.61, 0.46, 0.20, and 0.15, respectively. These correlations indicate that resilience demonstrates a strong inverse relationship with neuroticism and strong positive relationships with extraversion and conscientiousness (all $p<0.001$) (see Campbell-Sills et al., 2006).

Coping styles also predicted variance in resilience beyond the contributions of the personality traits mentioned above. Task-oriented coping was positively related to resilience and mediated the relationship between conscientiousness and resilience. Emotion-oriented coping was associated with low resilience. Examination of regression coefficients showed that both task-oriented coping and emotion oriented coping contributed significantly to the prediction of resilience. Resilience was shown to moderate the relationship between a form of childhood maltreatment (emotional neglect) and current psychiatric symptoms (Campbell-Sills et al., 2006).

Most remarkably, however, Connor and Davidson (2003) found that significant increases in CD-RISC scores were found for patients who showed significant overall clinical improvement, and the increase in resilience score was proportional to the increase in global improvement. These findings were remarkable for several reasons. CD-RISC scores were demonstrated to be sensitive to real changes in patient well-being, suggesting that improved resilience is related to patient improvement in other ways than symptom reduction. Also, findings indicated that resilience was subject to change resulting from pharmacotherapy and cognitive behavioral therapy.

Connor and Davidson (2003) hypothesized possible physiological pathways associated with their findings. First the hypothesis was offered that there are biologic aspects of resilience that may be affected by drug treatment and that the CD-RISC was tapping the subject's experience of these changes. Physiological underpinnings of changes associated with drug treatment were hypothesized as follows. Resilience is characterized by a response profile to major stress in which low baseline catecholaminergic activity is transformed into high catecholamine production, along with increased tissue-specific response (e.g., glucose levels) and an attenuated cortisol response (Dienstbier, 1991). The authors had shown previously that fluoxetine has an improving effect in PTSD (Connor et al., 1999). Connor et al. (1999) reported greater attenuation of stress responsivity with fluoxetine than with placebo, leading them to speculate that serotonergic antidepressants may have resilience-enhancing or "saliostatic" properties in the treatment of PTSD. It was also hypothesized that relationships exist between resilience and central serotonergic function (Andrews, Parker, & Barrett, 1998; Healey & Healey, 1998).

A large multicenter study of PTSD patients showed that relative to placebo, venlafaxine extended release (ER) produced significantly greater enhancement of resilience (Davidson et al., 2006). Davidson et al. found that significant differences between treatment and placebo groups in symptom severity occurred by week 4 whereas cognitive changes occurred between week 4 and week 12 suggesting that "saliostatic" effects of pharmacologic treatment take longer time to occur than improvement in core PTSD symptoms. The authors suggested further that that pharmacotherapy for PTSD with venlafaxine ER, as well as floroxatine as found previously, accomplishes more than symptom reduction through improvement of function and quality of life. Davidson et al. suggested that this effect might generalize across other antidepressants to the extent that physiological changes facilitated by drug treatment allowed cognitive changes to occur.

Davidson et al. (2005, 2008) extended this analysis with a study looking at improvement in patients with PTSD as reflected in effect size of changes at the item level of the CD-RISC as well as for the total score. Among the 25 items of the CD-RISC, 14 items showed the strongest effect sizes, arbitrarily taken as 0.25 or greater. Five of the items showing the most change reflected hardiness (items 7, 1, 14, 19, and 16). Three of the items showing the most change reflected tenacity (items 24, 12, and 11). Three of the items that were sensitive to change reflected belief in a benevolent world (items 3, 9, and 20), and three were difficult to classify (items 5, 13, and 15).

Factor Analytic Studies, 10 Item and 2 Item Versions

Additional research using the CD-RISC has indicated that the factor structure has varied according to setting. For instance, the original five factors have been supported in one Australian study of nurses (Gillespie, Chaboyer, & Walli, 2007).

However, in a US sample of community-dwelling older women, a four factor solution was observed. Factor 1 (9 items) included items related to goal orientation, tenacity, and personal control. Factor 2 (10 items) included tolerance for negative affect and adaptability. Factor 3 (4 items) included items on leadership and acting on a hunch. Factor 4 (2 items) involved spiritual orientation, (Lamond et al., 2008). Additionally, a Chinese study of the CD-RISC failed to verify the original factor structure through confirmatory factor analysis (CFA) and reported three factor solutions through exploratory factor analysis: Tenacity, Strength, and Optimism (Yu & Zhang, 2007). Singh and Yu (2010) found in a study of Indian college students that the data failed to replicate the 5-factor model obtained among American samples. These authors found that for this sample a 4 factor solution was easier to interpret and recommended that cross-cultural differences in the meaning of resilience needed to be considered.

Campbell-Sills and Stein (2007) conducted a reanalysis of the factor structure of the CD-RISC. First, they suggested that it should be determined whether the CD-RISC measures resilience as a unitary dimension or multiple latent dimensions. Second, if the CD-RISC has a multifactorial structure, it must be established that this structure is stable across independent samples and that each factor can be reliably and validly measured. These authors used a sequential approach with three independent samples that consisted of (a) an initial EFA, (b) replication of EFA findings in an independent sample, and (c) CFA which indicated that the CD-RISC had an unstable factor structure across two demographically equivalent samples. Based on the results of the two EFAs, they could not confidently specify a model for CFA that contained the full 25 items. Problems with the 25-item CD-RISC included (a) several items that displayed inconsistent loadings across the two EFAs (items 5, 15, 18, 23, and 25), (b) an item that had no salient loading in either EFA (item 20), (c) a factor that was consistently defined by too few items (faith), and (d) a factor that was consistently defined by four items but was difficult to interpret because it contained two disparate themes (social support/purpose).

Ten Item Version

Problems with stability of factor structure for the original scale led Campbell-Sills and Stein (2007) to propose a shorter version of the CD-RISC. They dropped all items that had either inconsistent or non-salient loadings, as well as items corresponding to factors that were poorly defined. Campbell-Sills and Stein (2007) repeated EFA in Samples 1 and 2 using this shorter version of the CD-RISC before conducting CFA that identified two predominant factors corresponding with "hardiness" and "tenacity" (the other two factors identified in the analysis, corresponding to "social support" and "faith" were weaker, and did not contribute items to the 10-item scale). A series of empirically driven modifications was made. The hardiness factor was defined by items 1, 4, 6–8, 14, 16, 17, and 19. The persistence factor was defined by items 10–12 and 24. The correlation of the hardiness and persistence factors was 0.63. The 10-item version of the CD-RISC scale combines scores on items 1 ("Able to adapt to change"), 4 ("Can deal with whatever comes"), 6 ("See the humorous side of things"), 7 ("Coping with stress strengthens"), 8 ("Tend to bounce back after illness or hardship"), 11 ("You can achieve your goals"), 14("Under pressure, focus and think clearly"), 16 ("Not easily discouraged by failure"), 17 ("Think of self as strongperson"), and 19 ("Can handle unpleasant feelings"). These authors reduced the two factor model to a one factor model of resilience for the 10 item version based on the finding that the items loading on the persistence factor were redundant, introducing error into the model. The abridged CD-RISC therefore contained only items that had consistent, salient loadings on the hardiness and persistence factors in the Sample 1 and Sample 2 EFAs.

Campbell-Sills and Stein (2007) conceded that it might be argued that their elimination of items resulted in important features of resilience being left out of the measure such as faith, social support, and self-efficacy. They acknowledged that the reasons for excluding them from the CD-RISC were primarily statistical in nature. It is possible that if each of these domains was represented by a sufficient number of items, they would emerge as reliable and valid dimensions of resilience (p. 1027). These authors concluded that rather than reflect negatively on the CD-RISC, the results of their investigation were positive in demonstrating that resilience can be reliably assessed with a subset of the CD-RISC items. These authors went on to use the CD-RISC-10 in future research arguing that the two instruments measured essentially the same thing as the original version (Campbell-Sills, Forde, & Stein, 2009).

A community study was conducted by Campbell-Sills et al. (2009) using the CD-RISC-10, in a nonrepresentative sample of community residents in the vicinity of New York City in the aftermath of 9/11 terrorist attack. Results suggested that approximately 11% of the variance in resilience as measured by the 10 item version was explained by demographic characteristics and an additional 2% of the variance in resilience was explained by history of childhood maltreatment. Salient demographic predictors included being female, having a lower education level and a lower level of income. The authors noted that (1) many other possible contributors to resilience were not measured in this study; and (2) 87% of variance in resilience was left unexplained, leaving much room for factors other than demographic characteristics and childhood maltreatment to "explain" a person's level of resilience. The authors also acknowledged that under-representation of minorities and administration of the CD-RISC-10 may have limited generalizability of their findings. The samples were homogeneous in terms of age and educational level and were predominantly Caucasian women, African American students were under-represented. In addition, some potentially important demographic features (e.g., income level) were not assessed.

Two Item Scale

A 2-item version of the CD-RISC scale was developed by Vaishnavi, Connor, and Davidson (2007). The 2-item CD-RISC version combined scores on items 1 ("Able to adapt to change") and 8 ("Tend to bounce back after illness or hardship"). These items were selected by the originators of the scale as etymologically capturing the essence of resilience, i.e., the ability to spring back and successfully adapt to change. The two items of the CD-RISC2 were thought by the authors to reflect resilience and thus were felt to likely overlap similar concepts such as "hardiness," "stress vulnerability," and "perceived stress." The authors reported that there are several limitations to this report. First, the CD-RISC2 items were chosen out of the full CD-RISC based on what items were thought to capture the essence of resilience, a subjective approach, rather than based on empirical criteria. Second, the CD-RISC2 assesses the characteristics of resilience, but does not assess the resiliency process or provide information about the underpinnings of resilience.

Discussion

The CD-RISC provides an example of an assessment tool developed in a research environment with a specific purpose of assessing improvements over and above symptom reduction in patients with PTSD associated with drug treatment. The item selection appears to have had a good theoretical basis. As the result of factor instability in equivalent but nonrepresentative samples, items were reduced from 25 to 10. It was acknowledged that the instability of factor structure might have been related to insufficient numbers of items covering various aspects of the original construct and that the reduction was guided by statistical rather than theoretical principles. It has been suggestion however, that factor structure differences would be expected in studies of groups that varied culturally and demographically. It is possible that factor analyses of samples that have been systematically selected to represent specific populations would render more structural stability within populations.

Acknowledgment Appreciation is expressed to Jonathan Davidson, second author of the CD-RISC for his assistance in preparing this chapter.

References

Alexander, C. (1998). *The Endurance: Shackleton's legendary Antarctic expedition*. New York: Knopf.

Andrews, W., Parker, G., & Barrett, E. (1998). The SSRI antidepressants: Exploring their "other" possible properties. *Journal of Affective Disorders, 49*, 141–144.

Campbell-Sills, L., Cohan, S. L., & Stein, M. B. (2006). Relationship of resilience to personality, coping and psychiatric symptoms in young adults. *Behavior, Research and Therapy, 44*, 585–599.

Campbell-Sills, L., Forde, D., & Stein, M. B. (2009). Demographic and childhood environmental predictors of resilience in a community sample. *Journal of Psychiatric Research, 43*, 1007–1012. doi:10:106/j.psychires.2009.01.013.

Campbell-Sills, L., & Stein, M. (2007). Psychometric analysis and refinement of the Connor-Davidson Resilience Scale (CD-RISC): validation of a 10-item-measure of resilience. *Journal of Traumatic Stress, 20*, 1019–1028.

Connor, K. M., & Davidson, J. R. (2003). Development of a new resilience scale: The Connor-Davidson Resilience Scale (CD-RISC). *Depression and Anxiety, 18*, 76–82.

Connor, K. M., Sutherland, S. M., Tupler, L. A., Churchill, L. E., Malik, M. L., & Davidson, J. R. T. (1999). Fluoxetine in posttraumatic stress disorder: A randomized, placebo-controlled trial. *The British Journal of Psychiatry, 175*, 17–22.

Davidson, J., Baldwin, D., Stein, D. J., Kuper, E., Benattia, I., Ahmed, S., et al. (2006). Treatment of posttraumatic stress disorder with venlafaxine extended release: A 6-month randomized, controlled trial. *Archives of General Psychiatry, 63*, 1158–1165.

Davidson, J. R., Payne, V. M., Connor, K. M., Foa, E. B., Rothbaum, B. O., Hertzberg, M. A., et al. (2005). Trauma, resilience and saliostasis: Effects of treatment in posttraumatic stress disorder. *International Clinical Psychopharmacology, 20*, 43–48.

Davidson, J. R. T., Baldwin, D. S., Stein, D. J., Petersen, R., Ahmed, S., Musgnung, J. L., Benattia, I., & Rothbaum, B. O., (2008). Effects of venlafaxine extended-release in post-traumatic stress disorder: an item analysis of the Connor-Davidson Resilience Scale (CD-RISC). *Int Clin Psychopharmacology, 23*: 299–303.

Dienstbier, R. A. (1991). Behavioral correlates of sympathoadrena reactivity: The toughness model. *Medicine and Science in Sports and Exercise, 23*, 846–852.

Gillespie, B. M., Chaboyer, W., & Walli, M. (2007). The influence of personal characteristics on the resilience of operating room nurses: A predictor study. *International Journal of Nursing Studies, 10*, 1016.

Healey, D., & Healey, H. (1998). The clinical pharmacologic profile of reboxetine: Does it involve the putative neurobiological substrates of wellbeing? *Journal of Affective Disorders, 51*, 313–322.

Kobasa, S. C. (1979). Stressful life events, personality, and health: An inquiry into hardiness. *Journal of Personality and Social Psychology, 37*, 1–11.

Lamond, A. J., Depp, C. A., Allison, M., Langer, R., Reichstadt, J., Moore, D. J., et al. (2008). Measurement and predictors of resilience among community-dwelling older women. *Journal of Psychiatric Research, 43*(2), 148–154. doi:10.1016/j.jpsychires.2008.03.007.

Lyons, J. (1991). Strategies for assessing the potential for positive adjustment following trauma. *Journal of Traumatic Stress, 4*, 93–111.

Rutter, M. (1985). Resilience in the face of adversity: Protective factors and resistance to psychiatric disorders. *The British Journal of Psychiatry, 147*, 598–611.

Singh, K., & Yu, X. (2010). Psychometric evaluation of the Connors-Davidson Resiliency Scale (CD-RISC) in a sample of Indian students. *Journal of Psychology, 1*(1), 20–30.

Vaishnavi, S., Connor, K., & Davidson, J. R. (2007). An abbreviated version of the Connor-Davidson Resilience Scale (CD-RISC), the CD-RISC2: Psychometric properties and applications in psychopharmacological trials. *Psychiatry Research, 152*, 293–297.

Yu, X., & Zhang, J. (2007). Factor analysis and psychometric evaluation of the Connor-Davidson Resilience Scale (CD RISC) with Chinese people. *Social Behaviour and Personality, 35*, 19–30.

13 The Foundations of Resilience: What Are the Critical Resources for Bouncing Back from Stress?

Bruce W. Smith, Emerson M. Epstein, J. Alexis Ortiz, Paulette J. Christopher, and Erin M. Tooley

Resilience has been defined in so many ways that it is in danger of losing its central place in examining and understanding the human experience of stress. Although resilience is universally referred to as something that is beneficial in relation to stress, there are several different kinds of positive phenomena that have been associated with it (Dyer & McGuinness, 1996). Definitions of resilience have included the ability to bounce back or recover from stress (Carver, 1998; Smith et al., 2008), adapting positively to stressful circumstances or difficulties (Luthar, Cicchetti, & Becker, 2000), not becoming ill or maintaining stability despite stress (Bonanno, 2004), and functioning above the norm in spite of stress or adversity (Tusaie & Dyer, 2004). The variety of ways of defining resilience has made it difficult both for lay people and for social scientists to clearly communicate about how to think about and cultivate resilience. The purpose of this chapter is to focus on a basic and central meaning of resilience as the ability to bounce back from stress and differentiate it from the personal and social resources that may serve as a foundation for it.

B.W. Smith, Ph.D. (✉) • E.M. Epstein • J.A. Ortiz
P.J. Christopher • E.M. Tooley
Department of Psychology, University of New Mexico, Albuquerque, NM 87131-1161, USA
e-mail: bwsmith@unm.edu

Defining Resilience

The original meaning of the English word resilience is "to bounce or spring back" (Simpson, 2005). The root word for the English word "resilience" is the word "resile," which means "to bounce or spring back" (from re- "back" + salire "to jump, leap"; Agnes, 2005). The typical dictionary definitions of resilience have included phrases that make it applicable to both the physical and the social sciences. The idea that a piece of metal may be able to spring back into shape or its original position is an example of resilience in an engineering context. The idea of a person being able to bounce back and recover strength, spirits, or humor after adversity, misfortune, or a stressful event is the gist of this idea of resilience in a human context. Thus, in psychological terms, the ability to bounce back or recover from stress is closest to the original meaning of the word "resilience" and its root in the word "resile."

However, resilience has come to be associated with several additional meanings including resistance to illness, positive adaptation, and even finding benefits and growth in the context and aftermath of stress. In distinguishing between the other meanings associated with resilience, it may be better to use different words or expressions for resistance to illness, adaptation to stress, and functioning above the norm in spite of stress. Carver (1998) provided a clear distinction between "resilience" as returning to the previous

S. Prince-Embury and D.H. Saklofske (eds.), *Resilience in Children, Adolescents, and Adults: Translating Research into Practice*, The Springer Series on Human Exceptionality,
DOI 10.1007/978-1-4614-4939-3_13, © Springer Science+Business Media New York 2013

level of functioning (e.g., bouncing back or recovery) and "thriving" as moving to a superior level of functioning following a stressful event. In addition, "stress adaptation" could be used for changing or making a positive adjustment to a new situation. Finally, it may be preferable to use a word like "resistance" (as in "stress resistance" or "resistance to illness") to refer to not becoming ill or showing any initial decrease in functioning during stress.

Measures of Resilience

Although several definitions of resilience have been proposed, the measures that have been associated with the word "resilience" have rarely targeted these definitions and have not specifically focused on the ability to bounce back from stress. For example, in the Connor–Davidson Resilience Scale (CD-RISC; Connor & Davidson, 2003), resilience is defined by the selective strengths or assets needed to help an individual survive adversity. Specifically, the CD-RISC measures the concepts of control, commitment, goal-orientation, self-esteem, adaptability, social skills, humor, strengthening through stress, and the endurance of pain. Similarly, the Resilience Scale (RS; Wagnild & Young, 1993) attempts to assess an individual's capacity to live a life worth living. Specifically, the RS measures five personal concepts including equanimity, perseverance, meaningfulness, self-reliance, and existential aloneness. Finally, the Resilience Scale for Adults (RSA; Friborg, Hjemdal, Rosenvinge, & Martinussen, 2003) measures factors that are thought to promote resilience in adults. The RSA specifically measures five factors that may promote resilience including personal competence, social competence, family coherence, social support, and personal structure.

Thus, rather than focusing on resilience as bouncing back from stress or any of the other more specific meanings that have been associated with resilience, most measures of resilience have attempted to assess an array of personal characteristics and social factors that may promote resilience. Because of the need to assess and better understand the specific meanings that has been associated with resilience, we developed the "Brief Resilience Scale" (BRS; Smith et al., 2008) in order to assess resilience as the ability to bounce back or recover from stress. While we realize that it is possible to make an argument for associating the word resilience with other specific meanings such as stress resistance, stress adaptation, and thriving and growth, we thought that having a measure of resilience as the ability to bounce back from stress may be a good place to start since it is the original and most basic meaning of the word "resilience."

One primary advantage of defining and assessing resilience in this more specific manner is that it makes it possible to clearly differentiate resilience as the ability to bounce back from the other factors that may promote it. After we developed the BRS, we thought that a logical next step in our research program was to examine its relationship with the potential personal and social resources that may be most likely to increase the ability to bounce back from stress. We also sought to assess resilience and potential resilience resources in a variety of populations: including those who are healthy individuals, patients facing the kinds of stress that call for resilience, and people facing other kinds of challenging situations. Our goal was to identify the personal and social resources that may be most important in providing the foundations for the ability to bounce back from stress. Thus, we now present the potential resources that we assessed and then the kind of samples in which we examined their relationship with resilience.

The Potential Resources for Resilience

What are the most important resources for the ability to bounce back from stress? Rather than including a laundry list of variables that may be related to general positive adaptation, our approach was to identify factors that have been empirically or can be conceptually linked to this specific definition of resilience. One of the most distinctive aspects of resilience as the ability to bounce back or recover from stress is that it involves a temporal dimension (Carver, 1998). That is, the process of bouncing back from stress may involve three stages: (1) actually confronting an event that is stressful, (2) orienting oneself towards a positive future outcome of the event, and (3) engaging in efforts to cope with it. As with most stage theories, we do not mean to imply that they always occur in this order or that people may go back and forth between them. However, we do think that people generally move through and master these stages in this order and that all three may be critical for the successfully bouncing back from a stressful event. In addition, many of the potentially important resources for resilience can be categorized by which of the above three stages that they best address and we thought it would be important to address each of them. Thus, we decided to identify the factors that may be relevant for each.

First, the ability to bounce back from stress may generally require actually confronting a stressful event. This may sound simple but may often be underestimated in theory and research regarding resilience (Hayes, Follete, & Linehan, 2004). While avoidance or denial may frequently be used to cushion the blow of a stressful event, over the long-term they may be counterproductive and prevent an individual from taking in all the information necessary for successfully recovering. Indeed, when faced with a traumatic event, avoidance may lead to the vicious cycle of both avoidance and reexperiencing that can breed and sustain posttraumatic stress disorder (Lanius et al., 2010). Recently developed mindfulness and acceptance-based interventions have focused more on this present-focused aspect of confronting a stressor than previously developed approaches (Hayes et al., 2004). Thus, we thought that the ability to pay attention to present moment experiences (Kabat-Zinn, 1990) and the ability to be clear about one's emotional experience (Feldman-Barrett, Gross, Christensen, & Benvenuto, 2001) may be important for enabling a person to confront a stressful experience and begin the process of bouncing back. To measure the first we used the Mindful Attention and Awareness Scale (MAAS; Brown & Ryan, 2003) and to measure the second we used the mood clarity subscale of the Trait Meta Mood Scale (Salovey, Mayer, Goldman, Turvey, & Palfai, 1995).

Second, the ability to bounce back from stress may generally require that an individual orients themselves towards a positive future outcome of the event. This may require both a sense of direction and purpose in life (Wong & Fry, 1998) and a sense of optimism that it is possible to move in the direction of achieving one's goals and this purpose (Scheier & Carver, 2001; Smith & Zautra, 2004). Frankl (1963) wrote about how valuable a sense of meaning and purpose and life was for enabling and motivating him to survive living in a concentration camp during WWII. We found that a sense of purpose in life was the most important factor in recovery for people who had total knee replacement surgery (Smith & Zautra, 2004) and others have found that purpose in life has been related to better adjustment to stress (Bonebright, Clay, & Ankenmann, 2000). Optimism, in the sense of the expectation of a successful outcome to a stressful event may be critical in giving people the confidence to begin to engage in efforts to cope with it rather than avoid or deny it (Scheier & Carver, 2003). Optimism has been associated with better mental and physical health in the aftermath of a variety of stressors including coronary artery bypass graft surgery and cancer (Andersson, 1996; Scheier et al., 1999; Schnoll, Knowles, & Harlow, 2002). Thus, because of the value of orienting oneself to a positive outcome to a stressful event, we included the Life Orientation Test-Revised (Scheier, Carver, & Bridges, 1994) to assess optimism and the purpose in life subscale of the Scales of Psychological Well-Being to assess a sense of meaning, purpose, and direction in life (Ryff & Keyes, 1995).

Third, the ability to recover from a stressful event involves efforts to actively engage in efforts to cope with it. The two factors that we thought may be most important here were an active approach to coping (Scheier & Carver, 2003) and the support of other people for the coping process (Cohen & Hoberman, 1983). Although a great challenge of studying coping has been to assess all of the different kinds of strategies that individuals use to cope with stress, researchers have consistently pointed to an overarching approach coping factor that may be best thought of as active coping (Smith & Zautra, 2008). The idea here is that recovery from a stressful event is more likely with an active approach to dealing with the event rather than passively accepting it or avoiding it. While an active approach to coping can be thought of as a personal resource, social support is the prime example of a social resource that may be particularly relevant for times of stressful events and thus for resilience in the face of stress. There is strong and consistent evidence that social support is related to better health and functioning in the context and the aftermath of a variety of kinds of stress (Cohen & Wills, 1985). Thus, we included measures of both active coping (Carver, 1997) and social support (Cohen, Mermelstein, Kamarck, & Hoberman, 1985; Sherbourne & Stewart, 1991) as resources that may be important for actively engaging in efforts to recover from a stressor.

We decided to include two additional potential resources that may not be as directly tied to one of the three temporal aspects of bouncing back from stress. First, we wanted to include a general measure of spirituality because of the evidence that religion may play an important role in coping with stress and in resilience (Banerjee & Pyles, 2004; Pargament, 1997). Rather than being tied to one of three temporal aspects, we view spirituality as a personal resource that may pervade, help to integrate, and operate in all three. Second, we wanted to include a measure of positive relationships with others as a second social resource that may not as specifically be tied to stress and coping but that may still be linked to the ability to bounce back from stress. We have found that positive relationships with other people may be a unique source of positive emotions (Smith & Zautra, 2008) and positive emotions have been experimentally linked to the ability to recover from stress (Tugade & Fredrickson, 2004). We also thought that positive relations may be related to all three temporal aspects rather than most directly tied to one.

Finally, we decided to include four important demographic factors because they may also be important resources for resilience and because we wanted to include them as control variables. The demographic factors that we included in our analyses were age, gender, education, and income. We thought that age may be related to an improved ability to bounce back from stress because of research showing that emotional regulation and health may improve with age (Scheibe & Carstensen, 2010). We thought that education and income may be related to higher resilience because of evidence that socioeconomic status is often related to better health and functioning (Adler et al., 1994). Finally, we were not sure how gender might be related to the ability to bounce back from stress but thought it would be important to include in order to help determine whether there may be gender differences.

Resilience in a Variety of Samples

Finally, we thought it may be important to examine the relationship between resilience and these potential resilience resources in a variety of individuals and samples. First, we thought it would be important to include healthy individuals and had assessed most of these variables in a large general sample of college undergraduates and in a sample of healthy adult women who served as a control group for a study of women with fibromyalgia. Second, we thought it could be particularly valuable to include patients whom are facing chronic health stressors where stress is high and where resilience may be critical. Thus, we included the sample of women with fibromyalgia and a sample of cardiac patients in a cardiac rehabilitation program. Third, we thought it would be also interesting to include individuals who were facing other kinds of stressors that were not related to health problems but that were voluntarily selected. Thus, we include a sample of first-generation college students (e.g., students without a parent who has attended any college) in their first year of college and a sample of urban firefighters who face both normal adult stressors and traumatic stressors on the job. We thought that this might provide us with important contrasts between what we will call "healthy," "patient," and "at-risk" individuals and also give us a larger total number of participants with which to examine our hypotheses.

Study Hypotheses

Our primary hypothesis was that the variables selected to assess each of the three aspects of the temporal dimension of bouncing back from stress would be related to the BRS. That is, we expected mindfulness and mood clarity to be related to resilience because they may enable a person to confront a stressful event (Brown & Ryan, 2003; Salovey et al., 1995), optimism and purpose in life to be related to resilience because they may be involved in orienting a person towards a successful outcome (Scheier & Carver, 2001; Smith & Zautra, 2004), and active coping and social support to be related to resilience because they are important for engaging in efforts to cope with stress (Cohen & Wills, 1985; Scheier & Carver, 2003). Our secondary hypothesis was that that spirituality (Pargament, 1997), positive relations with others (Smith & Zautra, 2008), age (Scheibe & Carstensen, 2010), income, and education (Adler et al., 1994) would be related to resilience. We had no specific hypothesis about whether resilience scores would vary by gender.

Method

Participants and Procedures

There were a total of 844 participants in the six samples included for this chapter. The samples can be divided into three categories that we will called be "patient" because they have a chronic health problem ($n=260$), "at-risk" because they have voluntarily selected a chronic and challenging stressor ($n=274$), or "healthy" because they neither have a chronic health problem or have selected a chronic and challenging stressor ($n=310$).

There were two healthy samples including college students (sample 1; $n=259$) and healthy adult women (sample 2; $n=51$). The healthy women are similar to other adult women samples with the exception that they had no chronic pain because they served as a control group for a study of women with fibromyalgia. The college students were recruited through the participant pool in the Department of Psychology at the University of New Mexico, Albuquerque, New Mexico. The healthy adult women were recruited through newspaper ads in Albuquerque, New Mexico.

There were two patient samples including women with fibromyalgia (sample 3, $n=32$) and cardiac patients in a cardiac rehabilitation program (sample 4; $n=228$). The women with fibromyalgia were recruited through newspaper ads and through physician's offices in the Albuquerque metropolitan area and all had their diagnoses confirmed by a physician. The cardiac patients were recruited through the New Heart, Inc. cardiac rehabilitation program in Albuquerque, New Mexico. The requirements for participating in the New Heart cardiac rehabilitation program include having had a myocardial infarction (MI), coronary artery bypass surgery (CABG), having a stent installed, having value repair or replacement, or having had a heart transplant.

There were two at-risk samples including first-generation college students (they did not have a parent who had attended any college) in their first year of college (sample 5; $n=151$) and urban firefighters (sample 6; $n=123$). The first-generation college students were all students at the University of New Mexico and were recruited through newspaper ads, the distribution of newsletters on the campus, and the through announcements in classes for first year students. The urban firefighters were members of the Albuquerque Fire Department and were recruited through newspaper ads, the distribution of newsletters to the fire departments, and emails on a listserv of all of the firefighters in the department.

Measures

The Brief Resilience Scale (BRS) and several demographic, personal, and social resources that may be related to the ability to bounce back from stress were assessed by a questionnaire in each of the six samples. Each of these measures is described below.

Resilience

Resilience was assessed using the Brief Resilience Scale (BRS; Smith et al., 2008) which was designed to capture the original and most basic meaning of resilience as the ability to bounce back or recover from stress (Agnes, 2005). The BRS includes six questions, with an equal number of positive and negatively worded items to reduce the effects of social desirability and positive/negative response bias. The following instructions were used to administer the BRS: "Please indicate the extent to which you agree with each of the following statements by using the following scale; 1 = strongly disagree, 2 = disagree, 3 = neutral, 4 = agree, 5 = strongly agree." The items on the BRS are as follows

1. I tend to bounce back quickly after hard times.
2. I have a hard time making it through stressful events (*R*).
3. It does not take me long to recover from a stressful event.
4. It is hard for me to snap back when something bad happens (*R*).
5. I usually come through difficult times with little trouble.
6. I tend to take a long time to get over set-backs in my life (*R*).

   R = reverse coded items.

The scores are calculated as the average of responses on all questions after reverse coding items 2, 4, and 6. The Cronbach's alphas for the BRS in samples 1–6 were 0.836, 0.902, 0.877, 0.798, 0.754, and 0.702.

Demographic Resources

The potential demographic resources assessed in all six samples were age, gender, and education. Income was assessed in all of the samples except the two college student samples (samples 1 and 5).

Personal Resources

Active Coping. The active coping subscale of the Brief COPE (Carver, 1997) was used to assess an active approach to coping with stress (e.g., "I take action to try to make the situation better"). The two items were scored on a 4-point scale from 0 = "I do not do this at all" to 3 = "I do this a lot." The active coping subscale was included in all six samples and the Cronbach's alphas for samples 1–6 were 0.621, 0.599, 0.538, 0.723, 0.614, and 0.467, respectively.

Mindfulness. The Mindful Attention Awareness Scale (MAAS; Brown & Ryan, 2003) was included in samples 1 and 6. The MAAS included 15 items (e.g., "I feel it difficult to stay focused on what's happening in the present," reverse scored) that were scored on a 6-point scale from 1 = "almost never" to 6 = "almost always." The Cronbach's alpha for the MAAS was 0.865 in sample 1 and 0.913 in sample 6.

Mood Clarity. The mood clarity subscale of the Trait Meta-Mood Scale (TMMS; Salovey et al., 1995) assessed the degree to which participants believe that they are clear about what they are feeling. There are 11 items (e.g., "I am rarely confused about how I feel," reverse coded) were scored on a 5-point scale from 1 = "strongly disagree" to 5 = "strongly agree." The mood clarity subscale was included in samples 1, 2, 3, and 6 and the Cronbach's alphas were 0.833, 0.765, 0.855, and 0.841, respectively.

Optimism. The tendency to have positive expectations about outcomes in the future was assessed by the Life Orientation Test Revised (LOTR; Scheier, Carver, & Bridges, 1994). There are six items ("I'm always optimistic about my future") that were scored on a 5-point scale from 1 = "strongly disagree" to 5 = "strongly agree." The LOTR was assessed in six samples and the Cronbach's alphas for samples 1–6 were 0.759, 0.870, 0.931, 0.787, 0.731, and 0.748, respectively.

Purpose in Life. The purpose in life subscale of the Scales of Psychological Well-Being (Ryff & Keyes, 1995) was included to assess the sense that life has a sense of meaning and purpose. The purpose in life subscale includes items (e.g., "I have a sense of purpose and direction in life") that were scored on a 6-point scale from 1 = "strongly disagree" to 6 = "strongly agree." The 3-item version of the purpose in life subscale was used in sample 4, and the 7-item version was used in samples 1, 2, 3, 5, and 6. The Cronbach's alphas for samples 1–6 were 0.697, 0.870, 0.901, 0.561, 0.814, and 0.641, respectively.

Spirituality. The measure used to assess spirituality included three items to assess religious service attendance, religious salience, and spiritual salience (Fetzer Institute, 1999). The items were scored on a 6-point scale (e.g., 0–5 range) with response anchors that varied according to the items. The Cronbach's alphas for samples 1–6 were 0.934, 0.981, 0.942, 0.790, 0.807, and 0.753, respectively.

Social Resources

Positive Relations. The positive relations with others subscale of the Scales of Psychological Well-Being (Ryff & Keyes, 1995) was included to assess the sense that life has a sense of meaning and purpose. The purpose in life subscale includes seven items (e.g., "I enjoy personal and mutual conversations with family members or friends") that were scored on a 6-point scale from 1 = "strongly disagree" to 6 = "strongly agree." The positive relations subscale was included in samples 1, 5, and 6 and the Cronbach's alphas were 0.705, 0.836, and 0.736, respectively.

Social Support. The Interpersonal Support Evaluation List (ISEL; Cohen et al., 1985) was used for samples 1, 5, and 6 and the MOS Social Support Survey (Sherbourne & Stewart, 1991) was used for the samples 2, 3, and 4. The ISEL has 12 items (e.g., "when I need suggestions on how to deal with personal problems, I know someone I can turn to") and the MOS measure has 20 items (e.g., "someone to turn to for suggestions about how to deal with a personal problem"). Both of the scales were scored on 0–4 scales to facilitate collapsing them for comparison across studies and samples. The Cronbach's alphas for the ISEL in samples 1, 5, and 6 were 0.888, 0.828, and 0.811, respectively. The Cronbach's alphas for the MOS measure in samples 2, 3, and 4 were 0.782, 0.977, and 0.930, respectively.

Statistical Analyses

Independent samples *t*-tests were conducted to examine the differences between the six samples on the measures of resilience and the potential demographic, personal, and social resilience resources. Correlation analyses were used to examine the relationship between resilience and the potential resources for resilience in each of the six samples and in all samples together. Multiple regression analyses were used to examine the relative importance of different resources in predicting resilience in each of the six samples and in all samples together. The alpha used as the cut-off for all statistical tests was $p < 0.05$.

Results

Descriptive Statistics and Comparisons of Means

Table 13.1 displays the descriptive statistics for the potential demographic, personal, and social resources for resilience in all six samples and in all of the samples combined. The overall sample of 844 was relatively evenly divided with 48% female. The healthy women and women with fibromyalgia samples were of course all women, the cardiac patients and urban firefighters had a majority of men, and the college student samples had a relatively larger proportion of women. All of the differences in the proportion female were significant except that between general college students and the first-generation college students and that between the healthy women and women with fibromyalgia.

The mean overall age was 37 years with the two college samples with a lower mean age, the cardiac patients with a higher mean age, and the women and urban firefighter samples in the middle. All of the differences between the samples in age were significant. The mean years of education was in the 12–15 years for all samples with the college students having the lowest mean scores. All of the differences were significant except the difference between the women with fibromyalgia and the cardiac patients. The mean incomes were in a similar $60,000–70,000 range for the healthy women, cardiac patients, and urban firefighters and lower at $45,530 for the women with fibromyalgia although none of the differences in income were significant.

The means for the personal resources generally followed the pattern of the healthy women

Table 13.1 Descriptive statistics for the study variables in each of the six samples and all samples combined[a]

	Healthy		Patient		At-risk		
	College students ($n=259$)	Healthy women ($n=51$)	Women with fibromyalgia ($n=32$)	Cardiac patients ($n=228$)	First generation ($n=151$)	Urban firefighters ($n=123$)	All samples ($n=844$)
Demographic resources							
Female (%)	64	100	100	27	56	7	48
Age (years)	21.08(4.26)	45.01(8.49)	49.99(6.30)	63.91(10.81)	18.42(0.99)	33.61(8.09)	36.60(20.01)
Education (years)	12.29(0.75)	15.33(2.92)	14.69(2.07)	14.73(2.78)	12.00(0.00)	13.29(1.38)	13.29(2.14)
Income ($1,000)	–	65.47(52.96)	45.53(47.57)	64.19(39.68)	–	61.47(11.92)	62.20(37.09)
Personal resources							
Active coping	2.31(0.65)	2.62(0.50)	2.14(0.70)	2.40(0.67)	2.10(0.68)	2.61(0.50)	2.35(0.66)
Optimism	3.65(0.64)	4.14(0.59)	3.36(0.89)	3.89(0.72)	3.64(0.66)	3.97(0.55)	3.78(0.69)
Purpose in life	4.19(0.70)	5.13(0.62)	4.21(1.10)	4.50(0.80)	4.57(0.82)	4.54(0.59)	4.26(0.79)
Spirituality	2.73(1.16)	2.73(1.14)	3.54(1.26)	3.24(1.61)	3.15(1.24)	2.54(1.10)	2.61(1.46)
Mood clarity	3.65(0.56)	3.81(0.46)	3.43(0.67)	–	–	3.86(0.50)	3.71(0.56)
Mindfulness	4.08(0.73)	–	–	–	–	4.39(0.85)	3.97(0.87)
Social resources							
Social support	3.38(0.54)	3.75(0.69)	3.31(0.75)	3.60(0.72)	3.41(0.51)	3.49(0.44)	3.47(0.64)
Positive relations	4.54(0.65)	–	–	–	4.68(0.92)	4.60(0.69)	4.59(0.75)
Resilience	3.56(0.67)	3.93(0.66)	3.18(0.90)	3.87(0.69)	3.54(0.63)	3.95(0.49)	3.70(0.68)

[a]Standard deviations are in parentheses

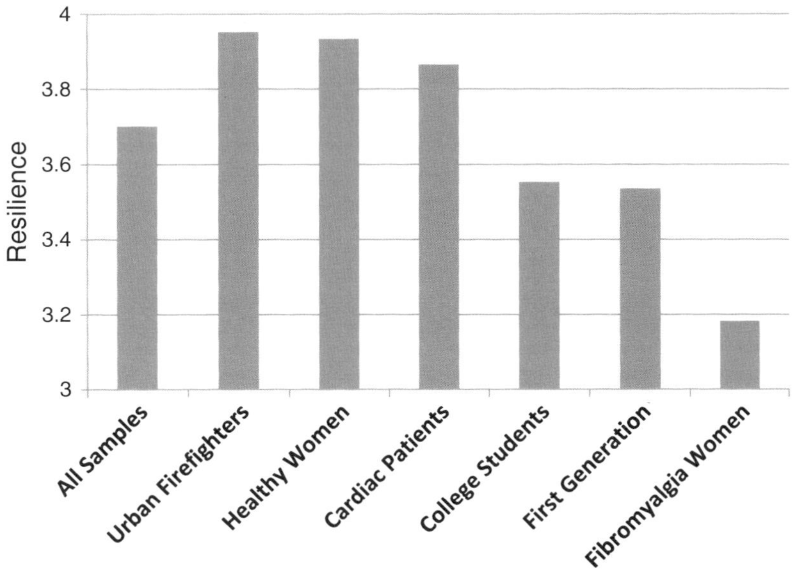

Fig. 13.1 Mean levels of resilience in all six samples and in each individual sample

and urban firefighters being the highest, the cardiac patients, college students and first-generation students being in the middle, and the women with fibromyalgia being the lowest. For active coping, the healthy women and urban firefighters were significantly higher than the general college students and cardiac patients who were significantly higher than the first-generation students and women with fibromyalgia. For optimism, the healthy women, urban firefighters, and cardiac patients were significantly higher than the general college students and first-generation college students, who were significantly higher than the women with fibromyalgia. For purpose in life, the healthy women were significantly higher than the first-generation students, urban firefighters, and cardiac patients who were significantly higher than the general college students and women with fibromyalgia. For spirituality, in contrast, the women with fibromyalgia were significantly higher than the cardiac patients and first-generation students who were significantly higher than the general college students, healthy women, and urban firefighters. For mood clarity, the healthy women and urban firefighters were significantly higher than the general college students who were significantly higher than the women with fibromyalgia. Finally, the urban firefighters were significantly higher on mindfulness than the general college students.

The patterns of significant differences in the social resources measures were similar to that of the personal resource measures for social support but not for the positive relations measure. For the MOS social support measure used with the healthy women, women with fibromyalgia, and cardiac patient samples, the only significant difference was that the healthy women were higher than the women with fibromyalgia. For the ISEL measure used with the general college student, first-generation, and urban firefighter samples, the only significant differences was that the urban firefighters were higher than the general college students. There were no significant differences in mean scores on the positive relations measure between the general college student, first-generation, and urban firefighter samples.

Finally, the mean scores for the BRS are displayed in Table 13.1 as well as in Fig. 13.1 because it is the focus of this chapter. The urban firefighters, healthy women, and cardiac patients were significantly higher than the general college students and first-generation students who were significantly higher than the women with

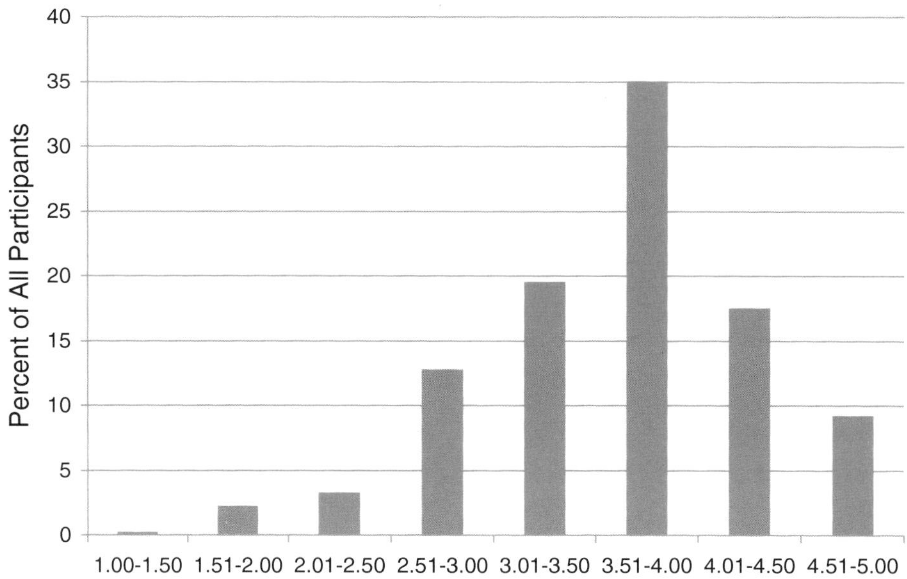

Fig. 13.2 Distribution of scores on the Brief Resilience Scale for all samples combined

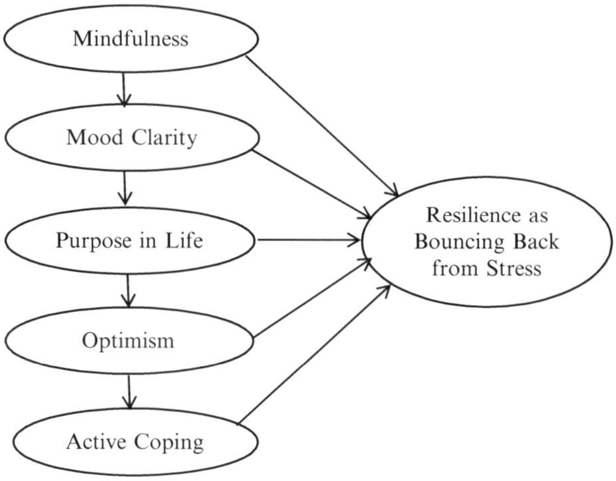

Fig. 13.3 Theoretical model of the effects of personal resources on resilience as bouncing back from stress

fibromyalgia. Thus, the samples can be thought of as being at three tiers regarding the ability to bounce back from stress with the urban firefighters, healthy women, and cardiac patients with a higher range of scores between 3.6 and 3.8, the two college student samples with a middle range of scores between 3.4 and 3.6, and the women with fibromyalgia with a mean score in the lower range with scores between 3.0 and 3.2.

Because this is the first report of the mean scores on the BRS in so many participants in a variety of samples, we present the range of scores in Fig. 13.2. As can be seen when viewing the figure, the distribution is nearly normal with a slight negative skew. Although researchers could select any one of these samples for comparison if they had a similar sample, we combined the samples since they include a range of healthy, patient, and at-risk participants. Because of the near normal distribution and the wide range of samples and participants, we suggest that the combined sample mean of 3.70 as an overall average resilience score. Because the standard deviation is nearly 0.70 (e.g., 0.68) and it is a conventional for one standard deviation to be a marker for high and low scores on a measure, we also suggest that scores below 3.00 be considered low and scores above 4.30 be considered high in resilience.

Correlations Between Resilience and the Potential Resilience Resources

Table 13.2 displays the zero-order correlations between the BRS and the potential resilience resources in each of the samples and in all of the samples combined. The general convention of describing $r=0.10$ as a small effect, $r=0.30$ as a medium effect, and $r=0.50$ as a large effect will be used in discussing the results. Age, education, and income were not correlated with resilience in any of the samples alone but had small positive relationships with greater resilience in all samples combined. Male gender had a small-to-moderate relationship with greater resilience in the general college student sample and in all of the samples combined.

As for the potential personal resources, all of the six potential personal resources were positive related to resilience when all of the samples were combined. However, there were large differences in the effect sizes and in how much each of these personal resources was related to resilience in each of the individual samples. Optimism and purpose in life were positively related with at least a medium effect size to resilience in all six samples and in all samples combined. Moreover, optimism had a very strong relationship with resilience in both patient samples ($r=0.701$ in the women with fibromyalgia and $r=0.743$ in the cardiac patients) and purpose in life had a very strong relationship with resilience in the women with fibromyalgia ($r=0.734$). Mood clarity had a strong positive relationship with resilience in three of the four samples in which it was assessed including a healthy sample (general college students), a patient sample (women with fibromyalgia), and an at-risk sample (urban firefighters). Mindfulness had a medium positive relationship with resilience in both of the samples (general college student and urban firefighter) in which it was assessed. Active coping had a medium positive relationship with resilience in four of the six samples in which it was assessed and a small or medium positive nonsignificant relationship with resilience in the other two samples. Finally, spirituality had only a small positive relationship with resilience in the cardiac patient sample and was not related to resilience in any of the other samples.

As for the potential social resources, both social support and positive relations had small-to-medium positive relationships with resilience when all of the samples were combined. Social support had small-to-medium positive relationships with resilience in five of the six samples and a small nonsignificant positive relationship with resilience in the healthy women sample. Positive relations had small-to-medium positive significant relationship with resilience in each of the three samples in which it was assessed.

An overall univariate perspective on the relative value of the potential resources might be gained by classifying them based on effect sizes in the analyses using all samples combined. Using this approach, optimism and mood clarity had strong positive relationships with resilience ($r=0.575$ and 0.486, respectively) and mindfulness, active coping, and purpose in life which had medium positive relationships with resilience (rs from 0.287 to 0.351), suggesting that these five personal resources may be some of the most important factors for resilience. In addition, male gender, positive relations, social support, age, and education had effects that were all in the small-to-medium sized range (rs from 0.162 to 0.231). Finally, income and spirituality had the smallest positive, but significant, relationships with resilience ($r=0.091$ and 0.102, respectively).

Table 13.2 Zero-order correlations between the Brief Resilience Scale and the potential resilience resources in each of the six samples and all samples combined[a]

	Healthy		Patient		At-risk		
	College students ($n=259$)	Healthy women ($n=51$)	Women with fibromyalgia ($n=32$)	Cardiac patients ($n=228$)	First generation ($n=151$)	Urban firefighters ($n=123$)	All samples ($n=844$)
Demographic resources							
Age	0.113^{+}	0.010	−0.123	0.097	−0.018	0.060	0.185^{**}
Male gender	0.260^{**}	–	–	0.099	0.124	0.058	0.231^{**}
Education	0.062	0.269^{+}	−0.044	0.081	–	−0.028	0.162^{**}
Income	–	−0.098	0.321^{+}	0.068	–	0.096	0.102^{*}
Personal resources							
Active coping	0.289^{**}	0.100	0.291	0.357^{**}	0.266^{**}	0.322^{**}	0.341^{**}
Mindfulness	0.328^{**}	–	–	–	–	0.308^{**}	0.351^{**}
Mood clarity	0.466^{**}	0.258^{+}	0.588^{**}	–	–	0.420^{**}	0.486^{**}
Optimism	0.443^{**}	0.358^{**}	0.701^{**}	0.743^{**}	0.458^{**}	0.353^{**}	0.575^{**}
Purpose in life	0.250^{**}	0.440^{**}	0.734^{**}	0.359^{**}	0.270^{**}	0.429^{**}	0.287^{**}
Spirituality	0.056	0.090	0.146	0.132^{**}	0.042	0.084	0.091^{*}
Social resources							
Positive relations	0.197^{**}	–	–	–	0.269^{**}	0.313^{**}	0.230^{**}
Social support	0.171^{**}	0.165	0.411^{*}	0.230^{**}	0.252^{**}	0.367^{**}	0.213^{**}

$^{+}p<0.10$
$^{*}p<0.05$
$^{**}p<0.01$

Multiple Regressions Predicting Resilience in Each of the Individual Samples

Table 13.3 displays the results of the multiple regression analyses predicting the BRS from the potential resilience resources in each of the six samples. In the general college student sample, male gender, active coping, mindfulness, mood clarity, and optimism were all significant predictors of resilience and the full model accounted for 40% of the variance in resilience scores. In the healthy women sample, there were no significant predictors of resilience probably due to the relatively small sample size and large number of predictors. However, there was a trend for purpose in life which had a medium effect in predicting greater resilience and the full model accounted for 30% of the variance. In the women with fibromyalgia sample, purpose in life had a very strong effect in predicting higher resilience and the full model accounted for 68% of the variance. In the cardiac patient sample, optimism had a very strong effect in predicting greater resilience and male gender and active coping also significant predictors of greater resilience with the full model accounting for 59% of the variance. In the first-generation sample, optimism and male gender were again significant predictors of greater resilience with the full model accounting for 26% of the variance. Finally, in the firefighter sample, purpose in life, mood clarity, and active coping had significant effects in predicting greater resilience with the full model accounting for 36% of the variance.

In summary, the potential demographic resources predicted resilience 3 out of the 19 possible times (16%), the potential personal resources predicted resilience 11 out of the 30 possible times (37%), and the potential social resources predicted resilience 0 out of the 9 possible times (0%). The potential resource that predicted resilience the greatest percentage of the time was male gender (75%), followed by optimism, active coping, mood clarity, and mindfulness (50%), and then by purpose in life (33%). Finally, the variance explained by the full model in the patient samples (68 and 59%) was generally higher than the variance explained in the healthy (40 and 30%) and at-risk (26 and 36%) samples. This difference was largely due to the strong effect of the purpose in life on resilience in the women with fibromyalgia and of optimism on resilience in the cardiac patient sample.

Multiple Regressions Predicting Resilience in Different Combinations of the Samples

Although all of the potential resources were not included in all six samples, several of the variables were included in all samples and we combined them to compare their effects with a larger overall sample size. We also examined each of the potential resources that were not included in all of the samples while controlling for the variables that were included in all of the samples. In addition, we created dummy variables to determine whether being in a patient or at-risk sample was related to higher or lower resilience scores. Thus, we created a "patient" variable where participants in samples 1, 2, 5, and 6 were coded "0" and those in the patient samples 3 and 4 (e.g., the women with fibromyalgia and the cardiac patients) were coded "1." Similarly, we created an "at-risk" variable where participants in samples 1, 2, 3, and 4 received a "0" and those in samples 5 and 6 (e.g., the first-generation students and the urban firefighters) were coded "1." Zero-order correlation analyses with the participants from all six samples combined showed that resilience was not related to being in an at-risk sample ($r = 0.022$, ns) but had a very small positive relationship with being in a patient sample ($r = 0.078$, $p < 0.05$).

Table 13.4 displays the results of each of the additional multiple regression analyses that we conducted with various combinations of the samples. The first column in Table 13.4 shows the multiple regression analysis with all of the variables that were included in all six samples. These analyses showed that optimism was a medium-to-strong predictor of greater resilience, while male gender, age, active coping, and purpose in life were small-to-medium predictors of greater

Table 13.3 Multiple regression analyses predicting the Brief Resilience Scale from the potential resilience resources in each of the six samples

	Healthy		Patient		At-risk	
	College students	Healthy women	Women with fibromyalgia	Cardiac patients	First generation	Urban firefighters
Demographic resources						
Age	0.003	0.149	−0.247	0.044	0.042	0.099
Male gender	0.219**	–	–	0.243**	0.188*	0.100
Education	0.075	0.250	−0.047	−0.014	–	−0.134
Income	–	−0.243	0.142	−0.032	–	0.062
Personal resources						
Active coping	0.158**	−0.202	−0.140	0.163**	0.075	0.205*
Mindfulness	0.169**	–	–	–	–	−0.112
Mood clarity	0.278**	0.011	0.248	–	–	0.239*
Optimism	0.289**	0.218	0.138	0.704**	0.361**	0.158
Purpose in life	−0.036	0.336+	0.642**	−0.036	0.107	0.257*
Spirituality	0.015	0.080	0.015	−0.006	−0.007	−0.103
Social resources						
Positive relations	−0.073	–	–	–	0.057	−0.104
Social support	0.019	−0.075	−0.183	0.043	0.040	0.213+
F	15.04**	1.84+	5.15**	31.95**	6.19**	5.03**
R^2	0.401	0.298	0.678	0.589	0.260	0.356

+$p<0.10$
*$p<0.05$
**$p<0.01$

Table 13.4 Multiple regression analyses predicting the Brief Resilience Scale in all samples with selected potential resilience resources as predictor variables

	All samples ($n=844$)	All samples with income ($n=435$)	All samples with mindfulness ($n=381$)	All samples with mood clarity ($n=465$)	All samples with positive relations ($n=532$)
Demographic resources					
Age		0.130*	0.049	0.077	0.055
Male gender	0.205**	0.195**	0.234**	0.236**	0.223**
Education	0.008	−0.029	0.030	0.043	0.011
Income	–	−0.005	–	–	–
Personal resources					
Active coping	0.130**	0.135**	0.169**	0.116**	0.144**
Mindfulness	–	–	0.163**	–	–
Mood clarity	–	–	–	0.257**	–
Optimism	0.449**	0.529**	0.317**	0.257**	0.340**
Purpose in life	0.087*	0.113*	0.036	0.111*	0.105*
Spirituality	−0.002	−0.005	−0.034	0.002	−0.028
Social resources					
Positive relations	–	–	–	–	−0.029
Social support	0.050+	0.048	0.034	−0.003	0.077
Sample type					
Patient	−0.088	−0.072	–	0.099	–
At-risk	−0.025	−0.049	−0.038	−0.058	–
F	15.04**	33.19**	30.10**	25.90**	24.96**
R^2	0.401	0.476	0.423	0.333	0.325

+$p<0.10$
*$p<0.05$
**$p<0.01$

resilience. The full model accounted for 40% of the total variance in resilience scores. The second column in Table 13.4 shows the results for these same variables with the addition of income which was included in all of the samples except the two college student samples. The results show that optimism was a strong predictor of greater resilience, while male gender, age, active coping, and purpose in life were again small-to-medium predictors of greater resilience. Income was not related to resilience and the full model accounted for 48% of the variance.

The third column in Table 13.4 shows the results for the original variables that were included in all six study plus mindfulness in the two studies in which it was assessed. The results show that optimism was a medium predictor of greater resilience while male gender, active coping, and mindfulness were small-to-medium predictors of greater resilience with the full model accounting for 42% of the variance. Similarly, the fourth column shows the results for the original variables plus mood clarity in the four studies in which it was assessed. Interestingly, the results show that optimism and mood clarity had identical small-to-medium effects in predicting greater resilience, while male gender also had a small-to-medium effect and active coping and purpose in life had small effects with the full model accounting for 33% of the variance. Finally, the fifth column shows the results for the original variables plus positive relations in the three studies in which it appears. The results show that optimism has a medium effect with male gender, active coping, and purpose in life having smaller effects in predicting greater resilience. Positive relations were not related to resilience and the full model accounted for 33% of the variance.

Overall, optimism, active coping, and male gender were consistent predictors of greater resilience across the different combinations of samples. In addition, purpose in life was related to greater resilience in all combinations except the one including mindfulness and mood clarity and mindfulness were related to greater resilience when combining the studies in which they were included and controlling for the variables included in all of the samples. Finally, being in a patient or at-risk sample, education, spirituality, social support, positive relations, and income were not related to resilience in any of the combinations of the samples.

Discussion

The purpose of this chapter was to examine the relationship between resilience as the ability to bounce back from stress and potential demographic, personal, and social resources for resilience. Our primary hypothesis was that the variables selected to assess each of the three aspects of the temporal dimension of resilience would be related to the BRS. These three stages include confronting a stressful event which was assessed by measures of mindfulness and mood clarity (Brown & Ryan, 2003; Feldman-Barrett et al., 2001; Kabat-Zinn, 1990; Salovey et al., 1995), orienting oneself towards a positive future outcome which assessed by measures of optimism and purpose in life (Ryff & Keyes, 1995; Scheier & Carver, 2001; Scheier, Carver, & Bridges, 1994; Smith & Zautra, 2004), and engaging in efforts to cope with the stressor which was assessed be measures of active coping and social support (Carver, 1997; Cohen et al., 1985; Scheier & Carver, 2003; Sherbourne & Stewart, 1991). Our secondary hypothesis was that spirituality, positive relations with others, age, income, and education would be related to greater resilience (Adler et al., 1994; Pargament, 1997). We will first discuss the results in relation to the combined samples and then how the results varied across the individual samples.

Resilience Resources in All Samples Combined

We found that our primary hypothesis was generally confirmed in that each of the six variables that we expected to be involved in the temporal aspects of resilience were correlated with resilience in the overall sample. Even when controlling for the other variables in the combined sample multiple regression analyses, all of these variables were significantly related to greater resilience except for social support in which there was a trend. The effect sizes for the correlations were large for optimism and mood clarity, medium for active coping, mindfulness, and purpose in life, and in the small-to-medium range for social support. The effects sizes for the multiple regression analyses were medium-to-large for optimism, medium for mood clarity, small for active coping, purpose in life, and mindfulness, and very small for social support. The findings suggest that optimism and mood clarity are the most important resources for resilience across all samples, while each of the other four resources appear important but less so.

We also found that our secondary hypothesis was confirmed in that age, education, income, spirituality, and positive relations were all correlated with greater resilience when the samples were combined. The correlations were small-to-medium for age and positive relations and small for income and spirituality. However, when controlling for other variables, only age was still significantly related to resilience and the effect size of the other three variables was almost zero. Also, although we made no predictions about gender, we found that male gender had a small-to-medium size zero-order correlation with resilience and a small-to-medium effect in predicting greater resilience when controlling for the other variables. Thus, both age and male gender are demographic factors that may be resources for resilience.

What are the implications of these findings for understanding the foundations of resilience? While the findings for age and male gender are noteworthy, we were most interested in personal and social resources for resilience that can be targeted in interventions. In addition, we particularly wanted to focus on factors that may address the temporal aspects of bouncing back from stress. Although our cross-sectional data cannot provide evidence for the temporal order in our model, we believe that our results general confirm that value of thinking about resilience from a temporal perspective and emphasize the value of mindfulness, mood clarity, active coping, purpose in life, and optimism in our revised model. While we did not want to discount the potentially important role of social resources or spirituality (Cohen & Wills, 1985; Pargament, 1997), we did want to develop a model based the resources that received the strongest empirical support. We suspect that both social relationships and different aspects and forms of spirituality may be involved in each of three stages but that their effects may not be as strong or direct, at least not in the samples that we studied.

Figure 13.1 presents a hypothetical model of the foundations for bouncing back for stress that may be consistent with findings. The arrows pointing from the column of resources displayed on the left side of the model to "resilience as bouncing back from stress" show that mindfulness, mood clarity, purpose in life, optimism, and active coping may all be important personal resources for resilience. The arrows descending vertically from one personal resource to the next are meant show that they may operate in a temporal sequence that general follows this order. Although our findings led us to include these five variables as important predictors of resilience and this order is consistent with our three stage model, the temporal sequence of the five variables presented in this hypothetical model can only be confirmed in additional research that assesses each variable at different time points.

With this in mind, we present our hypothetical model of how these five variables may affect each other in the temporal sequence shown in Fig. 13.1. First, the mindful attention to and awareness of present moment experience may enable a person to confront and fully take in all of the information available during the experience of a stressful event (Brown & Ryan, 2003; Kabat-Zinn, 1990). Second, mood clarity may enable a person to make sense of their emotional experience of the event in a way in which they can best understand how it affects them and what choices they can make about what to do next (Feldman-Barrett et al., 2001; Salovey et al., 1995). Third, purpose in life may help to orient the person (or keep the person oriented) to what is most important to them and provide motivation and direction for coping with the event (Frankl, 1963; Smith & Zautra, 2004). Fourth, optimism may enable the person to envision a positive outcome to the stressful event and help give them the confidence necessary to begin to engage in coping efforts

(Andersson, 1996; Scheier & Carver, 2003). Fifth, an active approach to coping involves actually engaging in the coping efforts that are may be necessary for bouncing back or recovery from the stressful event (Scheier & Carver, 2003; Smith & Zautra, 2008).

While these findings and this hypothetical model may be generally applicable to a variety of situations, we did want to comment on what we view as the most important differences that we found across samples in the relationship between the resilience resources and resilience; the amount of variance explained by the resilience resources in accounting for BRS score varied across samples, particularly with respect to optimism and purpose in life. The zero-order correlation for the relationship between optimism and resilience was very strong in both the women with fibromyalgia and in the cardiac patients and the correlation between purpose in life and resilience was very strong in the women with fibromyalgia. When controlling for the other variables in the multiple regression analyses, purpose in life was still a strong predictor of greater resilience in the women with fibromyalgia and optimism was still a strong predictor of greater resilience in cardiac patients. It is striking that both of these resources were selected because they were thought to contribute to orienting oneself towards a successful outcome. For patients in cardiac rehabilitation, optimism may be critical for giving a person the confidence for coming to the rehabilitation sessions and believing that it will be beneficial (Scheier et al., 1999). For women with fibromyalgia, a sense of purpose in life may be vital in motivating them to continue to get out of bed and search for ways to reduce the stress of having chronic pain (Smith & Zautra, 2004). Thus, for those facing a health challenge, the ability to orient themselves toward positive future outcomes through optimism and a sense of purpose in life may be particularly valuable.

While the main focus of this chapter was on examining the relationship between resources for resilience and resilience as measured by the BRS, we also presented descriptive data on the BRS in all samples combined and compared the mean of the BRS across individual samples. The fact that the distribution of resilience scores was nearly normal suggests that the measure can be used to identify people who are both high and low in resilience defined as the ability to bounce back from stress. Also, we found intriguing differences in the mean resilience scores across the six samples. The mean scores were generally distributed across three tiers with the urban firefighters, healthy women, and cardiac patients higher in resilience, the general college students and first-generation students in the middle range, and the women with fibromyalgia in the lower range. It is particularly interesting that one patient group (the cardiac patients) was in the higher resilience group, while the other was in the lower resilience group (the women with fibromyalgia). This raises important questions about the variability between chronic illnesses and about whether and how an illness may lead to reduced resilience or be occasions for growing or increasing resilience. It also may be true that lower levels of resilience could be predisposing factors for certain illnesses, especially stress-related disorders (Smith et al., 2010). The other notable finding about group differences in resilience scores is that both college student groups were lower than the urban firefighter, healthy women, and cardiac patient samples. It is possible that this difference could reflect the effects of age and experience, although other differences between the samples and cohort effects could also explain or could confound this interpretation.

Implications for Research and Clinical Work

This research represents an important initial step in examining the relationship between potential resilience resources and the BRS as a specific measure of resilience as the ability to bounce back from stress. A logical next step may be to examine the relationship between the same resilience resources and other measures of resilience to see if there are differences across measures. Another step may be to examine other potential resources that may appear to be theoretically important for different aspects or processes of resilience as targeted in different measures. Of course a primary limitation of the analyses presented in this chapter is that the data are cross-sectional. While we believe that our theory and data analyses are consistent with the resources we identified as being vital for resilience, longitudinal studies are necessary to provide evidence that the presence of these resources precedes and may truly help to make it possible for a person to bounce back from a stressful event.

A second important limitation of this study is the lack of evidence that the BRS, as a self-report measure of resilience, predicts actual "bouncing back" or recovery as evidenced by independent behavioral and physiological measures. The closest thing to this kind of evidence so far is that the BRS predicted greater habituation to heat and cold pain (Smith et al., 2009). Specifically, higher BRS scores were associated with greater adaptation to thermal pain across five trials when controlling for other personal and social factors such as neuroticism, optimism, and social support. However, there is much additional work that needs to be done to test the predictive validity of the BRS with other kinds of stressors and in relation to other potential markers of recovery from stress. The type of studies that could be most useful are those using the BRS to assess resilience before a stressful event and then determining whether BRS scores are related to improvement on the behavioral and physiological measures that are most initially affected by the stressor.

The research presented in this chapter also may have implications for clinical research and interventions. First of all, one way of further testing whether the resources identified here are important for bouncing back from stress would be to target one or more of these resources in an intervention and determine whether it increases resilience as assessed by the BRS and behavioral and physiological measures. Second, in clinical interventions that are aimed at enabling a person to recover from a stressful event or events, it might be valuable to include both the BRS and the others measures that we found to be most strongly related to it. This could be a way of both disentangling the temporal and causal order of the relationships and determining whether a change in the level of specific resources is associated with a change in resilience itself. Finally, we would suggest that people doing clinical work might pay attention to the three stages that we identified to determine whether they see them as being involved in the process of bouncing back from stress. The careful observation of the client experience and communication of this to clinical researchers would help to better determine whether and how people may use the resources we assessed to confront a stressor, orient to a successful outcome, and how much active coping may be necessarily in recovery from different kinds of stressors.

Conclusions

The purpose of this chapter was to present research to enable us to better understanding the foundations of the human experience of resilience. We were particularly interested in identifying what kind of personal and social resources may be critical to resilience as bouncing back or recovering from stress. We identified potential resilience resources based on a model of resilience that involves three stages of confronting a stressor, orienting to a positive outcome, and actively coping with the stressor. We examined resilience and these resilience resources in six samples including general college students, healthy adult women, women with fibromyalgia, cardiac patients, first-generation college students, and urban firefighters. Our results were consistent with our model in that the personal resources that targeted each of these stages were generally related to the resilience. Overall, we found that mindfulness, mood clarity, purpose in life, optimism, and active coping all appear to be important personal resources for bouncing back from stress as assessed by the BRS. Optimism and mood clarity had the strongest effect sizes across all samples and optimism and purpose in life had the strongest effects in the patient populations.

References

Adler, N. E., Boyce, T., Chesney, M. A., Cohen, S., Folkman, S., Kahn, R. L., et al. (1994). Socioeconomic status and health: The challenge of the gradient. *American Psychologist, 49*, 15–24.

Agnes, M. (Ed.). (2005). *Webster's new college dictionary*. Cleveland, OH: Wiley.

Andersson, G. (1996). The benefits of optimism: A metaanalysis review of the life orientation test. *Personality and Individual Differences, 21*, 719–725.

Banerjee, M. M., & Pyles, L. (2004). Spirituality: A source of resilience for African American women in the era of welfare reform. *Journal of Ethnic and Cultural Diversity in Social Work, 13*, 45–70.

Bonanno, G. A. (2004). Loss, trauma, and human resilience. *American Psychologist, 59*, 20–28.

Bonebright, C. A., Clay, D. L., & Ankenmann, R. D. (2000). The relationship with work-life conflict, life satisfaction, and purpose in life. *Journal of Counseling Psychology, 47*, 469–477.

Brown, K. W., & Ryan, R. M. (2003). The benefits of being present: Mindfulness and its role in psychological well-being. *Journal of Personality and Social Psychology, 84*, 822–848.

Carver, C. S. (1997). You want to measure coping but your protocol's too long: Consider the Brief COPE. *International Journal of Behavioral Medicine, 4*, 92–100.

Carver, C. S. (1998). Resilience and thriving: Issues, models, and linkages. *Journal of Social Issues, 54*, 245–266.

Cohen, S., Mermelstein, R., Kamarck, T., & Hoberman, H. (1985). Measuring the functional components of social support. In I. G. Sarason & B. R. Sarason (Eds.), *Social support: Theory, research and applications* (pp. 73–94). The Hague: Nijhoff.

Cohen, S., & Wills, T. A. (1985). Stress, social support, and the buffering hypothesis. *Psychological Bulletin, 98*, 310–357.

Connor, K. M., & Davidson, J. R. T. (2003). Development of a new resilience scale: The Connor–Davidson Resilience Scale (CD-RISC). *Depression and Anxiety, 18*, 76–82.

Dyer, J. G., & McGuinness, T. M. (1996). Resilience: Analysis of the concept. *Archives of Psychiatric Nursing, 10*, 276–282.

Feldman-Barrett, L., Gross, J., Christensen, T. C., & Benvenuto, M. (2001). Knowing what you're feeling and knowing what to do about it: Mapping the relation between emotion differentiation and emotion regulation. *Cognition and Emotion, 15*, 713–724.

Fetzer Institute. (1999). *Multidimensional measurement of religiousness/spirituality for use in health research: A report of the Fetzer Institute/National Institute on Aging Working Group*. Kalamazoo, MI: John E. Fetzer Institute.

Frankl, V. E. (1963). *Man's search for meaning*. New York, NY: Pocket.

Friborg, O., Hjemdal, O., Rosenvinge, J. H., & Martinussen, M. (2003). A new rating scale for adult resilience: What are the central protective resources behind healthy adjustment? *International Journal of Methods in Psychiatric Research, 12*, 65–76.

Hayes, S. C., Follette, V. M., & Linehan, M. M. (2004). *Mindfulness and acceptance: Expanding the cognitive-behavioral tradition*. New York, NY: Guilford.

Kabat-Zinn, J. (1990). *Full catastrophe living*. New York, NY: Delta.

Lanius, R. A., Vermetten, E., Loewenstein, R. J., Brand, B., Schmahl, C., Bremner, J. D., et al. (2010). Emotion modulation in PTSD: Clinical and neurobiological evidence for a dissociative subtype. *American Journal of Psychiatry, 167*, 640–647.

Luthar, S. S., Cicchetti, D., & Becker, B. (2000). The construct of resilience: A critical evaluation and guidelines for future work. *Child Development, 71*, 543–562.

Pargament, K. I. (1997). *The psychology of religion and coping: Theory, research, practice*. New York, NY: Guilford.

Ryff, C. D., & Keyes, C. L. M. (1995). The structure of psychological well-being revisited. *Journal of Personality and Social Psychology, 69*, 719–727.

Salovey, P., Mayer, J. D., Goldman, S. L., Turvey, C., & Palfai, T. P. (1995). Emotion attention, clarity, and repair: Exploring emotional intelligence using the Trait Meta Mood Scale. In J. W. Pennebaker (Ed.), *Emotion, disclosure, and health* (pp. 125–154). Washington, DC: American Psychological Association.

Scheibe, S., & Carstensen, L. L. (2010). Emotional aging: Recent findings and future trends. *Journal of Gerontology: Psychological Sciences, 65B*, 135–144.

Scheier, M. F., & Carver, C. S. (2001). Adapting to cancer: The importance of hope and purpose. In A. Baum & B. L. Anderson (Eds.), *Psychosocial interventions for cancer* (pp. 213–235). Washington, DC: American Psychological Association.

Scheier, M. F., & Carver, C. S. (2003). Self-regulatory processes and responses to health threats: Effects of optimism on well-being. In J. Suls & K. A. Wallston (Eds.), *Social psychological foundations of health and illness* (pp. 395–428). Oxford: Blackwell.

Scheier, M. F., Carver, C. S., & Bridges, M. W. (1994). Distinguishing optimism from neuroticism (and trait anxiety, self-mastery, and self-esteem): A reevaluation of the life orientation test. *Journal of Personality and Social Psychology, 67*(6), 1063–1078.

Scheier, M. F., Matthews, K. A., Owens, J. F., Schulz, R., Bridges, M. W., Magovern, G. J., et al. (1999). Optimism and rehospitalization after coronary artery bypass graft surgery. *Archives of Internal Medicine, 159*, 829–835.

Schnoll, R. A., Knowles, J. C., & Harlow, L. (2002). Correlates of adjustment among cancer survivors. *Journal of Psychosocial Oncology, 20*(1), 37–59.

Sherbourne, C. D., & Stewart, A. L. (1991). The MOS social support survey. *Social Science and Medicine, 32*, 705–714.

Simpson, J. (Ed.). (2005). Oxford English Dictionary (3rd ed.). New York, NY: Oxford University Press.

Smith, B. W., Dalen, J., Wiggins, K., Tooley, E., Christopher, P., & Bernard, J. (2008). The Brief Resilience Scale: Assessing the ability to bounce back. *International Journal of Behavioral Medicine, 15*, 194–200.

Smith, B. W., Papp, Z., Tooley, E. M., Montague, E. Q., Robinson, A. E., & Cosper, C. J. (2010). Traumatic events, perceived stress, and health in women with fibromyalgia and healthy controls. *Stress and Health, 26*, 83–93.

Smith, B. W., Tooley, E. M., Montague, E. Q., Robinson, A. E., Cosper, C. J., & Mullins, P. G. M. (2009). The role of resilience and purpose in life in habituation to heat and cold pain. *The Journal of Pain, 10*, 493–500.

Smith, B. W., & Zautra, A. J. (2004). The role of purpose in life in recovery from knee surgery. *International Journal of Behavioral Medicine, 11*, 197–202.

Smith, B. W., & Zautra, A. J. (2008). Vulnerability and resilience in women with arthritis: Test of a two-factor model. *Journal of Consulting and Clinical Psychology, 76*, 799–810.

Tugade, M. M., & Fredrickson, B. L. (2004). Resilient individuals use positive emotions to bounce back from negative emotional experiences. *Journal of Personality and Social Psychology, 86*, 320–333.

Tusaie, K., & Dyer, J. (2004). Resilience: A historical review of the construct. *Holistic Nursing Practice, 18*, 3–8.

Wagnild, G. M., & Young, H. M. (1993). Development and psychometric evaluation of the resilience scale. *Journal of Nursing Measurement, 1*, 165–178.

Wong, P. T. P., & Fry, P. S. (1998). *The human quest for meaning: A handbook of psychological research and clinical applications*. Mahwah, NJ: Lawrence Erlbaum.

14 Assessing Personal Resiliency in Young Adults: The Resiliency Scale for Children and Adolescents

Donald H. Saklofske, David W. Nordstokke, Sandra Prince-Embury, Tara Crumpler, Sarah Nugent, Ashley Vesely, and Yvonne Hindes

The Resiliency Scales for Children and Adolescents were developed to tap core underlying characteristics of personal resiliency in children and adolescents (RSCA; Prince-Embury, 2007). The theoretical and conceptual model underlying the original RSCA has been comprehensively described in Chap. 3 of this volume along with a summary of reliability and validity evidence accumulated thus far (Prince-Embury, 2013). Briefly, the original RSCA is a 64-item self-report questionnaire in which responses are given on a 5-point Likert rating scale. This chapter discusses the psychometric properties of two more recent versions of the RSCA that have been altered slightly for use with adults. RSCA-A is essentially the same as the RSCA with only two items altered to be more appropriate for adults. The RSCA-A-R includes eight additional items; four items were added to the Adaptability subscale and a four-item Meaning subscale was included. As with the original RSCA, items are divided into three global scales that are labeled *Sense of Mastery*, *Sense of Relatedness*, and *Emotional Reactivity* (Prince-Embury, 2007).

Discussions of resiliency in adults have inferred more complex mechanisms such as "ego" in the discussion of "ego resiliency" by Block and Block (1980), "meaning" as described by Frankl (1979), or "commitment" as discussed by Kobasa (1979). It was the intention of Prince-Embury (2007) in the design of the RSCA to tap underlying developmental systems (Masten, 2001) that would apply across developmental stages, with the understanding that these systems might be enhanced by more cognitive complexity and expressed in different ways across life stages. For this purpose, Prince-Embury has recently developed new Adaptability and Meaning items for addition to the Sense of Mastery Scale. The new Adaptability items assess the degree to which an individual uses a mindset that views life changes as chances to grow and obstacles as challenges to overcome. The new Meaning items

D.H. Saklofske, Ph.D. (✉) • A. Vesely
Department of Psychology, Social Science Centre, 7th Floor, The University of Western Ontario, London, Ontario, Canada N6A 5C2
e-mail: dsaklofs@uwo.ca

D.W. Nordstokke, Ph.D.
School and Applied Psychology Program, University of Calgary, Calgary, Alberta, Canada T2N 1N4

S. Prince-Embury, Ph.D.
Resiliency Institute of Allenhurst, LLC., 625 North Edgemere Drive, W. Allenhurst, NJ 07711, USA
e-mail: Sandraprince-embury@earthlink.net

T. Crumpler
Strengths in ADHD, Education Tower, University of Calgary, 2500 University Drive NW, Calgary, Alberta, Canada T2N 1N4

S. Nugent
Foothills Academy, 745—37th Street N.W., Calgary, Alberta, Canada T2N 4T1

Y. Hindes, Ph.D.
University of Calgary, Calgary, Alberta, Canada T2N 1N4

S. Prince-Embury and D.H. Saklofske (eds.), *Resilience in Children, Adolescents, and Adults: Translating Research into Practice*, The Springer Series on Human Exceptionality, DOI 10.1007/978-1-4614-4939-3_14, © Springer Science+Business Media New York 2013

focus on describing various ways in which an individual might search for sense of meaning in hardships that are encountered.

Adaptability was chosen as an area to expand consistent with Block and Block's (1980) definition of ego resiliency as the capacity to adjust control of emotions to fit most appropriately with presenting circumstances. Adaptability is represented in the original RSCA in a manner more appropriate to children and adolescents by the degree to which they can learn from their mistakes and the degree to which they can let others help when needed. Prince-Embury enhanced this subscale with items more appropriate to adults such as conceptualizing hardships as opportunities for new learning and growth. Meaning making was introduced by the inclusion of a new subscale that specifically suggested different ways that adults find meaning in hardship within larger contexts such as belief system or religious orientation.

This chapter addresses three broad issues. First, the RSCA in its modified form will be applied with young adult samples to test the applicability of the RSCA with a young adult population. For this purpose multiple samples will be employed and multiple analyses,including confirmatory factor analysis, reliability analyses, and correlational analyses, conducted to examine the validity and reliability of the RSCA in an adult sample. The criteria of applicability for young adults will include the following: whether the factor structure of the RSCA-A and RSCA-A-R are acceptable and consistent with that of the earlier version, whether the alpha coefficients for the scales and subscales are acceptable, and whether relationship with other theoretically related variables are acceptable and in the predicted direction. Secondly, the added value of new items will be evaluated with the criteria being whether new items add to the reliability and validity of the scales.

The third issue addressed in this chapter is expansion of validity evidence for the RSCA-A and RSCA-A-R. According to the theoretical formulations and operational definitions of resiliency, persons scoring high on, for example, self-report measures of psychological well being, or low on anxiety and high on adaptive coping strategies, would be seen as being more resilient than those scoring in the opposite direction. This chapter explores the relationship between personal resiliency as measured by the RSCA-A and RSCA-A-R with other measures of psychological well-being, psychological flourishing, emotional intelligence, factors of personality, positive and negative emotion, and student motivation and amotivation.

In pursuit of the above three intentions, this chapter will present findings from several studies of university students that focused on identifying the characteristics of students reporting a high degree of well-being and satisfaction versus those who did not. In particular, the adult versions of the RSCA were administered to students in each of the reported studies. All participants were from three studies conducted at the University of Calgary, Canada and represented a cross sampling of university undergraduates from most faculties and programs over three semesters of a 2-year period. The first sample of 274 students was comprised of 78 males and 196 females with a mean age of 21.79 years (standard deviation of 6.05). The second sample of 361 students was comprised of 102 males and 259 females with a mean age of 20.63 years (standard deviation of 4.26). The third sample including 390 students included 104 males and 286 females with a mean age of 21.55 years (standard deviation of 5.64). This resulted in a total sample size of 1025 with 284 males and 741 females. However there are a few instances where the *N*s are slightly less because the participant did not fully complete one of the measures. This sample information is summarized in Table 14.1.

For both the modeling and reliability determinations of the scales, data were split by test version.

Table 14.1 Description of three studies with undergraduate samples

Term of study	Mean age (years)	SD	M	F
Winter 2009	21.79	6.05	78	196
Fall 2009	20.63	4.26	102	259
Winter 2010	21.55	5.64	104	286

Note. Average 2 years university

The first two data collection periods used the RSCA-A. This is a minimally modified version that only slightly changed the wording to make it more relevant to adolescents and adults, hence the addition of the A. A total of 635 participants were used in the reliability analyses and model testing. The third data collection period used the two variations of the original scale now referred to as the RSCA-A-R to provide data for 390 participants. This version of the scale added four more Adaptability items as well as a new subscale labeled Meaning. These data were used in the both reliability analyses and model testing employing confirmatory factor analysis.

Construct Validity: Confirmatory Factor Analyses

The modeling approach to investigate the factoral structures of the RSCA-A and the RSCA-A-R utilized a confirmatory factor analysis (CFA) framework analyzed by LISREL 8.80. The method of estimation used in all models was maximum likelihood (ML). The indices that were used to assess the fit of the models were the Chi-square test, the adjusted goodness of fit index (AGFI), the root mean square error of approximation (RMSEA), the non-normed fit index (NNFI), and the comparative fit index (CFI).

Several models were tested during this phase of the study and all are shown in Table 14.2. The first series of CFA models combined the data from the first two studies using the RSCA-A data ($n=635$) and tested one, two, and three factor solutions, similar to that found in the test manual. The results support the three factor structure as the best fitting model for the data.

The next series of CFA analyses tested one, two, and three factor solutions for the modified RSCA-A-R ($n=390$) that included the four new items added to the Adaptability Scale and the Meaning Scale. However, the first set of models investigated one, two, and three factor solutions using only the original items included in the RSCA-A. The fit indices for this series of models are also presented in Table 14.2 and once again, it is evident that the three factor model is the best fitting replicating the finding from the first sample. Next was a series of CFA models that included the eight new items added to the RSCA-A-R. In line with the previous CFA models, one, two, and three factor solutions were investigated. The results of these models once again confirmed

Table 14.2 Goodness-of-fit statistics for confirmatory factor analysis of different models

Model	χ^2	df	p	AGFI	RMSEA	NNFI	CFI
Winter/Fall 2009 (N= 535)							
One factor	578.17	35	<0.001	0.76	0.156	0.84	0.88
Two factor	267.19	34	<0.001	0.87	0.104	0.93	0.94
Three factor	171.68	32	<0.01	0.91	0.083	0.95	0.96
Winter 2010 original scale (N=390)							
One factor	470.31	35	<0.001	0.66	0.191	0.81	0.85
Two factor	192.87	34	<0.001	0.84	0.117	0.92	0.94
Three factor	129.03	32	<0.01	0.88	0.094	0.94	0.96
Winter 2010 with eight new items (N=390)							
One factor	543.89	44	<0.001	0.67	0.18	0.83	0.86
Two factor	339.66	43	<0.001	0.79	0.133	0.91	0.93
Three factor	155.64	41	<0.01	0.89	0.085	0.96	0.97
Winter 2010 with four new Adaptability items (N=390)							
One factor	577.84	35	<0.001	0.64	0.2	0.81	0.85
Two factor	310.35	34	<0.001	0.78	0.145	0.9	0.92
Three factor	135.97	32	<0.01	0.89	0.091	0.95	0.97

Note. *AGFI* adjusted goodness of fit index, *RMSEA* root means square error of approximation, *NNFI* non-normed fit index, *CFI* comparative fit index that a three factor solution offered the best fit for the data. The final series of CFA models tested the factor structure of the RSCA-A-R with only the inclusion of the four new items that were added to the Adaptability Scale. Once again, one, two, and three factor solutions were investigated. The result of these models shown in Table 14.2 again provide strong support for the three factor model having the best fit for the data.

Reliabilities of the RSCA Factors and Subscales

The internal consistency reliabilities of the RSCA-A and the RSCA-A-R were investigated by calculating coefficient alphas for each of the global scales and subscales. Table 14.3 illustrates the reliability coefficients for the RSCA-A data. It can be seen that the coefficient alpha values for the scales and subscales are 0.70 and above for all of the scales and 0.89 and above for the three global scales. Table 14.3 also presents the reliability coefficients for the RSCA-A-R data. It includes coefficient alpha values for the Adaptability Scale with the four new items, and also the alpha values for the four new Meaning items. It can be seen that all reliability estimates are >0.70 for the subscales and >0.91 for the global scale scores. As well, the reliability for the Sense of Mastery Scale and the Adaptability subscale were improved with the addition of the new Adaptability items.

Criterion Validity Studies

As shown above, the RSCA-A and RSCA-A-R, with the addition of both Adaptability and Meaning items, show both good construct validity as reflected in the CFA results and satisfactory reliability estimates at both the factor and subscale levels. To further demonstrate that the scale has good criterion validity, other scales that would be expected to be theoretically and empirically linked to resiliency were administered in various combinations in the three studies.

The first validity study was conducted with the fall and winter 2009 samples. As a preliminary analysis, The *Ego-Resiliency Scale* (Block & Kremen, 1996) was administered to 179 students in this cohort. This scale was one of the first to assess personal resiliency in adults.

Table 14.3 Reliability of the RSCA—coefficient alphas

	Winter/fall 2010	
Scales	α	α
Sense of Mastery: original scale	0.89	0.89
New Meaning facet and Adaptability items		0.92
New Adaptability items		0.91
Optimism	0.84	0.83
Self-efficacy	0.84	0.85
Adaptability—original scale	0.66	0.74
Adaptability with four new items		0.83
Four new Meaning items		0.71
Sense of Relatedness	0.92	0.93
Trust	0.84	0.86
Support	0.84	0.83
Comfort	0.84	0.86
Tolerance	0.77	0.80
Emotional Reactivity	0.90	0.91
Sensitivity	0.82	0.78
Recovery	0.70	0.77
Impairment	0.88	0.90

Table 14.4 Correlations from fall and winter 2009 datasets

RSCA-A	PSYCH FL[a]	SWL[a]	SPANE[a]	Trait EI[b]	SWL[b]
Mastery	0.72**	0.57**	0.63**	0.71**	0.57**
Optimism	0.65**	0.53**	0.59**	0.64**	0.59**
Self-efficacy	0.58**	0.42**	0.51**	0.62**	0.47**
Adaptability	0.53**	0.49**	0.45**	0.43**	0.27**
Relatedness	0.66**	0.59**	0.58**	0.62**	0.51**
Trust	0.61**	0.50**	0.49**	0.55**	0.50**
Support	0.54**	0.55**	0.52**	0.55**	0.52**
Comfort	0.52**	0.43**	0.37**	0.52**	0.33**
Tolerance	0.42**	0.38**	0.45**	0.46**	0.34**
Emotional Reactivity	−0.33**	−0.34**	−0.49**	−0.28**	−0.59**
Sensitivity	−0.14	−0.17*	−0.36**	−0.49**	−0.24**
Recovery	−0.31**	−0.31**	−0.46**	−0.33**	−0.32**
Impairment	−0.35**	−0.33**	−0.41**	−0.52**	−0.17*

Note. *Psych Flour.* Psychological Flourishing Scale, *SWL* satisfaction with life, *SPANE* Scale of Positive and Negative Experience, *EI* emotional intelligence
[a]Winter 2009 dataset
[b]Fall 2009 dataset
*$p<0.05$
**$p<0.01$

Here resiliency is defined as the "capacity of the individual to effectively modulate and monitor an ever-changing complex of desires and reality constraints" (Block & Kremen, 1996, p. 359). The 14 items on this scale are scored using on a 4-point Likert scale, with high scores indicating higher levels of resilience. As expected, the Ego-Resiliency Scale showed moderate and significant ($p<0.01$) positive correlations with the RSCA-A Mastery (0.60) and Relatedness (0.57) factors and a significant negative correlation with Emotional Reactivity (−0.37).

Several further scales tapping constructs that have been linked with resiliency were then administered to either or both of the 2009 samples to extend this phase of the validity analyses. The *Psychological Flourishing* Scale is an eight-item scale that assesses an individual's functioning in areas of positive relationships, feelings of competence, and having meaning and purpose in life (Diener et al., 2009). Items are responded to on a 7-point Likert scale, and high scores reflect an individual with many psychological strengths and resources. One of the most often used brief scales in positive psychology studies is the *Satisfaction With Life Scale* (Diener, Emmons, Larsen, & Griffin, 1985). This measure evaluates an individual's self-evaluated satisfaction with life as a whole including life domains such as health or finances. It is a five-item scale that employs a 7-point Likert rating system, with high scores indicating higher levels of absolute as well as relative life satisfaction. The growing interest in emotional intelligence and its important position in studies of psychological health and wellness led to the inclusion of the *Trait Emotional Intelligence Questionnaire: Adult Short Form* (*TEi-Que ASF*). This 30-item self-report questionnaire was derived from the long form of the TEI-Que (Petrides & Furnham, 2004). Items are responded to on a 7-point Likert scale and provide an overall trait emotional intelligence score. Finally, the *Scale of Positive and Negative Experience* (SPANE) was employed to measure Positive and Negative Feelings. It is a 12-item adjective questionnaire that yields three separate subscales: Positive Feelings, Negative Feelings, and affect balance (Diener et al., 2009). Respondents use a 5-point Likert scale to describe how often they have experienced specific feelings in the past month.

Correlations between the above listed scales and the three broad factors and subscales of the RSCA-A are shown in Table 14.4. As predicted,

Table 14.5 Correlations from winter 2010 dataset

RSCA-A-R	Trait EI	SWL	EXTRA.	AGREE.	CONSC.	EMOT.	OPEN.
Mastery	0.73**	0.49**	0.37**	0.11*	0.38**	0.49**	0.34**
Optimism	0.64**	0.50**	0.37**	0.11*	0.31**	0.38**	0.25**
Self-efficacy	0.65**	0.33**	0.28**	0.02	0.40**	0.47**	0.38**
Adaptability	0.63**	0.35**	0.63**	0.12*	0.29**	0.41**	0.33**
Meaningfulness	0.33**	0.22**	0.15**	0.12*	0.16**	0.23**	0.04
Relatedness	0.66**	0.47**	0.49**	0.30**	0.21**	0.38**	0.25**
Trust	0.59**	0.42**	0.45**	0.31**	0.18**	0.34**	0.19**
Support	0.52**	0.46**	0.31**	0.15**	0.18**	0.27**	0.12**
Comfort	0.54**	0.26**	0.61**	0.24**	0.11*	0.30**	0.29**
Tolerance	0.52**	0.38**	0.28**	0.27**	0.21*	0.35**	0.25**
Emotional Reactivity	−0.61**	−0.30**	−0.14**	−0.27**	−0.27**	−0.63**	−0.17**
Sensitivity	−0.47**	−0.23**	−0.07	−0.32**	−0.16**	−0.63**	−0.09
Recovery	−0.44**	−0.26**	−0.12*	−0.16**	−0.18**	−0.40**	−0.09
Impairment	−0.57**	−0.26**	−0.15*	−0.21**	−0.28**	−0.55**	−0.12*

Note. *Trait EI* trait emotional intelligence, *SWL* satisfaction with life, 1–5 Big Five personality, *EXTRA*. Extraversion, *EMOT*. Emotional Stability/Neuroticism, *OPEN*. Openness to Experience, *AGREE*. Agreeableness, *CONSC*. Conscientiousness
*$p<0.05$
**$p<0.01$

Mastery and Relatedness are moderately to highly positively correlated with all scales. Again, as would be expected, Emotional Reactivity shows a smaller but negative relationship with these same measures. These results certainly support the contention that resiliency, and the RSCA-A, has a strong connection with self-reported psychological health and wellness. For example, emotional intelligence has been linked with well-being, adjustment, physical health, and success in the workplace (Stough, Saklofske, & Parker, 2009). The finding that EI very closely aligns with Mastery and Relatedness, including the subscales of these two resiliency factors, suggests that resiliency may be an overarching construct that reflects and describes the impact on persons that these various other factors may have. As an additional look, the SPANE positive and negative feeling subscales were correlated with the three RSCA factors. These results add further support to the significant relationship between Positive Feelings and Mastery (0.63) and Relatedness (0.59) in contrast to the negative correlations between Negative Feelings and Mastery (−0.45) and Relatedness (−0.40). Also confirming the expected relationship is the positive correlation of Emotional Reactivity with Negative Feelings (0.51) compared to a negative relationship with Positive Feelings (−0.32).

Moving to the 2010 dataset, the RSCA-A was revised to include the additional Adaptability items as well as add the new Meaningfulness subscale. To determine if the relationships observed with the earlier dataset were supported, it was decided to re-administer both the TEIQue and the SWL scales because of the theoretical and empirical links with resiliency. The same scales were again employed here. Added also was a measure of the "Big Five" personality factor model not only because of the relationship observed between, for example, EI and personality, but also because personality and temperament are clearly both linked with resiliency (Saklofske & Nordstokke, 2011). Given the number of measures already included on the full questionnaire administered to students, it was decided to use a short measure to assess personality. The *Ten-Item Personality Inventory* (TIPI; Gosling, Rentfrow, & Swann, 2003) was selected to use with this cohort. This is a brief self-report measure that assesses the Big-Five personality dimensions of Openness to Experience, Conscientiousness, Extraversion, Agreeableness, and Emotional Stability. Respondents indicate on a 7-point Likert scale to what extent they agree that each pair of characteristics applies to them.

The results reported in Table 14.5 for the revised version of the RSCA are in line with those shown in Table 14.4 for both SWL and EI. This provides compelling support for the view that positive characteristics such as EI and self-reported evaluations of one's sense of well-being are very much related to human resiliency. Of interest is that the newly added Meaningfulness subscale showed the lowest relationship of all the Mastery subscales with SWL and EI and may require some further development as a component of both overall resiliency and mastery.

The results of these validity studies both support the RSCA-A and RSCA-A-R as measures of resiliency and further elaborate our understanding of resiliency. The personality measures representing the Big Five personality structure show that these factors are variously correlated with the three resiliency factors and subscales. The connection between personality and psychological health and wellness as well as psychopathology is well established (Boyle, Saklofske, & Matthews, 2008a; Boyle, Saklofske, & Matthews, 2008b). In particular extraversion–introversion and Neuroticism-Emotional Stability have been linked with a wide range of social and emotional behaviors (Saklofske, Eysenck, Eysenck, Stelmack, & Revelle, 2012) that may be viewed as reflecting resiliency. Also as predicted, correlations between the RSCA-A-R and most of these variables were significant and in the predicted direction. Positive correlations between Trait EI and SWL and Mastery and Relatedness were consistent with findings reported above in the 2009 samples. The relationship between emotional intelligence and Sense of Mastery warrant special attention in being the most strongly related variables of those assessed (0.73). This strong relationship highlights the nature of emotional intelligence as a competency, although the causal basis of the correlation cannot be determined by this analysis. It is interesting to note that the Meaning subscale did not relate as highly to this variable or to any of the other variables tapped in this analysis, again questioning the value added by this subscale, at least in its current form.

On the other hand, relationships between the RSCA-A-R and the Big Five personality measures were relatively weaker although still significant and in the predicted direction. These findings suggest that personal resiliency as assessed by the RSCA-A-R overlaps with but is not a personality trait as assessed by the Big Five measure employed in this analysis. This idea is consistent with the formulation of Prince-Embury (2007) and Masten (2006) that resiliency is not a trait but a dynamic process that varies across time and circumstance. That said, there are two interesting areas of overlap between Big Five personality factors and subscales of the RSCA-A-R that are consistent with the definitions of two of the factors and provide criterion validity for several subscales. The Extraversion factor correlates strongly with the Adaptability subscale of the RSCA-A-R Sense of Mastery Scale (0.63) and the Comfort subscale of the Sense of Relatedness Scale (0.61). These relationships are stronger than the relationships between Extraversion and the more global Mastery and Relatedness Scales. These rather specific relationships make sense when considered from the perspective of the personality factor. Extraversion is commonly conceptualized to be at least in part based on comfort and flexibility in relating to others.

Criterion validity is also provided for the Emotional Reactivity Scale and the Sensitivity subscale as shown in the strong negative correlations between this scale and subscale and the Emotional Stability Factor (both −0.63). These relationships are consistent with the notion that emotional instability may be manifested by an oversensitivity to potentially stressful life events.

To add yet another piece of evidence to support the contention that resiliency is linked with positive characteristics, behaviors, and beliefs, the *Single Item Self-esteem Scale* that purports to evaluate self-esteem was responded to by this cohort of students. Developed by Robins, Hendin, and Trzesniewski (2001), this one-item scale is rated on a 5-point Likert scale. Whether using the original RSCA or the modified versions that included the eight-new items on the Mastery Scale, self-esteem correlated 0.51 with Sense of Mastery. Relatedness and Emotional Reactivity correlated 0.39 and −0.30, respectively, with this single item self-reported measure of self-esteem. These findings are consistent with those reported

Table 14.6 Correlations with motivation from the winter 2010 dataset

	Intrinsic motivation			Extrinsic motivation			Amotivation
RSCA-A-R	IMTK	IMTA	IMES	EMID	EMIN	EMER	AMOT
Mastery	0.25**	0.28**	0.08	0.25**	0.10	0.01	−0.33**
Relatedness	0.11*	0.13*	−0.01	0.21**	0.06	0.07	−0.25**
Emotional Reactivity	−0.06	0.03	0.12*	−0.30**	0.20**	0.13*	0.23**

Note. *IMTK* intrinsic motivation to know, *IMTA* intrinsic motivation to accomplish, *IMES* intrinsic motivation to experience stimulation, *EMID* identified regulation, *EMIN* introjected regulation, *EMER* external regulation, *AMOT* amotivation
*$p<0.05$
**$p<0.01$

in Chap. 3 of this volume (Prince-Embury, 2013) that Sense of Mastery was highly positively correlated with two independent assessments of self-esteem for children and adolescents (0.60 through 0.80).

A last set of results come from the *Academic Motivation Scale* (AMS: Vallerand et al., 1992). As will be discussed below, resiliency would appear to be part of the complex of characteristics that underlies successful university performance. This scale is comprised of 28 items set in a questionnaire format and designed to measure different motivational orientations in college students. Items are responded to using a 7-point Likert scale. The AMS is divided into seven subscales with three of these assessing *extrinsic motivation*, three assessing *intrinsic motivation*, and a final subscale which measures *amotivation*. While it was not expected that resiliency would be so highly correlated with student motivation, one apparent finding is the positive correlation between Emotional Reactivity and amotivation along with a negative correlation between Sense of Mastery and Relatedness and amotivation (Table 14.6).

Discussion

Confirmatory factor analyses for the combined fall and winter 2009 sample was consistent in supporting a three factor solution as the best fit for the responses to the RSCA-A and RSCA-A-R. This finding supports the existing structure of the RSCA and the underlying theoretical constructs. However, this fit was not as good as the fit reported for younger samples in the RSCA manual. The RMSA was 0.083 as compared to 0.05–0.07 (Prince-Embury, 2007) and elsewhere 0.03–0.07 (Prince-Embury & Courville, 2008a; Prince-Embury & Courville, 2008b). This suggests the possibility that resiliency factors for young adults might be slightly more interrelated than for younger samples. However, it is noted that for the 2010 sample the three factor fit was slightly better with the new items added than without the new items (see Table 14.2).

Reliability for RSCA-A and RSCA-A-R scales and subscales were consistent across college samples and with those found in younger samples reported in the RSCA manual (Prince-Embury, 2007). Reliability evidence was good to excellent for global scale scores and adequate to good for subscale scores. Reliability evidence was stronger for the Adaptability subscale with the new items added (alpha = 0.74, alpha = 0.83) and for the Sense of Mastery Scale with Adaptability and Meaning items added (alpha = 0.91 and 0.92). The new Meaning subscale yielded an alpha of 0.71 but did not seem to increase reliability of the overall Sense of Mastery Scale.

Validity evidence was strong for all three of the RSCA-A and RSCA-A-R global scales and subscales across a variety of positive health and well-being scales. Sense of Mastery was most strongly correlated with the *Psychological Flourishing* (0.72) and trait emotional intelligence (0.71). The subscale most highly correlated with these scales was Sense of "Optimism" (0.65,

0.64). Overlap with Big Five personality factors were fairly specific suggesting that personal resiliency as defined by the RSCA-A-R is not a personality trait as assessed by the Big Five but more a set of competencies expressed partly through emotional intelligence and influenced by specific personality factors such as extraversion (e.g., comfort and adaptability) and emotional stability which is related to higher sensitivity as manifested in Emotional Stability. These findings suggest that personal resiliency is a multifaceted competency which may be influenced by underlying temperament factors.

Findings regarding student motivation suggest that all three aspects of personal resiliency assessed by the RSCA-A-R are more related to inhibiting motivation than they are to increasing motivation and these correlations are relatively small. This is consistent with the idea that personal resiliency is a support to ordinary functioning in ordinary circumstances and not necessarily a boost to ordinary functioning. These factors would come into play for motivation in their absence. Thus low Sense of Mastery and low Sense of Relatedness might slightly impede motivation as would higher Emotional Reactivity.

Limitations of the study include the following. This study extends the application of the original RSCA-A-R upward to young adults who are attending university in Canada. For this reason, the findings, although consistent with earlier findings in the US normative samples still need to be extended to other adult samples to ensure the generalizability of results across age groups and countries. Also, university students might be assumed to be a predominantly nonclinical and not a specifically at risk population. In this respect the findings reported here are untested in adult samples experiencing identified trauma or illness. The modifications of the original RSCA introduced here may apply to young adults but may not generalize to those in middle or older adulthood. For example, the Sense of Meaning subscale might have more salience in an older, chronically ill or at-risk sample. Additional studies will need to be conducted to understand application of the RSCA to other adult populations.

Conclusions

1. The RSCA-A and the RSCA-A-R are applicable for use with young adults as shown by consistency of factor structure, reliability estimates, and correlations with validity measures.
2. The addition of the four Adaptability items to the previous Adaptability subscale appears to improves the validity and reliability of this scale and the Sense of Mastery global scale.
3. The addition of the Meaning subscale does not appear to add value to the RSCA-A, at least in its current form. This may be because of the few items offered to cover a complex construct. In an effort to keep the number of items down and to preserve the relative simplicity of the original RSCA we suggest dropping the Meaning subscale until it can be tested in other adult samples.
4. Findings presented here suggest that personal resiliency is not a personality trait but rather a set of competencies that are influenced by underlying temperament qualities of comfort with others, flexibility and sensitivity.
5. Findings presented here suggest that aspects of personal resiliency do not necessarily increase personal motivation in college students but rather support normal functioning and are more notable in their absence by decreasing motivation. For this reason the RSCA-A might be most useful for screening for lack of Motivation in young adult college samples in contrast to predicting those who will excel.

References

Block, J. H., & Block, J. (1980). The role of ego-control and ego-resiliency in the organization of behavior. In W. A. Collins (Ed.), *Development of cognition, affect, and social relations. The Minnesota symposia on child psychology* (Vol. 13, pp. 39–101). Hillsdale, NJ: Lawrence Erlbaum.

Block, J., & Kremen, A. M. (1996). IQ and ego-resiliency: Conceptual and empirical connections and separateness. *Journal of Personality and Social Psychology, 70*, 349–361.

Boyle, G., Matthews, G., & Saklofske, D. H. (2008a). *The sage handbook of personality theory and assessment.*

Vol. 1: Personality theories and models. London: Sage.

Boyle, G., Matthews, G., & Saklofske, D. H. (2008b). *The sage handbook of personality theory and assessment. Vol. 2: Personality measurement and testing*. London: Sage.

Diener, E., Emmons, R. A., Larsen, R. J., & Griffin, S. (1985). *The Satisfaction with Life Scale. Journal of Personality Assessment, 49*, 71–75.

Diener, E., Wirtz, D., Tov, W., Kim-Prieto, C., Choi. D., Oishi, S., & Biswas-Diener, R. (2009). *New measures of well-being: Flourishing and positive and negative feelings. Social Indicators Research, 39*, 247–266.

Frankl, V. (1979). *Man's search for meaning*. New York, NY: Simon & Schuster.

Gosling, S. D., Rentfrow, P. J., & Swann, W. B., Jr. (2003). A very brief measure of the Big-Five personality domains. *Journal of Research in Personality, 37*, 504–528.

Kobasa, S. C. (1979). Stressful life events, personality, and health: An inquiry into hardiness. *Journal of Personality and Social Psychology, 37*, 1–11.

Masten, A. S. (2001). Ordinary magic: Resilience processes in development. *American Psychologist, 56*(3), 227–238.

Masten, A. S. (2006). Developmental psychopathology: Pathways to the future. International Journal of Behavioral Development, 31, 47–54.

Pavot, W., & Diener, E. (1993). Review of the satisfaction with life scale. *Psychological Assessment, 5*(2), 164–172.

Petrides, K. V., & Furnham, A. (2004). *Technical manual of the Trait Emotional Intelligence Questionnaire (TEIQue)*. London: University of London, Institute of Education.

Prince-Embury, S. (2007). *Resiliency Scales for Children and Adolescents: Profiles of personal strength*. San Antonio, TX: Harcourt Assessment, Inc.

Prince-Embury, S., & Courville, T. (2008a). Comparison of one, two and three factor models of personal resilience using the Resiliency Scales for Children and Adolescents. *Canadian Journal of School Psychology, 23*, 11–25.

Prince-Embury, S., & Courville, T. (2008b). Measurement Invariance of the Resiliency Scales for Children and Adolescents with respect to sex and age cohorts. *Canadian Journal of School Psychology, 23*, 26–40.

Prince-Embury, S. (2013). Resiliency scales for children and adolescents (RSCA): Theory, research and clinical application. In S. Prince-Embury & D.H. Saklofske (Eds.), *Resilience in Children, Adolescents, and Adults: Translating Research into Practice* (pp. 19–44). New York, Springer.

Robins, R. W., Hendin, H. M., & Trzesniewski, K. H. (2001). Measuring global self-esteem: Construct validation of a single item measure and the Rosenberg Self-esteem Scale. *Personality and Social Psychology Bulletin, 27*, 151–161.

Saklofske, D. H., & Nordstokke, D. (2011). *The relationship of the RSCA with personality and motivation measures in Canadian young adult samples*. Paper presented at the Society for Personality Assessment, March, Boston.

Saklofske, D. H., Eysenck, H. J., Eysenck, S. B. G., Stelmack, R., & Revelle, W. (2012). *Extraversion introversion. In V. S. Ramachandran (Ed.), Encyclopedia of human behavior (2nd ed.) (Vol 2)*. pp. 150–159. London: Elsevier.

Stough, C., Saklofske, D. H., & Parker, J. (Eds.). (2009). *Assessing emotional intelligence: Theory, research and applications*. New York, NY: Springer.

Vallerand, R. J., Pelletier, L. G., Blais, M. R., Brière, N. M., Senécal, C. B., & Vallières, E. F. (1992). The Academic Motivation Scale: A measure of intrinsic, extrinsic, and amotivation in education. *Educational and Psychological Measurement, 52*, 1003–1017.

Exploring Adolescent Resilience Through the Lens of Core Self-Evaluations

15

Diane Cardenas Elliott, Pamela Kaliski, Jeremy Burrus, and Richard D. Roberts

> I don't think of myself as a poor deprived ghetto girl who made good. I think of myself as somebody who from an early age knew I was responsible for myself, and I had to make good.
>
> Oprah Winfrey

Oprah Winfrey's lifetime accomplishments are impressive by any measure. Named one of *Time* magazine's 100 most influential people of the twentieth century, she hosted one of the world's most watched television shows for 24 years (Academy of Achievement, 2011). She is also a film producer, runs her own magazine and cable television station, and was nominated for an Academy Award for her role in the movie *The Color Purple*. She has variously been the highest-paid performer on television, the richest self-made woman in America, and the richest African-American of the twenty-first century.

Oprah Winfrey's success is doubly impressive when the facts of her childhood are taken into consideration. She was born into poverty. From the time she was 9 years old until she was 13, she was sexually abused by family members. At age 14, she became pregnant and gave birth to a premature baby, who died shortly after birth. Clearly, there is something about Oprah Winfrey that has allowed her to thrive in the face of challenges that occurred during her childhood and adolescence. That something can be called resilience, and it is our contention that at least part of the reason she has been so resilient is that she has a steadfast belief in her capability and worthiness as a person. In short, she has what is known in scientific circles as a positive *Core Self-evaluation* (e.g., Erez & Judge, 2001; Judge, 2009; Judge, Erez, Bono, & Thoresen, 2002, 2003).

In this chapter, we provide a brief overview of resilience and the role it plays in adolescents' lives. Next, we propose a construct that reflects one's own perception of capability and worthiness as a person—core self-evaluations. Core self-evaluation is a higher-order construct consisting of the shared variance of many of the individual characteristics associated with resilience (see "Individual Characteristics" discussion below). As such, the introduction of the core

We thank Patrick Kyllonen, Bobby Naemi, John Sabatini, and Franklin Zaromb for comments on an earlier draft of this manuscript and Anthony Betancourt, Daniel Howard, and Mary Lucas for supporting the preparation of this chapter. All statements expressed in this chapter are the author's and do not reflect the official opinions or policies of the any of the authors host affiliations.

D.C. Elliott, Ph.D. • J. Burrus, Ph.D.
Educational Testing Service, Center for Academic and Workforce Readiness and Success,
Rosedale Road MS 18E, Princeton, NJ 08541, USA
e-mail: delliott@ets.org; jburrus@ets.org

P. Kaliski, Ph.D.
The College Board, 661 Penn Street, Suite B, Newtown, PA 18940, USA
e-mail: pkaliski@collegeboard.org

R.D. Roberts, Ph.D. (✉)
Educational Testing Service, Center for Academic and Workforce Readiness and Success, R&D,
Rosedale Road MS 18E, Princeton, NJ 08541, USA
e-mail: rroberts@ets.org

S. Prince-Embury and D.H. Saklofske (eds.), *Resilience in Children, Adolescents, and Adults: Translating Research into Practice*, The Springer Series on Human Exceptionality,
DOI 10.1007/978-1-4614-4939-3_15, © Springer Science+Business Media New York 2013

self-evaluation construct represents a proposed synthesis of the individual predictors of resilience. This synthesis should help advance the study of the individual characteristics that predict resilience by leading researchers to focus on one overarching trait that predicts resilience rather than several highly related traits, thus allowing related lines of research to "speak" to one another.

It is our contention that core self-evaluations are an essential and fundamental component of resilience. To support our argument, we also include initial results of an analysis investigating the relationship between core self-evaluations and a variety of educational outcomes related to, and impacted by, resiliency. Finally, we close with a brief discussion of the results of this study, highlight some interventions that follow on from these findings, and offer some future research directions.

Resilience: An Overview

Resilience, a complex psychosocial phenomenon generally describing a level of adaptability that allows individuals to survive and thrive in adverse conditions (Dent & Cameron, 2003), is becoming one of the most prominent and significant constructs in contemporary psychology (see, e.g., Armstrong, Birnit-Lefcovitch, & Unger, 2005; Luthar, Cicchetti, & Becker, 2000). Its importance is supported by early longitudinal research on children and adolescents, which showed that there exists a subset of individuals who are able to become successful and healthy adults despite being raised under unfavorable circumstances. More specifically, resilience has been defined as "a process of, or capacity for, or the outcome of, successful adaptation despite challenging and threatening circumstances" (Garmezy & Masten, 1991, p. 459). Similarly, Werner (1982; 1993) has used resilience to describe those children and adolescents who successfully cope with a range of social and biological risk factors.

Originally, research on resilient individuals examined how a range of risk factors (e.g., poverty, parental mental illness, family dysfunction, catastrophic life events) were related to negative developmental outcomes, resulting in identification of risk factors associated with maladaptive behavior (Richardson, 2002; Werner & Smith, 1992). Consensus has grown in the field recently that personality operates as a "self-righting mechanism," (Werner & Smith, 1992, p. 202) allowing the individual to continually adapt to her/his environment (Benard, 1991). Furthermore, the findings from longitudinal research have prompted a shift in resilience research. As many of the chapters in this book attest, research centers on "protective" factors (i.e., characteristics, qualities, and environmental factors) that promote resiliency (Benard, 1991; Garmezy, 1991; Hjemdal, Friborg, Stiles, Rosenvinge, & Martinussen, 2006; Rhule, McMahon, Spieker, & Munson, 2006; Werner & Smith, 1992). Broadly, these protective factors are qualities that modify, ameliorate, and cushion an individual from the worst effects of adverse experiences to help them survive and cope in spite of being disadvantaged relative to those in the reference population (e.g., Armstrong et al., 2005; Dent & Cameron, 2003; Garmezy & Masten, 1991; Rutter, 1985). The intersection of research on resilience, adolescent development, and educational outcomes has produced literature classifying protective factors into three main categories: home environment, community environment (which we will discuss together), and individual characteristics (e.g., Benard, 1991; Dent & Cameron, 2003).

Environmental Factors

Longitudinal studies tracking individuals in high risk environments have shown that resilience is governed by a dynamic interaction between protective factors within an individual and the larger environmental context (see Werner & Smith, 1992). Home, school, and community environments are integral to resilience in that they serve as protective buffers and ameliorate adverse conditions. For instance, school and community programs often offer services that develop social and emotional competencies, problem solving, and leadership skills, which serve as protective factors associated with resilience (see, e.g., Bell, 2001; Brooks, 2006; Durlak, Weissberg, Dymnicki, Taylor, & Schellinger, 2011; Edwards, Mumford, & Serra-Roldan, 2007; Zeidner, Roberts, & Matthews, 2002). Similarly, research studies have suggested that the existence of both a close bond and positive, appropriate relationship with at least one adult is critical to the development of resilience in children and adolescents (Armstrong et al., 2005; Benard, 1991; Fonaghy, Steele, Steele, Higgett, & Target, 1994; Harvard Mental Health Letter, 2006; Rhule et al., 2006). In fact, in his longitudinal study of resilient children, Rutter (1985) found that even in extremely distressed homes, a warm, stable, and supportive relationship with one parent was a significant protective factor. If the presence of a caring adult is not available within the home environment, schools and community organizations are important resources from which adolescents can develop a caring relationship with an adult. Thus, Werner and Smith's (1989) longitudinal study found that the presence of an influential teacher who served as a counselor, confidant, and role model was critical for resiliency in children and adolescents. The presence of a caring adult is crucial to the development of resilience because such a supportive relationship can help instill empathy for others, a sense of confidence, and self-esteem in adolescents (Werner & Smith, 1992). Furthermore, adults can offer guidance, insight, and positive support promoting locus of control, self-efficacy, and individual responsibility (Benard, 1991; Weissberg & Elias, 1993). In short, home and community environments are important for resilience because they reinforce individual characteristics associated with resiliency (Brooks, 2006; Dent & Cameron, 2003; Edwards et al., 2007).

Individual Characteristics

Research suggests that there exists a common core of protective individual and dispositional characteristics (i.e., traits) in resilient individuals (Werner & Smith, 1992). General intelligence appears to be one of the most significant protective individual characteristics (e.g., Brooks, 2006; Kitano & Lewis, 2005; Osofsky & Thompson, 2000) helping individuals reframe challenges and reappraise difficult situations (see, e.g., Werner, 2000). However, since intelligence only accounts for part of the variance in important life outcomes (such as school performance and life satisfaction), resilience research has also concentrated on other core individual protective factors. For example, self-efficacy, self-esteem, and self-concept are traits associated with resilience (Brooks, 2006; Edwards et al., 2007; Rhule et al., 2006; Rutter, 1985; Rutter, Maughan, Mortimore, Ouston, & Smith, 1979; Werner & Smith, 1992). Rutter's (1985) early work investigating youth with mentally ill parents found that a belief in one's own capabilities, or personal self-efficacy, was instrumental in the development of resilience. In addition, Werner and Smith (1992) tracked children living in impoverished and troubled family environments longitudinally and found that resilient children and adolescents had positive self-concepts and a high sense of self-esteem.

A sense of personal control is also associated with resiliency in adolescents (e.g., Edwards et al., 2007; Harvard Mental Health Letter, 2006; Werner, 2000). Experience in successfully overcoming adverse situations provides adolescents with a repertoire of problem-solving skills that help them actively counteract adversity, giving them a greater sense of control in their lives (Kitano & Lewis, 2005; Rutter, 1985). Other psychosocial traits associated with resiliency in adolescents include impulse control (e.g., Rhule et al., 2006; Werner, 1990, 2000), social competence (e.g., Armstrong et al., 2005; Benard, 1991; Kitano & Lewis, 2005; Rutter, 1985; Werner, 1990, 2000), good communication skills (e.g., Kitano & Lewis, 2005), resourcefulness (e.g., Armstrong et al., 2005; Werner, 1990, 2000), a sense of autonomy (e.g., Benard, 1991; Rhule et al., 2006), a sense of responsibility (Brooks, 2006; Werner, 2000), the ability to harness social support from peers, family, and teachers (Armstrong et al., 2005; Masten, Garmezy, Tellegen, Pellegrini, Larkin, & Larsen, 1988), and the capacity to identify and select positive role models (Edwards et al., 2007; Garmezy & Masten, 1991).

Resilience is also associated with coping with life stressors (Kitano & Lewis, 2005; Werner, 2000). Coping can be thought of as the behavioral, emotional, cognitive, or physiological processes that occur in response to stressful situations (see, e.g., Lazarus & Folkman, 1984). The predominant view of coping is that people tend to deal with stressful situations in one of three ways:

1. *Problem-focused coping*. In these situations, the individual attempts to find and resolve the root cause of the stressors.
2. *Emotion-focused coping*. In these situations, the individual focuses upon emotional responses to the stressor.
3. *Avoidant coping*. In these situations, the individual avoids the stressor as much as possible (see Folkman & Moskowitz, 2004; Parker & Endler, 1996; Zeidner, Matthews, & Roberts, 2006 for various overviews of the coping literature).

Research suggests that problem-focused coping is generally the most effective strategy in most situations, avoidant coping tends to result in increased stress and negative outcomes, while findings for emotion-focused coping are mixed (see, e.g., Aspinwall & Taylor, 1992; MacCann, Fogarty, Zeidner, & Roberts, 2011; Zeidner & Saklofske, 1996). Dumont and Provost (1999) examined the coping strategies of a group of close to 300 adolescents of various ages and found resilient adolescents engaged in more problem-focused coping strategies (such as issue confrontation and proactive problem solving), encouraging resolution of the dilemma more than emotion-focused coping strategies (which encouraged distancing and a lack of social support).

In the research discussed above, traits such as self-esteem, self-efficacy, empowerment, and positive outlook on life are associated with resilience in adolescence. Generally, these characteristics are studied in isolation with little consideration given as to how they might overlap, both conceptually and empirically. Recent research in the field of industrial-organizational psychology, however, has begun to identify a set of interrelated characteristics that have a common core and that hold promise in understanding how resilience is formed and strengthened. Taken together, these characteristics form a construct known as Core Self-Evaluations (e.g., Erez & Judge, 2001; Judge, 2009; Judge et al., 2002, 2003), which we believe is integral to providing a better understanding of resilience. Relevant research on core self-evaluations and resilience follows.

Core Self-Evaluations: A New Lens for Resilience Research?

The core self-evaluations construct is defined as a higher-order trait consisting of the variance shared by four constructs that are highly related, if not identical, to some of the protective factors associated with resilience (i.e., self-esteem, self-efficacy, self-concept, and personal control). The four constructs comprising core self-evaluations are

1. *Self-esteem*, the overall value that one places on oneself as a person (Harter, 1990).
2. *Generalized self-efficacy*, an evaluation of how well one can perform across a variety of tasks and situations (Locke, McClear, & Knight, 1996).
3. *Emotional stability* (often caste misleadingly in the current literature as its opposite pole, neuroticism), the tendency to have a positive cognitive/explanatory style and to focus on positive (rather than negative) aspects of the self (Watson, 2000).
4. *Locus of control*, a belief system where the individual internalizes the causes of events in one's life; making the individual see events as being contingent on their own behavior (Rotter, 1966).

In essence, each construct reflects how capable, worthy, and effective a person feels (Judge et al., 2003). In terms of resiliency, one should be able to better deal with adversity if she or he feels highly capable and effective in handling the situation, and worthy enough to deserve the resulting rewards.

Individually, these constructs represent some of the most often studied constructs in the field of psychology. In fact, a PsychINFO search conducted by Judge et al. (2002) found that more than 50,000 papers on these constructs have been published, with over 30,000 more published in the intervening period. Furthermore, the vast majority of these papers describe studies that consider only the influence of a single construct, and in the rare case that more than one of these constructs was included in a study, the relationship between these constructs was usually not investigated. Evidence suggests, however, that these constructs are common indicators of a more basic evaluation of oneself, and as such, any attempt to study these constructs separately might be an example of the *jangle fallacy* (i.e., the tendency for researchers to create labels for "new constructs" that are in reality nearly identical to constructs that already exist [see Kelley, 1927]).

Core Self-Evaluations: Empirical Findings

Judge and his colleagues have conducted several studies demonstrating that these four constructs are highly interrelated and can be considered to represent one construct called core self-evaluations (e.g., Erez & Judge, 2001; Judge, 2009; Judge et al., 2002, 2003). A meta-analysis of studies that included at least two of the constructs found an average correlation of 0.60 among the four constructs (Judge et al., 2002). The correlations of emotional stability, self-esteem, and self-efficacy were particularly strong, ranging from 0.62 to 0.85. Furthermore, several studies employing confirmatory factor analysis have indicated that the four constructs consistently share salient loadings on one common factor, with factor loadings generally ranging from 0.55 to 0.85 (e.g., Judge, Locke, Durham, & Kluger, 1998). Although the relationships of these constructs do not reach unity, the evidence is highly suggestive that there is considerable overlap among them. Judge (2009) describes this well

> This does not mean that there is no meaningful variance attributable to the individual traits. Many survey items that measure self-esteem (e.g., "I take a positive attitude towards myself"), for example, are not necessarily inter-changeable with items that measure locus of control ("My life is determined by my own actions"). There is some uniqueness to the measures of self-esteem and locus of control. However, these measures have something important in common that explains why these measures are correlated, and that is what we call core self-evaluations (p. 59).

In summary, the factor structure of core self-evaluations appears to be higher-order; that is, the shared variance between the four first-order factors of self-esteem, locus of control, self-efficacy, and emotional stability is large enough to indicate that one higher-order factor circumscribes this domain. Put another way, core self-evaluations are multi-faceted, but enough variance exists to be accounted for by one higher-order factor.

In samples of college students and working adults, core self-evaluations have been shown to predict important outcomes related to resilience. For example, controlling for personality variables such as agreeableness, conscientiousness, and extraversion, core self-evaluations were related to general life stress and strain for college students, and work-related stress and strain in working adults (Judge et al., 2002). Importantly, self-esteem, self-efficacy, and locus of control tended not to provide incremental validity to the prediction of stress and strain when the general factor was controlled for, although neuroticism did tend to have much additional predictive utility.

More recently, two studies found that core self-evaluations also related to the frequency of experiencing stressful situations (Kammeyer-Mueller, Judge, & Scott, 2009). First, a meta-analysis revealed that those with positive core self-evaluations tend to experience less stress and strain than those with negative core self-evaluations. Second, a diary study in which participants were surveyed every day for 2 weeks found that those with positive core self-evaluations tended to experience less stress than those with negative core self-evaluations and that the relationship between stress and strain was weaker for those with positive core self-evaluations. Collectively these findings suggest that when those with positive core self-evaluations experience stressful situations, they are sufficiently resilient to cope with the situation without suffering extreme emotional and physical exhaustion.

Consistent with this proposition, studies have also found that core self-evaluations are related to coping style. Recall from our previous discussion that people tend to cope with stressful situations in one of three ways (i.e., problem-focused, emotion-focused, and avoidant coping), and that problem-focused coping is generally the most effective strategy and avoidant coping the least. Accordingly, Kammeyer-Mueller et al.'s (2009) meta-analysis found that people with positive core self-evaluations practiced more problem-focused coping, while those with negative core self-evaluations used emotion-focused and avoidant coping strategies. In the diary study, once again those with positive core self-evaluations tended to practice less avoidant coping. However, there was only a weak relationship with problem-focused coping, and core self-evaluations were actually positively correlated with emotion-focused coping. Thus, although the relationship of core self-evaluations with a productive coping style is somewhat equivocal, at minimum, this research provides convincing evidence that those with positive core self-evaluations avoid coping in nonproductive ways.

If core self-evaluations are related to a person's ability to be resilient in the face of challenge, these evaluations should also be related to outcomes that are generally reflective of resilient behaviors. In both worker and student samples, evidence is beginning to mount that this is indeed the case. In workforce research, a study of employees of a veteran's health care system found that core self-evaluations were related to job burnout, with a standardized path coefficient of –0.30, suggesting that those with positive core self-evaluations were better able to handle job-related stress than those with negative core self-evaluations (Best, Stapleton, & Downey, 2005). In another study, core self-evaluations were also related to workers' responses to the stress of receiving disappointing work evaluations (Bono & Colbert, 2005). That is, participants' work performance was rated by both themselves and their work colleagues (supervisors, coworkers, and direct reports). When self-ratings exceeded other ratings (e.g., when colleagues rated work performance lower than did participants), those with positive core self-evaluations responded with increased commitment to their goals, whereas when self-ratings exceeded other ratings, those with negative core self-evaluations responded to this discrepancy with decreased commitment to their goals.

Less systematic research has been conducted on student samples, although there are at least two studies that suggest that student core self-evaluations are associated with resilience-related outcomes. In one laboratory study, college students were asked to solve ten anagrams, two of which were unsolvable (Erez & Judge, 2001). To the extent that resilient individuals display steadfast determination in the face of challenge, those who persist while attempting to solve an (unbeknownst to them) unsolvable problem can be said to be demonstrating resiliency. In line with this view, core self-evaluations were positively and significantly correlated with time spent attempting to solve the anagrams ($r = 0.24$).

In another study employing student samples, data on 7,724 participants were obtained from the National Longitudinal Survey of Youth (see Judge & Hurst, 2007). Participants were first interviewed in 1979 when they were 14–22 years old and then interviewed on a yearly basis until 1994. After 1994 they were interviewed every-other year until 2002. Included in data collection were variables that corresponded to core self-evaluations, family socioeconomic status (SES)-related variables (e.g., parental education, family poverty status), demographic characteristics, and income (as measured in 2002). Judge and Hurst predicted 2002 participant income from their 1979 core self-evaluations and family variables, controlling for demographic characteristics. Results revealed an interaction between core self-evaluations and SES. Specifically, those with positive core self-evaluations had higher predicted incomes than those with negative core self-evaluations, and this difference was greatest for those with high socioeconomic status. The authors explain these findings by stating that those with positive core self-evaluations better capitalize on advantage. Although the data support this claim, it also supports the claim that positive core self-evaluations help people remain resilient in the face of challenge. For example, people with positive core self-evaluations who experienced childhood poverty had a predicted

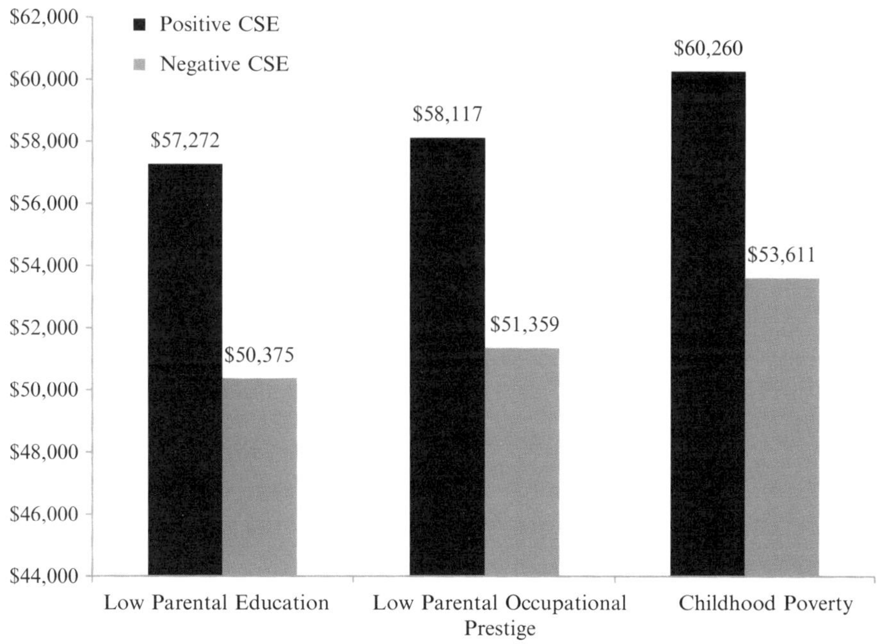

Fig. 15.1 Core self-evaluation and the ability to overcome childhood obstacles (adapted from Judge & Hurst, 2007). *Note*: Dollar amounts indicate predicted 2002 income from core self-evaluation assessed in 1979, controlling for demographic characteristics. *CSE* core self-evaluation

2002 income of $60,268, whereas people with negative core self-evaluations who experienced childhood poverty had a predicted 2002 income of $53,611. Figure 15.1 displays this result, along with similar results for low parental education and low parental occupational prestige.

Although the preceding two examples involved student samples, very little, if any, work has been conducted on core self-evaluations in adolescent samples. One tangentially related study consisted of a reanalysis of 2003 Program for International Student Assessment (PISA) data predicting math achievement from math self-efficacy, math anxiety (similar to neuroticism, the opposite pole of emotional stability), and math self-concept for 260,000 ninth grade students from 41 countries (Vieluf, Lee, & Kyllonen, 2009). In this study, the average correlation of these three constructs was 0.50. Of the variables tested in this study (PISA samples 12–15 academic-related psychosocial variables), a factor made up of these three constructs was the best predictor of math achievement. It is unclear, however, in this study whether these "core self-evaluations" variables predict math achievement because they reflect resilience or because they themselves are a proxy for math achievement.

Despite the lack of research on core self-evaluations in non-adult samples, we have every reason to believe that this construct applies to children and adolescents, as well; as each of the individual components of core self-evaluations has been studied extensively in these populations. In fact, some form of meta-analysis has been conducted on the incidence of each of the four components of core self-evaluations in children and adolescents: emotional stability (Roberts, Walton, & Viechtbauer, 2006), locus of control (Twenge, Zhang, & Im, 2004), self-efficacy (Holden, Moncher, Schinke, & Barker, 1990), and self-esteem (Twenge & Campbell, 2001). If each of the individual constructs can be measured in children and adolescents, then we should also be able to measure the higher-order core self-evaluations construct in the same population. Furthermore, the fact that each of these constructs can be measured in children suggests that core self-evaluations are formed very early in life.

Table 15.1 Summary of hierarchical multiple regression analyses

	Life satisfaction	CSE SSPC	Stress	CSE SSPC	Depression	CSE SSPC	Anxiety	CSE SSPC
Model 1 R^2	0.29		0.07		0.16		0.05	
Model 2 R^2	0.55	0.26	0.15	0.08	0.41	0.25	0.13	0.08

Notes: Model 1 = hierarchical multiple regression including four personality traits (Agreeableness, Conscientiousness, Extraversion, Openness,) and intelligence. Model 2 includes core self-evaluations
All changes in R^2 from Model 1 to Model 2 significant at $p < 0.05$
CSE SSPC core self-evaluations squared semi-partial correlation. This indicates the proportion of variance core self-evaluations explains in the criterion above and beyond the other predictors

An Empirical Demonstration of the Importance of Core Self-Evaluations in a High School Sample

Recently, we have attempted to bridge what we perceive as a gap in the literature and explore core self-evaluations more directly (Burrus, Elliott, Kaliski, & Roberts, in preparation). In one of the studies reported by Burrus et al. (in preparation), 49 freshman, 78 sophomores, 73 juniors, and 74 seniors from a private high school completed a battery of assessments, which included scales measuring three of the four components of core self-evaluations. Students completed a self-esteem scale (Rosenberg, 1965; e.g., "On the whole, I am satisfied with myself"), a generalized self-efficacy scale (Schwarzer & Jerusalem, 1995; "I am certain that I can accomplish my goals"), and a measure of emotional stability (Benet-Martinez & John, 1998; e.g., "I see myself as someone who gets nervous easily" [reverse-keyed]). A measure of locus of control was not included in the assessment battery. Additionally, students completed assessments of the four remaining factors of the Big Five model of personality (Agreeableness, Conscientiousness, Extraversion, and Openness to Experience) (Benet-Martinez & John, 1998), which were used as controls in the analysis. As a control for intelligence, student Secondary School Admission Test (SSAT) percentiles were used.

Student responses to these assessments were used to predict stress, depression, anxiety, and life satisfaction. Stress, depression, and anxiety were measured with the Depression Anxiety Stress Scales (DASS; Lovibond & Lovibond, 1995; e.g., "I felt that I was rather touchy" [stress], "I couldn't seem to experience any positive feeling at all" [depression], "I felt that I was using a lot of nervous energy" [anxiety]). Finally, life satisfaction was assessed with the Students' Life Satisfaction Scale (SLSS; Huebner, 1995; e.g., "My life is going well").

Consistent with the method of Judge and his colleagues, we formed a core self-evaluations score by conducting principal components analysis on the items measuring the three core self-evaluations constructs. A factor score was created by multiplying items by the factor weights associated with the first principal component. For each outcome, we then conducted a hierarchical multiple regression analysis consisting of two steps. At the first step, personality and intelligence were entered. At the second step, the core self-evaluations variable was entered, to determine if this variable explains a practically and statistically significant amount of variance above and beyond personality and intelligence.

This analysis revealed the core self-evaluations are indeed related to outcomes typically associated with resilience in adolescents. For stress, depression, anxiety, and life satisfaction, core self-evaluations explained variance over and above personality and intelligence. Effects were moderate to large in size. Specifically, for life satisfaction and depression, the core self-evaluations variable explained a large amount of variance according to Cohen's (1988) benchmarks: 25% of the variance was explained uniquely by core self-evaluations for both life satisfaction and depression, while for anxiety and stress, a moderate effect size was found (8% of the variance was explained uniquely by core self-evaluations). A brief summary of these regression analyses are included in Table 15.1.

In sum, in the Burrus et al. (in preparation) study, adolescents with positive core self-evaluations felt less stress, anxiety, and depression and were more satisfied with their lives than adolescents with negative core self-evaluations. Notably, these were students from the same school, taking roughly the same classes, and participating in roughly the same extracurricular activities. Indeed, because many of them live on campus, they were likely experiencing similar life obstacles. Given these conditions, the results are consistent with the proposition that positive core self-evaluations are a trait of resilient adolescents.

Some Limitations of Burrus et al. (in preparation). Regarding the conditions of their adolescence, students in our study were very "un-Oprah-like." For the most part, these are students from high socioeconomic status families. As such, the results from our study are likely attenuated by the fact that our sample of students simply has not faced the types of obstacles more common to people less fortunate. Also, because they came from a relatively prestigious academic institution, it is likely that these students are higher than average in core self-evaluations, further attenuating our results. Thus, we would predict stronger results if our study were conducted with a sample more representative of the "typical" adolescent.

Another limitation is that, unlike most studies of core self-evaluations, we did not have a locus of control measure. However, this may not be as big a problem as it might appear at first blush. Locus of control tends to have the weakest relationship with the other three core self-evaluation traits (Judge et al., 2002). Additionally, locus of control tends to be less highly predictive of criteria measures than the other traits. Judge et al. (2002) state that part of the problem may be the lower reliabilities that tend to plague locus of control measures. As such, it may be the case that the addition of locus of control to our study may not have contributed much in the way of prediction.

How Might Positive Core Self-evaluations Lead to Resilience? How do positive core self-evaluations lead to resilience? In the current study, we did not have data available to investigate possible mechanisms that explain the link between core self-evaluations and life satisfaction, stress, anxiety, and depression. A return to the Kammeyer-Mueller et al. (2009) research discussed above on core self-evaluations and coping may be informative. Recall that they found that those with positive core self-evaluations experienced less stress and strain, and were less likely to employ a maladaptive coping style, than those with negative core self-evaluations. It is possible that, because adolescents with positive core self-evaluations in our study likely possessed the belief that they could effectively deal with any challenging situation that would arise, they simply felt less stress in response to such situations. Furthermore, when they did experience stress, they were less likely to use an avoidant-coping style in dealing with it. The use of productive coping styles would tend to lead to more positive life outcomes, and thus possibly greater life satisfaction. Of course, each of these suppositions is an empirically testable hypothesis, and are, we suggest, directions for future research.

Core Self-Evaluations and Remediation: A Draft Blueprint

One of the advantages of viewing resilience through the lens of core self-evaluations lay in the research that has been conducted showing that core self-evaluations can be remediated. In short, interventions can be designed to improve core self-evaluations as a means towards enhancing adolescents' resilience. Before we discuss interventions, however, a point is in order about the malleability of traits such as core self-evaluations. Although researchers previously believed that traits tend to be fixed (especially after age 30; Costa & McCrae, 1997), more recent research has found that traits do indeed change. For example, meta-analysis has demonstrated that personality traits changes over the entire course of the lifespan (Roberts et al., 2006), and a recent study found personality maturation in children and adolescents in the Netherlands (Klimstra, Hale, Raaijmakers, Branje, & Meeus, 2009). Certainly, traits do change, and this leaves open the possibility that purposeful change through intervention can be effective.

In particular, interventions aimed at improving self-esteem, self-efficacy, and locus of control are particularly salient to enhancing core self-evaluations and resilience. Below, we briefly discuss five interventions that we feel are especially relevant for building resilience. The principles include creating positive self-evaluations, reinforcing effort, modeling, creating facilitative attributions, and self-exploration.

1. *Creating Positive Self-evaluations*. The first principle is to help adolescents create a positive self-evaluation of their skills and abilities. One way to do this is to have students first pursue goals that are moderately challenging but that can be accomplished to ensure that they develop some history of previous success. Next, to help link new problems to old successes, when attempting a new, and more difficult task, adolescents should be prompted to think how this new work is related to the work they already succeeded at, and how this new work can be accomplished using the same techniques that they have previously used. Finally, adolescents should be periodically asked to assess their progress by answering questions such as, "How much better are you at overcoming this kind of challenge than you were at the beginning of the school year?"

   One intervention, which benefits all students, includes changes to the delivery of curriculum. Curricula can enhance self-efficacy when individuals are given the opportunity to master progressively difficult tasks and model more advanced peers (Bandura, 1997). For instance, Svinivki & McKeachie (2006) has suggested that faculty offer frequent short tests rather than a cumulative midterm or final exam, which offers students multiple chances to master course content. Further, frequent testing ensures students who do not initially perform well have the chance to improve their content understanding throughout the course of the semester. Since self-efficacy perceptions are cyclical in nature, multiple opportunities to have mastery experiences can have positive and long-lasting effects on students' self beliefs. For example, Meece, Blumfield, & Hoyle (1988) found that mastery goals were positively related to fifth and sixth grade students' perception of their academic ability.
2. *Reinforcing Effort*. Interventions aimed at increasing self-esteem and self-efficacy can also focus on reinforcing effort rather than focusing solely on success or failure (Brooks, 2006). This principle is related to the previous principle in that those creating interventions can begin to reinforce effort by first giving adolescents challenging tasks that they can succeed at and by providing them with feedback at each step of the learning process. Feedback should emphasize praising adolescents for trying hard to accomplish a task more than praising adolescents for successfully completing a task (keeping in mind that praise should be specific to a task). However, when adolescents master a task, they should be given a more difficult one, and then once again feedback should emphasize praising effort for attempting to accomplish this new task. This should be done because adolescents may begin to assume that they do not need to try hard at what they are doing if they continue to be praised for completing tasks that are too easy for them (e.g., Schunk, 1991).
3. *Modeling*. Another principle for increasing self-efficacy is to make use of modeling by peers (Bandura, 1986, 1997). Self-efficacy is likely to increase when adolescents see others who are very similar to them succeed in the face of challenge. In this case, the student might tell themselves, "If he/she can do it, and he/she is like me, then I can do it too." Peer models can model both goal attainment and how to appropriately cope with stressful situations. Interventions can be created that ask student to take advantage of peer modeling through many means. This includes asking adolescents to work in groups at school that are composed both of adolescents who have high self-efficacy and those who have low self-efficacy, and by giving adolescents information about exemplary people (e.g., Oprah) who were resilient in facing challenges similar to their own.

For example, peer or collaborative learning may be a useful tool for promoting self-efficacy perceptions (Schunk, 1987). Peer learning encourages opportunities for students to develop relationships and receive encouragement from high achieving peers (Brooks, 2006). Furthermore, collaborative learning enables students who are shy or lack confidence to discuss their ideas in a small group setting garnering support their before speaking to the larger class thereby encouraging classroom engagement and enhancing students' sense of personal agency (Brooks, 2006; Learning First Alliance, 2001). These successful encounters produce confidence which strengthen self-efficacy perceptions.

4. *Facilitative Attributions.* Attributions are explanations for the causes of events, and adolescents can attribute the events that happen to them to many different sources, with some attributions more conducive to building self-efficacy, and thus resilience, than others. Facilitative attributions are those that explain successes as caused by abilities that were brought about by effort and persistence. When one makes a facilitative attribution for a failure, however, they do not explain this failure as a lack of ability. Those interested in designing interventions to encourage facilitative attributions can do so by helping adolescents stress this attribution style throughout the day, reminding them that success is most often a function of effort. It is likely that this attribution style will have to be practiced and reinforced over a long time period before it becomes a fully ingrained and regularly practice attributional style, especially for adolescents already low in self-efficacy.
5. *Self-exploration.* Some research suggests self-esteem is the result of social rejection (e.g., Rao, 1994) and accordingly improvements to self-esteem can be linked to perceptions of social success (Feldman & Elliott, 1990). Within an educational context, social success can be derived through academic success, athletic ability, and social belonging (Feldman & Elliott, 1990). Therefore, one way to improve self-esteem is to provide children and adolescents opportunities to explore a variety of academic, athletic, and social activities in low stakes environments. Exposure to a wide berth of activities promotes better self-understanding and gives students the change to gauge their skills in new arenas. Success and enjoyment derived from participation in distinct activities can help students find a social and/or academic niche and result in improved sense of self-esteem. In addition, development of a social niche can also expose students to caring adults and peers, which is critical to the development of resilience.

One particular resiliency training program, the Penn Resiliency Project (Positive Psychology Center, 2011), focuses in part on helping children create positive self-evaluations and facilitative attributions. This 12 lesson program includes lessons to help students identify negative self-talk and develop more optimistic alternatives to negative and pessimistic self-talk. Such exercises may work to promote resilience through improving student self-esteem, locus of control, and emotional stability. A recent meta-analysis has found that children who participated in this program reported moderately fewer depressive symptoms than control group children after 12 months (Brunwasser, Gillham, & Kim, 2009).

Other interventions could be designed to also increase self-esteem, increase emotional stability, and increase locus of control. The principles of self-efficacy interventions described above should also be effective in helping design interventions of self-concept and locus of control. The challenge, then, is to create interventions to successfully reduce neuroticism, surely no small challenge. We suggest that the literature on reducing anxiety may be useful in designing such interventions. For example, techniques such as systematic desensitization, cognitive restructuring, and relaxation training have been shown to be useful in reducing test anxiety (Ergene, 2003; Zeidner, 1998). Similar intervention techniques could be combined with self-efficacy interventions to create a comprehensive core self-evaluations intervention system.

Conclusion

> Believe in yourself! Have faith in your abilities! Without a humble but reasonable confidence in your own powers you cannot be successful or happy.
>
> Norman Vincent Peale

We would be willing to place a rather large bet that Oprah Winfrey, based on her own experiences as an adolescent, agrees with this quote from Norman Vincent Peale. Although we believe that he probably overstated his case, our findings suggest that to an extent he may have been correct. Adolescents with positive core self-evaluations, what could be called "reasonable confidence in your own powers," were indeed happier than those with negative core self-evaluations. They were also less prone to stress, anxiety, and depression. One interpretation of these results is that these adolescents, like Oprah, were resilient.

The core self-evaluations concept is a new one to the study of resilience in adolescents. We believe that it holds promise in both synthesizing a number of research literatures and in providing a parsimonious account of the individual factors associated with resilience. Feeling that one is capable, effective, and worthy can give an adolescent the strength to be confident in the face of challenge and to bounce back from adversity. Resilience is defined as, "the power or ability to return to the original form, position, etc., after being bent, compressed, or stretched; elasticity" (Dictionary.com, 2011). If core self-evaluations are the "original form" to which one returns after being stretched or compressed by a stressful situation, then having a strong core self-evaluation is perhaps the most essential component of resilience.

References

Academy of Achievement. (2011). *Oprah Winfrey Biography*. Retrieved May 20, 2011, from http://www.achievement.org/autodoc/page/win0bio-1

Armstrong, M. I., Birnit-Lefcovitch, S., & Unger, M. T. (2005). Pathways between social support, family well being, quality of parenting, and child resilience: What we know. *Journal of Child and Family Studies, 14*(2), 269–281.

Aspinwall, L. G., & Taylor, S. E. (1992). Modeling cognitive adaptation: A longitudinal investigation of the impact of individual differences and coping on college adjustment and performance. *Journal of Personality and Social Psychology, 63*, 989–1003.

Bandura, A. (1986). *Social foundations of thought and action: A social cognitive theory*. Upper Saddle River, NJ: Prentice-Hall, Inc.

Bandura, A. (1997). *Self-efficacy: The exercise of control*. New York, NY: W. H. Freeman.

Bell, C. C. (2001). Cultivating resiliency in youth. *Journal of Adolescent Health, 29*, 375–381.

Benard, B. (1991). *Fostering resiliency in kids: Protective factors in the family, school, and community*. San Francisco, CA: Far West Laboratory for Educational Research and Development. ED 335 781.

Benet-Martinez, V., & John, O. P. (1998). Los Cinco Grandes across cultures and ethnic groups: Multitrait multimethod analyses of the Big Five in Spanish and English. *Journal of Personality and Social Psychology, 75*, 729–750.

Best, R. G., Stapleton, L. M., & Downey, R. G. (2005). Core self-evaluations and job burnout: The test of alternative models. *Journal of Occupational Health Psychology, 10*, 441–451.

Bono, J. E., & Colbert, A. E. (2005). Understanding responses to multisource feedback: The role of core self-evaluations. *Personnel Psychology, 58*, 171–203.

Brooks, J. A. (2006). Strengthening resilience in children and youths: Maximizing opportunities through the schools. *Children & Schools, 28*, 69–76.

Brunwasser, S. M., Gillham, J. E., & Kim, E. S. (2009). A meta-analytic review of the Penn Resiliency Program's effect on depressive symptoms. *Journal of Consulting and Clinical Psychology, 77*, 1042–1054.

Burrus, J., Elliott, D. C., Kaliski, P., & Roberts, R. D. (in preparation). Core self-evaluations, stress, and coping in adolescents.

Cohen, J. (1988). *Statistical power analysis for the behavioral sciences*. Hillsdale, NJ: Erlbaum.

Costa, P. T., & McCrae, R. R. (1997). Longitudinal stability of adult personality. In R. Hogan, J. Johnson, & S. Briggs (Eds.), *Handbook of personality psychology* (pp. 269–292). San Diego, CA: Academic.

Dent, R. J., & Cameron, S. R. (2003). Developing resilience in children who are in public care: The educational psychology perspective. *Educational Psychology in Practice, 19*, 3–19.

Dictionary.com (2011). *Resilience*. Retrieved June 1, 2011, http://dictionary.reference.com/browse/resilience

Dumont, M., & Provost, M. A. (1999). Resilience in adolescents: Protective role of social support, coping strategies, self-esteem, and social activities on experience of stress, and depression. *Journal of Youth and Adolescence, 28*, 343–363.

Durlak, J. A., Weissberg, R. P., Dymnicki, A. B., Taylor, R. D., & Schellinger, K. B. (2011). The impact of enhancing students' social and emotional learning: A meta analysis of school based universal interventions. *Child Development, 82*, 405–432.

Edwards, O. W., Mumford, V. E., & Serra-Roldan, R. (2007). A positive youth development model for students considered at-risk. *School Psychology International, 28*, 29–45.

Erez, A., & Judge, T. A. (2001). Relationship of core self-evaluations to goal setting, motivation, and performance. *Journal of Applied Psychology, 86*, 1270–1279.

Ergene, T. (2003). Effective interventions on test anxiety reduction: A meta-analysis. *School Psychology International, 24*, 313–328.

Feldman, S., & Elliott, G. (1990). Adolescence: Path to a productive life or a diminished future? *Carnegie Quarterly, 35*, 1–13.

Folkman, S., & Moskowitz, J. T. (2004). Coping: Pitfalls and promise. *Annual Review of Psychology, 55*, 745–774.

Fonaghy, P., Steele, M., Steele, H., Higgett, A., & Target, M. (1994). The Emanuel Miller Memorial Lecture, 1992: The theory and practice of resilience. *Journal of Child Psychology and Psychiatry, 35*, 231–257.

Garmezy, N. (1991). Resiliency and vulnerability to adverse developmental outcomes associated with poverty. *American Behavioral Scientist, 34*, 416–430.

Garmezy, N., & Masten, A. S. (1991). The protective role of competence indicators in children at risk. In E. M. Cummings, A. L. Greene, & K. H. Karraker (Eds.), *Life-span developmental psychology: Perspectives on stress and coping* (pp. 151–174). Mahwah, NJ: Lawrence Erlbaum Publishers.

Harter, S. (1990). Causes, correlates, and the functional role of global self-worth: A life span perspective. In R. J. Sternberg & J. Kolligan Jr. (Eds.), *Competence considered* (pp. 67–97). New Haven, CT: Yale University Press.

Harvard Mental Health Letter. (2006). *Resilience*. Retrieved June 9, 2011, from http://www.health.harvard.edu/

Hjemdal, O., Friborg, O., Stiles, T. C., Rosenvinge, J. H., & Martinussen, M. (2006). Resilience predicting psychiatric symptoms: A prospective study of protective factors and their role in adjustment to stressful life events. *Clinical Psychology and Psychotherapy, 13*, 194–201.

Holden, G. W., Moncher, M. S., Schinke, S. P., & Barker, K. M. (1990). Self-efficacy of children and adolescents: A meta-analysis. *Psychological Reports, 66*, 1044–1046.

Huebner, E. S. (1995). The adolescents' life satisfaction scale: An assessment of psychometric properties with black and white elementary school adolescents. *Social Indicators Research, 34*, 315–323.

Judge, T. A. (2009). Core self-evaluations and work success. *Current Directions in Psychological Science, 18*, 58–62.

Judge, T. A., Erez, A., Bono, J. E., & Thoresen, C. J. (2002). Are measures of self-esteem, neuroticism, locus of control, and generalized self-efficacy indicators of a common core construct? *Journal of Personality and Social Psychology, 83*, 693–710.

Judge, T. A., Erez, A., Bono, J. E., & Thoresen, C. J. (2003). The Core Self-evaluations Scale (CSES): Development of a measure. *Personnel Psychology, 56*, 303–331.

Judge, T. A., & Hurst, C. (2007). Capitalizing on one's advantages: Role of core self-evaluations. *Journal of Applied Psychology, 92*, 1212–1227.

Judge, T. A., Locke, E. A., Durham, C. C., & Kluger, A. N. (1998). Dispositional effects on job and life satisfaction: The role of core evaluations. *Journal of Applied Psychology, 83*, 17–34.

Kammeyer-Mueller, J. D., Judge, T. A., & Scott, B. A. (2009). The role of core self-evaluations in the coping process. *Journal of Applied Psychology, 94*, 177–195.

Kelley, E. L. (1927). *Interpretation of educational measurements*. Yonkers, NY: World.

Kitano, M. K., & Lewis, R. B. (2005). Resilience and coping: Implications for gifted children and youth at risk. *Roeper Review, 27*, 200–205.

Klimstra, T. A., Hale, W. W., Raaijmakers, Q. A., Branje, S. J., & Meeus, W. H. (2009). Maturation of personality in adolescence. *Journal of Personality and Social Psychology, 96*, 898–912.

Lazarus, R. S., & Folkman, S. (1984). *Stress, appraisal, and coping*. New York, NY: Springer.

Learning First Alliance. (2001). *Every child learning: Safe and supportive schools*. Retrieved June 7, 2011, from http://www.learningfirst.org

Locke, E. A., McClear, K., & Knight, D. (1996). Self-esteem and work. *International Review of Industrial/Organizational Psychology, 11*, 1–32.

Lovibond, P. F., & Lovibond, S. H. (1995). The structure of negative emotional states: Comparison of the Depression Anxiety Stress Scales (DASS) with the Beck Depression and Anxiety Inventories. *Behaviour Research & Therapy, 33*, 335–343.

Luthar, S. S., Cicchetti, D., & Becker, B. (2000). Research on resilience: Response to commentaries. *Child Development, 71*, 573–575.

MacCann, C., Fogarty, G. J., Zeidner, M., & Roberts, R. D. (2011). Coping mediates the relationship between emotional intelligence (EI) and academic achievement. *Contemporary Educational Psychology, 36*, 60–70.

Masten, A. S., Garmezy, N., Tellegen, A., Pellegrini, D. S., Larkin, K., & Larsen, A. (1988). Competence and stress in school children. *Journal of Child Psychology and Psychiatry, 29*, 745–764.

Meece, J. L., Blumenfeld, P. C., & Hoyle, R. H. (1988). Students' goal orientations and cognitive engagement in classroom activities. *Journal of Educational Psychology, 80*, 514–523.

Osofsky, J. D., & Thompson, M. D. (2000). Adaptive and maladaptive parenting: Perspectives on risk and protective factors. In J. P. Shonkoff & S. J. Meisels (Eds.), *Handbook of early childhood intervention* (2nd ed., pp. 54–75). New York, NY: Cambridge University Press.

Parker, J. D. A., & Endler, N. S. (1996). Coping and defense: An historical over-view. In M. Zeidner & N. S. Endler (Eds.), *Handbook of coping: Theory, research, applications* (pp. 3–23). New York, NY: John Wiley & Sons.

Positive Psychology Center. (2011). *Resilience Research in Children*. Retrieved July 14, 2011, from http://www.ppc.sas.upenn.edu/prpsum.htm

Rao, U. (1994). Adolescent depression may lead to depression later in life. *The Brown University Child and Adolescent Behavior Letter, 10*, 3.

Rhule, D. M., McMahon, R. J., Spieker, S. J., & Munson, J. A. (2006). Positive adjustment and associated protective factors in children of adolescent mothers. *Journal of Child and Family Studies, 15*, 231–251.

Richardson, G. E. (2002). The meta-theory of resilience and resiliency. *Journal of Clinical Psychology, 58*, 307–321.

Roberts, B. W., Walton, K., & Viechtbauer, W. (2006). Patterns of mean-level change in personality traits across the life course: A meta-analysis of longitudinal studies. *Psychological Bulletin, 132*, 1–25.

Rosenberg, M. (1965). *Society and the adolescent self-image*. Princeton, NJ: Princeton University Press.

Rotter, J. B. (1966). Generalized expectancies for internal versus external control of reinforcement. *Psychological Monographs, 80* (Whole No. 609).

Rutter, M. (1985). Resilience in the face of adversity: Protective factors and resistance to psychiatric disorder. *British Journal of Psychiatry, 147*, 598–611.

Rutter, M., Maughan, B., Mortimore, P., Ouston, J., & Smith, A. (1979). *Fifteen thousand hours*. Cambridge: Harvard University Press.

Schunk, D. H. (1987). Peer models and children's behavioral change. *Review of Educational Research, 57*, 149–174.

Schunk, D. H. (1991). Self-efficacy and academic motivation. *Educational Psychologist, 26*, 207–231.

Schwarzer, R., & Jerusalem, M. (1995). Generalized Self-Efficacy scale. In J. Weinman, S. Wright, & M. Johnston (Eds.), *Measures in health psychology: A user's portfolio. Causal and control beliefs* (pp. 35–37). Windsor, UK: NFER-NELSON.

Svinivki, M., & McKeachie, W. J. (2006). *McKeachie's teaching tips: Strategies, research, and theory for college and university teachers*. Belmont, CA: Wadsworth, Cengage Learning.

Twenge, J. M., & Campbell, W. K. (2001). Age and birth cohort differences in self-esteem: A cross-temporal meta-analysis. *Personality and Social Psychology Review, 5*, 321–344.

Twenge, J. M., Zhang, L., & Im, C. (2004). It's beyond my control: A cross-temporal meta-analysis of increasing externality in locus of control, 1960–2002. *Personality and Social Psychology Review, 8*, 308–319.

Vieluf, S., Lee, J., Kyllonen, P. (2009). *The predictive power of variables from the PISA2003 student questionnaire*. QEG(0910)5a.doc, QEG meeting Offenbach, Germany, October 19–21, 2009.

Watson, D. (2000). *Mood and temperament*. New York, NY: Guilford.

Weissberg, R. P., & Elias, M. J. (1993). Enhancing young people's social competence and health behavior. *Applied and Preventative Psychology, 3*, 179–190.

Werner, E. E. (1982). *Vulnerable but invincible: A longitudinal study of resilient children and youth*. New York, NY: McGraw-Hill.

Werner, E. E. (1990). Protective factors and individual resilience. In S. J. Meisels & M. Shonkoff (Eds.), *Handbook of early intervention* (pp. 97–116). New York, NY: Cambridge University Press.

Werner, E. E. (1993). Risk, resilience, and recovery: Perspectives from the Kauai Longitudinal Study. *Development and Psychopathology, 5*, 503–515.

Werner, E. E. (2000). Protective factors and individual resilience. In J. P. Shonkoff & S. J. Meisels (Eds.), *Handbook of early childhood intervention* (2nd ed., pp. 115–132). New York, NY: Cambridge University Press.

Werner, E., & Smith, R. (1989). *Vulnerable but invincible: A longitudinal study of resilient children and youth*. New York, NY: Adams, Bannister, and Cox.

Werner, E., & Smith, R. (1992). *Overcoming the odds: High-risk children from birth to adulthood*. New York, NY: Cornell University Press.

Zeidner, M. (1998). *Test anxiety: The state of the art*. New York: Plenum Press.

Zeidner, M., Matthews, G., & Roberts, R. D. (2006). Emotional intelligence, adaptation, and coping. In J. Ciarrochi, J. Forgas, & J. D. Mayer (Eds.), *Emotional intelligence in everyday life: A scientific inquiry* (2nd ed., pp. 100–125). Philadelphia, PA: Psychology Press.

Zeidner, M., Roberts, R. D., & Matthews, G. (2002). Can emotional intelligence (EI) be schooled? A critical review. *Educational Psychologist, 37*, 215–231.

Zeidner, M., & Saklofske, D. (1996). Adaptive and maladaptive coping. In M. Zeidner & N. Endler (Eds.), *Handbook of coping: Theory, research, applications* (pp. 505–531). New York, NY: Wiley.

Resilience Revisited: Toward an Expanding Understanding of Post-disaster Adaptation

16

Raymond F. Hanbury and Monica J. Indart

Introduction

Over the course of the past two decades, the impact of global disasters and complex emergencies has increasingly become a part of inter-disciplinary dialogue. Economic, political, biopsychosocial, and sociocultural aspects of large-scale events have drawn attention to the widespread and long-term consequences of such events (Calhoun & Tedeschi, 1998). These events are broadly classified into categories that reflect their precipitants, which from a psychosocial perspective can be understood as "sources of suffering." These sources include the following events: natural disasters (e.g., tornadoes, wild fires, floods, hurricanes, earthquakes); technological disasters (air crashes, nuclear power plant accidents); disasters of human intent (bombings, terrorist attacks); interpersonal violence (domestic violence, child abuse, sexual assault, school or workplace violence, homicide, torture); sudden traumatic loss (serious or fatal motor vehicle accidents, suicide); serious medical illness; war, combat, and civil conflicts; and lastly what is described within an international context as complex emergencies (e.g., the current famine in Somalia, which combines the consequences of natural disaster (drought), with civil conflict (the murderous actions of the militant group Al-Shabab) within the context of a geopolitical region ravaged by decades of civil unrest, lack of governance, and limited public health infrastructure).

Without question, these events result in human suffering across the life span and across the world. Yet, despite such enormous tragedy and suffering, studies of such events consistently reveal "sources of strength," i.e., human stories that reflect a capacity for not simply coping with, enduring and recovering from trauma, but the possibility of healing and transformation. Thus, from every region of the world, every disaster, emergency, and traumatic event encountered, we repeatedly witness the human capacity for *resilience*.

This chapter will review the current status of the literature on resilience as it applies to the human capacity to effectively cope with such adverse events. The focus will be on adult resilience as a distinct response to more extreme adverse events. The broad range of adjustment patterns manifested by survivors of potentially traumatic events (PTEs) is well-documented, with responses that reflect stress resistance and resilience to acute distress and the more infrequently occurring long-term

R.F. Hanbury, Ph.D., A.B.P.P. (✉)
Department of Psychiatry, Jersey Shore University Medical Center, Private Practice, Behavioral Medicine, Trauma and Police Psychology, State Director Trauma Response Team, 2640 Highway 70, Bldg. 7A Suite 202, Manasquan, NJ 08736-2609, USA
e-mail: hanburypsy@aol.com

M.J. Indart, Ph.D.
Department of Clinical Psychology, Rutgers University, Graduate School of Applied and Professional Psychology, Private Practice, 152 Frelinghuysen Road Piscataway, Maplewood, NJ 08854, USA
e-mail: mjmindart@yahoo.com

S. Prince-Embury and D.H. Saklofske (eds.), *Resilience in Children, Adolescents, and Adults: Translating Research into Practice*, The Springer Series on Human Exceptionality,
DOI 10.1007/978-1-4614-4939-3_16, © Springer Science+Business Media New York 2013

maladjustment (Bonanno, 2004; Bonanno, Brewin, Kaniasty, & Greca, 2010).

Current empirical research reflects a growing awareness that too much attention has been devoted to the negative outcomes of exposure to PTEs (e.g., posttraumatic stress disorder (PTSD), depression, substance abuse, etc.), while neglecting what may represent the most common or frequent response to exposure to PTEs: resilience (Bonanno, 2004; Bonanno et al., 2010; Reich, Zautra, & Hall, 2010). A final potential outcome to such adversity is *posttraumatic growth*. Coined by Tedeschi and Calhoun, posttraumatic growth represents a trajectory of response distinct from resilience (Tedeschi & Calhoun, 1995). These response patterns will be briefly reviewed in the following section which focuses on an overview of outcomes to PTEs.

Trauma and Its Aftermath: The Range of Human Response

The DSM-IV-TR provides a list of PTEs which were included in the introduction to this chapter as examples of event categories. Some of these categories will be briefly reviewed in this section. Natural disasters are the most common type of disaster in the USA and worldwide. Fires, floods, hurricanes, tornadoes, tsunamis, volcanic eruptions, and other events can occur more frequently than other types of disasters. Therefore, more is known about the psychological outcomes of natural disasters than any other type of event. These disasters can be defined as large scale and affecting a large number of people. Most of these tragedies are environmental events causing massive numbers of injuries, deaths, and loss of possessions and homes.

The term technological disaster incorporates many different types of dangerous events. Transportation accidents, such as air or rail disasters, as well as high profile events such as the loss of a space shuttle, accidents at chemical plants, oil refineries, or nuclear power plants are considered technological disasters. Included in this category would be two recent events that received widespread media attention and will provide unique opportunities for study by disaster and emergency service professionals from various disciplines for years to come. The Deepwater Horizon/BP gulf oil spill in 2010 resulted from human error, and highlighted the critical factors of human intention, social support safety nets, and a rapid and competent response in tracking the trajectory of response and recovery. In March 2011, Japan experienced an unprecedented combination of events, when an earthquake off the Pacific coast of Tohoku triggered a tsunami, which in turn resulted in the meltdown of at least four nuclear reactors in the Fukushima nuclear power plant. Although the earthquake and tsunami resulted in immediate loss of life, it was the nuclear power plant disaster that received the most public attention and citizen concern.

Mass interpersonal violence or disasters of human intention involve large number of casualties and huge numbers of injuries. Although the USA had been largely "protected" from such events historically, the past two decades have unfortunately brought the impact of two large-scale events into our consciousness: the Oklahoma City bombing in 1995 and the terrorist attacks on the World Trade Center in 2001. At the time of the writing of this chapter, the authors have recently had occasion to witness first-hand the long-term sequelae of terrorism on a larger scale as the nation remembers and mourns 10 years after the attacks. Much of the empirical findings related to the continued consequences of these events have been chronicled in the recent edition of the Journal of Traumatic Stress (International Society of Traumatic Stress Studies, October 2011); however, the personal narratives of those who suffered and responded will continue to be heard for months to come. The last section of this chapter will include the authors' reflections on their work after 9/11 as well as other disasters.

Although the United States' introduction to terrorism within its national borders is relatively recent, history is replete with examples of how suffering is inflicted upon one group by another, for reasons both simple and complex. From the Holocaust to the Rwandan genocide to the systemic slaughter of 5.4 million Congolese citizens since 1998 giving rise to the Darfur genocide, the world bears witness to hate and violence writ large on a global scale. These most extreme events, categorized variously as genocides, complex emergencies, or disasters of human intention, all share the particular psychological fingerprint of the unique suffering that results when humans turns against one another on a massive scale. As we advance our understanding of the human capacity for evil through avenues such as genocide studies, however, we also further our appreciation for the human capacity for strength, endurance, and even generosity through the current focus upon resilience studies.

Lastly, other interpersonal violence events include situations as diverse as intimate partner violence, child abuse, rape and sexual assault, torture, shootings, stabbings, school, and workplace violence. Again, the common denominator in these situations is the presence of human intention to do harm. The well-documented finding that events of human intention bear particularly pernicious consequences for those affected is an accepted aspect of intervention planning. Such events may often involve distress and dysfunction, require intervention over a longer period of time, and result in groups of individuals who may require specialized trauma-focused treatment, in contrast to the more universal intervention of Psychological First Aid (PFA) that is typically provided for natural disaster survivors. Additionally, these events result in specialized affected populations: first responders. Emergency workers, a category which includes such diverse professions as law enforcement, firefighters, paramedics and medical examiner teams, as well as public health professionals (physicians and nurses), mental health professionals and clergy, are typically identified as a "special population" in many all hazards disaster plans. These individuals respond to local events as well as large-scale national and even international events, the latter as exemplified by the deployment of many local urban search and rescue teams to Port-au-Prince after the January 2010 earthquake in Haiti. Because of the intensity and proximity of their exposure to the traumatic event, these professional groups are considered to be at greater risk for more complicated adjustment reactions, all other factors being equal. Of particular relevance for this chapter is the recent inclusion of mental health professionals who respond to such events as more front-line "first responders," reflecting a recognition of their unique exposure to certain psychosocial occupational risks (Fullerton, Ursano, & Wang, 2004). Additionally, psychotherapists who provide treatment for trauma survivors are considered vulnerable to such psychosocial hazards and may be at greater risk for development of vicarious traumatization (Pearlman & Saakvitne, 1995).

As previously mentioned, clinical and research attention has largely focused on the sequelae of exposure to PTEs, and within this framework, an even more exclusive focus on the negative outcomes of exposure, particularly prevalence of PTSD. Ironically, this intense focus upon PTSD has given rise to the current wave of resilience research. This "third wave" of trauma-focused studies examines a broader spectrum of adaptational trajectories (Bonanno et al., 2010; Bonanno & Mancini, 2012; Yehuda & Flory, 2007), reflecting the rich tradition of research on individual differences, and the essential heterogeneity of human response (Dickstein, Suvak, Litz, & Adler, 2010).

Resilience Redefined

The recent surge in research related in the concept of resilience, and related interventions highlights the difficulties that arise from the is many definitions of resilience. Much information on resilience has come from developmental psychopathology, where initially researchers tried to identify general characteristics associated with resilient recovery from stressors: resourcefulness, hardiness, self-efficacy, and flexibility (Luthar & Cicchetti, 2000; Luthar, 2006). The American Psychological Association Task Force on Promoting Resilience to Terrorism defines resilience as "the process of adapting well in the force of adversity, trauma, tragedy, threats, or even significant sources of stress." It cites many studies showing that the primary factors in resilience are (1) caring relationships within and outside the family that create love and trust, provide role models, and encourage and reassure; (2) the capacity to make realistic plans and implement them; (3) self-confidence; (4) communication and problem-solving skills; and (5) the capacity to manage emotions (Watson, Ritchie, Demer, Bartone, & Pfefferbaum, 2006). A statement that is generally accepted is that resilience is ordinary and common ("ordinary magic") and derives from the basic human ability to adapt to new situations (Masten, 2001).

Resiliency is the term applied to individuals who were exposed to trauma and risk factors but are able to overcome psychological and physical trauma (Werner, 2001). According to Dass-Brailsford (2007) resiliency is an ability to successfully overcome physical and psychological trauma. Research has shown that the capacity of social support enhances coping abilities and increases resilience and hardiness during times of stress, crisis, or trauma (Kessler, Sonnega, Bromet, Hughes, & Nelson, 1995). Winfield (1994) also describes resilience as an interaction between the characteristics of the individual and the environment. Resilience is a person's ability not only to cope with, survive, and bounce back from difficult and traumatic experiences and situations but also to grow and develop psychologically and emotionally (Walsh, 1998). Fraser (1998) proposes that clinicians should consistently view a crisis as a catalyst for individuals experiencing growth and development beyond a precrisis level of functioning.

Definitions of resilience include protective factors. Masten, Best, and Garmezy (1990) define resilience as "the process of, capacity for, or outcome of successful adaptation despite challenging or threatening circumstances." They identify three circumstances that can demonstrate resilience: (1) overcoming the odds, (2) sustained competence under adversity, and (3) recovery from trauma (Singer, 2005). Luthar (1993) uses the phrase "protective factors" to identify factors that are present in high risk children who exhibit positive rather than negative adjustment. Cummings, Davies, and Campbell (2000) cite Garmezy's (1991) three-part framework of protective factors.

1. *Dispositional attributes within the child*, including temperament, personality traits, gender, coping styles, locus of control, and self-esteem.
2. *Family characteristics*, including family cohesion and warmth, positive parent–child relationships, and harmonious inter-parental relations; and
3. *Domains of extra familial contexts*, including the availability of a positive adult figure (e.g., teacher), positive school experiences academically and socially, and safe, supportive neighborhoods (p. 143).

Further refining the constructs of adaptation to stress and traumatic stress the notion of "stress resistance" has emerged as a way of describing those individuals who may not exhibit any change in functioning or increased distress after exposure to a stressor. This emerging concept of stress resistance requires greater empirical examination to identify it as a distinct trajectory from resilience, however. As a point of distinction, resilient individuals may exhibit an initial decremental response, followed by an accelerated or positive recovery (Steinberg, 2004). Whether these two response patterns represent qualitatively distinct adaptational trajectories or merely incremental quantitative differences remains to be determined.

According to Luthar and Cicchetti (2000) resilience is oftentimes considered "multidimensional" with different characteristics expressed variably across many areas of the individual's life. These authors further describe these "resilient trajectories" as possibly being uneven. Essentially this means that an individual can function in a satisfactory manner in a particular area of life such as on the job or in school but experience inadequate performance in other aspects of life like family relationships. Luthar and Cicchetti (2000) advocate for defining resilience as a state, not a trait. They recommend using the phrase "resilient trajectory or adaptation" explaining that these trajectories vary across situations and within individuals at different times.

Bonanno (2004) defined resilience as "the ability of adults in otherwise normal circumstances who are exposed to an isolated and potentially highly disruptive event such as the death of a close relation or a violent or life-threatening situation to maintain relatively stable healthy levels of psychological and physical functioning … as well as the capacity for generative experiences and positive emotions." One does need to keep in mind that even though an individual is resilient, they too may manifest some form of stress reaction. Such signs of a stress reaction are generally short lasting and they do continue to function.

Zautra, Hall, and Murray (2010) state that "resilience is best defined as an outcome of successful adaptation to adversity. Characterization of the person and situation may identify resilient processes, but only if they lead to healthier outcomes following stressful circumstances." They also point out that there are two components that need to be considered when talking about resilience. These areas are recovery and sustainability. Recovery refers to how well individuals will "bounce back and recover fully from challenge" (Masten, 2001; Rutter, 1987). This recovery includes the ability to return to a state of equilibrium psychologically, physiologically, and socially. Being able to move forward in a time of adversity is the sustainability of health and psychological well-being (Bonnano, 2004). Resilience has been recently seen across our country with all the natural disasters that have occurred in the various states with tornadoes, flooding, and wildfires. There were examples of individuals caring and helping neighbors and a spirit of being able to face the challenges ahead of them. This adaptive response has been demonstrated many times, not only as individuals helping individuals, but entire communities that were affected able to connect and bond as an collective. This collective courage was observed by each of the authors throughout the different disasters and traumatic events to which we responded. This was also evidenced by the media coverage of all the tragedies witnessed by us.

Other theoretical constructs interact with resilience, including hardiness, coping, self-efficacy, posttraumatic recovery, posttraumatic growth, and biological processes related to resilience (Watson, Ritchie, Demer, Bartone, & Pfefferbaum, 2006). As an example, hardiness is a characteristic that has been shown to neutralize the negative effects of stress (Holgersen, Klockner, Boe, Weisaeth, & Holen, 2011; Zautra, Hall, & Murray, 2008; Waysman, Schwarzwald, & Soloman, 2001). Researchers suggest that individuals employ multiple strengths fostering resilient recovery, which include having a belief they can change a stressor; have strong support networks; view stress as a surmountable challenge; focus on positive aspects of trauma; and are not prone to using behavioral disengagement to confront stress (Kobasa, Maddi, & Kahn, 1982; Maddi & Hightower, 1999; Waysman et al., 2001).

Coping self-efficacy is defined as "the perception of one's capability for managing stressful or threatening environmental demands" (Watson, Ritchie, Demer, Bartone, & Pfefferbaum, 2006). In the aftermath of disasters, Benight et al. (1999) recommend that individuals learn new problem-solving skills and set achievable goals. Bonanno (2004) reports that recovery from traumatic stress is aided by social support and seeing oneself as a survivor rather than a victim. Calhoun and Tedeschi (2001) reported that positive adaptation has been called posttraumatic growth. They put this growth in three domains: changed sense of self, changed relationships, and changed philosophy of life. In the same publication, these authors emphasized that with resilience trajectories, reports of growth do not mean the absence of pain or distress. Another factor relating to resilience is the biological components. Evidence indicates that review of stress resistance and resilience must include psychological, environmental, social factors, and biological mechanisms and processes (Layne, Warren, Watson, & Shaleu, 2007).

Emphasizing that resilience is common and derives from the basic human ability to adapt to new situations (Masten, 2001), we move toward current conceptualizations of adult resilience. Resilience is generally considered to be multidimensional (Luthar & Cicchetti, 2000) with different characteristics expressed variably across many areas of the individual's life (e.g., family, job). These "resilient trajectories may be uneven" (Luthar & Cicchetti, 2000; Tusaie & Dyer, 2004) as an individual following a traumatic event may be able to perform tasks and responsibilities in an appropriate and adequate manner, such as conducting business as usual at work, but upon returning home may be withdraw from family members. Many researchers conclude that resilience is not a fixed attribute but a type of "functional trajectory" dependent on circumstances and individual variations in response to risk. Luthar and Cicchetti (2000) thus define resilience as a "state, not a trait" and suggest using the term "resilient trajectory or adaptation" rather than resiliency. They point out that "these trajectories vary across situations and within individuals at different times." Essentially one may see an individual demonstrate a behavior that is functional in one aspect of their life, such as work, and see an emotional detachment in their personal life with their family members.

Social support plays a strong role in the arena of resilience and recovery. It is well recognized that support from these networks are often sought more than mental health professionals. The overlapping and interacting factors in the support system and recovery environment include family, school, work, friends, religion, culture, and community. Webb (2001) points out "the concept of culture encompasses the beliefs, morals, values, customs, world view, behaviors, and communication styles that are socially transmitted and held in common by a group and to which the group's members are expected to conform." Culture can shape the experience and consequences of disaster exposure. As we have seen in the field, there can be striking ethnic disparities for use of mental health services. These disparities may partially be attributable to the stigma of illness that often accompanies seeking help, as well as distrust, a sense of shame, or and/guilt that are not uncommon responses to crisis and disasters. Lastly, further efforts must be made to offer psychosocial assistance that is experienced as helpful by various cultural communities, including making services safe and accessible to immigrants, refugees and undocumented community members.

The literature consistently highlights the capacity of social support to enhance coping abilities and to increase resilience and hardiness during times of trauma. These are theoretical constructs that overlap with resilience. For example, hardiness is a characteristic that can neutralize the negative effects of stress. Hardy individuals often employ multiple strengths that foster recovery. Kobasa et al. (1982) and Waysman et al. (2001) refer to some of these strengths as "individuals seek help and build large support networks and reframe their experiences more positively; belief they can change a stressor or recover from its detrimental effects—focus selectively on the positive effects of a trauma; view themselves as controlling their fate, are committed to meaningful goals, and view stress as a surmountable challenge—and, are less likely to use behavioral disengagement, denial, and alcohol to confront stress and more likely to try to solve problems."

Other Factors Contributing to Resilience

Coping self-efficacy which can be defined as the perception of one's capability for managing stressful or threatening environmental demands. The capacity for optimism and social support is mediated through the survivor's confidence in their own restorative capabilities.

Posttraumatic recovery following traumatic stress is promoted by a sense of relationship and social support, the perception that the social milieu accepts one's reaction, and seeing oneself as a survivor rather than a victim (Bonanno, 2006; Lyons, 1991).

Posttraumatic growth is seen as positive adaptation and return to adequate functioning following trauma. Calhoun and Tedeschi (2001) define this concept through examining it both in relation to trauma-related disorders (e.g., PTSD), as well as distinct entity that follows an entirely different trajectory. Thus, posttraumatic growth is understood as not simply quantitatively different than PTSD, but qualitatively different. Five domains of posttraumatic growth are identified: personal strength, new possibilities, relating to others, appreciation of life, and spiritual change. As part of his continued refinement of the construct, Tedechi emphasizes the essential paradoxes embedded in traumatic experience: loss and gain, support and individual strength, control and lack of control, grief and gratitude, and vulnerability and strength (Tedeschi, 2012). Caution here is not to minimize the burdens and challenges but rather to appreciate the nuanced paradoxes of experience.

Neurobiological Response Related to Resilience

The focus of this chapter is not to provide a comprehensive overview of the psychobiology of trauma but rather to identify the critical pathways by which traumatic and resilience responses traverse the mind and body. These critical pathways are controlled by the hypothalamus, brainstem, limbic system, and the neocortex. When we talk about resilience, it must include psychological, environmental, social and biological factors. The natural response of systems exposed to trauma is an attempt to maintain system stability or homeostasis. Sterling and Eyer (1998) coined the term "allostasis" regarding an individual's efforts to maintain stability and adapt to stressors and keep in the state of homeostasis. In times of stress, the brain responds by releasing catecholamines and hormones which help the person cope with the stressors.

During stressful events, the body releases hormones or glucocorticoids, including epinephrine or adrenaline, norepinephrine, and cortisol. When stressed, one experiences changes in brain structure and neurological functioning (Debiec & LeDoux, 2004). Brain imaging studies reveal a hyperactivation of the amygdala and a hypoactivation of the medical prefrontal regions in response to fearful stimuli (Shin et al., 2004). The fight or flight response is triggered by the release of hormones critical for survival in the brain and body.

As aspect of this biological component is the connection to health. Hughes (2003) defines health as the absence of illness and pathology. This definition of health is "the harmonious integration of mind, body, and spirit within a responsive community." Health status is a multidimensional construct that refers to an individual's biological regulation, the presence or absence of organic pathology, symptom perception, and physical function (Wilson & Cleary, 1995). Individuals who have been exposed to traumatic stressors may have adverse physical health outcomes, including poor self-reported health status, a greater number of self-reported medical problems, increased morbidity and mortality, and greater service utilization (Friedman & Schnurr, 1995). Evidence of the relationship between trauma exposure and self-reported health problems comes from large samples of civilians, veterans, and military personnel (Flett, Kazantzis, Long, MacDonald, & Millar, 2002), sexual assault victims (Golding, 1996), adults who experienced childhood trauma (Felitti et al., 1998), and older adults (Higgins & Follette, 2002).

There are aspects or characteristics of a traumatic event or disaster that may escalate the stress level for individuals. Some of these factors include lack of warning, the suddenness of the event, the type of disaster (natural, technological, etc.), the scale or scope of event, degree and extent of loss and damage, individual's proximity to the event, duration of the incident, differences in severity of the traumatic event, and the amount of exposure to the actual event (Everly, 1995).

Though most of the trauma and disaster work of the authors have been with adults, they certainly have encountered numerous events that have involved children. There is one aspect of the psychology of working with traumatized children that needs to be mentioned. Rescue work with traumatized children often evokes several core psychological processes such as it potentiates motivating forces which at times can be more intense in the helper's personality, intensifies identification with the victim and/or the victim's family, and there can be a breakdown of natural defenses. These factors can lead to the rescuer becoming overwhelmed by their own emotional reactions to the scene, the victims, and the survivors (Dyregrov, 1995). This is where the concept and practice of self-care becomes so necessary and essential so that we as responders can continue to perform our tasks. We always need to keep in mind that being aware of one's own needs and meeting them allows us to function in our roles of helper.

According to O'Leary and Ickovics (1995) there are three possible outcomes following the challenge of trauma, namely survival, recovery, or thriving. They report that individuals who survive "never regain their previous level of functioning." Individuals who recover "regain homeostasis and return to their previous level of functioning" and those who thrive are individuals who have the "ability to go beyond the original level of psychosocial functioning to grow vigorously, even flourish." The personal resources that enhance thriving include hardiness, active coping, sense of coherence, optimism, and a sense of humor (Freidman, 1991; Carver et al., 1993). Given that in one's life, change is unavoidable and often times is essential for adaptation it stands to reason that humans, as biological organisms, would have some innate capacity for recovery and thriving. Tedeschi and Calhoun (1995) considered change as the result of coping with an "unexpected and uncontrollable trauma." They also saw change as growth. The nature of the trauma and the strategies and techniques used to cope with it may vary among different types of traumatic events.

Calhoun and Tedeschi (1998) refer to the growth that survivors of trauma can have as posttraumatic growth. They address the role of the clinician in this process as being one who "needs to be open to this possibility of growth, help the survivors discover meaning in the traumatic event, and be open to discuss spiritual issues with the survivors."

Fostering resilience can be enhanced in different ways and have different outcomes. The American Psychological Association has fact sheets online for building resilience on its self-help website (http://www.apahelpcenter.org). Some of the steps for improving resilience, based on empirical data, include make connections, avoid seeing trauma as insurmountable, accept change as part of life, increase social support, maintain a hopeful outlook, keep things in perspective—to mention a few of these facts. There are interventions, resources, and capacity-building interventions that can be utilized in the process of enhancing. Most of these interventions include preparation and prevention as a way to inoculate individuals against trauma. Training programs for learned optimism, a cornerstone of positive psychology models, are one of the emerging models for capacity building interventions (Seligman and Peterson, 2003). These resiliency-based intervention models enable survivors to retain a sense of efficacy and control during traumatic situations, as well as educate individuals in specific adaptive coping strategies.

Reflections on Resilience

The authors conclude this chapter with brief comments regarding their respective experiences in the field, taking a "lessons learned" approach to understanding resilience from examples and encounters.

The second author's experiences working in the field reflects a lifelong learning curve that reveals both the essential strength of the human spirit, as well as the limits of resilience. For the purposes of this brief chapter, these experiences will be limited to an examination of the acute aftermath of the World Trade Center attacks, and long-term work with Rwandan genocide survivors through cocreating interventions with local NGOs in Rwanda, a nation that can teach the world a thing or two about suffering and the strength that remains.

In the immediate and acute aftermath of the 9/11 terrorist attacks, we did not need psychologists to tell us that "resilience was the default position." Most of us lived this resilience each day. We did it reflexively. We were resilient because we did not know what else to do, because there was no other option. Those of who worked in the family assistance center that was established at Liberty State Park in New Jersey worked long hours, with days and weeks melting together. We did not talk about promoting resilience. We simply tried to get through each day, each tragic story, each encounter with another devastated family. We encouraged human connection whenever and wherever possible. We quietly honored the strength we witnessed. We focused on what it meant to operationalize the construct "compassionate presence." All the things we thought we knew how to do, that we were trained to do, suddenly felt inadequate in the face of such enormous shock, and as the months passed, profound grief. Our teams met for daily briefings and debriefings (debriefings as in general information and support sharing sessions, not the CISD model). We put one foot in front of the other, psychologically speaking. Although I had worked in disaster and crisis response efforts previous to 9/11, in retrospect I recognize that this event marked my first real encounter with resilience as a distinct psychological entity. Each day, I looked into the face of a bewildered, terrified, grieving family member, who each day, found the strength to seek information and connection. It was their strength that gave me the courage to show up the next day. These encounters represented "resilience in motion," resilience as natural and automatic a part of life as breathing. The families, and our teams, spontaneously embraced resilience—without awareness, without guidance, without "best practice guidelines"—we did so because there was simply nothing else to be done.

The second "lessons learned" experience comes from longer-term work with survivors of the Rwanda genocide. In 1994, over 800,000 Tutsi's and moderate Hutu's were slaughtered in one of the most vicious and systematic ethnic cleansing acts in history. The women and children bore a particular burden of suffering. Identified as "vulnerable populations," and manifesting several "risk factors" for trauma-spectrum disorders, many of the affected women and children provided text book examples of the adaptational trajectories described by Bonanno et al. (2010). Seventeen years postgenocide, recovery is evident in abundance; indeed, Rwanda is hailed today for its ability to rebuild itself as a nation in the aftermath of unspeakable levels of horror and devastation. Within this context of a national recovery trajectory, however, lie individual stories of both chronicity and resilience (there are few examples of delayed onset distress, as would be expected from such massive and horrific violence). The story of the Rwandese I have been privileged to work with reflect an often neglected detail in the resilience literature: resilience and continued distress/dysfunction are not mutually exclusive.

For many Rwandese I work, socialize and live with during the weeks I spend each year in Rwanda, sorrow and suffering, resilience, and reconstruction are daily companions. Individually and collectively, the Rwandese women and children I work with speak of sources of strength that are familiar to disaster researchers: social support/connectedness (family and community bonds), and self/community efficacy (belief in their capacity to endure and survive). Factors that receive less attention, however, reflect the subtle, nuanced nature of transformation: safety and hope. Repeatedly, many Rwandese talk of the need for social justice, the rule of law, and a sense of collective order as necessary ingredients for resilience to be manifested. Ask Rwandese children what they would like to be when they grow up, and many answer that they seek to become judges and journalists. Why? "Because the world needs to know the truth in order to maintain order, and the truth can only be known when justice is present in everyday life." (direct quote, 18-year-old Rwandese girl, parents and most of family killed in genocide). Lesson #1: Resilience requires a basic sense of safety, in broad and specific measures. Ask Rwandese women genocide survivors what they believe has contributed to their survival, and many answer with expected responses of faith in God, focus upon raising their children. Yet listen again with patience and gentle curiosity, and a different answer emerges: "Believing that this could be the last genocide, that the world may learn a lesson from Rwanda, and hope that our suffering may leave the world a better place for our children." (composite response from a women's group). Lesson #2: Hope can be leveraged to foster resilience.

These are the lessons of the resilience trajectory. Lying side by side with this trajectory is the chronicity trajectory of suffering, distress and in some cases, disorder. Many of the Rwandese continue to suffer from depression, anxiety, trauma reactions, and national sense of prolonged grief. Seventeen years postgenocide, many of the Rwandese I speak with are not resigned to live with these experiences, but rather accept them as now part of their life, part of their psyche, part of their community. The chronicity of suffering does not diminish the resilience, yet the resilience does not necessarily mitigate the suffering. Lesson #3: Resilience has its limits.

The authors have responded to many of the same disasters, such as the 9/11 terrorist attacks, floods, and hurricanes in our state, as well as having been a provider or responder to some very unique experiences, such as longer-term work with local NGOs in Rwanda (second author) and deployment to Louisiana for Katrina (first author). The first author reflects upon these experiences with several observations. A question frequently asked of mental health responders relates to the impact of such tragedies upon responders. The authors have been trained in this field of disaster response in order to be as prepared as possible to know what to expect about human response across the life span. It is also essential to have knowledge about strategies and guidelines for reducing threat impact and promoting self-resilient behaviors. Being in the field, there are always challenges. There is a sense of functioning on auto-pilot when on such deployments. Needless to say, responders oftentimes confront massive death and destruction (terrorist attacks on 9/11, flooding with Katrina, deaths from malnutrition or malaria in east Africa, genocide in Rwanda and Congo) and it is fair to say that one's view of life does change. It leaves one to think of one's vulnerability, mortality, and the fragility of life. Yet being able to provide such mental health and psychosocial services, particularly on a volunteer basis, strengthens one's sense of compassion, caring, and altruism. In short, it provides a true "lesson learned" on an essential principle of resilience: giving to others in need may be one of the best strategies for promoting resilience.

As we write this chapter, we have reached the commemoration of the tenth anniversary of the September 11, 2001 display of dispiriting hatred and shocking violence that took 2,987 human lives. It left one faced with the need to face unspeakable inhumanity. This was not just a day to remember but a period of time which was actually months of events that occurred raising the fear of more terrorist attacks. These subsequent events included the anthrax attacks, the American Airlines plane crash in Queens, and the ongoing threat of additional terrorist activities.

Having been activated and deployed within a very short period of time after the attack, one can still vividly recall the details of the many weeks and months witnessing the extremely high level of emotions we encountered working with the rescuers, survivors, and family members looking for and waiting for news of their loved ones. The first assignment was to be assigned to Newark International Airport, which was closed, to work with the Port Authority Police who knew they had lost many of their colleagues. At approximately 2 AM Wednesday when the river crossing were opened for responders, we were transported to Ground Zero. We were introduced to the shocking and unbelievable devastation of the several stories of twisted steel and concrete of the two towers. The sense of loss, the carnage and destruction was numbing. Knowing the vast number of lives lost, one quickly realized the sacredness of this site. The only way to try to describe was that it was surreal. Even though the task at hand was overwhelming, there was the sense that there were people working feverishly to rescue and recover those that were there when attacked. It was clear to us that we too had a role to play, to put our training into practice and initially address the needs of the responders. As was mentioned earlier, one went into the response mode or auto-pilot which was in effect for the duration of each shift. This of course was intertwined with emotions of sadness, disbelief, and thoughts of the death of so many innocent people especially when one might take a break and ponder the images before us but having the feeling of sustaining hope, compassion, and resiliency.

There are sights, sounds, and smells of that tragic day that will never be forgotten—just as the memory of the tremendous loss of human life. Some of these include the monochrome of gray ash covering blocks, the burning odor of fire and death, and the sounds of silence when the remains of a firefighter or police officer was found and the color guard accompanying the body as they left the site. As time progressed, the daunting tasks, and responsibilities changed. Our efforts initially were focused on the responders. We would then be at different locations trying to provide comfort, assistance, and information available to the family members regarding their loved ones who were victims of this tragedy. We were at the Family Assistance Center in New Jersey, collaborating with the various agencies stationed there to help families with the reporting process. When it was deemed safe, families were transported to Ground Zero by ferry where they could pay their respects to their loved ones. There was clearly a human awareness of death but one really gained strength watching these individuals try to cope with the psychological impact and the reality of their losses as a result of that horrific day. During those days, the concept of just how short life can be and how mortality and vulnerability comes to the forefront. This tragic day also demonstrated the altruistic tendencies that exist in so many people.

As a second example for the first author of personal involvement in a major national disaster was the Hurricane Katrina. Upon arrival in Louisiana, the devastation that existed as a result of the flooding was overwhelming. Towns were literally washed away, people were left without homes, possessions, and in many cases, loved ones. This too at times was an example that seemed to allow feelings that we were not doing enough for the individuals effected by the flood waters. Our role in this disaster was to assist with providing medical and psychological care since Louisiana's infrastructure was totally destroyed and nonexistent. There were no hospitals, clinics, or medicines. Many of their own medical professionals were victims and lost everything. Being there a few weeks, you left with a feeling that the resilience trajectory and determination of the people of the different Parishes would be the factor that would help them cope with the impact and consequences of this disaster and that they would be survivors.

There is also a need to understand the intense, emotionally tumultuous and at times paradoxical reactions that accompany disaster and crisis response, requiring a regular focus on mindful awareness and maintaining self-care. Examining the many tragic events to which the authors have been deployed, the concept of adapting to the adversities and tragedies is the roadway to reach the point of being resilient, ready for the next call out whenever that may occur. This self-care practice allows one to move toward healing by disciplining oneself to reflect and talk about the experiences, feelings, and emotions attached to these disasters. Relying upon strong social support systems, better considered as the responders own attachment figures who can ensure that responders are safe and cared for, enable the responders to perform their tasks and responsibilities to their full capabilities. Having the ability to maintain contact with one's own personal family connections enhances the energy to do the assigned job. In these respects, technology provides one of the best systems to maintain connection. Additionally, always being aware of one's limitations is critical, maintaining that crucial balance of assisting survivors while nurturing oneself. Learning more about, and from, such tragic events presents a clear juxtaposition of loss and growth—disasters and resilience. The authors have each had unique experiences that characterize posttraumatic growth—the personal development that comes from immersion in such tragedies and leads to positive healing and further expansion of a robust and compassionate self. Following the principle that *everyone* is impacted by disasters and traumas is important, but with proper preparation and training, one does not need to be traumatized by the events. Knowing oneself, including having an awareness of one's self-confidence, good communication and coping skills, strong connections, attachments, and support systems, and implementing good self-care techniques, can help make such deployments a source of not just resilience, but transformation as well, allowing one to thrive, accomplish more and value a life well-lived.

Conclusions

Resilience is one of those terms that has many variations in definitions as we have shown in this chapter. As we have attempted to demonstrate, resilience focuses on the recovery trajectory from adversities and traumatic events and the human capacity to rebound from such events. The objective is to return to the prior level of functioning before the disaster and even move beyond that point. As Reich et al. (2010) point out, "the resilience paradigm suggest that healthy reactions to risk factors are the norm, not the unusual reaction for individuals and communities." Yet despite the conceptual abundance of resilience related literature, there is little empirical evidence examining resilience building techniques and their effectiveness as early interventions for post-distress distress. What is key in this field of trauma and disaster, is that mental health responders realize that they too are vulnerable and mortal and need a place and time to reflect on the impact that these events have on us.

References

Benight, C., Ironsen, G., Klebe, K., Carver, C., Wynings, C., & Burnett, K. (1999). Coping self-efficacy as a predictor of psychological distress following a national disaster: A casual model analysis. *Anxiety, Stress, and Coping, 12*, 107–126.

Bonanno, G. A. (2006). Is complicated grief a valid construct? *Clinical Psychology: Science and Practice, 13*, 129–134.

Bonnano, G. A. (2004). Loss, trauma, and human resilience. Have we underestimated the human capacity to thrive after extremely aversive events? *American Psychologist, 59*(1), 20–28.

Bonanno, G. A., & Mancini, A. D. (2012). Beyond resilience: Mapping the heterogeneity of response to potential trauma. *Psychological Trauma: Theory, Research, Practice and Policy, 4*, 74–83.

Bonanno, G. A., Brewin, C. R., Kaniasty, K., & La Greca, A. M. (2010). Weighing the costs of disaster: Consequences, risks and resilience in individuals, families and communities. *Psychological Science in the Public Interest, 11*, 1–49.

Calhoun, L. G., & Tedeschi, R. G. (1998). Posttraumatic growth: Future directions. In R. G. Tedeschi, C. L. Park, & L. G. Calhoun (Eds.), *Posttraumatic growth: Positive changes in the aftermath of crisis*. New Jersey: Lawrence Erlbaum Associates, Inc.

Calhoun, L. G., & Tedeschi, R. G. (2001). *Posttraumatic growth: The positive lessons of loss*. Washington, DC: American Psychological Association.

Carver, C. S., Pozo, C., Harris, S. D., Noreiga, V., Scheier, M. F., Robinson, D. S., et al. (1993). How coping mediates the effect of optimism on distress: A study of women with early stage heart cancer. *Journal of Personality and Social Psychology, 65*, 375–390.

Cummings, E. M., Davies, P. T., & Campbell, B. S. (2000). *Developmental psychopathology and family process: Theory, research and clinical implications*. New York: Guilford Press.

Dass-Brailsford, P. (2007). *A practical approach to trauma: Empowering interventions*. California: Sage.

Debiec, J., & Ledoux, J. (2004). Fear and the brain. *Social Research, 71*(4), 807–818.

Dickstein, B. D., Suvak, M., Litz, B. T. & Adler, A. B. (2010). Heterogeneity in the course of posttraumatic stress disorder: Trajectories of symptomatology. *Journal of Traumatic Stress, 23*, 331–339.

Dyregrov, A. (1995). Effects of traumatized children on the rescuer. In G. Everly (Ed.), *Innovations in disaster and trauma psychology: Applications in emergency services and disaster response*. Maryland: Chervon Publishing Corporation.

Everly, G. (1995). Traumatic stress as a consequence of emergency and disaster response. In G. Everly (Ed.), *Innovations in disaster and trauma psychology; applications in emergency services and disaster response*. Maryland: Chervon Publishing Corporation.

Felitti, V. J., Anda, R. F., Norenberg, D., Williamson, D. F., Spitz, A. M., & Edwards, V. (1998). Relationship of childhood abuse and household dysfunction to many of the leading courses of death in adults. *American Journal of Preventive Medicine, 14*, 245–258.

Flett, R. A., Kazantzis, N., Long, N. R., Macdonald, C., & Millar, M. (2002). Traumatic events and physical health in a New Zealand community sample. *Journal of Traumatic Stress, 15*, 303–312.

Fraser, M. W. (1998). Aggressive behavior in childhood and early adolescence: An ecological-developmental perspective on youth violence. In E. M. Freeman, C. G. Franklin, R. Fong, G. L. Shaffer, & E. M. Timberlake (Eds.), *Multisystem skills and interventions in school social work practice* (pp. 83–102). Washington, DC: NASW Press.

Freidman, H. S. (1991). *The self- healing personality. Why some people achieve health and others succumb to illness*. New York: Henry Holt.

Friedman, M. J., & Schnurr, P. P. (1995). The relationship between PTSD, trauma, and physical health. In M. J. Friedman, D. S. Charney, & A. Y. Deutch (Eds.), *Neurobiological and clinical consequences of stress: From normal adaptation to PTSD*. Philadelphia: Lippincott-Raven.

Fullerton, C. S., Ursano, R. J., & Wang, L. (2004). Acute stress disorder, posttraumatic stress disorder, and depression in disaster or rescue workers. *The American Journal of Psychiatry, 161*, 1370–1376.

Garmezy, N. (1991). Resilience in children's adaptation to negative life events and stressed environments. *Pediatrics. 20*, 459–466.

Golding, J. M. (1996). Sexual assault history and women's reproductive and sexual health. *Psychology of Women Quarterly, 20*, 101–121.

Higgins, A. B., & Follette, V. M. (2002). Frequency and impact of interpersonal trauma in older women. *Journal of Clinical Geropsychology, 8*, 215–226.

Holgersen, K. H., Klöckner, C. A., Jakob Boe, H., Weisæth, L. and Holen, A. (2011). Disaster survivors in their third decade: Trajectories of initial stress responses and long-term course of mental health. *Journal of Traumatic Stress, 24*, 334–341.

Hughes, R. (2003). *Resilience: Health in a new key*. Phoenix: St. Luke's Health Initiative.

Kessler, R. C., Sonnega, A., Bromet, E., Hughes, M., & Nelson, C. B. (1995). Posttraumatic stress disorder in the National Comorbidity Survey. *Archives of General Psychiatry, 52*, 1048–1060.

Kobasa, S. C., Maddi, S. R., & Kahn, S. (1982). Hardiness and health: A prospective study. *Journal of Personality and Social Psychology, 42*(1), 168–177.

Layne, C., Warren, J., Watson, P., & Shaleu, A. (2007). Risk, vulnerability, resistance, and resilience: Toward an integrative conceptualization of posttraumatic adaptation. In M. Friedman, T. Keane, & P. Resnick (Eds.), *Handbook of PTSD: Science and practice*. New York: Guilford Press.

Luthar, S. S. (1993). Methodological and conceptual issues in research on childhood resilience. *Journal of Child Psychology and Psychiatry, 34*, 441–453.

Luthar, S. (2006). Resilience in development: A synthesis of research across five decades. In D. Cicchetti & D. J. Cohen (Eds.), *Developmental psychopathology: Risks, disorders, and adaptation* (2nd ed., pp. 739–795). New York: Wiley.

Luthar, S. S., & Cicchetti, D. (2000). The construct of resilience: Implications for interventions and social phobias. *Development and Psychopathology, 12*, 857–885.

Lyons, J. A. (1991). Strategies for assessing the potential for positive adjustment following trauma. *Journal of Traumatic Stress, 4*(1), 93–111.

Maddi, S. R., & Hightower, M. (1999). Hardiness and optimism as expressed in coping pattern. *Journal of Consulting Psychology, 51*, 95–105.

Masten, A. S. (2001). Ordinary magic: Resilience processes in development. *American Psychologist, 56*(3), 227–238.

Masten, A. S., Best, K., & Garmezy, N. (1990). Resilience and development: Contributions from the study of children who overcome adversity. *Development and Psychopathology, 2*, 425–444.

O'Leary, V. E., & Ickovics, J. R. (1995). Resilience and thriving in response to challenge: An opportunity for a paradigm shift in women's health. *Women's Health, 1*, 121–142.

Pearlman, L. A., & Saakvitne, K. W. (1995). *Trauma and the therapist: Countertransference and vicarious traumatization in psychotherapy with incest survivors*. New York: Norton.

Reich, J., Zautra, A., & Hall, J. (Eds.). (2010). *Handbook of adult resilience*. New York: The Guilford Press.

Rutter, M. (1987). Psychosocial resilience and protective mechanisms. *The American Journal of Orthopsychiatry, 57*, 316–331.

Seligman, M. E. P., & Peterson, C. (2003). Positive clinical psychology. In L. G. Aspinwall & V. M. Staudinger (Eds.), *A psychology of human strengths: Fundamental questions and future directions for a positive psychology*. Washington, DC: American Psychological Association.

Shin, L. M., Orr, S. P., Carson, M. A., Rauch, S. L., Macklin, M. L., & Lasko, N. B. (2004). Regional cerebral blood flow in the amygdala and medial prefrontal cortex during traumatic imagery in male and female Vietnam veterans with PTSD. *Archives of General Psychiatry, 61*, 168–176.

Singer, J. (2005). Child and adolescent psychiatric emergencies: Mobile crisis response. In A. Roberts (Ed.), *Crisis intervention handbook* (3rd ed., pp. 319–361). New York: Oxford Press.

Steinberg, A. (2004). *A conceptual framework for stress – related concepts and community resilience.* Paper presented at the National Center for Child Traumatic Stress, University of California, Los Angeles.

Sterling, P., & Eyer, J. (1998). Allostasis. A new paradigm to explain arousal pathology. In S. Fisher & J. Reason (Eds.), *Handbook of life stress, cognition and health*. Oxford: Wiley.

Tedeschi, R. G., & Calhoun, L. G. (1995). *Trauma and transformation: Growing in the aftermath of suffering*. California: Sage.

Tusaie, K., & Dyer, J. (2004). Resilience: A historical review of the construct. *Holistic Nurse Practitioner, 18*, 3–8.

Wash, F. (1998). Strengthening family resilence. New York: Guilford Press.

Watson, P., Ritchie, E., Demer, J., Bartone, P., & Pfefferbaum, B. (2006). Improving resilience trajectories following mass violence and disaster. In E. Ritchie, P. Watson, & M. Friedman (Eds.), *Intervention following mass violence and disasters: Strategies for mental health practice*. New York: The Guilford Press.

Waysman, M., Schwarzwald, J., & Soloman, Z. (2001). Hardiness: An examination of its relationship with positive and negative long term changes following trauma. *Journal of Traumatic Stress, 14*(1), 531–548.

Webb, N. B. (2001). *Culturally diverse parent-child and family relationships: A guide for social workers and other practitioners*. New York: Columbia University Press.

Werner, E. E. (2001). *Journeys of childhood to mid-life: Risk, resilience and recovery*. New York: Cornell University Press.

Wilson, I. B., & Cleary, P. D. (1995). Linking clinical variables with health-related quality of life. *Journal of the American Medical Association, 273*, 59–65.

Winfield, L. F. (1994). *Developing resilience in urban youth*. Urban Monograph Series. Oak Brook, IL: North Central Regional Educational Laboratory.

Yehuda, R., & Flory, J. D. (2007). Differentiating biological correlates of risk, PTSD and resilience following trauma exposure. *Journal of Traumatic Stress, 20*, 435–447.

Zautra, A. J., Hall, A. J., & Murray, K. E. (2008). Resilience: A new integrative approach to health and mental health research. *Health Psychology Review, 2*, 41–64.

Zautra, A. J., Hall, J. S., & Murray, K. E. (2010). Resilience: A new definition of health for people and communities. In J. Reich, A. Zautra, & J. Hall (Eds.), *Handbook of adult resilience*. New York: Guilford Press.

17 Community-Level Resiliency Intervention in a Post-disaster Environment: The Three Mile Island Health and Environmental Information Series—Theoretical Assumptions, Implementation, and Participant Response

Sandra Prince-Embury

This chapter presents a case illustration of a community-level resiliency intervention in a post-disaster environment. The intervention described was the Three Mile Island Health and Environmental Information Series, a community course developed to provide information pertaining to unanswered questions which had remained among TMI community members since the March 28, 1979 nuclear accident at the Three Mile Island nuclear generating facility. This intervention is described within the context of unique post-disaster psychosocial circumstances in the community at that time which contributed to chronic stress. These conditions included lack of clear, understandable information about the accident and its aftermath as well as loss of faith in experts associated with conflicting and incomplete information delivered by officials at the time of the accident. This experience has been referred to as an "information crisis" in the literature.

Also described are the assumptions underlying the design of the intervention; that delivering of understandable information by credible experts would foster resilience in this community by addressing the "information crisis" created in the aftermath of the accident; and that loss of faith in experts might be ameliorated by community participation in the selection of the topics and credible experts to discuss them. The intentions of the community course were the following: (1) to reduce the stressors of risk-related information by delivering the information in a manner designed to minimize emotional reactivity; (2) to restore a sense of mastery by providing understandable information that could be used by community members in processing their experience and making informed decisions; and (3) to restore a sense of relatedness in the community members who attended the course by providing direct personal access to experts who delivered credible information in a way that was understandable to the lay public. Overview of the series proposes a model for the delivery of understandable information, in a manner that is mindful of potential stress and lowered credibility under conditions of uncertainty in the aftermath of technological disaster.

Please do not cite without permission of the author.

S. Prince-Embury, Ph.D. (✉)
Resiliency Institute of Allenhurst, LLC,
625 North Edgemere Drive, West Allenhurst,
NJ 07711, USA
e-mail: sandraprince-embury@earthlink.net

Critical Resiliency Constructs

As mentioned previously in this volume, definitions of resiliency have been numerous and research has operated at different levels of analysis, each with its own language and caveats.

S. Prince-Embury and D.H. Saklofske (eds.), *Resilience in Children, Adolescents, and Adults: Translating Research into Practice*, The Springer Series on Human Exceptionality,
DOI 10.1007/978-1-4614-4939-3_17, © Springer Science+Business Media New York 2013

Among these definitions of resilience there are a number of shared features all relating to human strengths, some type of disruption and growth, adaptive coping, and positive outcomes following exposure to adversity (e.g., Bonanno, 2004; Connor & Davidson, 2003; Friborg, Hjemdal, Rosenvinge & Martinussen, 2003; Masten, 2001; Masten et al., 2003; Richardson, 2002). Much of the empirically based research reflects a developmental perspective, examining the adaptive capacities of individuals faced with personally experienced adversities or traumas. However, as Masten and Obradovic (2008) point out … "Threat of catastrophe looms over the beginning of the 21st century, including massive disasters in the form of terrorist attacks, wars, a tsunami, hurricanes, and outbreaks of disease. The mass media are saturated with stories of a possible flu pandemic and global warming, along with reports of ongoing genocide, terrorism, and natural disaster events." These authors suggest further that it is imperative for scientists concerned with adaptive systems in many disciplines to consider what is known and what needs to be known that could inform efforts to prevent or ameliorate the consequences of disaster and promote recovery. Masten and Obradovic suggested the following regarding consideration of resilience in the face of disaster (2008).

> "In the event of a flu pandemic, bioterrorism, a natural disaster, or any other large-scale catastrophe, the best surveillance, equipment, communication systems, antiviral supplies, military, and emergency services in the world will not be effective without equal attention to the issues posed by human behavior under conditions of life-threatening danger to children and families. The adaptive systems for positive human adaptation and development, legacies of biological and cultural evolution, must be considered and enjoined to promote resilience."

Fundamental Adaptive Systems for Human Resilience

Many protective factors have been identified as contributing to resilience. It has also been recognized that the importance of these factors vary depending on the individual's stage of development and the nature of the adversity(s) that are faced. With that caveat, Masten and Obradovic (2008) and others have identified basic, core, adaptive systems that have repeatedly been related to resilience in children and adolescence (Masten & Coatsworth, 1998; Masten & Gewirtz, 2006; Masten, Burt, & Coatsworth, 2006; Wright and Masten 2001) and adults (Bonanno, 2004; Charney, 2004). Following is a brief consideration of four of these adaptive systems with comments about how they might relate in the aftermath of technological disaster.

Attachment and Sense of Relatedness

In a review of resilience studies, Luthar (2006:780) concluded the following: "Resilience rests, fundamentally, on relationships." The pioneers in the field noted the essential role of human attachments in resilience, and every major review since that time has upheld their observations. Beginning in early development, the attachment figure provides a child with a secure base for reassurance under threat, and when conditions are relaxed, with the confidence to venture out to explore and learn about the world. Separation from attachment figures can cause extreme anxiety to the point of panic, particularly when a threat is perceived, and loss can induce profound grief. Sensitive attachment figures also serve a powerful regulatory function, up- or down-regulating stress and arousal or containing impulses. The presence of a secure-base attachment figure has been shown to moderate stress in threatening situations for infants and toddlers. Disaster may present a threat at the "attachment" level by separating family members, disrupting contact between family members, and obscuring information about the safety among family members. In such circumstances locator systems and means for communication among family members are critical.

Masten and Obradovic (2008) suggest that "All planning for disaster must account for the attachment system and how such relationships are likely to motivate behavior and provide for a sense of security." In the vicinity of TMI, findings of loss of faith in experts (Prince-Embury &

Rooney, 1987a, 1987b) might be interpreted within this framework, whereby officials and experts who were relied upon to safeguard the community were lost as credible bases of security and replaced by a sudden realization among community members that they were on their own to interpret complex risk information which was beyond their understanding and training.

For purposes of discussion we may distinguish between "attachment" which refers to the psychological process that occurs in early childhood and "relatedness" which exist in many forms throughout the course of development. At the community level, the aftermath of disaster may disrupt "relatedness" by polarizing community members from each other. For example, many of those in the vicinity of the TMI plant worked at the plant and were out of work for as long as the nuclear facility was shut down. For these workers, finding alternative work that paid as well was not likely. On the other hand members of the community who did not have a family member employed by the nuclear facility were diametrically opposed, wanting the plant to remain shut down. These circumstances contributed to fractures in the community, fewer sources of support, and heightened stress in community members who suddenly found themselves at odds with their neighbors.

Agency, Self-Efficacy, and the Mastery Motivation System

As noted by Robert White (1959) in his classic paper on competence and the mastery motivation system, human beings are motivated to adapt to the environment and to experience reward for perceived success. Albert Bandura (1997) elaborated on this system in his empirical work and theory concerning self-efficacy. People with a positive view of their own efficacy will exert more effort to succeed and are more likely to persist in the face of adversity. People who persist are more likely to succeed, which reinforces efforts to adapt. Thus, individuals who overcome adversity report more positive views of their own effectiveness and self-worth, express more confidence about success, and experience pleasure in doing well. The mastery motivation system can be extinguished by prolonged exposure to unresponsive environments or uncontrollable events, which was noted in learned helplessness experiments (Seligman, 1975). Disaster, presents a threat to human sense of agency, mastery, and control on many levels. Disaster by definition is an overwhelming life-threatening circumstance that overwhelms one's resources to control outcome. The type of disaster and its aftermath influences the extent of this effect. Prior to the TMI accident, sense of mastery over the safety of community members in the vicinity of Three Mile Island had been deferred to the expertise of the experts and local officials who has assured them that there was little if any chance of an accident. The occurrence of the accident and associated conflicting information disrupted this sense of mastery. If the experts and officials had been wrong then who was in charge of their safety? Confronted with this dilemma community members were forced to confront the realization that they did not have the expertise to protect themselves or to monitor the level of their safety. Remaining conditions of uncertainty about actual amounts of radiation released during and after the accident and possible health effects further obstructed a sense of mastery over possible consequences. Within this context, many area residents were motivated to seek information for themselves, forming citizens groups, conducting their own informal surveys and studies, and seeking experts who were considered credible. It was within the context of these community efforts that the TMI Public Health and Environmental Information Series was developed.

Central Nervous Systems for Problem-Solving and Information Processing

Under conditions of high threat or adversity, the ability to continue thinking and planning effectively is characteristic of resilience; good intellectual skills show protective effects for children and adults dealing with adversity (Luthar, 2006;

Masten, 2001). Intelligent behavior is influenced not only by past development, learning, and experience but also by current arousal level, stress, fatigue, illness, injury, motivation, values, emotions, and in general a good information-processing system. It is also important to remember that information processing requires good quality information to process. Absence of information or the presence of unclear, ambiguous or conflicting information in the presence of disaster would impair individuals and the community collectively to process information effectively. It is likely that absence of clear, credible information in the aftermath of the TMI accident obstructed the ability of community members to effectively process information for problem solving. This ability to effectively process information may have been further compromised by chronic arousal and emotional reactivity sustained by conditions of uncertainty in the community.

Regulatory Systems for Controlling Arousal, Affect, Attention, and Action

Overcoming adversity often calls on self-regulation skills to continue functioning effectively under highly stressful or arousing circumstances. Many aspects of voluntary self-control, e.g., voluntary self-restraint and resolving conflicts between competing feelings, thoughts, and behaviors, are associated with higher competence as well as better adaptation during and following adversity and trauma (Masten & Abradovic, 2006; Masten & Coatsworth, 1998). Fear and anxiety, along with other negative emotions presented by disaster and its aftermath, can influence human self-control systems and the quality of executive functioning including information processing in the aftermath of crisis. High levels of arousal can interfere with decision making, working memory, and other forms of executive functioning. The degree to which one can manage arousal and direct the resources at hand are likely to play a critical role in disaster response and resilience.

In the past, decisions to withhold information from the public in the face of disaster have been justified by the intention of not creating panic. However, this approach has often backfired when eventually conflicting information is released, resulting in loss of credibility for the information source and loss of faith in experts among the receiving community. Research in the vicinity of TMI following the accident has substantiated the presence of emotional arousal or heightened emotional reactivity. It is likely that this arousal in addition to incomplete and conflicting information dissemination obstructed information processing.

The Nature of Disaster

As is the case for defining "resilience," the definition of disaster is not a simple matter. The literature on disaster research and interventions is extensive and beyond the scope of this chapter. Therefore a brief discussion relevant to this chapter follows. Disasters have been traditionally considered according to the extent of damage done and the extent to which that damage exceeds the ability of the impacted community to cope. Trainer and Bolin (1976) defined disasters as abrupt, unanticipated events that produce severe disruption and a need for relocation. Consideration of resiliency in the face of disaster is informed by consideration of the characteristics of the disaster. Protective factors that facilitate resiliency may differ across type of disaster, and whether the intervention is during, immediately after, or in the aftermath of the disaster. Identified aspects of disaster critical for planning interventions include but are not limited to the following.

a. *Extent of raw physical loss/or threat of loss of life and/or property*
b. *Predictable* versus *unpredictable*
c. *Sudden* vs. *gradual*
d. *Clear end point* versus *no clear end point*
e. *Natural* versus *man-made*
f. *Visible* versus *invisible consequences*

Multiple Consequences

The more elements of loss, change, lack of control, and uncertainty introduced by the disaster the more potential psychological difficulty it presents. Disaster impact includes immediate and prolonged danger to self and others, loss of homes and possessions, relocation in an unpredictable fashion. The number of negative consequences and the cumulative effect will vary across individuals and their specific circumstances.

Man-Made Elements

For the purpose of this chapter we will limit our discussion to the aftermath of man-made technological disaster. In man-made disasters there is frequently an assumed element of intentional neglect which is likely to engender more anger and prolonged bitterness. As in Buffalo creek, if there is perception that "those in charge or the experts" knew ahead of time and did not prevent or make adequate provisions for disaster this creates another powerful dimension of disaster aftermath; intense anger and blame at those who are perceived to have been negligent or in some way irresponsible. For some this experience is a profound disillusionment or loss of faith that can undermine one's sense of well-being and sense of control. For those who already have lost faith and are skeptical of the intentions of others, such an event serves to confirm the distrust that already exists for them.

Invisible Consequences

One characteristic of man-made disasters is that the threat of danger is often posed by invisible consequences such as radiation or other air-borne toxic substances. The lack of ability of community members to see or monitor radiation levels on their own presents ongoing circumstances of uncertainty. This was the case in the aftermath of Three Mile Island where there had been conflicting reports of how much radiation had been released and continued to be released during cleanup, along with an inability to monitor this. Absence of the ability to see the threat would certainly obstruct effective information processing, thus undermining the community's ability to experience mastery in the situation. The psychological need for visible consequences is illustrated by the persistence of one community member in finding and recording mutated plants in the vicinity of the Three Mile Island facility to document that there had been some effect.

Lack of a Clear end Point

In circumstances when there is a clear end point, people can begin to recover. When there is no clear end point it is harder to deal with because conditions of uncertainty are prolonged, closure is prevented and steps toward recovery are delayed. In the aftermath of the Three Mile Island accident, there was extended cleanup of the damage Unit 2 reactor that took many years to complete. Included in this process was the illegal release of 43,000 Ci of radioactive Kryton-85 between June and July of 1980. The evaporation of 2.3 million gallons of accident-generated radioactive water which began in December 1990 despite legal objections by a local community organization (TMIA). This evaporation was completed on October 28, 1993 resulting in the release of 658 Ci of tritium over a 3-year period. Thus in addition to uncertainty about what radiation levels had been released at the time of the accident, there was continued uncertainty about the levels of radiation being released during cleanup.

Re-Traumatization

When disaster conditions are prolonged, or when there is not a clear emergency plan in effect victims are subject to re-traumatization. As in Katrina, when expected help did not come for some, or perceived promises were not kept, those who felt that they were in the clear may have experienced additional traumatization. In the aftermath of the Three Mile Island accident residents were confronted with potential sources of re-traumatization. Public statements after the accident suggested that radiation releases and health effects were minimal with the implication that those who thought otherwise were "malcontents." In addition, community members faced restart of the Unit 1 undamaged reactor which had been shut down since the time of the accident. It is likely that both of these circumstances may have added stress onto an already stressed community (Prince-Embury & Rooney, 1988).

A poignant example of reminders of the accident is illustrated in the words of one Middletown resident interviewed by this author. This mother spoke of the panic experienced by a young child in her home when she saw steam boiling on her mother's stove. Neither the mother nor the child had recognized that the steam on the stove was associated with the frequent images on TV of the reactors releasing steam during the TMI accident.

Three Mile Island Nuclear Accident

The accident at Unit II of the Three Mile Island Nuclear Generating Facility during which there was a partial core meltdown had presented a life crisis for the residents of the neighboring vicinity, the full extent of which had not been completely determined at the time of the conception of this course. At the onset of the accident which began March 28, 1979, area residents faced threat of a hydrogen explosion and radiation release were confronted with conflicting information, and, in some instances, were instructed to evacuate their homes, (Baum, Gatchel, & Schaeffer, 1983; Bromet, 1980; Dohrenwend, Dohrenwend, Kasl, & Warheit, 1979; Houts, Cleary, & Hu, 1988; Houts & Goldhaber, 1981). TMI-1 had been in operation since September 1974 but TMI-2 had only been online since December 1978, or 90 days prior to the accident. Since the accident, conflicting information had remained about the dose estimates of ionizing radiation released at that time, leaving many area residents with uncertainty about the possibility of health and genetic effects that might eventually develop (Lindy & Lindy, 1985).

During the 1979 accident, the nuclear power station at Three Mile Island experienced a pump malfunction leading to exposure of the core, melting of fuel rods, release of radioactive emissions, and spilling of radioactive water on the reactor building floor. For several days release of incomplete, inconsistent and contradictory information by responsible officials created an information crisis and loss of faith in the credibility of these officials. An example of the information provided at the time of the accident is expressed in the press conference of Lt. Governor William Scranton of Pennsylvania, released on March 28, 1979, 4:30 p.m.

> "This is an update on the incident at Three-Mile Island Nuclear Power plant today. This situation is more complex than the company first led us to believe. We are taking more tests. And at this point, we believe there is still no danger to public health. Metropolitan Edison has given you and us conflicting information. We just concluded a meeting with the company officials and hope this briefing will clear up most of your questions. There has been a release of radioactivity into the environment. The magnitude of this release is still being determined, but there is no evidence yet that it has resulted in the presence of dangerous levels. The company has informed us that from about 11 a.m. until about 1:30 p.m., Three-Mile Island discharged into the air, steam that contained detectable amounts of radiation."

Subsequently, 140,000 residents evacuated when women and children were advised by the governor to do so after earlier reassurances that conditions were safe.

Baum et al. (1983) found chronically elevated levels of stress in TMI area residents as long as 6 years after the accident and related this to the unique circumstances of man-made disasters including loss of credibility of responsible authorities and remaining conditions of uncertainty. In addition, Davidson, Baum, and Collins (1982) found that TMI area residents reported greater feelings of helplessness and less perceived control over their environment than did control subjects and that this appeared to contribute to ongoing stress among TMI residents. Additional studies of Middletown residents, revealed a relationship between perceived TMI threat and perceived lack of control and loss of faith in experts among residents in the vicinity after the accident (Prince-Embury & Rooney, 1987a, 1987b, 1988). Lack of control was associated with greater perceived threat among area residents consistent with prevailing theory. This finding held primarily for recent arrivers however. Among those present at the time of the accident, loss of faith in experts was more significantly related to lack of perceived control than was threat. Prince-Embury and Rooney (1987a, 1987b) concluded that a profound loss of faith in experts had been a significant psychological impact of the accident for area residents present at the time and that loss of faith had supplanted perceived threat as a psychological concomitant of perception of control.

Additional research by Prince-Embury and Rooney (1987a, 1987b) surveyed a stratified random sample of Middletown residents to determine the extent of interest in information associated with the accident. This survey indicated that 79% were interested in information on cancer detection and treatment; 58% were interested in radiation monitoring and 56% were interested in information on the epidemiological distribution of cancer in the area. This level of interest in information related to TMI substantiated the need for the Information Series.

The Three Mile Island Public Health and Environmental Information Series

Four years after the TMI accident, the author of this chapter began collaboration with a small group of community activists representing a number of community organizations, for the purpose of addressing issues remaining in the aftermath of the TMI accident that might have been contributing to continued elevated stress cited above. The Three Mile Island Public Health and Environmental Information Series was the result of this collaboration. The intentions of this community course were the following: (1) to reduce the stressors of ambiguous information related to the TMI accident by identifying and delivering relevant information in a manner designed to minimize emotional reactivity; (2) to restore a sense of mastery by providing understandable information to be used by community members in processing their experience and making informed decisions; (3) to restore sense of relatedness in the community members who attended the course by providing direct personal access to experts who delivered credible information in a way that was understandable to the lay public. The proposal was approved by the TMI Public Health Fund and the course was implemented. Description of the course as conceptualized in the original proposal follows.

The Three Mile Island Health and Environmental Information Series was a unique intervention offered in Middletown, PA, for members of the community who 6 years earlier had experienced technological disaster emanating from the 1979 accident at the Three Mile Island Nuclear generating facility. The series was designed by the author of this chapter in collaboration with activist members of the community organization TMI-PIRC who identified the areas of unanswered questions and experts who were perceived by the community as credible and unbiased. The author of this chapter developed the proposal and rationale for the community course and obtained funding from the TMI Public Health Fund for the intervention. The series began in February of 1985 and extended for 12 weeks. The design and implementation of this course is of interest for the following reasons: it presented information of scientific complexity to community members; it presented information for which there remained several unanswered questions pertaining to potential hazard; it was presented to a population that was highly polarized on issues pertaining to the TMI accident; and it was presented at a time when the community faced imminent restart of the plant which many viewed as increasing potential hazard in the community. Restart of TMI-1 was imminent, despite a vote on May 18, 1982 in which voters in Cumberland, Dauphin and Lebanon counties voted by a 2–1 margin in a non-binding referendum to oppose the restart of Unit 1.

Questions had been raised as to whether community members could understand information of a highly scientific/technical nature, whether information which contained uncertainty could be presented to a technologically impacted population without increasing stress, whether information could be received by a politically polarized community in the face of a major environmental change in a way that was perceived as credible.

Underlying Assumption Regarding Understandability, Stress, and Perceived Credibility

The development of the TMI course was based on three of theoretical assumptions. First, access to information related to possible adverse circumstances is sought by impacted community members and can be delivered in a format and manner that increases the experience of understanding by the lay public. Secondly, intervention in a stressed population should not be avoided because of possible stress reactions but should take this possible effect into account so as to not elevate stress unnecessarily. Such an intervention should address the potential for heightened emotional reactivity and should be designed to minimize the possibility that heightened reactivity will interfere with adequate information processing. Thirdly, an intervention delivered in a stressed population should be sensitive to and address sources of lowered credibility such as perceived and unexplained discrepancies between expert opinions.

Access to Information about Possible Negative Circumstances

Whether or not individuals prefer information about possible threat conditions has been a matter of considerable theoretical and empirical interest (Averill & Rosenn, 1972; Averill, O'Brien, & DeWitt, 1977; Berlyne, 1960; Calvert-Boyanowsky & Leventhal, 1960; Miller & Mangan, 1983; Monat, 1976; Monat, Averill, & Lazarus, 1972). According to the information seeking model, when faced with uncertainty, people and animals seek information and strive for certainty (Berlyne). In an earlier study Prince-Embury and Rooney (1987a, 1987b) had found that 56–79% of a stratified random sample of Middletown residents expressed interest in information on radiation epidemiology and cancer 5 years after the accident. These authors also found that interest in information was significantly correlated with worry about these topics among area residents. Assumptions prevalent at the time of the course were that stressed individuals do not desire information about adverse circumstances particularly if this information does not increase predictability. Miller & Mangan (1983) addressing this issue found that delivery of information which matches the information seeking style of the individual minimized anxiety while that which does not match increases it. The TMI series was based on the assumption that part of the healing process in the aftermath of technological disaster was the availability of accurate, reliable, and understandable information in a way that allows individuals to pace information intake consistent with their ability to integrate information into a meaningful context. It was recognized, however, that complete healing of a community from the traumatic elements of such an event would not occur from one time limited intervention.

Attention to Emotional Reactivity in Stressed Populations

Davidson and Baum (1980) identified members of a sample of TMI residents as manifesting symptoms of posttraumatic stress. Researchers have noted that one aspect of posttraumatic stress state is hypervigilance or the ability to continue to respond to stimuli with emotional intensity appropriate only to emergency situations (Kardiner, 1941; Krystal, 1978; Vanderkolk, 1987). McCurdy (1943) identified events that are "near-miss" catastrophes, such as the TMI accident, as critical determinants of hypervigilance.

Previous research suggests that hypervigilance interferes with an individual's ability to assess situations calmly as well as the ability to process information appropriately. Specifically, hypervigilance has been described as impairing cognitive functioning by constricting cognition with premature closure, restricting range of attention, narrowing range of perceived alternatives, reduction in immediate memory, and fostering of simplistic ideas, (George, 1974; Hamilton, 1975; Janis, 1971; Janis & Leventhal, 1968; Janis & Mann, 1977). Thus residents at TMI who might remain hypervigilant were seen as possibly less capable of processing information accurately and completely. Among the factors most frequently implicated as antecedents of hypervigilant reactions are lack of perceived control over dangerous events and lack of preparatory information about what is to be expected (Epstein, 1973; Janis; Monat et al., 1972). The TMI course was designed mindful of potential interference by hypervigilance in the information processing by course participants.

Attention to Potentially Perceived Discrepancies

Reports of incidents during and following the TMI accident suggest that the situation had lent itself to cognitive contradiction in that area residents were given contradictory messages during and after the accident; local radio stations had reported safe conditions, cable stations at a distance were reporting warnings; officials were offering reassuring messages to be followed by emergency evacuation instructions (Lindy & Lindy, 1985; Walsh, 1988). The origin of theoretical concern about congruence of reality and expectation is found in the theory of cognitive dissonance offered by Festinger (1957). According to Festinger, dissonance refers to cognitive contradiction which is associated with discomfort and drive toward consistency. It was hypothesized that sensitivity to information inconsistency remained in the postaccident environment and might be relevant to the delivery of new information. The TMI course design took into account the possible negative effects of perceived contradiction and inconsistency among course presenters.

TMI Course Structure

Discussion of the TMI course begins with aspects of the course which were intended to address the theoretical assumptions discussed above and unique psychosocial circumstances present in the community at the time.

Providing Access to Information and Increased Understanding

The relationship between individual interest in information, individual coping styles in seeking information and providing an appropriate structure for this to occur is complex and involves many levels of intervention. Step one was determining the need for such as intervention, appropriate content, and format. This was done in collaboration with interested community members of diverse backgrounds. Step two was providing a vehicle for information delivery. The design of the TMI series required finding appropriate sponsors for such a project, documenting the need and structuring the intervention that would allow for maximum individual access and understanding. The TMI course came into being at that time due to the unique convergence of a variety of significant ingredients including supporting empirical research (Prince-Embury & Rooney, 1987a, 1987b), significant community pressure, the involvement of different institutions of equal power and visibility, the availability of expertise, financial resources, sponsorships by a neutral institution of higher learning, and the involvement of a municipal court judge in the administration of the TMI Public Health Fund and perhaps most important, community involvement in the planning and implementation of the course. Also the inception and implementation of the TMI course predated enactment of the "right to know" legislation but was consistent with the intention of this evolving legislation. Step three was a complex collaborative process involving community members, representatives of the various institutions and scientist consultants. This step was based on the assumption that any intervention addressing the knowledge gap between community and experts would benefit from collaboration between these groups in the planning stage.

Step four was maximizing ease of access. Ease of access to information was assured by adequate advertising for the course, providing the course free of charge and in an accessible location. Individual differences in style of coping were accommodated by having frequency of attendance voluntary. In addition, videotapes of the

Series were created and made accessible to those who for individual reasons were unable to attend the course itself. Step five was providing information that was understandable. Increased potential for individual understanding of information was addressed in preliminary instruction to scientist presenters to express concepts in lay language. Increased potential for individual understanding was also addressed in the format of each session which provided the second hour for dialogue and individual's questions to the speaker. This format was implemented to address the specific questions of individuals so that they might integrate the information into a context that was understandable to them. It was also believed that information received in an interactive fashion could be more readily adjusted to the unique needs of the individuals.

Structure for Managing Emotional Reactivity to Lessen the Possibility of Increased Stress as an Obstacle to Understanding

The series was based on the assumption that communication of information in an environment of intense polarization on different sides of the nuclear power debate (Walsh, 1988) must in some way address the possibility of intense emotionality among course participants. Ground rules were developed by this author to maximize the likelihood of information flow and comprehension by minimizing or controlling emotional reactivity. The specific ground rules were read to participants at the beginning of each session and were presented in the form of a mutually agreed upon verbal contract for participation in the sessions. Additional mechanisms for managing emotional reactivity included the following. Break times between the first and second half of each session and following each session allowed informal debriefing to occur. The opportunity to express questions and comments to the speaker in a formal way during the second half of each session served also as a tension release. The coordinator of the series, a psychologist, and two psychology graduate students were available to individuals who wanted to express concerns individually.

Structure for Managing Uncertainty and Perceived Discrepancy in Expert Opinion as Sources of Lowered Credibility

Informal observation and community collaboration revealed that at the time of the accident and afterwards members of the Three Mile Island community were confronted with discrepancies between reports of experts and between official statements. This was associated with a significant loss of credibility attributed to official statements. This lack of perceived credibility of information was associated with a significant loss of faith in experts and demoralization (Dohrenwend et al., 1979; Prince-Embury & Rooney, 1987a, 1987b). Lack of credibility was addressed in the choice of credible scientist presenters and in designing the structure of sessions. The choice of scientist experts included national experts in their areas of expertise, who were knowledgeable about areas of uncertainty and disagreement in their field and could discuss this openly. Furthermore, many of these individuals were identified by a panel of scientist commissioned by the Three Mile Island Public Health Fund, as politically neutral on potentially controversial issues relevant to their areas of expertise. In addition, dialogue periods in each session allowed attendees to ask questions to clarify points of uncertainty or perceived inconsistency.

Specific Ground Rules

Ground rules addressing tolerance of disagreement respecting the opinions of others, managing ones own emotions and anticipating uncertainty were stated at the beginning of each session.

Ground rule A: It was stated that the mission of the course was conveyance of information not agreement among participants; that participants held varied opinions and perspectives and that each person was asked to respect the right of all others to hold a different opinion. Furthermore, course participants were asked to treat each other and speakers with respect. The specific request that participants acknowledge and accept diversity in opinion was intended to prepare participants with a more realistic expectation for the series so that emotional reactivity would not be aroused by discrepancies between expectation and reality.

Ground rule B: It was acknowledged that some of the topics to be presented might be stressful for some participants. It was asked that each participant be responsible for controlling their own emotional reaction so that it would not prevent them from hearing the information presented, or lead them to treat anyone else with disrespect. This ground rule was intended to clarify that information presented was not designed to assuage emotion and might be stressful. This ground rule also addressed expectations by predicting elevated stress. It was believed that anticipation of stress would allow participants to prepare for this with the suggestion of possible control of emotions as a positive act.

Ground rule C: it was stated that the purpose of the series was to give information that was understandable but that everyone's questions would not necessarily be answered either because the answer was not available or perhaps because the answer was not yet known. The distinction between what was known and what was unknown was an important message throughout the course. Previous guarantees of certainty and the inability to fulfill this promise had been a source of disappointment and disillusionment within this community. Ground rule C was based on the assumption that unwarranted expectation of certainty would lead to disappointment and distrust, whereas an expectation of incomplete knowledge would prepare participants more realistically for what they would receive.

Course Content

The series was divided into three segments to address three areas of interest expressed by area residents. Each segment was divided into several individual sessions addressing different aspects of the topic. Basic explanations of relevant concepts and general issues were presented earlier in sequence. Topics and questions relevant to TMI specifically were presented in the middle or towards the end of each segment. The following is a list of topics in the order that they occurred in the series.

Session 1: Overview of the series "Introduction to Health effects and radiation epidemiology."
Session 2: "Radiation in the environment, basic concepts, definitions and findings."
Session 3: "Three Mile Island Accident Dose Assessment: What we know and what we don't know."
Session 4: "Radiation monitoring, basic concepts, methods and understanding results."
Session 5: "Overview of Health Effects of Radiation."
Session 6: "Cancer, basic concepts and relationship to immunological functioning."
Session 7: "Radiation related cancer and treatment."
Session 8: "Stress and immunological functioning the Three Mile Island area."
Session 9: "Local facilities for cancer early detection and treatment."
Session 10: "Overview of basic concepts of epidemiology and application in the community."
Session 11: "Health Findings in the Three Mile Island Area and ongoing studies."
Session 12: "Community/Expert Collaboration in the Assessment of Health Effects."

Post-course Participant Analysis

Description

Although total attendance of the series was 278, this represented repeated attendance by some of a group of 117 distinct individuals who attended the series one or more times. Average attendance of the 12 sessions in the TMI series was slightly over 47 persons per session. Attendance ranged from a high of 80 persons at session 3 which addressed dose assessments of radiation released at the time of the TMI accident, to a low of 12 persons at session 10 addressing basic concepts of epidemiology and application in the community. Seventy-one percent of participants had lived in the Middletown area at the time of the accident, 36% had evacuated at that time, 35% had not; 51% were male, 49% were females; 62% were parents, 38% were not; 49.8% reported some college or more. The average age of course participants was 41 years. Course attendees represented a variety of professional and educational backgrounds including homemakers (12%), teachers (12%), nurses (4%), engineers and environmental scientist (10%), pipefitters and laborers (5%), lobbyist (1%), activists (10%); retired individuals (8), employees of the US Environmental Protection Agency, the US Nuclear Regulatory Commission, and the Pennsylvania State Health Department (5%), mental health professionals (4%), students (6%), clerical/sales (10%), and (15%) occupation unaccounted for. Course participants as a group were not representative of the general population in the area. They were younger, better educated, reported less worry about TMI issues and reported slightly less faith in experts than a normative sample of TMI area residents (see Prince-Embury, 1991 for a discussion of these differences).

Participants Responses

Open-ended questionnaires were distributed to participants to allow them to record their responses. This included an open-ended questionnaire distributed in the 5th and 12th sessions; midway through the series and at the end. In addition, self-reported assessment of information attributes as perceived by participants was conducted in each session (Prince-Embury, 1992a, 1992b). It should be noted that assessment of participant response was not the primary mission of the project and was offered to participants to do on a voluntary basis. Therefore, attitudes of participants prior to participation have not been assessed and variations among participants across sessions have not been controlled for. Therefore findings are offered as suggestive rather than conclusive.

Regarding reliability of information, the percentage of respondents rating the information as reliable ranged from 56% to 95% across sessions with a median of 87%. The percentage of respondents reporting that they understood the material ranged from 89% to 100%. The percentage of respondents reporting that their questions had been addressed ranged from 56% to 89% across sessions with a median of 82%. The percentage of individuals reporting that their questions had been answered ranged from 44% to 80% with a median frequency of 70%.

These results suggest that the TMI Series was most successful in bringing the public information that was understandable, moderately successful in presenting information that was perceived as reliable and in addressing specific questions. The series was least successful but adequate in answering these questions.

Participants surveyed in the 5th and 12th sessions of the course were asked whether the sessions had led to new thoughts or behaviors and whether questions remained. During session 5, 58% of respondents reported that information presented in the session had led to new thoughts or behaviors for them. Thirty-six percent reported specifically, change in increased understanding. Other individual responses included: concern about existing physical conditions, increased information seeking, learning new ways of appreciating research on radiation, greater respect for scientists and their efforts, and a need to be more prepared for the unknown.

During the 12th session 17% of the individuals responded that the Series had led to new thoughts or behaviors for them. Eighty percent reported increased understanding. Others mentioned increased awareness that scientists were still seeking answers or specific facts they had learned about radiation or cancer. A majority of respondents, 75% responded that they still had unanswered questions pertaining to radiation. It should be noted that participant self-reports of increased understanding or learning about specific topics were not objectively measured, as evaluation of participants was not in keeping with the mission of the series. Therefore reported understanding reflected the subjective experience of the participants.

Assessment of information attributes revealed that participant subjective experience of understandability across all sessions was ($X=0.98$) on a scale of 0–1, a rating which was higher than other rated information attributes. In addition, subjective experience of understandability of information was slightly but significantly related to a lower level of psychological symptoms reported by participants in the course accounting for 3% of the variability in symptoms. Subjective experience of reliability of information received the second highest rating ($X=0.82$) across all sessions, on a scale of 0–1. (For a more complete description of an assessment of information attributes see Prince-Embury, 1992a, 1992b).

Conclusions Based on Participant Responses

Analysis of participants' responses suggested that community members can experience increased understanding of highly technical topics. Participants reported the subjective experience of increased understanding of the material presented in the Series supporting the initial assumption that the TMI course could be designed to enable participants to have this experience. This finding was consistent with findings that participants rated the information presented at each session to be very understandable (Prince-Embury, 1992a, 1992b). However, it is important to note that increased understandability reported by course participants was not synonymous with answered questions. Participants appeared to be aware that they still were lacking in objective knowledge of the topics presented. Seventy-five percent of respondents reported that they still had unanswered questions about radiation. Assessment of the degree that their specific questions had been answered in each session received the lowest rating ($X=0.76$) on a scale of 0–1.

An unanticipated finding of this study was that reliable information that acknowledges conditions of uncertainty may be associated with decreased perception of control. A stepwise hierarchical multiple regression analysis revealed that perceived reliability of information was negatively related to perceived control accounting for 5% of the variance in this variable. (Prince-Embury, 1992a, 1992b). Some insight about this finding may be revealed in the words of one course participant who reported the following; "at the time of the accident some experts said they didn't know, but people thought they were lying. It's what they didn't know that you thought they did know that's scary." Thus, increased belief in experts who acknowledged uncertainty was associated with less perceived control. The words of one course participant might reflect the experience of others. "It is scary to find out how much the scientists themselves don't really know, but at the same time it is reassuring because it fits with what I have been experiencing and explains some of the contradictory information we have been getting." This statement demonstrates how one person, a homemaker had come to terms with uncertainty and experienced a sense of closure by having this uncertainty acknowledged by trusted experts.

Technical topics associated with some uncertainty can be presented in an environmentally impacted community without raising stress level.

Regarding impact of the information series on level of psychological stress, findings reported elsewhere suggest that the average level of stress did not increase across the duration of the Series, across all participants of all sessions or considering only repeat attendees. Participants were asked to indicate the degree of worry about their most pressing question before and after the session pertaining to that question. Comparison of these pre- and postsession degrees of worry indicated no significant change. Also, self-reported understanding was slightly related to a lower level of psychological symptoms (Prince-Embury, 1992a, 1992b), suggesting that the experience of greater understanding is related to lower levels of psychological stress. However, due to the lack of systematic controls these findings are suggestive rather than conclusive. Regarding credibility of information, rated reliability of information was moderately high and comments made by participants reflected an increased appreciation for "the other side" for experts who were investigating unanswered questions as well as moderate belief in the credibility of information provided. These comments are optimistic in a community that had experienced intense polarization up to that point. Similarly, a survey of the expert speakers following the course indicated that they were surprised at the knowledgeable questions asked by attendees, enjoyed the experience more that they thought they would and said they would participate again in such a course for lay participants.

In summary, responses to open ended questions and informal observations suggested the following.

1. Some course participants expressed the fact that this had been the first time that they had been presented with objective information that was designed for them and not motivated by vested interests designed either to persuade, alarm, or allay their fears.
2. Course participants representing diverse viewpoints in a highly polarized community were able to participate alongside each other in a non-adversarial learning experience in a way that had not been customary in this highly polarized community.
3. Course participants, particularly those who attended multiple sessions expressed increased appreciation for the complexity of the topics presented by the speakers, more receptive to the idea that not all of their questions were immediately answerable and with an increased appreciation for those who might contribute to the long-term clarification of unanswered questions in the community.
4. Invited scientist/expert speakers, some initially wary of public response, grappled with the task of making complex scientific tasks more comprehensible to the public and in most cases reported success in that endeavor.

General Conclusions

Overall, the above description provides a case example of dissemination of information in an environmentally impacted polarized community with findings suggestive of who might attend and how they might respond. Also illustrated is how a community intervention may be designed based on unique needs and remaining stressors in the aftermath of technological disaster and at the same time designed to bolster the collective resilience of the community. It is recognized, however, that the Three Mile Public Health and Environmental Information Series occurred 26 years ago and much has changed since that time. For example, access to information has been greatly increased by prevalent access to the internet in homes of technologically developed societies. However, the possibility of technological disaster is ever present as evidenced by the recent disaster in the Japanese nuclear reactor at Fukushima. In addition, increased threat of terrorist attacks has increased the environment of uncertainty worldwide. For this reason consideration of information dissemination as a means of fostering resiliency in the aftermath of technological disaster or under pervasive conditions of uncertainty remains a valid pursuit.

The importance of communicating accurately about risks was persuasively expressed by Baruch Fischhoff in the Special Issue of the American Psychologist titled 9/11: 10 years later (Fischhoff, 2011). "Psychological Research has essential roles to play in identifying the public's information needs, designing responsive communications and evaluating their success. Fulfilling these roles requires policies that treat two-way communication as central." (p.520).

Fischhoff warns against obstacles to this pursuit such as underestimating the public's ability to learn and make decisions, a tendency seen in the myth of panic and popular accounts of human frailty. In this article Fischhoff identifies steps to be taken in creating communications about risks of terror (or anything else). Some of these steps may be summarized as follows. Identify the information most relevant to helping audience members make decisions. Identify subject matter experts, who can ensure fidelity to the best available technological knowledge. Draft communications in precise and comprehensive form. Assure the maintenance of respectful, two-way communications channels. To the extent that the Three Mile Island Health and Environmental Information Series followed these steps in 1985, it provided an early model for threat-related communication.

Ongoing Examples of Resilience in the TMI Community

Although this chapter has focused on the TMI Health and Environmental Information Series as an example of a post-disaster intervention aimed at fostering resilience through information clarification and dissemination, other more remarkable examples of resilience are ongoing in the TMI vicinity. One example is the establishment of a citizen-based radiation monitoring system. In 1992, Eric Epstein, acting as a private citizen, reached an agreement with the GPU Nuclear and the Nuclear Regulatory Commission, resulting in the training of and funding for the EFMR Monitoring group, a citizens group organized for the purpose of ongoing monitoring of radiation in the vicinity of TMI (Epstein, 2005; Epstein, 2011, personal communication). In the opinion of this author this outcome represents a significant act of sustaining sense of mastery and safety in the aftermath of a technological disaster characterized by loss of faith in experts, invisible threat, and remaining conditions of uncertainty.

References

Averill, J. R., O'Brien, L., & DeWitt, G. W. (1977). The influence of response effectiveness on the preference for warning and on physiological stress reactions. *Journal of Personality, 45*, 396–418.

Averill, J. R., & Rosenn, M. (1972). Vigilant and nonvigilant coping strategies and psych- physiological stress reactions during the anticipation of an electric shock. *Journal of Personality and Social Psychology, 23*, 128–141.

Bandura, A. (1997). *Self-efficacy: The exercise of control*. New York: Freeman.

Baum, A., Gatchel, R., & Schaeffer, N. (1983). Emotion, behavior and physiological effects of chronic stress at Three Mile Island. *Journal of Consulting and Clinical Psychology, 51*, 656–672.

Berlyne, D. E. (1960). *Conflict arousal and curiosity*. New York: McGraw Hill.

Bonanno, G. A. (2004). Have we underestimated the human capacity to thrive after extremely aversive events? *The American Psychologist, 59*(1), 20–28.

Bromet, E. (1980). *Three Mile Island: Mental health findings*. Pittsburgh, PA: Western Psychiatric Institute and Clinic and the University of Pittsburgh.

Calvert-Boyanowsky, J., & Leventhal, H. (1960). The role of information in attenuating behavioral response to stress: A reinterpretation of the misattribution phenomenon. *Journal of Personality and Social Psychology, 32*, 214–221.

Charney, D. (2004). Psychobiological mechanisms of resilience and vulnerability: Implications for successful adaptation to extreme stress. *The American Journal of Psychiatry, 161*, 195–216.

Connor, K. M., & Davidson, J. R. T. (2003). Development of a new resilience scale: The Connor-Davidson resilience scale (CD-RISC). *Depression and Anxiety, 18*, 76–82.

Davidson, L., & Baum, A. (1980). Chronic stress and post-traumatic stress disorders. *Journal of Consulting and Clinical Psychology, 54*, 303–308.

Davidson L, Baum A, Collins D. (1982) Stress and control-related problems at Three Mile Island. *Journal of Applied Social Psychology, 12*, 349–59.

Dohrenwend, B. P., Dohrenwend, B. S., Kasl, S. V., & Warheit, G. J. (1979). *Report of the task force on behavioral effects of the president's commission on the accident at Three Mile Island*. Washington, DC: U.S. Government Printing Office.

Epstein, S. (1973). Expectancy and magnitude of reaction to a noxious. *Psychophysiology, 10*, 100–107.

Epstein, E. (2005) Biennial report of the EFMR monitoring group. (TIAA-Alert, self-publication).

Festinger, L. (1957). A theory of cognitive dissonance. Evanston, IL: Row, Peterson.

Fischhoff, B. (2011). Communicating about the risks of terrorism (or anything else). *The American Psychologist, 66*(6), 520–531.

Friborg, O., Hjemdal, O., Rosenvinge, J. H., & Martinussen, M. (2003). A new rating scale for adult resilience: What are the central protective resources behind healthy adjustment? *International Journal of Methods in Psychiatric Research, 12*, 65–76.

George, A. (1974). Adaptation to stress in political decision making. The individual, small group and organizational content. In G. V. Coelho, D. A. Hamberg, & J. E. Adams (Eds.), *Coping and adaptation*. New York: Basic Books.

Hamilton, V. (1975). Socialization and information processing: A capacity model of anxiety- induced performance deficits. In I. G. Sarason & C. O. Speilberger (Eds.), *Stress & anxiety* (Vol. 2). Washington, DC: Hemisphere.

Houts, P. S., Cleary, P. O., & Hu, T.-W. (1988). *The Three Mile Island crisis: Psychological, Social and economic impacts on the surrounding population* (p. 32). University Park and London: The Pennsylvania State University Press.

Houts, P. S., & Goldhaber, N. K. (1981). Psychological and social effects on the population surrounding Three Mile Island after the nuclear accident. In S. Majumdar (Ed.), *Energy, environment and the economy*. Philadelphia, PA: Pennsylvania Academy of Science.

Janis, I. L. (1971). *Stress & frustration*. New York: Hartcourt.

Janis, I. L., & Leventhal, H. (1968). Human reactions to stress. In E. Borgatta & W. Lambert (Eds.), *Handbook of personality theory and research*. Chicago, IL: Rand McNally.

Janis, I. L., & Mann, L. (1977). *Decision making*. New York: The Free Press.

Kardiner, A. (1941). *The traumatic neuroses of war*. New York: P. B. Hoeber.

Krystal, H. (1978). Trauma and effects. *Psychonalytical Study of the Child, 33*, 81–116.

Lindy, J. D., & Lindy, J. G. (1985). Observation in the media and disaster recovery period. In J. Laube &

S. A. Murphy (Eds.), *Perspectives on disaster recovery* (pp. 295–303). Norwalk, CT: Appleton.

Luthar, S. S. (2006). Resilience in development: A synthesis of research across five decades. In D. Cicchetti & D. J. Cohen (Eds.), *Developmental psychopathology, volume 3. Risk, disorder, and adaptation* (2nd ed., pp. 739–795). New York: Wiley.

Masten, A. S. (2001). Ordinary magic: Resilience processes in development. *The American Psychologist, 56*, 227–238.

Masten, A. S., Burt, K. B., & Coatsworth, J. D. (2006). Competence and psychopathology in development. In D. Cicchetti & D. Cohen (Eds.), *Handbook of developmental psychopathology* (2nd ed., Vol. 3, pp. 696–738). New York: Wiley.

Masten, A. S., & Coatsworth, J. D. (1998). The development of competence in favorable and unfavorable environments: Lessons from research on successful children. *The American Psychologist, 53*, 205–220.

Masten, A. S., & Gewirtz, A. H. (2006). Vulnerability and resilience in early child development. In K. McCartney & D. A. Phillips (Eds.), *Handbook of early childhood development* (pp. 22–43). Malden, MA: Blackwell.

Masten, A. S., & Obradovic, J. (2008). Disaster preparation and recovery: Lessons from research on resilience in human development. *Ecology and Society, 13*(1), 9.

McCurdy, J. (1943). *The structure of morale*. New York: Macmillan.

Miller, I. M., & Mangan, C. E. (1983). Interacting effects of information and coping style in adaptation to gynecology and stress: Should the doctor tell all? *Journal of Personality and Social Psychology, 45*(1), 223–236.

Monat, A. (1976). Temporal uncertainty, anticipation time, and cognitive coping under threat. *Journal of Human Stress, 2*, 32–43.

Monat, A., Averill, J. R., & Lazarus, R. S. (1972). Anticipatory stress and coping reactions under various conditions of uncertainty. *Journal of Personality and Social Psychology, 24*, 237–252.

Prince-Embury, S. (1991). Information seekers in the aftermath of technological disaster. *Journal of Applied Social Psychology, 21*(7), 569–584.

Prince-Embury, S. (1992a). Psychological symptoms as related to cognitive appraisals and demographic differences among information seekers in the aftermath of technological disaster. *Journal of Applied Social Psychology, 22*(1), 38–54.

Prince-Embury, S. (1992b). Information attributes as related to psychological symptoms and perceived control among information seekers in the aftermath of technological disaster. *Journal of Applied Social Psychology, 22*(14), 1148–1159.

Prince-Embury, S., & Rooney, J. (1987a). Perception of control and faith in experts among residents in the vicinity of Three Mile Island. *Journal of Applied Social Psychology, 17*(11), 953–968.

Prince-Embury, S., & Rooney, J. (1987b). Interest in information as a function of worry and perceived control in the aftermath of nuclear disaster. *International Quarterly of Community Health Education, 8*(1), 33–49.

Prince-Embury, S., & Rooney, J. (1988). Psychological symptoms of residents in the aftermath of the Three Mile Island nuclear accident and restart. *The Journal of Social Psychology, 128*, 779–790.

Richardson, G. E. (2002). The metatheory of resilience and resiliency. *Journal of Clinical Psychology, 58*, 307–321.

Seligman, M. (1975). *Learned helplessness: A theory for the age of personal control*. Oxford: New York.

Trainer, P., & Bolin, R. (1976). Persistent effects of disasters on daily activities: A cross- cultural comparison. *Mass Emergencies, 2*, 279–290.

Vanderkolk, K. (1987). *Psychological trauma*. Washington, DC: American Psychiatric Press.

Walsh, E. (1988). *Democracy in the shadows*. New York: Greenwood Press.

White, R. W. (1959). Motivation reconsidered: The concept of competence. *Psychological Review, 66*, 297–333.

Wright, M. O., & Masten, A. S. (2005). Resilience processes in development: Fostering positive adaptation in the context of adversity. In S. Goldstein & R. Brooks (Eds.), *Handbook of resilience in children* (pp. 17–37). New York: Kluwer Academic/Plenum Press.

Part IV

Resilience, Cultural and Systemic Issues

A Measure of Resilience with Contextual Sensitivity—The CYRM-28: Exploring the Tension Between Homogeneity and Heterogeneity in Resilience Theory and Research

18

Michael Ungar and Linda Liebenberg

In this chapter, we build on three propositions regarding the concept of resilience. First, we understand resilience to refer to *coping under stress*, and therefore a description of populations who do well when facing adversity. The term is not the same as the processes that contribute to positive development across an entire population, nor the everyday qualities that promote well-being. In fact research shows that the mechanisms that are protective under stress operate differently depending on the amount of adversity individuals and their families or communities experience (Rutter, 2009; Ungar, 2011). An external asset such as a mentor is going to account for far more of the change in a child's development trajectory if the child has been exposed to severe and persistent neglect (Gilligan, 1999; Larson, 2006), just as an internal asset like persistence is more advantageous to a child whose schools are inadequately funded, or if she is excluded because of cultural norms regarding gender and education (Shin, Daly, & Vera, 2007).

Second, because most of what we know about resilience (positive coping under stress) is almost entirely based on studies and clinical experience with populations in what Kagitçibasi (2007) has referred to as the "Minority World," the concept of resilience requires *further study across contexts and cultures*. The Minority World are the numerically small numbers of people who live in relatively advantaged contexts in western democracies, often of European descent. It excludes new immigrants and indigenous peoples in western countries, and the vast majority of the world's population who have not participated in the development of theory concerned with optimal human development. There is a growing body of research that suggests that western psychological sciences have erred in presenting the external validation of their theories, including theories of resilience. We assume that the ideas we export from the Minority World to the Majority World will be valid. We share what we know but seldom do research to identify and then import back to the Minority World processes that may better explain contextually relevant outcomes for populations that live in adverse environments. For example, the ubiquitous study of first year psychology students at universities should be discounted as valid if solely on the basis of their class privilege and the tautology of defining successful development by their adherence to educational goals. In other words, how we define

M. Ungar, Ph.D. • L. Liebenberg, Ph.D. (✉)
Resilience Research Centre, Dalhousie University, 6420 Coburg Road, PO Box 15000, Halifax, NS, Canada B3H 4R2
e-mail: michael.ungar@dal.ca; linda.liebenberg@dal.ca

S. Prince-Embury and D.H. Saklofske (eds.), *Resilience in Children, Adolescents, and Adults: Translating Research into Practice*, The Springer Series on Human Exceptionality,
DOI 10.1007/978-1-4614-4939-3_18, © Springer Science+Business Media New York 2013

successful development needs to be negotiated with those whose voices are not yet represented in the literature.

Third, because the study of resilience necessarily requires the description and subsequent quantification of unnamed, or indigenous, processes, the development of a measure of resilience requires *both a review of the existing literature and qualitative inquiry* that documents the lives of those who are not well-represented in that literature. There is a need to consider epistemological questions regarding the production of knowledge: specifically, how and by whom is our understanding of resilience generated? To this end the Child and Youth Resilience Measure (CYRM), discussed in detail in this chapter, reflects the perspectives of an international partnership of researchers and clinicians that includes a great many participants from Majority World contexts.

With these three propositions before us, the Resilience Research Centre set out to develop a measure of resilience that addressed all three. While original development of a measure was a collaboration across 14 international research sites, its recent validation includes studies with Aboriginal and non-Aboriginal youth in Canada and New Zealand, youth in countries like South Africa, Colombia, and China, as well as youth living in poverty or marginalized by family breakdown, exposure to violence and other challenges in Minority World (USA, Canada) contexts. In order for young people to have been selected into the validation studies, they must have been judged by their communities to be exposed to heightened levels of adversity that distinguished them from other children. More than 100 researchers are now using the CYRM in studies ranging from investigations with children with physical disabilities in India, deinstitutionalized children in Ethiopia, Aboriginal children at risk of suicide in Canada, and Californian youth who are disengaged from their communities. In this chapter we report briefly on the development and validation of a 28-item version of the CYRM and reflect on the measure's application. A shortened version with 12 items has also been adapted from the original and is being validated as a tool to screen children at risk for conduct disorder and delinquency.

A More Ecological Definition of Resilience

In his work over half a century, Boris Cyrulnik (2008) has described *resiliency* as a set of personal characteristics found among children who grow like dandelions amid rubble. Building his theory on the narratives of people who survive war and other trauma, he and many others have focused on what we can change in individuals to make them hardier in dangerous environments. The emphasis on individual growth is worthwhile, but when viewed ecologically, it may make us overlook evidence that shows that changing the environment accounts for far more of the developmental gains of a population at risk than individual factors. Orphan-friendly communities, for example, that create conditions in which children who require support receive the caring they need, are likely to protect the majority of young people under their care regardless of an individual child's motivation to change (Skovdal & Campbell, 2010). In this regard, Lerner (2006) has hypothesized that resilience reflects the interaction between individuals and their context. Neither the individual nor the context predicts positive development. It is the interactional processes that are protective. To reflect what Ungar (2011) describes as a "decentered" approach to resilience, meaning one that does not overemphasize individual agency, but rather retains a strong focus on both the individual and contextual forces that seed growth, resilience can be defined as a person's successful navigation towards the resources necessary to sustain well-being, and the negotiations with those who control resources for these to be provided in ways that are culturally meaningful (Ungar, 2008). This definition of resilience suggests that resilience is not just the capacity of the child to navigate in dangerous environments but also the capacity of the environment to provide all the resources the child needs in appropriate ways. In practice, this means resilience depends as much or more on the capacity of families, schools, communities, and governments to provide what children need as on children's individual qualities alone.

However, individual assets like persistence, an internal locus of control, and a sense of humor, as described in the work of Prince-Embury and Steer (2010) and others (Donnon & Hammond, 2007) are an essential part of the individual × environment processes associated with resilience. Evidence of this association is abundant in studies showing that children with specific qualities tend to do better in dangerous environments, tend to suffer less depression or signs of PTSD following exposure to violence, tend to remain engaged with school and prosocial peers, and avoid drugs when these personal qualities are well formed (Phelps et al., 2007; Wingo et al., 2010). All of these patterns are powerful predictors of an association between individual qualities and developmental outcomes.

Building on these theoretical components of resilience, the CYRM reflects a collection of these qualities, measuring the individual's perception of their own assets as well as experience of their environment. Though a self-report measure, the implication of many of the questions is that the environment must be supportive and facilitate the availability and accessibility of the protective processes required to make individuals flourish. In other words, community values regarding education and social welfare, and government policy that supports children's mental well-being, recreation, and access to treatment are all aspects of a resilient social ecology that make it more likely children facing adversity do well.

Development of an Ecologically Sensitive Measure of Resilience

The full story of the development of the CYRM is detailed in a number of previous publications by the authors (Ungar & Liebenberg, 2005, 2009, 2011; Ungar et al., 2008; Liebenberg, Ungar, & Van de Vijver, 2012), though a few points are particularly important to the purposes of this volume. The CYRM was the result of a 14-site, 11-country pilot study of resilience in which advisory groups from each community contributed to the development of the questions. Items emerged from focus group interviews with youth and adults at each site. Only after local communities had suggested items for inclusion on the measure was a survey of the literature done. Face-to-face meetings of all team members in 2003 helped to identify the most useful 58 items to be piloted with youth known to be facing significant levels of adversity as defined by members of local advisory committees. Though this introduced to the initial pilot sample great heterogeneity, it also helped the research team to identify common aspects of resilience that demonstrated construct validity across all 14 sites. A minimum of 60 youth participated in each site; the total sample included 1,451 youth (aged 12–21). The measure was translated where necessary before administration (for a detailed discussion of this process, see Ungar & Liebenberg, 2011). While the team did follow a process of back-translation (Brislin, 1970) the emphasis was on translation of the intended meaning of each item, rather than on a literal translation. Because of the goals of translation the principal investigator worked with research teams to explore possible translations of questions and negotiate on final versions. Negotiation and discussion between members of the international team took place when during translation items were found to be complex (e.g., multiple meanings in the course of translation) or troubling (e.g., questions with a lack of cultural sensitivity, such as those relating to sexual behavior and drug use).

Analyses of the original 58 questions administered across all 14 sites included an exploratory factor analysis (EFA) (varimax orthogonal rotation) on all 58 items with all 1,451 youth. This initial step allowed us to identify four groupings of youth, using logical sorts by research site. These groups included boys and girls from minority world settings (southern Canada, Florida, USA), girls from all majority world sites (Aboriginal communities in northern Canada, Colombia, the Gambia, Tanzania, South Africa, Palestine, Israel, India, Russia, and China), and two groupings of boys from majority world sites: those from communities considered to have high levels of social cohesion (Palestine, Russia, China, the Gambia, India, Israel, and Tanzania) and those from communities considered to have low levels of social cohesion (Colombia, South Africa, and Northern Canada) as judged by the studies local advisors.

A second set of analyses were then conducted on the data using each of the four groupings of youth. This allowed us to reduce the measure's length and select 25 items which were most likely to predict resilience. Specifically, nonresponse rates of 10% or higher, low variance, and the communality criterion (using a cut off value of 0.45) were used to remove 11 poorly performing items. We then conducted further EFAs on the remaining items for all four groupings of youth as well as the total sample. Using an unrotated factors analysis we were able to determine which items were of most significance to youth in each of the four subgroups, as well as the sample as a whole. Only those items which loaded with sufficient strength (0.30 or higher) on the first factor for each of the five analyses were retained. Several of these questions were modified slightly to correct errors in wording or where a question was addressing more than one aspect of resilience, resulting in a final measure with 28 items. Of importance is that while initial items and the pilot sample were both heterogeneous, the 25 items selected for inclusion were those identified through this series of exploratory factor analyses as being most significant to youth across all sites. A second face-to-face meeting of all team members in 2005 allowed the team to reach consensus on items contained in the final version of the measure, rewording and splitting questions until consensus was achieved on the selection of the final 28 items.

Qualitative data collection, concurrent with the development of the CYRM, provided further validation of the construct of resilience in each research site. In total 89 interviews were conducted with youth (Ungar et al., 2007). Seven themes, or tensions, in the data emerged that were associated with resilience across all research sites: access to material resources, cultural adherence, identity, power and control, relationships, social justice, and social cohesion (including religious affiliation). Combined, the qualitative and quantitative data confirmed that a great deal of what young people understood as resilience across many different cultures was related to both individual qualities and the quality of their families, schools, communities, and cultures. The data also showed both the heterogeneity and homogeneity in how these concepts were understood and the importance youth attached to them.

A second wave of international research has allowed us to continue validation of the CYRM.[1] Using Canadian data on 497 concurrent users of multiple services (aged 12–21), we have identified three subscales of the CYRM, using an EFA with oblique rotation (Direct Oblimin): individual, relational, and contextual. We then conducted an EFA again using oblique rotation (Direct Oblimin) to support mean clustering of items within each factor of the model. In this way we have been able to establish that items related to individual components include personal skills, peer support and social skills; caregiver components include psychological caregiving and physical caregiving; and contextual components include educational, cultural, and spiritual components. This structure was then confirmed with an additional sample of 410 multiple service using youth. Of note is that the data set was split into visible minority and visible majority youth, accounting for cultural variation in the analysis. Multigroup confirmatory factor analysis showed high invariance and model stability across the two groups (measurement residuals model :$\chi^2(53, N=410)=98.00, p<.001$; TLI=0.957; CFI=0.979; RMSEA=0.046) (Liebenberg et al, 2012).

Adding 192 vulnerable youth from South Africa and 581 from New Zealand to the Canadian sample, we have been able to further confirm high invariance of the three subscales and their constellations of questions across cultures and contexts (structural covariance model: $\chi^2(51, N=1{,}270)=135.97$, $p<.000$; TLI=0.757; CFI=0.743; RMSEA=0.080). Cronbach alpha values for the three scales across the three research sites are satisfactory (see Table 18.1). Concurrent validity of the CYRM-28 is yet to be established. Validation of the measure across additional cultures continues.

[1] We have also been able to establish reproducibility agreement for the CYRM-28. A subsample of 53 youth who completed the measure approximately 3 weeks apart provided test–retest data. Interclass Correlation Coefficients (absolute agreement) showed satisfactory psychometric properties for the measure (ranging from 0.583 to 0.773). Furthermore, paired sample t-tests showed no significant differences between Time 1 and Time 2.

Table 18.1 Cronbach alpha values of CYRM-28 subscales

	Individual (11 items)	Relational (7 items)	Contextual (10 items)
Canada (n=410)	0.789	0.830	0.817
New Zealand (n=581)	0.772	0.773	0.747
South Africa (n=192)	0.807	0.813	0.810

The CYRM-28 as an Ecological Measure of Resilience

The CYRM-28 is a measure that accounts for indigenous processes across a multitude of sites addressing the errors noted earlier (e.g., cultural bias) that are evident in many discussions of resilience. The measure is also unique in that its content is heavily weighted towards contextual and relational components of resilience, while still accounting for individual factors.

The individual factors subscale allows researchers to understand individual characteristics associated with resilience in terms of both personal resources such as capacity to complete tasks and ability to solve problems constructively. It also provides information on a youth's capacity to interact with others, assessing social skills (such as "I know how to behave in different social situations") and interaction with peers ("I feel supported by my friends").

Relational elements in the CYRM explore micro-systemic interactions between young people and their parents or primary caregivers. The subscale provides information on both physical ("My caregivers watch me closely") and psychological ("I feel safe when I am with my caregivers") aspects of relationships. These relational processes are well studied in the resilience literature as mediating the impact of risk on developmental trajectories (Bonanno, Westphal, & Mancini, 2011; Easterbrooks, Chaudhuri, Bartlett, & Copeman, 2011).

Finally, the CYRM asks a series of questions regarding young people's experiences of their context and culture. In this regard, the measure assesses the quality of processes that depend on the quality of the meso-, exo-, and macro-systems, including spiritual, educational, and cultural components of these systems.

It is noteworthy that rather than exploring each separate aspect of the three subscales, the CYRM explores constellations of questions within each subscale, with no one element assumed to be the most predictive of positive development. Because of this, studies of resilience may use the CYRM as an overall assessment of the likelihood for resilience to occur and more detailed measures of individual qualities to assess more thoroughly research questions related to aspects of personal agency or coping strategy.

As the CYRM is a self-report measure, it does not objectively assess the functionality of each system with which the young person interacts, only the individual's experience of elements of those systems that are known to be protective under stress. A thorough study of resilience should include a detailed examination of how well different systems function individually and together. For example, in a study of school engagement, Shernoff and Schmidt (2008) found that paradoxically young people who were the most disadvantaged and often perceived as least likely to attend class were the ones who reported the highest sense of engagement at school. Such nuanced patterns of the processes associated with coping under adversity require that studies be designed to capture the interactions between stressors, resilience, and individual qualities. The CYRM assesses only the individual's experience of belonging at school (a quality of resilience noted by all our international partners) but not the quality of the school itself. The challenge, therefore, is to be able to know where to attribute causality. As Bottrell and Armstrong's (2012) work illustrates, a child's engagement with educators is not an individual quality alone and also strongly influenced by school, community, and cultural factors. It is likely that changes in systemic elements of the child's environment can account for far more change in a child's behavior than efforts to change the child (Bronfenbrenner & Morris, 2006; Cicchetti, 2010).

Clinical and Community Applications for an Ecological Measure of Resilience

The CYRMs focus on both individual and ecological factors makes it ideally suited to the assessment of the resources individuals have and the likelihood they will experience the support they need to cope under adversity. In this regard, the CYRM reflects a growing understanding of resilience as more than individual qualities. For example, personal qualities like persistence and agency can manifest in ways that may not be socially normative. Many studies of youth in economic and political contexts of poverty, injustice, and social oppression show that young people who survive best are those who exploit opportunities that are available to them, even if their patterns of behavior (e.g., delinquency, early school leaving) appear to further disadvantage them (Bottrell, 2009; Ng-Mak, Salzinger, Feldman, & Stueve, 2010). For example, gang involvement may be protective to the child without other means of feeling secure in his community (Taylor et al., 2002); alcohol use (Ziervogel, Ahmed, Fisher, & Robertson, 1997), or early sexual initiation may be preferred as rites of passage into adulthood (Moffitt, Caspi, Rutter, & Silva, 2001); children's participation in the labor force may bring with it social and economic gains that exceed what they can expect at school (Liborio & Ungar, 2010).

It is important to note that the CYRM does not distinguish between prosocial and non-normative means of accessing personal and social resources. It avoids value-laden language about behaviors that are expected of young people such as having hobbies or their selection of peers. What are good activities or good friends is not the issue. It is the act of keeping one's self busy and engaged with others which is understood as important to survival. Assets are thought of as generic, though specific qualities like a sense of belonging at school ("I feel I belong at my school" and "Getting an education is important to me") rather than academic achievement were identified as a universal prosocial behavior across the entire sample.

These examples show what longitudinal studies of at-risk populations of children have repeatedly proven: that a nurturing environment like a safe neighborhood, good schools, and secure attachments to caregivers account for more of the variation in children's developmental trajectories than individual qualities of the child alone (Sroufe, Egeland, Carlson, & Collins, 2005).

The quality of the nurturing environments children experience, however, shows both homogeneity and heterogeneity across contexts and cultures. For example, in Feldman and Masalha's (2007) study of parenting practices and children's developmental outcomes among Israeli and Arab families, it was shown that social support plays a larger role in the lives of Arab parents where there are more traditional extended family living arrangements and lower father involvement in parenting tasks. In contrast, Israeli adults raising children showed more attunement to their children but experienced more problems resolving multiple roles of family and work life. Despite these differences, the overall picture is of similarities across both groups with threats to maternal well-being like depression putting the child at risk, while parental well-being was associated with better coping under stress. Feldman and Masalha write "In both societies, maternal depression was related to infant observed and reported difficult temperament, infant negative emotionality correlated with lower parental sensitivity, marital satisfaction was associated with higher social support, social support was related to higher sensitivity, and maternal depression correlated with lower marital satisfaction" (p. 13). The same risks and protective processes are relevant to each group but they affect parenting practices differently. Culture shapes the cognitions and behaviors associated with each factor. Of course, factors like social support and sensitivity to children can be considered common to most ethnoracial populations. The tension, then, is between common factors that all people experience and the unique patterns which shape how each factor becomes meaningful.

We will return to this point again later, but it is important to consider how much resilience is a latent quality of the individual (resiliency), or a latent quality of the individual triggered by a facilitative environment, or a quality of the environment itself that seeds the possibility for most children to succeed despite the adversity they experience. A thoughtful read of the research suggests that resilience is most likely to occur when environments are well designed to meet children's needs, trigger the expression of capacities they have, or provide opportunities for children to develop new capacities when personal strengths are lacking.

The Differential Impact of Resilience-Related Processes Depends on the Risks That Are Present

While the factors that contribute to a positive psychological disposition or other functional outcome have been shown to be relatively common across populations, aspects of human cognition and behavior that support positive development may not function in the same way for more stressed individuals. The selection of items for the CYRM reflect this specificity, with the assets that are measured those which are most relevant to populations facing high levels of stress. Research shows once again that we make two conceptual errors when we equate the findings from positive psychology (which does not address the confounding effect of stress exposure) with those from studies of resilience. We mistakenly assume through study design and measurement that, regardless of level of adversity, some behaviors are functionally bad and some cognitions and coping styles demonstrably good. The principle of differential impact suggests otherwise.

To illustrate, McMahon and Luthar (2007) studied 361 mother–child dyads where the mothers were being treated for drug abusing behavior and coping with life in the inner city. They showed that the relationship between a child's responsibility to care for their mother, perform household chores and provide instrumental support, in general showed a curvilinear relationship with psychological distress. In cases where the mother was evidently facing psychological challenges, extremely high and low levels of responsibility for the child, compromised parent–child relationships and was associated with alienation from school. Moderate levels of emotional caretaking by the child of the mother, however, was associated with less psychological distress on the part of the child, less alienation from school and better functioning relationships between the child and parent. It would seem that the expectation that the child contribute (allowing themselves to become parentified) in a situation where there was clearly a need to help was validating of the child, protecting the child's sense of well-being and social functioning. This same pattern would not hold true for children under less stress where patterns of parentification in which children are obligated to take over the executive functions of their caregivers produces psychological damage (Hooper, Marotta, & Lanthier, 2008). In other words, under stress a pattern of behavior that may be maladaptive at lower levels of risk exposure may be facilitative of positive development in more stressful environments. We call this phenomena the differential impact of processes associated with resilience.

The second problem which arises when we mistake promotive factors that support an entire population's mental well-being (like self-efficacy) for protective processes associated with resilience under stress (like making a contribution to the care of a parent) is that we may overlook factors that predict positive development for those populations under stress, but which have little or no relevance to populations that are not under stress. For example, while a divorce disadvantages all children to some degree, most grow up relatively unscathed by the experience (Greene, Anderson, Hetherinton, Gorgatch, & DeGarmo, 2003). But children who were living with parents where there was emotional or physical abuse between family members may experience divorce as a protective factor. Their lives after divorce are functionally better. In this case, a protective process can only be understood as good or bad when we appreciate the context of adversity in which it occurs.

Context and Culture Influence Which Protective Processes Matter Most

While the principle of differential impact suggests that we need to pay attention to the environment and its interactions with individuals, it is the quality of that environment (the broader sociopolitical, cultural, and economic context) that determines which protective processes are most likely to be associated with resilience. Researchers who use the CYRM are encouraged to also assess the level of resources available to young people in their communities. The factors that are most protective will reflect the values held by those who are most influential in a young person's life, including members of their families, schools, and broader communities. For example, military service in the USA has been shown to be a protective factor for delinquent young men (Laub & Sampson, 2003). Regular church attendance is associated in some contexts with less delinquency (Benson, 2003). Mother's education predicts a number of child behaviors like school completion and the delay of early pregnancy (Werner & Smith, 1992). In each case, it is the value placed on a particular behavior and the resources made available to a child in a particular context that make it more or less likely a child succeeds. Furthermore, aspects of context and culture intersect. In a study of anonymous disclosures of abuse by adolescents who had participated in violence prevention programming provided by the Canadian Red Cross, Ungar, Barter, McConnell, Tutty, and Fairholm (2009) found that abused children took advantage of the supports they were provided to disclose slowly over time. No single pattern suited both boys and girls, nor did older and younger children disclose in the same ways. Mandatory reporting laws, which were designed to ensure children's safety by obligating community members to report suspected abuse to authorities, might actually threaten children's sense of autonomy and make them more hesitant to disclose if disclosure is perceived as leading to out-of-home placement. Thus, in a social context where child abuse is taken very seriously, children may experience a protective process like mandatory reporting as a potential risk.

As the above example shows, there are many factors to consider when assessing the potential benefits of a protective process. Gender is one such contextual variable that shapes how resilience is experienced. To illustrate, Spencer, Zimet, Aalsma, and Orr (2002) found in their longitudinal study of teens who answered a coital status questionnaire that participants who self-identified as virgins at Time 1 differed by gender in terms of future behavior. Boys with higher self-esteem at Time 1 were more likely to initiate sexual intercourse by Time 2. Girls showed the reverse pattern; those with lower self-esteem at Time 1 reported still being virgins at Time 2. Spencer et al. conclude that "girls with low self-esteem may initiate coitus to feel better about themselves, to provide themselves with intimacy, a sense of maturity, or to rebel against conventional norms concerning early sexual activity… [but] early sexual initiation for boys may be seen as a badge of honor that is celebrated within peer culture. Thus, those boys who have higher self-esteem and are more self-confident may be more likely to find willing partners than boys with low self-esteem who remain virgins" (p. 583). If one of our ways to assess resilience among youth is whether they engage in processes that delay early sexual initiation then we see that gender (and culture) influence whether a protective process like this is functionally the same for all children, or just girls, or just girls with low self-esteem. A young woman who chooses to become sexually active to cope with diminished self-esteem may, however, be demonstrating an unconventional pattern of resilience that is meaningful to her but not to others in her wider community.

Patterns like this highlight the nuanced differences noticeable in studies of protective factors typical of resilience (in this case, delayed sexual initiation). Contextual norms, gender, and individual qualities like self-esteem (and the availability of the resources required to grow it) combine to determine whether a behavior contributes to well-being. Other studies of class and race differences among young women who become sexually active suggest that these factors too may determine whether this particular behavior is meaningful and protective in contexts where there is heightened risk (Saewyc & Edinburgh, 2010).

One of the most well-studied aspects of context as it relates to unique patterns of resilience is culture. Culture is a commonly held set of values, beliefs, and identifications among individuals who reify these as everyday practices (Berry, 1979). The co-construction of what is a meaningful expression of resilience, then, reflects the relative power of those who share a common culture. Typically, those individuals who are most at risk have the weakest voices when it comes to deciding what is and is not an indicator of adaptive coping. At what point does dropping out of school make more sense to a child who is racially marginalized than remaining in school and suffering the debilitating effects of racism (Dei, Massuca, McIsaac, & Zine, 1997)? And why do first generation immigrants who do not acculturate report better mental health than those who do (Grant et al., 2004)? These examples suggest that culture matters a great deal when determining the developmental path of a child and how they will experience the protective factors that are provided to them. Cultural outsiders frequently misperceive resistance among cultural minorities as a lack of adaptability when in fact culturally specific modes of coping may be protective in threatening environments.

To illustrate this point, Nguyen-Gillham (2008) conducted a qualitative study with 321 grade 11 Palestinian youth. These young people describe resilience in a unique way as social suffering: "The Palestinian concept of *samud*—a determination to exist through being steadfast and rooted to the land—is at the heart of resilience. Within a Palestinian context, suffering and endurance have to be interpreted at both an individual and collective level. The construct of resilience goes beyond an individualistic interpretation: resilience is (re)constituted as a wider collective and social representation of what it means to endure" (p. 292). Though the themes these youth raised, like the value they place on supportive relationships, the need to keep life as normal as possible, political participation, education, and optimism are values shared with other youth, including Israelis (Shamai & Kimhi, 2006), there are culturally specific ways that these resources combine with a sense of purposeful suffering in a context of political struggle.

How, then, can a group both resemble the dominant culture and still show unique patterns of coping? And how can we design measures like the CYRM to capture this low invariance? Among research that has investigated culturally specific understandings of resilience-related phenomena there has been a tendency to overlook the contagion effect of the dominant culture on subpopulations that are embedded therein (Dana, 2008). How much ethnoracial minorities become a part of the dominant culture is an important consideration in assessing the influence of cultural norms and practices. While we tend to focus on differences between cultural groups, we seldom if ever know how closely each ethnoracial population is influenced by dominant culture expectations and practices. Herein lies the challenge when understanding resilience across contexts and cultures: there is a need to appreciate the tension between the sameness between groups and differences between groups, as well as between individuals in these groups.

Conclusion

Defining resilience as a quality of individuals places most of the responsibility for growth on vulnerable people who face significant adversity. A shift in focus to a more ecological understanding of resilience helps us to identify the complex weave of protective processes that both prevent risk exposure and build the capacities associated with positive development. Measuring this complex association between environment and individuals is difficult, especially when the goal is to avoid the cultural bias or presuppositions of what is and is not adaptive functioning. Life histories are often told from the perspective of the individual who appears more resilient than others and often highlights what these individuals did to improve their lives. A more detailed examination of lives lived well can usually identify a number of facilitators of a child's personal success, including individual mentors, institutional supports, and social policies that make resources available and accessible. When resilience is understood as first and foremost a quality of the environment, and second, a quality of the individual who exploits that environment as best they can, then helping professionals, politicians, communities, and families become implicated in making resilience more likely to occur.

References

Benson, P. L. (2003). Developmental assets and asset-building community: Conceptual and empirical foundations. In R. Lerner & P. L. Benson (Eds.), *Developmental assets and asset-building communities: Implications for research, policy, and practice* (pp. 19–46). New York, NY: Kluwer.

Berry, J. W. (1979). A cultural ecology of social behavior. *Advances in Experimental Social Psychology, 12*, 177–206.

Bonanno, G. A., Westphal, M., & Mancini, A. D. (2011). Resilience to loss and potential trauma. *Annual Review of Clinical Psychology, 7*, 511–535.

Bottrell, D. (2009). Understanding 'marginal' perspectives: Towards a social theory of resilience. *Qualitative Social Work, 8*(3), 321–340.

Bottrell, D., & Armstrong, D. (2012). Local resources and distal decisions: The political ecology of resilience. In M. Ungar (Ed.), *The social ecology of resilience: A handbook of theory and practice* (pp. 247–264). New York, NY: Springer.

Brislin, R. W. (1970). Back-translation for cross-cultural research. *Journal of Cross-Cultural Psychology, 1*, 185–216.

Bronfenbrenner, U., & Morris, P. A. (2006). The bioecological model of human development. In R. M. Lerner & W. Damon (Eds.), *Handbook of child psychology* (6th ed., pp. 793–828). Hoboken, NH: Wiley.

Cicchetti, D. (2010). A developmental psychopathology perspective on bipolar disorder. In D. J. Miklowitz & D. Cicchetti (Eds.), *Understanding bipolar disorder: A developmental psychopathology perspective* (pp. 1–32). New York, NY: Guilford.

Cyrulnik, B. (2008). Children in war and their resiliences. In H. Parens, H. P. Blum, & S. Akhtar (Eds.), *The unbroken soul: Tragedy, trauma, and resilience* (pp. 23–36). Lanham, MD: Jason Aronson.

Dana, R. H. (2008). Clincial diagnosis in multicultural populations. In L. A. Suzuki & J. G. Ponterotto (Eds.), *Handbook of multicultural assessment: Clinical, psychological, and educational applications* (3rd ed., pp. 107–131). New York, NY: Wiley.

Dei, G. J. S., Massuca, J., McIsaac, E., & Zine, J. (1997). *Reconstructing 'drop-out': A critical ethnography of the dynamics of Black students' disengagement from school*. Toronto, ON: University of Toronto Press.

Donnon, T., & Hammond, W. (2007). Understanding the relationships between resiliency and bullying in adolescence: An assessment of youth resiliency from five urban junior high schools. *Child and Adolescent Psychiatric Clinics of North America, 16*(2), 449–472.

Easterbrooks, M. A., Chaudhuri, J. H., Bartlett, J. D., & Copeman, A. (2011). Resilience in parenting among young mothers: Family and ecological risks and opportunities. *Children and Youth Services Review, 33*, 42–50.

Feldman, R., & Masalha, S. (2007). The role of culture in moderating the links between early ecological risk and young children's adaptation. *Development and Psychopathology, 19*, 1–21.

Gilligan, R. (1999). Enhancing the resilience of children and young people in public care by mentoring their talents and interests. *Child and Family Social Work, 4*, 187–196.

Grant, B. F., Stinson, F. S., Hasin, D. S., Dawson, D. A., Chou, S. P., & Anderson, K. (2004). Immigration and lifetime prevalence of DSM-IV psychiatric disorders among Mexican Americans and non-Hispanic Whites in the United States: Results from the national epidemiologic survey on alcohol and related conditions. *Archives of General Psychiatry, 61*(12), 1226–1233.

Greene, S. M., Anderson, E. R., Hetherinton, E. M., Gorgatch, M. S., & DeGarmo, D. S. (2003). Risk and resilience after divorce. In F. Walsh (Ed.), *Normal family processes* (3rd ed., pp. 96–120). New York, NY: Guilford.

Hooper, L. M., Marotta, S. A., & Lanthier, R. P. (2008). Predictors of growth and distress following childhood parentification: A retrospective exploratory study. *Journal of Child and Family Studies, 17*, 693–705.

Kagitçibasi, C. (2007). *Family, self, and human development across cultures: Theory and applications* (2nd ed.). Mahwah, NJ: Lawrence Erlbaum.

Larson, R. (2006). Positive youth development, wilful adolescents, and mentoring. *Journal of Community Psychology, 34*(6), 677–689.

Laub, J. H., & Sampson, R. J. (2003). *Shared beginnings, divergent lives: Delinquent boys to age 70*. Cambridge, MA: Harvard University Press.

Lerner, R. M. (2006). Resilience as an attribute of the developmental system: Comments on the papers of professors Masten & Wachs. In B. M. Lester, A. S. Masten, & B. McEwen (Eds.), *Resilience in children* (pp. 40–51). Boston, MA: Blackwell.

Liborio, R., & Ungar, M. (2010). Children's perspectives on their economic activity as a pathway to resilience. *Children and Society, 24*, 326–338.

Liebenberg, L., Ungar, M., and Van de Vijver, F. R. R. (2012). Validation of the Child and Youth Resilience Measure-28 (CYRM-28) Among Canadian Youth with Complex Needs. *Research on Social Work Practice, 22*(2), 219–226. doi: 10.1177/1049731511428619.

McMahon, T. J., & Luthar, S. S. (2007). Defining characteristics and potential consequences of caretaking burden among children living in urban poverty. *American Journal of Orthopsychiatry, 77*(2), 267–281.

Moffitt, T. E., Caspi, A., Rutter, M., & Silva, P. A. (2001). *Sex differences in antisocial behaviour*. Cambridge: Cambridge University Press.

Ng-Mak, D. S., Salzinger, S., Feldman, R. S., & Stueve, C. A. (2010). Pathologic adaptation to community violence among inner-city youth. *American Journal of Orthopsychiatry, 74*(2), 196–2008. doi:10.1037/0002-9432.74.2.196.

Nguyen-Gillham, V. (2008). Normalising the abnormal: Palestinian youth and the contradictions of resilience in protracted conflict. *Health and Social Care in the Community, 16*(3), 291–298.

Phelps, E:, Balsano, A. B., Fay, K., Peltz, J. S., Zimmerman, S. M., Lerner, R. M., et al. (2007). Nuances in early adolescent developmental trajectories of positive and problematic/risk behaviors: Findings from the 4-H study of positive youth development. *Resilience. Monograph for the Child and Adolescent Psychiatry Clinics of North America, 16*(2), 437–448.

Prince-Embury, S., & Steer, R. A. (2010). Profiles of personal resiliency for normative and clinical samples of youth assessed by the Resiliency Scales for Children and Adolescents. *Journal of Psychoeducational Assessment, 28*(4), 303–314.

Rutter, M. (2009). Understanding and testing risk mechanisms for mental disorders. *Journal of Child Psychology and Psychiatry, 50*(1–2), 44–52.

Saewyc, E. M., & Edinburgh, L. D. (2010). Restoring healthy developmental trajectories for sexually exploited young runaway girls: Fostering protective factors and reducing risk behaviors. *Journal of Adolescent Health, 46*, 180–188.

Shamai, M., & Kimhi, S. (2006). Exposure to threat of war and terror, political attitudes, stress, and life satisfaction among teenagers in Israel. *Journal of Adolescence, 29*, 165–176.

Shernoff, D. J., & Schmidt, J. A. (2008). Further evidence of an engagement achievement paradox among U.S. high school students. *Journal of Youth and Adolescence, 37*, 564–580.

Shin, R., Daly, B., & Vera, E. (2007). The relationships of peer norms, ethnic identity, and peer support to school engagement in urban youth. *Professional School Counseling, 10*(4), 379–388.

Skovdal, M., & Campbell, C. (2010). Orphan competent communities: A framework for community analysis and action. *Vulnerable Children and Youth Studies, 5*(1), 19–30.

Spencer, J. M., Zimet, G. D., Aalsma, M. C., & Orr, D. P. (2002). Self-esteem as a predictor of initiation of coitus in early adolescents. *Pediatrics, 109*(4), 581–584.

Sroufe, L. A., Egeland, B., Carlson, E. A., & Collins, W. A. (2005). *The development of the person: The Minnesota study of risk and adaptation from birth to adulthood*. New York, NY: Guilford.

Taylor, C. S., Lerner, R. M., von Eye, A., Balsano, A. B., Dowling, E. M., Anderson, P. M., et al. (2002). Individual and ecological assets and positive developmental trajectories among gang and community-based organization youth. In R. M. Lerner, C. S. Taylor, & A. Von Eye (Eds.), *Pathways to positive development among diverse youth* (pp. 57–72). New York, NY: Jossey-Bass.

Ungar, M. (2008). Resilience across cultures. *British Journal of Social Work, 38*(2), 218–35.

Ungar, M. (2011). *Counseling in challenging contexts: Working with individuals and families across clinical and community settings*. Belmont, CA: Brooks/Cole.

Ungar, M., Barter, K., McConnell, S., Tutty, L., & Fairholm, J. (2009). Patterns of disclosure among youth. *Qualitative Social Work, 8*(3), 341–356.

Ungar, M., Brown, M., Liebenberg, L., Othman, R., Kwong, W. M., Armstrong, M., et al. (2007). Unique pathways to resilience across cultures. *Adolescence, 42*(166), 287–310.

Ungar, M., & Liebenberg, L. (2005). The International Resilience Project: A mixed methods approach to the study of resilience across cultures. In M. Ungar (Ed.), *Handbook for working with children and youth: Pathways to resilience across cultures and contexts* (pp. 211–226). Thousand Oaks, CA: Sage.

Ungar, M., & Liebenberg, L. (2009). Cross-cultural consultation leading to the development of a valid measure of youth resilience: The International Resilience Project. *Studia Psychologica, 51*(2–3), 259–268.

Ungar, M., & Liebenberg, L. (2011). Assessing resilience across cultures using mixed-methods: Construction of the child and youth resilience measure-28. *Journal of Mixed Methods Research, 5*(2), 126–149.

Ungar, M., Liebenberg, L., Boothroyd, R., Kwong, W. M., Lee, T. Y., Leblanc, J., et al. (2008). The study of youth resilience across cultures: Lessons from a pilot study of measurement development. *Research in Human Development, 5*(3), 166–180.

Werner, E. E., & Smith, R. S. (1992). *Overcoming the odds: High risk children from birth to adulthood*. Ithaca, NY: Cornel University Press.

Wingo, A. P., Wrenn, G., Pelletier, T., Gutman, A. R., Bradley, B., & Ressler, K. J. (2010). Moderating effects of resilience on depression in individuals with a history of childhood abuse or trauma exposure. *Journal of Affective Disorders, 126*, 411–414.

Ziervogel, C. F., Ahmed, N., Fisher, A. J., & Robertson, B. A. (1997). Alcohol misuse in South African male adolescents: A qualitative investigation. *International Quarterly of Community Health Education, 17*(1), 25–41.

19 Resilience in Kenyan Youth Living in the Slums and Suburbs of Nairobi: An Exploratory and Descriptive Study

Beverly Tignor and Sandra Prince-Embury

"Resilience" in psychology is the positive capacity of people to cope with stress and adversity. This coping may result in the individual "bouncing back" to a previous state of normal functioning, or using the experience of exposure to adversity to produce a "steeling effect" and function better than expected (much like an inoculation gives one the capacity to cope well with future exposure to disease) (Masten, 2009). Resilience is most commonly understood as a process and not a trait of an individual which is more typically referred to as resiliency (Masten, 2001). Most research now shows that resilience is the result of individuals interacting with their environments and the processes that either promote well-being or protect them against the overwhelming influence of risk factors. These processes combine the influence of individual coping strategies, with support by families, schools, and communities.

Cross-cultural consideration of resilience or personal resiliency adds conceptual complexity to the understanding of this process (Ungar, 2008; Ungar et al., 2008; Ungar & Liebenberg, 2005). For example, what constitutes adversity and what constitutes positive outcome? Some researchers have identified characteristics of coping with abuse situations that may be adaptive although not necessarily considered optimal (Obradović, Bush, Stamperdahl, Adlerm, & Boyce, 2010). Circumstances in many areas of the world would constitute hardship experienced by all residents relative to US standards, home of many studies of resilience/resiliency. What constitutes positive outcome in these circumstances? Strength and achievement-based assessments of positive outcome used in the USA might not be within reach in other more impoverished regions. International studies focusing on impoverished or failed states often focus on the absence of conflict, starvation, genocide, HIV, and radicalization as positive outcomes.

The current study focuses on the assessment of personal resiliency as experienced by 83 youth between the ages of 9 and 18 living in the slums and middle class of Nairobi, the capital of Kenya. This study is descriptive in nature and begins by comparing subjectively experienced personal resiliency reported by the Nairobi youth with norms based on a representative sample of youth in the USA. The experience of personal resiliency is assessed using the *Resiliency Scales for Children and Adolescents* (RSCA, Prince-Embury, 2007). The RSCA was chosen in that it is based on three core developmental processes, sense of mastery, sense of relatedness, and emotional reactivity with the belief that core developmental processes may be shared cross-culturally, although specific

B. Tignor, Ph.D. (✉)
Private Practice, 14 West main St, Menham, NJ 07945, USA
e-mail: beverly.tignor@comcast.net

S. Prince-Embury, Ph.D.
Resiliency Institute of Allenhurst, LLC, 625 North Edgemere Drive, West Allenhurst, NJ 07711, USA
e-mail: sandraprince-embury@earthlink.net

S. Prince-Embury and D.H. Saklofske (eds.), *Resilience in Children, Adolescents, and Adults: Translating Research into Practice*, The Springer Series on Human Exceptionality,
DOI 10.1007/978-1-4614-4939-3_19, © Springer Science+Business Media New York 2013

competencies and achievements associated with these processes may differ across cultures. The RSCA has been employed previously with youth in South African (Van Wyk 2011), China (Cui, Teng, Li, & Oei, 2010), Brazil (Jordani, 2008), and Lebanon (Ayyash-Abdo & Sanchez-Ruiz, 2011). Ann Masten (2001) has described resiliency as ordinary magic, which consists of basic developmental processes that are part of human development (Masten, 2001). The three factor structure of the RSCA has been shown to be robust when compared to other factor structures and across age and gender in the USA (Prince-Embury & Courville, 2008a, 2008b) and across culture (Cui et al., 2010).

This study is exploratory in nature as the RSCA has not been previously administered in Kenya and no norms exist specifically for this country. Personal resiliency as assessed by the RSCA is examined relative to location of testing, gender, ethnic affiliation, and experience of genocide. The relationship between the three global scales for Nairobi youth is compared with the relationship between these scales for US youth. Cluster analyses identifying three characteristic profiles of personal resiliency are described and case examples are provided for each profile. An example of change in personal resiliency of one young victim of genocide is described after 6 months of support by a helping organization.

Socioeconomic Background of Nairobi

Risk conditions or adversities for many Nairobi youth are complex, multi-faceted, and in most cases cumulative stemming from such factors as death and loss of close family members due to the widespread HIV/AIDS epidemic, recent post-election violence and genocide, extreme poverty including lack of sanitation and safety in growing urban slums, homelessness and refugee status, tribal practices involving female genital mutilation and early marriage, as well as rape, emotional and physical abuse of children and youth.

Kenya faces many challenges that result in limited resources for its population. Rapid population growth plus declining economic performance has translated into less income per person. More than half (55%) of people live below Kenya's poverty line, up from 48% in 1990. In 2006, 58% lived on less than $2 a day (CIA, World fact Book, 2009). With a Human Development Index (HDI) of 0.470 in 2010, Kenya is classified in the low human development category, ranked 128 out of 169 countries (ECHO, 2011).

Demographics of the Area Studied

Nairobi is the capital and largest city in Kenya and all of East Africa, with a current population made up of 42 different ethnic groups totaling more than 3,017,000 people, and a growth rate of 6.9% per year. Nairobi became the capital of British East Africa in1907, replacing Mombassa, and then became the capital of independent Kenya, annexing nearby territories for future growth. Close to the equator and occupying a land area of 260 square miles, Nairobi is situated in southern Kenya adjacent to the eastern edge of the Rift valley, at an elevation of 5,889 ft above sea level (Mitullah, 2003). Nairobi is a culturally diverse cosmopolitan city, with all the major Kenyan ethnic groups represented. The largest group in Nairobi and nationally is Kikuyu, who make up 22% of the total Kenyan population, and whose traditional home area borders Nairobi. The second largest group is Luhya (14%), followed closely by Luo (12%), Kalenjin (12%), Kamba (11%), Kisii (6%), Meru (6 %), and other African, Asian, Arab, and European ethnic groups (15%) (Kenya-Ethnic Groups, 2010).

Refugees in Kenya

There are 412,000 registered refugees and asylum seekers in Kenya, with 6,000–7,000 new arrivals each month (Refugees International, 2010). Many more are not reported. The majority are from Somalia, but refugees who have fled conflicts in other neighboring countries such as Sudan and Ethiopia are also represented. Refugees, as represented by a number of youth in the current study, have been able to connect with relatives living in middle-class neighborhoods or in the poorer Eastleigh section of Nairobi, often referred to as "little Mogadishu" (Goldenberg, 2006) where Somalis have lived for more than 100 years. Here the 100,000 residents exist with a burgeoning unemployment rate because Kenya has strict refugee laws which do not permit them to work legally, so that many find casual jobs in the informal sector. Because of the high population density and the fact that living closely in one neighborhood is a priority for the refugee community, Kenyan landlords can charge high rental fees, although buildings are in bad condition with inadequate sanitary facilities. Children play in the heavily polluted streets as there are no parks or recreation areas (Herz, 2008). In addition, 8,000 Southern Sudanese refugees live in Nairobi (Mutambo, 2011). While the Somali refugees have managed to engage in businesses in the informal economy, their priority is to acquire an education, which is viewed as instrumental to self-development. Xenophobia and discriminative urban refugee policies preclude their admission into public elementary schools, while most private schools are unaffordable (Karanja, 2010). We have several Sudanese and a smaller number of Somali refugees in the sample.

Racial and Ethnic Tensions

While disputes over land had occurred long before the arrival of the Europeans, British explorers, missionaries, anthropologists, and colonialists increased existing tensions and created new ones by favoring certain groups over others. As Nairobi grew, native Kenyan ethnic groups remained at the bottom of the food chain with respect to jobs, land, and general living conditions compared to European, Asian, Arab, and other groups living in the region. Following independence in 1963, the ruling Kenyan elite encouraged ethnic division, alleging the ethnic superiority of certain groups in order to divide and weaken the power of the people so that the ruler's power would not be challenged (Wamwere, 2003). Widespread genocide following independence after colonial rule has been common in Africa, and even women and religious leaders have been caught up in it. Since 1963, more than five million Africans have died from civil wars created by politically motivated ethnic bias, inequality, and the struggle for resources to meet basic human needs.

The most recent violence pertinent to our study occurred in the aftermath of the 2007 presidential election when the Luo candidate Raila Odinga was said to have lost to the incumbent president Mwai Kibaki, a Kikuyu. Fueled by long-standing tensions over land, economic opportunity, and access to power, the political crisis turned into a violent ethnic one in 2008 when more than 1,000 people were killed and over 304,000 Kenyans displaced (CBC news, 2008). In Kisumu, the former home of one of our displaced orphans, thousands of Luo rioters swept across the city exacting revengeon innocent citizens for similar acts of violence enacted by a Kikuyu mob the day before (Gettleman, 2008).

Life in the Slums

While there is a wide variety of standards of living in Nairobi and a growing middle class, most of the population is poor and about half live in slum areas which cover 5 % of the total city area. At least 73 % of adult slum dwellers are living on less than $1.5 dollars per day. The growth of the slums has resulted from a variety of factors, historical and contemporary. During the colonial period, large-scale government sanctioned segregation along racial lines divided the city into four distinct sectors: north and west marked the European sector, east and southeast marked the African area, north and east was the Asian sector, with a second small Asian sector southeast to south, later bounded by the national parks (Olima, 2001). Unemployment, underemployment, and increased population in rural areas lead to migration into the city. Mathare Valley to the east of the city and Kibera to the west form the largest uncontrolled urban settlements in the city.

Mathare is a collection of slums in Nairobi with a population of about 500,000 people.

The population density is reported to be 460 people per hectare or 2.47 acres (Mitullah, 2003). Discrimination, especially along ethnic lines, exists within the slums, with a few dominant ethnic groups living together in specific areas. Neighborhood victimization of other groups is common.

Most slums are located on sites not planned for housing and residents are exposed to dehumanizing conditions. Women and young girls, in particular, are exposed to daily threats of violence including potential rape when attempting to use limited common toilet and bathing facilities (Amnesty International, 2010). Different forms of pollution, including both human and industrial waste, may cause serious illness or death, and medical treatment is either not available or not a viable option. General lack of effective policing and security, exclusion from social services and healthcare, combined with unemployment and poverty results in a high prevalence of crime and victimization. Crime, especially against women, goes widely unpunished and contributes to the cycle of poverty (Amnesty International, 2010). Perpetrators are mostly unemployed male youth or men, acting individually or as a part of groups or gangs. Violence in connection with forced evictions is also common.

Youth living in slum areas have no privacy or freedom at home as households are often unable to meet their basic needs (Mitullah, 2003). Many move into the streets where they are further exposed to violent behavior and suffer psychological trauma. According to Low (1998), 60,000 children at that time lived on the streets in Nairobi, with the number increasing exponentially. Many youth in the study were once living on the streets.

Children are often exploited sexually for commercial purposes. Child prostitution is an emerging phenomenon in Kenya (Mwangi, 2003). An increasing number of children enter prostitution as a means of survival. It was not possible to determine how many of the youth in this study might have lived on the streets because of the stigma attached to admitting this. With the death of parents due to the HIV/Aids epidemic, many of these children are orphans raising younger siblings. Others are from families facing conflicts or too poor to care for them. The percentage of people infected with HIV is highest in the slums, with the highest prevalence among young women age 15–24 (5.6 %), four times higher than among young men (1.4 %) (United Nations General Assembly Special Session on HIV and AIDS, Country Report-Kenya, 2010, p. 7). Ethnic violence is, also, more common in the slums than in middle or high income areas of Nairobi (Warah, 2008). Following the presidential election in 2007, politicians created ethnic tension for political gain.

The Middle Class in Nairobi

Ten percent of the population of Nairobi is middle class. These tend to be people who are college educated, live in a home with a gate around it for protection from theft and other crime, and can afford to send their children to school and college. Kenya is said to be one of the most unequal societies in the world. Ten percent of the country's 35 million people control 42 % of the nation's wealth (Warah, 2008). More than half of the children in our study were living and attending school in a middleclass setting (i.e., Komarack, the orphanage, and Neema high school). However, many of these children were from very poor families, having been moved into a middle-class setting through support from local Christian organizations. The rest were living in the slum area of Eastleigh or Mathare N.

Violence Against Children

Other forms of violence are also a regular part of Kenyan children's everyday experience. Almost all children in Africa are exposed to some form of physical, sexual, and psychological abuse in the home at school and in the community. Ninety nine percent of children in Kenya reported having experienced some form of physical abuse; 26 % of girls reported having been victims of rape (The African Child Policy Forum, 2010). In many schools, not only in the slums, teachers may use caning, slapping, and whipping to maintain classroom discipline and to punish children for poor academic performance (Human Rights Watch, 1999). Similar practices are often condoned and used at home.

Methods

Participants

A total of 83 Kenyan youth participated in the study, 40 males and 43 females between the ages of 9 and 18, from locations around or within very poor to middle-class areas of Nairobi. Forty-nine of eighty-three youth (59 %) participating in the study lived and attended school in a middle-class setting. However, many of these youth were originally from the slums. Less than half of these students might actually qualify as middle class. The remaining 34 youth lived in the slum, either in Mathere North or Eastleigh. Five different schools were represented including the Tumaini elementary School in the North Mathare slum, Eastleigh Technical School bounded by the East Mathare slum, the By Grace Children's Home in a lower middle income area of Ngong Hills, Neema High School near North Mathare, and the middle class By Grace Komarack Academy.

The study began as a humanitarian effort in July of 2010 through the Foundation for Peace, with the request for a psychological screening of the 18 children living in the By Grace Children's Home, a small Christian orphanage to the west of Nairobi in the Ngong Hills. Many of the children were actual orphans who had watched their parents' die of HIV/AIDS, while others still had a single living parent who could not afford to sustain them. Several youth in the orphanage had siblings who had died of AIDS, and four had tested positive for AIDS themselves, either as a result of rape or other acquired means. One was a victim of genocide. Others were suffering from Post-traumatic Stress Disorder related to prior sexual abuse or death of a close relative. Most had been displaced multiple times from their original village homes outside of Nairobi. The children represent several of the major tribes of Kenya including the majority from the Kikuyu tribe followed by Kamba, and then one child each from Luhya, Luo, Maasai, or Embu tribe, plus three children of mixed tribal origin. Psychological reports were prepared for these 18 children by the first author and recommendations were given to teachers at the By Grace Home. The decision was made to expand the testing to other Nairobi locations.

Foundation for Peace also sets up free medical clinics in the Mathare North (area one) slum, held within a local church but open to anyone living in the surrounding area. The pastor of the church arranged for the examiner to meet with teachers and screen children in the neighborhood elementary school, the Tumaini School. Eighteen students between the ages of 9 and 14 were evaluated there, plus 3 teenage girls, ages 15–18, who lived nearby and volunteered to participate in the study. Of the 14,000 people who live in Area One, Luo is the dominant tribe followed by Luhya, but there are also Agikuyu, Kamba, and Kisii.

A brief search of the neighborhood during the 2-day weekend medical clinic turned up no teenage boys in the 15–18 year-old age group, and individuals questioned stated that boys more than girls tended leave their families, drop out of school, and search for employment in other areas whenever possible. This is the first year that students from Tumaini School sat for the national exam, a necessary step to entering secondary school. Those who do not make it to secondary schools because of poor performance or inability to pay school fees are absorbed into Jua Kali sector (informal industries) where they are trained as they work, become unskilled laborers, or simply idle in the streets, abuse drugs, and join criminal gangs. Possibly there is a 3–4 age to grade discrepancy with many of the boys in particular, suggesting time out of school. It is not known what they were doing before being reintegrated into school at Komarack and Eastleigh. Older boys at Neema Boarding School were not tested due to the age limit-only girls fit the 15–18-year profile at Neema, and so the sample from there is girls for that reason.

With help from leaders of the local community, the Neema High School was located and the examiner transported by volunteer driver over dusty, unpaved roads to a small suburban area about 15 min outside of Mathare North. Neema is a privately funded day and boarding school for teens rescued from the difficult living conditions and poor family situations in the nearby slums. Those from the most desperate circumstances stay at Neema as boarding students. These were the students who were asked to participate in the present study. Of the group, all of the male students who presented exceeded the test age of 18, and so were excluded, leaving eight female students between the ages of 15 and 18. Of the students tested, tribal origins included three Luhya, Three Kikuyu, and two from the Luo tribe. Slum areas represented include Kariobangi North and South, Elderst, Saika, Zimmerman, and Mathare North.

The search for male participants in the 15–18-year age range resulted in a visit to the Eastleigh Technical School, part of the Eastleigh Community Center, located within the grounds of the Eastleigh Presbyterian Church. Eastleigh, located in the eastern part of Nairobi, is 1 of 16 areas in the Mathare Valley slum area. It has a very large Somali immigrant population, and many of the inhabitants are refugees. The lengths of the programs are designed for completion in less than a year, so that students may begin paid employment in the community as soon as possible. Since many of the students have family obligations, the shorter training period has resulted in a far smaller drop-out rate. Programs include everything from dressmaking and culinary arts to pottery design and auto-mechanics. Seven male and five female students from the Eastleigh School participated in the study.

A middle-class community sample was arranged through local community contacts. By Grace Komarack Academy is a private, Christian elementary and high school, with both day and boarding students located in a suburban area 15 km southeast of the Nairobi central business district. Twenty-four students, 12 males and 12 females, between the ages of 9 and 17 participated in the study. Although the school is Christian, a number of students attending are Muslim and several are refugees who have been out of school for some time, and require special tutoring to catch up, improve their English reading and writing skills, and fit in with the general population of students. Special religious accommodations are, also, made for the Muslim students, so that they may return home at customary prayer times during the day and then return to school. The length of the school day is purposefully long, extending into the evening hours, and encompasses academic, social, and sports activities as well as study time and homework assistance as needed. Of the 24 students participating, 6 were from the Sudan, and 2 from Somalia. Local tribes represented in order of prevalence included Kamba, Luo, Kikuyu, Luhya, Masai, Taita, and Kisii.

Measures

One testing instrument was used in this study, standardized on child and adolescent samples representative of the US population in terms of age, ethnicity, sex, and parent education level. *The Resiliency Scales for Children and Adolescents*, developed and written by second author Sandra Prince-Embury, 2007), are designed to systematically identify and quantify core personal qualities of resiliency in youth, as expressed in their own words about their own experience. Resiliency reflects the degree to which an individual's personal resources match or exceed their reactivity to internal and external stress. The results may be used for the purpose of education, screening, prevention, and counseling. The *Sense of Mastery* Scale, comprised of 20 items, is intended to measure a youth's experience of mastery as derived from three subscales. These include *Optimism*, an individual's expectation of a positive outcome, *Self-Efficacy*, designed to reflect persistence and flexible problem solving, and *Adaptability*, which reflects one's ability to acknowledge mistakes and to accept help from others. The *Sense of Relatedness* Scale, consisting of 24 items, taps different aspects of relatedness from the youth's point of view, including *Trust*, the experience of intimacy and ability to feel accepted as oneself in relation to others, *Support*, perceived access to support, *Comfort*, social ease, calm, ability to meet and make friends, and *Tolerance*, or the ability to risk expressing one's own opinion with others who might differ while still remaining in the relationship. The *Emotional Reactivity* Scale, with 20 items, measures *Sensitivity*, the ease with which emotional buttons may be triggered, *Recovery*, a youth's perception of the length of time it takes to return to normal functioning, and *Impairment*, which attempts to differentiate the degree of impairment experienced from emotionally arousing circumstances. The scale also includes a measure of the youth's overall resources, the Resource Index score. This score is derived from the standardized average of the Sense of Mastery *T* score and Sense of Relatedness *T* score. In addition, a measure of the youth's overall vulnerability to stress is indicated by the Vulnerability Index score. The Vulnerability Index is the standardized difference between the Resource Index and the Emotional Reactivity *T* scores.

Clinical Interviews

Each child at the orphanage was interviewed individually and privately by the first author with the help of the psychologist interpreter as needed. Due to time constraints, It was not possible to conduct individual interviews at the time of testing in other locations. Subsequent interviews with each child were handled by one specific teacher at both the Tumaini School and BY Grace Academy Komarack, and the results of those interviews with each child were written down in separate reports and sent to the head research psychologist as confidential email attachments.

Procedures

All tests were administered and hand scored by the first author, a licensed clinical psychologist with more than 30 years of experience working with children and youth. The same translator, an American graduate student in psychology, raised in the Nairobi area, served in all three major locations (By Grace Children's Home, By Grace Komarack Academy, and Tumaini School). A young adult volunteer from African Enterprise, with excellent English and Swahili skills, translated at Neema school, while a teacher from the Eastleigh Technical School familiar with the youth there translated in that location. Youth from the two latter schools were teenagers who could converse and comprehend quite well in both English and Swahili, and the translators were used mainly to assure consistency throughout the five locations.

All participants were told that they would be taking a test which could be used to help identify their personal strengths; there were no correct or incorrect answers, and the only right answer was the one that felt right to them. In the group settings, children were encouraged to do their own work, and seated far enough apart to make this possible. The test directions and each item of the test were read first in English and then translated into Swahili. The children were tested individually at the Orphanage, and in small groups of not more than 6–12 students in all other locations. The children were monitored closely to assure that they understood each question, wrote their name, age, tribe, and grade clearly on their answer sheet, and answered each question on the correct line.

Children in the orphanage were interviewed and then tested individually. Children in all other settings received the Resiliency Scales only. Due to time limitations, students at By Grace Komarack Academy and Tumaini School were individually interviewed subsequently by either the Head Teacher or the designated lead teacher in each setting. Results of the individual interviews were then forwarded to the first author.

Analysis

Analysis of the Nairobi sample was conducted by total sample, location, ethnic affiliation, and experience of genocide. Coefficient alphas were computed for the RSCA global scores and subscale scores to compare internal consistency of the scale scores in the Nairobi Sample with those in the USA. RSCA mean scores are compared with frequency of scores found in the US normative sample (Prince-Embury, 2007; Prince-Embury & Courville, 2008a, 2008b). ANOVAs were used to determine whether there were any significant differences in RSCA global scale, Index or subscale scores across location, gender, and ethnic affiliation. Correlation analyses were used to compare interrelatedness of the three global RSCA scales with those found for the US normative sample. Cluster Analyses were conducted to determine characteristic RSCA personal resiliency profiles for the Nairobi sample and youth representing each cluster group are described. Finally, a followup administration of the RSCA to one youth after 6 months of support by the helping organization is described to highlight the assessment of positive changes.

Results

RSCA Scores for the Nairobi Sample Compared with US Norms

Prior to other analyses, alpha coefficients were computed for the RSCA global scale and subscale scores in the Nairobi sample to estimate internal consistency for this group. Alpha coefficients for the three global scale scores were found to be adequate to good for the Nairobi sample: Sense of Mastery (0.70), Sense of Relatedness (0.74), and Emotional Reactivity (0.80). Although these alphas are lower than those for the US sample, they are adequate for use with the Nairobi sample. Comparable alpha coefficient values were found by Van Wyk (2011) for a sample of 487 South African youth; Sense of Mastery (0.74), Sense of Relatedness (0.83), and Emotional Reactivity (0.76). These alpha coefficients are lower than those found for the USA, China, and Brazil.

Table 19.1 Score rankings based on resiliency scale *T* score ranges

Ranking	*T* score ranges
High average	≥60
Above average	56–59
Average	46–55
Below average	41–45
Low	≤40

Table 19.1 displays the RSCA score ranges based on the US normative samples (see Prince-Embury, 2007, RSCA technical manual). Table 19.2 displays mean RSCA global and index scores for the total Nairobi sample as well as frequency of scores above and below average as compared with frequency of these scores found in the US normative sample.

Mean scores for Nairobi youth on Sense of Mastery, Sense of Relatedness and the Resource Index scores were all in the below average range as compared with the US normative rankings indicated in Table 19.1. Comparison of the percentage of Nairobi youth scoring below average in Sense of Mastery, Sense of Relatedness and Resources (60–64 %) was twice as large as the percentage of US youth scoring in the below average range on these variables (30–31 %). On the other hand, the percentage of Nairobi youth scoring in the above average range on these variables (1–8 %) was much smaller than the percentage of US youth scoring in the above average range (30–31 %) (Prince-Embury, 2007). These findings support the hypothesis that the majority of Nairobi youth in this sample experienced less protective strength or resources as compared with the US normative sample (see RSCA technical manual for description of US sample). The Nairobi youth mean score for Emotional Reactivity was within the average range (*T*54) and the Vulnerability Index score was slightly above the average range (*T*56) compared to the US norms. However, the percentage of Nairobi youth scoring in the above average range on both of these variables (46–60 %) is larger than the percentage of US youth in the normative sample scoring in the above average range on these variables (26–27 %).

Table 19.2 Mean RSCA Index and Scale scores for Nairobi Sample and frequency below and above average as compared to US Sample (*T* scores are rounded for ease of interpretation)

Scale or index	*N*	Mean	SD	% Below average or low Nairobi	% Below average or low USA	% Above average or high Nairobi	% Above average or high USA
Mast_T	83	45	7.13	60	31	8	30
Relat_T	83	43	6.94	64	30	1	31
React_T	83	54	8.53	17	37	46	27
Res_T	83	43	6.92	63	30	5	30
Vuln_T	83	56	6.06	5	33	60	26

Table 19.3 Comparison of Nairobi youth by gender on RSCA index and scale scores

	Sex	*N*	Mean	Standard deviation	Standard error mean
Vuln_T	Male	40	55	6.33	1.00
	Female	43	58	5.62	0.86
Res_T	Male	40	44	5.93	0.94
	Female	43	42	7.71	1.18
Mast_T	Male	40	45	6.04	0.96
	Female	43	44	8.02	1.22
Relat_T	Male	40	43	6.22	0.98
	Female	43	42	7.53	1.15
React_T	Male	40	53	9.24	1.46
	Female	43	55	7.73	1.18

Gender

Table 19.3 displays means, standard deviations and standard error for the RSCA global scale scores and Index scores by gender for the Nairobi sample. Results using *t*-tests indicated no significant gender differences on RSCA global scale or Index scores, although there was a nonsignificant trend for females to report lower Resources and higher Emotional Reactivity. Both male and female youth reported below average Resource Index scores (*T*44, *T*42), Sense of Mastery (*T*45, *T*44), and Sense of Relatedness Scale (*T*43, *T*42) scores. Emotional Reactivity was in the average range for both males and females (*T*53, *T*55). Vulnerability Index scores were in the average range for males (*T*55) but in the above average range (*T*58) for females. Examination at the subscale level found that females scored significantly lower on Trust (Sense of Relatedness) and significantly higher on Recovery (emotional Reactivity) than males ($p<0.05$).

Location

The next analysis looked at the RSCA global scale, index scores and subscale scores across locations where the youth had been tested: Tumaini School (Mathare N., area 1,slum area), By Grace Children's Home (The Orphanage), By Grace Komarack Academy (The Middle Class sample), Eastleigh (Technical School teens 15–18, ungraded as to year, most programs are for less than 1 year), and Neema High School (Teen boarding school for kids from severe slum areas) and four students from other locations. Analysis of variance across location indicated no significant differences between scores of youth tested in these different locations at the RSCA Index, scale or subscale level.

An examination of RSCA scores in Table 19.4 suggests uniformity of results across location. The Resource Index scores were below average compared with US norms (*T*40–*T*45) with the Tumaini group scoring the lowest (*T*40). The Sense of Mastery Scale score was low average

Table 19.4 RSCA Global Scale Scores and Index Score Means and SD's across Testing Location

	By grace home			Eastleigh			Komarack			Neema			Tumaini		
RSCA scale	*N*	*M*	SD	*N*	*M*	SD	*N*	*M*	SD	*N*	*M*	SD	*N*	*M*	SD
Mastery	17	45	8.17	12	46	6.57	24	46	9	8	46	3.66	18	43	5.29
Relatedness	17	42	7.71	12	44	5.12	24	44	7.51	8	44	7.59	18	39	6.19
Reactivity	17	54	6.61	12	53	9.03	24	57	8.74	8	55	8.64	18	51	9.88
Resource	17	43	7.98	12	45	5.65	24	44	8.47	8	45	5.01	18	40	5.24
Vulnerability	17	57	6.7	12	55	6.86	24	57	6.53	8	56	3.42	18	56	6.08
% of sample	20			14			29			10			22		

(*T* scores are rounded)

for two groups (*T*46) and below average for the rest (*T*45) with the Tumaini group scoring the lowest (*T*43). The Sense of Relatedness Scale score was the lowest score across locations (*T*39–*T*44). All mean Sense of Relatedness Scale scores were in the below average range with the exception of the Tumaini group for which mean Sense of Relatedness was in the low range (*T*39) when compared with the US normative sample. Emotional Reactivity and Vulnerability scores were highest for youth in the Komarack sample with both of these scores in the above average range (*T*56, *T*57).

Figure 19.4 displays *n* size, means, and standard deviations for youth at each location.

Analysis by Tribe or Ethnicity

Analysis of Variance of RSCA Index, global scale or subscale scores by Ethnicity (tribe) revealed no significant differences between groups on any measures (see Fig. 19.5). This may be partly accounted for by the fact that the groups were very small with one group having only four members. Also, ethnicity was identified for only 67 of the 83 youth in the sample so that 19 % of the sample was unidentified. Fifteen percent of the sample were youth of mixed ethnic origin or were the only representative of a specific ethnicity and were not included in the analysis. The percentage of the six ethnic groups, for which there were four or more participants in the sample are identified in Table 19.5. The percentage of each of these six groups in this sample is close to their national percentage with the exception of the Sudanese who were over represented. The following ethnicities included in the total sample but not in this analysis were the following: Embu (1), Maasai (1), Meru (1), Somali (2), Nandi (1), Taita (1), Mijikenda (1).

Of those studied the Sudanese, a refugee group scored the highest in Vulnerability (*T*62) and Emotional Reactivity (*T*60). The Kikuyu and Kisii youth scored within the average range on all measures. The Luhya and Luo youth score above average in Vulnerability and below average in Sense of Mastery. These differences suggest trends although they were not significant.

Victims of Genocide

Eleven youth, four females and seven males, were documented victims of genocide. Eight of these youth are from Komarack. All of the Sudanese (6 total) and all of the Somalis (2), 1 Kikuyu from Tumaini School, 2 mixed tribes from the orphanage, 1 Kikuyu/Luo, and 1 Mbere, Embu are included in this sample. Genocide victims' mean RSCA global scale scores are reported below by gender and for the total sample of 11. Female Mastery and Relatedness Scale scores are in the low range and Emotional Reactivity is in the above average range. Males are in the average range except for Relatedness which is below average. Although conclusions cannot be made from this small sample, it appears that females faired worse in these circumstances (Table 19.6).

Table 19.5 RSCA index and scale scores by tribe/ethnicity

Tribe/ethinicity Nat %	% of total sample	Vuln_T	Res_T	Mast_T	Relat_T	React_T
Kamba11%	Mean	56	43	43	44	54
	N/(10 %)	8	8	8	8	8
	Standard deviation	5.50	8.53	9.22	8.02	7.95
Kikuyu 22 %	Mean	54	46	47	45	53
	N/(19 %)	16	16	16	16	16
	Standard deviation	7.22	6.25	6.39	7.61	9.73
Kisii 6 %	Mean	55	45	45	45	53
	N/(5 %)	4	4	4	4	4
	Standard deviation	3.56	3.74	4.32	3.20	8.14
Luhya14 %	Mean	57	43	46	41	55
	N/(10 %)	8	8	8	8	8
	Standard deviation	4.43	4.55	6.56	2.80	7.36
Luo13 %	Mean	57	41	45	39	52
	N/(12 %)	10	10	10	10	10
	Standard deviation	4.42	8.23	8.83	6.27	8.92
Sudanese <1 %	Mean	62	40	42	39	60
	N/(7 %)	6	6	6	6	6
	Standard deviation	4.32	6.85	7.34	6.01	5.35
Total	Mean	56	43	45	42	54
	N/(63 %)	52	52	52	52	52
	Standard deviation	5.75	6.77	7.25	6.80	8.39

T scores were rounded for ease of interpretation

Table 19.6 RSCA scale score means for Nairobi youth victims of genocide

Gender		Mast_T	Relat_T	React_T
F	Mean	34	33	57
	N	4	4	4
	Standard deviation	9.52	8.96	7.14
M	Mean	48	42	51
	N	7	7	7
	Standard deviation	6.64	7.27	13.75
Total	Mean	43	39	53
	N	11	11	11
	Standard deviation	10.13	8.84	11.70

Inter-Relatedness of Emotional Reactivity, Sense of Mastery, and Sense of Relatedness

Comparison of Pearson's correlations of Emotional Reactivity and Sense of Mastery and Sense of Relatedness Scale scores for the Nairobi youth sample and US normative sample suggest some differences. For the Nairobi sample, a significant positive correlation was found between Sense of Relatedness and Emotional Reactivity Scale scores ($r=0.22$; $p<0.05$) and close to zero nonsignificant relationship between Sense of Mastery and Emotional Reactivity. These results differ from the US sample for which both Sense of Mastery and Sense of Relatedness are significantly negatively related to Emotional Reactivity ($r=-0.42$, -0.33; $p<0.01$) (Prince-Embury, 2007). This finding suggests that unlike in the US where Sense of Mastery and Sense of

Relatedness might have slight buffering effects, this is not the case for this sample of Nairobi youth. For Nairobi youth Sense of Mastery appears to be disconnected with Emotional Reactivity and Sense of Relatedness may be related to higher Emotional Reactivity. However, similar to the US sample there was a strong positive correlation between the two resource measures Sense of Mastery and Sense of Relatedness ($r=0.63$; $p<0.01$) (US Correlation, $r=0.70$; $p<0.01$; Prince-Embury, 2010). This finding suggests that a positive correlation between Sense of Mastery and Sense of Relatedness is robust cross-culturally, whereas the relationship between these and Emotional Reactivity may not be. The same correlational analysis was run by gender in the Nairobi sample yielding the following results. For males there were no significant correlations between Emotional Reactivity and either Sense of Mastery or Sense of Relatedness. There was however a significant positive correlation between Sense of Mastery and Sense of Relatedness for males ($r=0.56$; $p<0.01$). For females there was also a significant positive correlation between Sense of Mastery and Sense of Relatedness ($r=0.70$; $p<0.01$) and no association between Sense of Mastery and Emotional Reactivity. For females on the other hand there was a significant positive correlation between Sense of Relatedness and Emotional Reactivity ($r=0.31$; $p<0.05$), suggesting that this relationship held only for females in the Nairobi sample. Examination of this relationship at the subscale level revealed that this was accounted for by a significant positive correlation between Sense of Trust and Emotional Reactivity ($r=0.31$; $p<0.05$). An examination of scatter plots assured that these correlations were not due to outliers.

In contrast, for the US standardization sample Emotional Reactivity was significantly negatively correlated with both Sense of Mastery ($r=-0.42$; $p<0.01$), Sense of Relatedness ($r=-0.33$; $p<0.01$), suggesting that these perceived resources may have a slight buffering effect on emotional reactivity for US youth (Prince-Embury, 2007). Similar to Nairobi youth Sense of Mastery and Sense of Relatedness were positively correlated for US youth in the standardization sample ($r=0.70$; $p<0.01$). When the US sample was analyzed by gender these associations held up for both males and females (Prince-Embury, 2010).

Profile Analysis

Profile Analysis using the SPSS two step cluster analysis method controlling for 25 % noise factor yielded three clusters that best characterized the Kenyan sample. Table 19.7 presents mean RSCA scale scores revealed for each of three clusters and the percentage of the sample classified within each cluster.

Resiliency Profiles of these three clusters are pictured in Fig. 19.1 (RSCA Resiliency Profiles have also been determined for the US stratified normative sample see Prince-Embury & Steer, 2010). Below is a brief description of the demographics of each cluster and an illustrative case vignette.

Cluster 1 represented less than a quarter (23 %) of the Nairobi sample and was the most resilient of the profiles identified using the RSCA. Youth in this cluster group were characterized by Sense of Mastery, Sense of Relatedness, and Emotional Reactivity Scale scores within the average range representing adequate personal resiliency as assessed by the RSCA. Youth in this cluster manifested adequate resources and minimal vulnerability with a mean Resource Index score of *T*51 and Vulnerability of *T*49. This cluster was made up of more males (12) than females (7), consisted of youth from Komarack (6) and Eastleigh (5) and eight other youth from mixed locations.

Cluster 2 represented the largest portion of the sample (52 %) and was characterized by Mastery and Relatedness Scale scores in the below average range and Emotional Reactivity in the above average range. This group reports

Table 19.7 Resiliency clusters of Nairobi sample

Cluster			Mastery		Relatedness		Reactivity	
	N	%	*M*	SD	*M*	SD	*M*	SD
1	19	23	53	5.39	49	4.02	50	8.41
2	43	52	44	4.21	44	4.03	59	5.56
3	21	25	38	6.49	33	4.55	48	6.91
Total	83		45	7.13	43	6.94	54	8.53

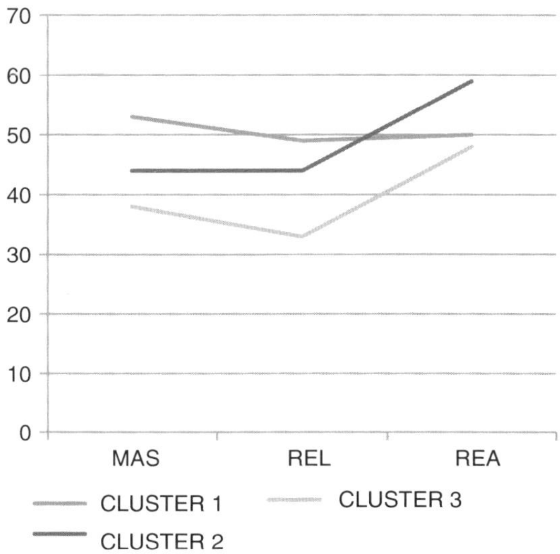

Fig. 19.1 RSCA clusters identified for Nairobi sample

below average Resources (*T*44) and above average Vulnerability (*T*59). This cluster was made up of slightly more females (23) than males (19), consisted mainly of youth from Komarack (13) and the By Grace Orphanage Home (9) and a smaller amount from several other locations.

Cluster 3 which represented a quarter (25 %) of the sample, scored in the very low range in Sense of Mastery and Sense of Relatedness and in the average range in Emotional Reactivity. This group is characterized as having extremely low Resources (*T*35) and above average Vulnerability (*T*58). This cluster was made up of slightly more females (12) than males (9), and consisted most of youth from Tumaini (8) (the majority from Tumaini School). Below are illustrative case vignettes representing each of the RSCA Profiles described above.

Case Vignette, Cluster 1: Kevin

Mastery, Relatedness, Emotional Reactivity in the Average Range

Kevin lived in Eastleigh, a Nairobi slum area which is predominantly inhabited by Somali refugees and their extended families, although a scattering of indigenous Kenyan ethnic groups also coexist within the community. Although Christianity is the predominant religion in Kenya, it is not in Eastleigh where most residents are Muslim. Nonetheless, The Eastleigh Presbyterian Church borders the community, separated by a large protective wall which surrounds the church and grounds. Within the property of the church is the Eastleigh Community Center and elementary school, supported by the church and welcoming neighborhood children and youth of any faith or ethnic background.

Kevin's RSCA Profile is illustrated in Fig. 19.2. His global scale scores are all within the average range: Sense of Mastery *T*53, Sense of Relatedness *T*51, and Emotional Reactivity *T*53. Examination at the subscale level indicated that all of Kevin's subscale scores are within the average range as well. Kevin's highest Sense of Mastery subscale score was Adaptability. Kevin reported that he can always ask for help when he needs it and can let others help him when he needs to. Kevin's highest Sense of Relatedness Subscale score was Comfort with others. Kevin reported that he can make friends easily, feels calm with people, and likes people. Kevin's strongest Emotional Reactivity subscale score was Recover; he reported that he recovers quickly when upset. In these respects Kevin's profile is consistent with youth manifesting adequate resiliency in the USA.

Kevin was first seen by the first author 5 years earlier as a young teen as he worked on a church sponsored mission project, where he participated with other Kenyan and American volunteers in constructing a heavy brick wall which separated the church property from the Eastleigh Community. This was to become the back sustaining wall of the new, local HIV/AIDs clinic. Kevin is currently an 18-year-old male student, who studies auto-mechanics at the Eastleigh Community Center Technical School, also located on the grounds of the Eastleigh Presbyterian Church. The stated goal of the community center is to restore lost hope to the vulnerable.

Kevin's program will allow him to graduate and find employment in less than a year. Currently, he works odd hour retail jobs selling local goods, making barely enough to sustain himself and his younger brother. Through organized community support and the effort of caring people at the

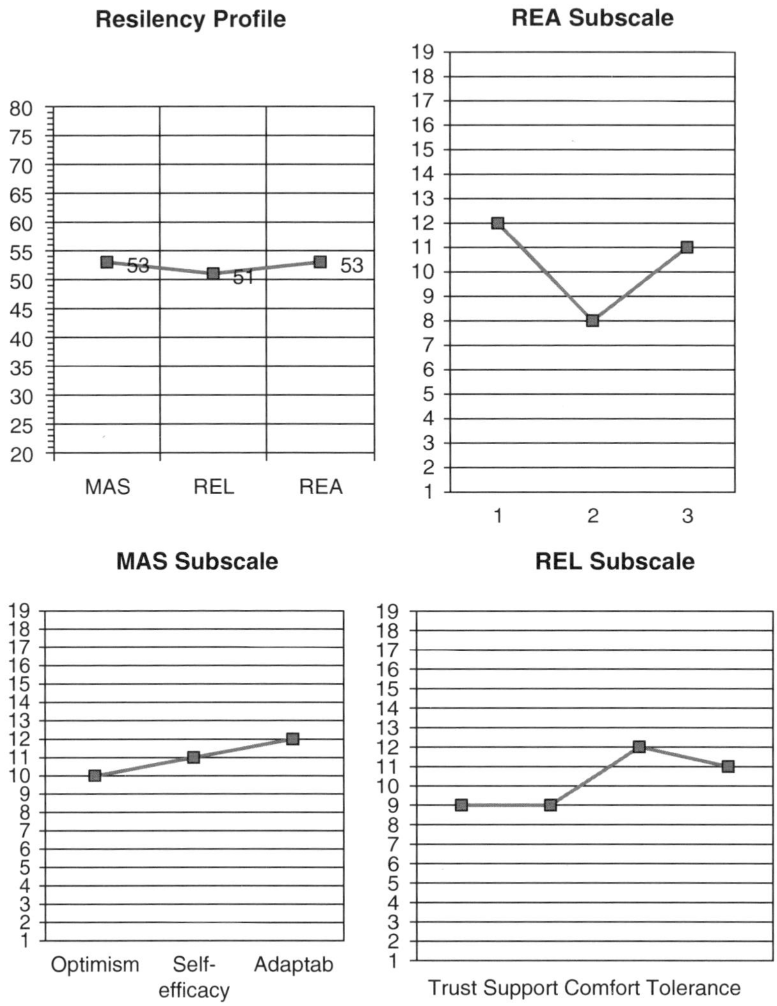

Fig. 19.2 Kevin's RSCA profile and subscale profiles

community center, the technical school program provides economic opportunity and guidance which have helped Kevin to experience the Sense of Mastery and Sense of Relatedness that he now reports.

Case Vignette, Cluster 2: Mark

Mastery and Relatedness Below Average, Above Average Emotional Reactivity

Mark is an almost 13-year-old boy whose RSCA scores placed him in Cluster 2. Mark's Resource Index score *T*36 was low and his Vulnerability Index score was high (*T*63) which in the USA would identify him as a youth who might be at risk (Prince-Embury, 2010). His Emotional Reactivity Score *T*60 is high, Sense of Mastery Scale score *T*41 is below average, and Sense of Relatedness Scale Score *T*36 is low. Examination of Mark's Emotional Reactivity subscale scores indicated that they were all high with Impairment being the highest. Items on the Impairment subscale endorsed by Mark included statements that he gets so upset that he cannot stand how he feels, that when upset he reacts without thinking, and that when upset he hurts himself. These responses are also indicators of psychological risk.

On the other hand, Mark's strengths as indicated on the RSCA are that his Mastery subscale score for Sense of Optimism was in the average range as was his Sense of Tolerance on the Relatedness Scale. Mark reported that he can frequently make good things happen and can do things well. Graphic representations of Marks RSCA profiles are presented below.

Mark came to the orphanage 3 years earlier following the death of his mother from HIV/AIDs. He never knew his father. Mark watched his mother waste away slowly from AIDs, and became so emotionally distressed that he asked to be buried with her. He has suffered from recurrent dreams of someone coming to kill him at night and has had two suicide attempts since her death. His relatedness skills were poor and he could not adjust successfully to the orphanage, running away on more than one occasion. He is now living with his maternal aunt and attends the By Grace Komarack Academy. Mark's original home was in a farming district "up country" where he learned to speak Swahili. His most trusted person is his grandfather, and he has fond early memories of his life on the farm. With encouragement by the examiner, Mark was able to visualize himself there with his grandparents as a young boy, helping in the fields where they grew bananas, mangos, passion fruit, and oranges. Several cousins still live in the farming community, and he hopes to visit them during December school vacation. At his school in Komarack, Mark is struggling to maintain a C+average. His English skills are not as good as the other students, and he will need to stay at school during the August holidays for tutoring. He likes his new school and current living situation, but continues to have difficulty concentrating as "things from the past" keep interfering with lessons being taught. His schedule is busy with classes in English, Swahili, French, mathematics, social studies, science, computer keyboarding, and sports activities. Mark enjoys soccer and describes himself as a fast runner. His future goal is to become a businessman and work in a bank. Mark appears to be suffering with Post-Traumatic Stress Disorder which is consistent with his high Emotional Reactivity Score. His emotional reactivity continues to interfere with his Sense of Mastery and Sense of Relatedness, although some positive earlier experience provide him with some optimistic attitudes.

Case Vignette, Cluster 3: Ruth

Very Low Range in Mastery and Relatedness, Average Range Emotional Reactivity

Ruth, a 14-year-old girl is originally from Kisumu, a port city in western Kenya, where she was cared for by an older sister after having been orphaned at age 6 following the death of her mother. She is of mixed tribal origin, part Luo and part Kikuyu. She became a victim of genocide in 2008, following the presidential election, when mob violence spread to her neighborhood, and rioting Luo's began killing local residents and burning their homes. Then age 12, Ruth fled with her sister, arriving by train in Nairobi, where they sought out an older brother who was believed to be living somewhere in the Kibera slum. The brother was never located and, soon after, the sister also departed, leaving Ruth to fend for herself on the streets of Nairobi. She began begging to survive, and eventually was taken to a children's shelter in Mathare North. Near to the shelter, Ruth found the small tin roofed building of the Living Word Church and began to attend services. There she met some of the children from the By Grace Children's Home who were attending Sunday School and services. She came to the medical clinics sponsored by the Foundation for Peace, and sang with the volunteers as people waited to be seen by the doctors.

One week later, she asked the chief of the children's shelter for enough money for bus fare to the By Grace Home, and not knowing whether she could be accepted, showed up on the doorstep where she was met by the children and the director. An evaluation followed, and she was accepted after official approval and release from the shelter where she recently resided.

Ruth was 14-and-a-half when she came to the orphanage, and emotionally depleted after living on her own with no family contact and no means of support for more than a year.

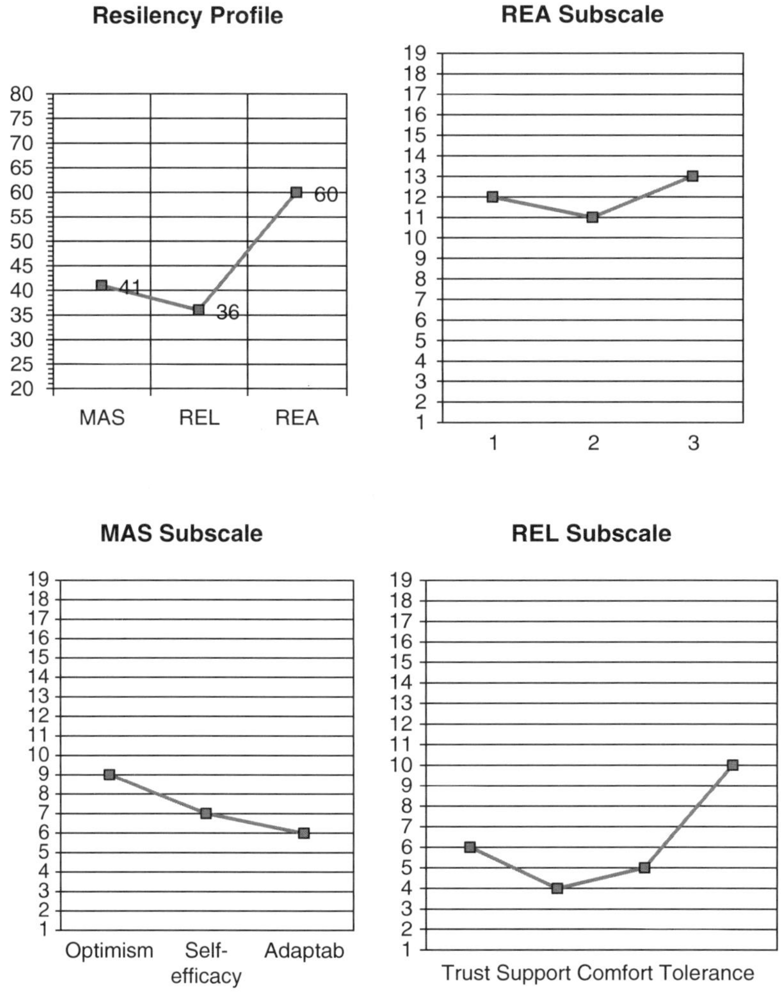

Fig. 19.3 Mark's RSCA profile and subscale scale profiles

Ruth's initial Resiliency Scores reflected her condition at the time, with a Vulnerability Index score of *T*65, in the very high range. Ruth's Resource Index score of *T*20, Sense of Mastery Scale score of *T*22, Sense of Relatedness Scale score *T*21 were in the very low range, and Emotional Reactivity Scale score of *T*48 was in the average range. These RSCA scores indicate high vulnerability due to very low perceived personal resources. Profiles of Ruth's RSCA Index, scale and subscale scores are shown in Fig. 19.3. In Ruth's case her perception matched her reality. Ruth's scores are not unlike those of other children tested who live in the slum conditions of Mathare North. Ruth's relative strength according to this protocol is her average level of emotional reactivity with Sensitivity, Recovery, and Impairment all in the average ranges. Examination of Ruth's Mastery subscale scores were all low as were her Sense of Relatedness subscale scores, see graph below. Her lowest subscale score was Sense of Support which was consistent with what her experience had been up to that time (Fig. 19.4).

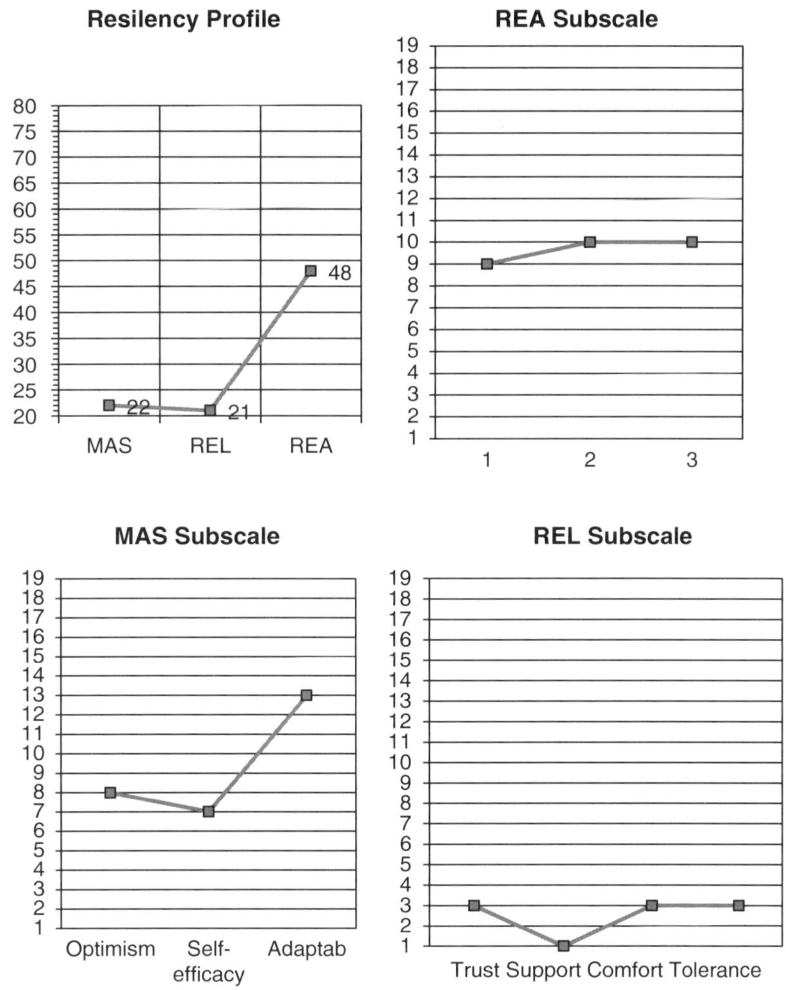

Fig. 19.4 Ruth's RSCA profile and subscale scale profiles, first testing

Examination of Ruth's responses to individual items, however, suggested that she maintained personal strength in spite of her experience. On the Sense of Mastery Scale, Ruth responded that she almost always "could let others help her when she needed to," and that "her life would be happy." On the Sense of Relatedness Scale Ruth responded that people almost always liked her and that she liked people. These responses indicated that although she had been exposed to genocide, the experienced had not soured her ability to like people. Ruth also indicated that she was capable of letting others see her real feelings and that she could tell people when she disagreed with them. These responses indicated that Ruth had maintained some resiliency in spite of her experiences. These indicators of personal strength in spite of harsh experiences are consistent with Ruth's ability to reach out and seek support and shelter at the By Grace Home. Ruth's RSCA Profile is consistent with the idea that the subjective experience of personal resiliency is a combination of the youth's strengths and their actual experience.

Evidence of Improvement with Intervention

Ruth was retested in January, 6 months after coming to the By Grace Children's Home. Living in a stable home environment where she was able to return to school, and knew that her basic needs

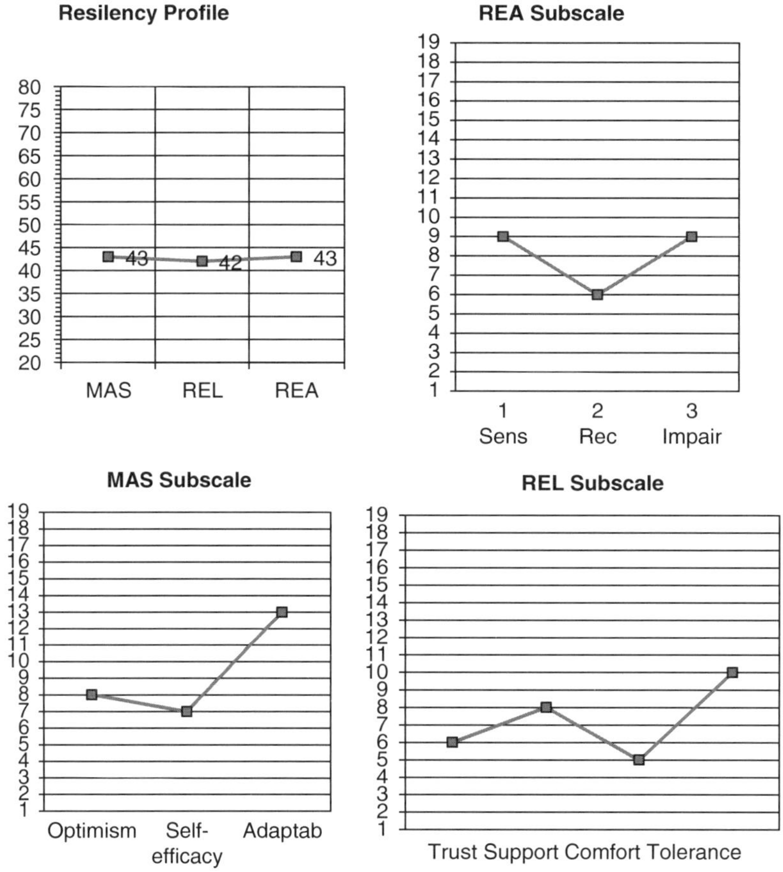

Fig. 19.5 Ruth's RSCA profile and subscale scale profiles, second testing 6 months later

for safety, food, and shelter would be met on a daily basis helped her to recover some of her basic personal strengths. At this time Ruth's Sense of Mastery (*T*43) and Sense of Relatedness (*T*42) Scale scores are still below average but closer to normal. However, these scores represents an increase of 20 points on each of these global scales. Subscale and scale score changes of five or more points are considered to be significant (Prince-Embury, personal communication). Examination of scores at the subscale level indicates improvement; Sense of Mastery subscale scores Optimism and Self-Efficacy were now in the average range and her Adaptability subscale score was high. Ruth's Sense of Support and Tolerance subscale scores of the Sense of Relatedness Scale were in the average range, while her Sense of Trust and Comfort subscale scores remained below average. Although it may still be difficult for Ruth to trust others fully, she has begun to make a few friends. Emotional Reactivity is now below average (*T*44), and her Vulnerability Index score (*T*51) is in the average range (Fig. 19.5).

With sponsorship support, Ruth now enjoys knitting as a hobby, loves to sing and has frequent opportunities to do so with other children at the Home. Her excellent English skills and learning aptitude have helped her to excel at school, and she can look forward to completing eighth grade at her current school, and then moving on to high school and possibly college. Ruth is a good example of what can happen when a child is faced with severe adversity, and then offered hope through the provision of a stable, loving, supportive environment. Ruth is also an example of the resilient youth identified by Emmy Werner who were able to seek out the support of adults outside of their immediate family (Werner & Smith, 1982, 1992).

Discussion

In this exploratory study, it was anticipated that poverty conditions and possible exposure to complex trauma in the daily lives of children growing up in and around Nairobi, Kenya would result in less protective strength or resources and increased vulnerability to stress compared to children in the US normative sample. The results of the study supported this hypothesis. Mean scores for Nairobi youth on Sense of Mastery, Sense of Relatedness, and the Resource Index were in the below average range relative to the US normative sample, whereas Vulnerability Index score was in the above average range. In addition, the percentage of Nairobi youth scoring below average in Sense of Mastery, Sense of Relatedness and Resources (60–64 %) was twice as large as the percentage of US youth scoring in the below average range on these variables (30–31 %). On the other hand, the percentage of Nairobi youth scoring above the average range on these variables (1–8 %) was much smaller than the percentage of US youth scoring in the above average range (30–31 %).

A second finding addressed the relationship between Sense of Mastery, Sense of Relatedness, and Emotional Reactivity. In the Nairobi female sample, there was a significant positive correlation between Sense of Relatedness and Emotional reactivity ($p < 0.05$) and close to zero relationship between Sense of Mastery and Emotional Reactivity. These results differ from the US sample for which both Sense of Mastery and Sense of Relatedness are significantly negatively related to Emotional Reactivity. This finding suggests that unlike in the USA where Sense of Mastery and Relatedness might have slight buffering effects, this is not the case for this sample of Nairobi youth. For Nairobi youth, Sense of Mastery appears to be disconnected from Emotional Reactivity and Sense of Relatedness may be related to higher Emotional Reactivity for females. However, similar to the US sample there was a strong positive correlation between the two resource measures Sense of Mastery and Sense of Relatedness. Interpretations of these findings require further study. It is possible that in the circumstances of the Nairobi where resources are in reality unavailable, low resource scores reflect the reality and that reactivity in the average range represents a positive adaptation to these circumstances as in the case of Ruth. On the other hand in the case of high emotional reactivity and less than average resources, this may reflect circumstances where resources are unable to buffer youth's emotional reactivity in the case of Mark. The positive correlation between trust and emotional reactivity may represent a coping strategy for some of the Nairobi females of reduced trust of others as a defense against being hurt emotionally. Obradović et al. (2010) refer to decreased engagement as an adaptive strategy in circumstances of abuse.

Although there were no significant gender differences on the three major resiliency scales viewed separately, there was a nonsignificant trend for females to report lower resources and higher emotional reactivity than males. Emotional Reactivity and Vulnerability Index scores were in the average range for males but in the above average range for females (*T*56, *T*58).

Examination at the subscale level found that females scored significantly lower on Trust and significantly higher on Recovery than males ($p < 0.05$). Female victims of genocide had scores on Mastery and Relatedness in the very low range (*T*34; *T*33) and in the above average range on Emotional Reactivity (*T*57), whereas males scored in the average range except for Relatedness which was below average (*T*42).

Analysis by location was not significant in the present study. This may be due to the relatively small *n* size for some locations and the degree of fluidity between locations when this was seen by the helping agencies' school or orphanage directors as of benefit to a specific child's needs. For example, the orphanage accepted children from the slum areas, and, sometimes, sent children to live and attend school in the middle-class community at By Grace Komarack Academy.

There were no significant differences on the RSCA between the various tribes or ethnic groups in the study also possibly due to small *n*-size for some groups. Negative ethnicity or the promotion of hatred among ethnic groups in Kenya, however, has been a long-term problem. Looking at mean scores, it is interesting to note that the Kikuyus, the dominant group in terms of numbers and political power also had the highest Sense of Mastery scores, while the Luos, the opposing group in the last presidential election, with more limited access to power, had lower than average Sense of Relatedness scores.

The cluster analysis identified three groups of youth according to similarity in their personal resiliency profiles. Youth in Cluster 1 reported Mastery, Relatedness, and Emotional Reactivity scores in the average range and consisted of several youth from the Middle Class Sample attending By Grace Komarack Academy, with a smaller number from Eastleigh Technical School and the By Grace Children's home. These children received the most support from helping organizations and benefitted most from the help they received. The youth in vignette 1, for example, had been known to the system and the first author for at least 5 years. In contrast, Ruth described in vignette 3 was the most vulnerable of the sample and had just recently been introduced to the system. When Ruth was retested in 6 months, her scores on the RSCA had improved, again suggesting the positive effect of the support that had been provided to her.

Youth in Cluster 2 reported Sense of Mastery and Relatedness in the below average range with above average Emotional Reactivity. Several of these youth are from By Grace Komarack Academy and the By Grace Children's Home. Many have experienced a variety of traumatic events including acts of genocide, rape, and the slow painful death of close relatives from HIV/AIDS and other conditions. Mark described in vignette 2, clearly suffers from PTSD, and were it not for the help and support he did receive might have taken his own life.

Youth in Cluster 3 include several from Tumaini School in the Mathare North slum area, living under the worst conditions, scored in the very low range on Sense of Mastery and Relatedness, with average scores on Emotional Reactivity, suggesting adaptation to low resource circumstances.

Limitations of the Study

1. The impact of trauma experienced by each child was difficult to assess due to the complexity and variety of traumas experienced, time constraints of the examiner and difficulty assessing the presence of trauma. A follow-up study should include a standardized measure of the trauma experienced by each child from the child's point of view.
2. Children were not all interviewed by the same person in different settings. Therefore information such as ethnic affiliation was missing for some of the participants. The first author who is an experienced clinical psychologist interviewed all children individually in the orphanage. A head teacher or lead teacher interviewed each child at By Grace Komarack Academy and Tumaini School subsequent to Resiliency Scale administration and forwarded the results to the author. It was not possible due to time constraints to conduct interviews with youth at Eastleigh Technical School or Neema High School.
3. It was not possible to accurately assess sexual abuse in all locations. Accurate data was obtained from the orphanage where children received a physical evaluation by a nurse prior to the study and were then interviewed at the time of the study by the psychologist examiner. Sexual abuse, HIV/AIDS, and emotional issues are not topics openly discussed in Kenya. Several children interviewed individually told the examiner that this was the first time anyone had ever asked them to speak about their feelings regarding their traumatic experiences. Some children found it difficult to describe their experiences, as in the case of

a young girl who was raped coming home from school at age seven.

4. Since the sample was located by helping organizations, the children in the sample were known to the helping agencies as opposed to outside the range of the helping agencies, homeless and on the street. For this reason the sample in the study may be considered to have more access to support than other unidentified youth in the Nairobi slums. Therefore the youth in this study may be those that are not in the worst circumstances in the slums of Nairobi.
5. The sample was drawn in Nairobi without a systematic effort to be representative of Nairobi, other parts of Kenya or Kenya as a country. Although ethnic affiliation was close to representation of Kenya, we cannot be assured that this sample is representative of Kenya or Nairobi but rather only of the Nairobi sample considered in the study.
6. Although estimated reliability of the RSCA global scales was adequate, it was lower than that found in US samples. This suggests that the meaning underlying the three constructs may differ for these youth as suggested by Ungar. Underlying meaning of personal resiliency in Kenyan youth requires additional qualitative study and the addition of other assessment tools.

Conclusions

In summary findings that perceived resources of Sense of Mastery and Sense of Relatedness are below average for the Nairobi sample tested are consistent with the reality that conditions of these youth are low in resources. In fact one might have expected the perceived resources of these youth to be lower on average than they were. This finding might be due to the fact that most of these youth had been identified and had had varying degrees of support by helping organizations. This suggestion is supported by the fact that the youth described in vignette 1 (most resilient) had been known to the system and the first author for at least 5 years. Similarly, Ruth, described in vignette 3, was the most vulnerable of the sample and she had just recently been introduced to the system. When Ruth was retested in 6 months her scores on the RSCA had improved, again suggesting the positive effect of the support that had been provided to her. Although not systematically tested in this study, length of time in contact with helping agencies and the ability of the youth to seek out and use this support may reflect the underlying aspects of resiliency in this sample. The significant changes reported by Ruth underline the idea that personal resiliency as expressed in responses to the RSCA reflects the subjective experience of the youth but is not an attribute or trait of the individual. Also suggested is the notion that even in extremely adverse conditions, personal resiliency in youth is modifiable with realistic changes in their circumstances.

References

Amnesty International. (2010). Insecurity and indignity, women's experiences in the slums of Nairobi, Kenya. *Amnesty International*. July, 2010, pp. 1–40. Index:AFR 32/002/2010.

Ayyash-Abdo, H., & Sanchez-Ruiz, M. J. (2011). Resilience, hope, and personality among Lebanese adolescents. Unpublished manuscript.

CBC news. (2008). *Kenya's death toll from violence*. Retrieved May 5, 2011 from http://www.cbc.ca/news/world/story/2008/02/05/kenya-violence.html.

Cui, L., Teng, X., Li, X., & Oei, T. P. S. (2010). The factor structure and psychometric properties of the resiliency scale in Chinese undergraduates. *European Journal of Psychological Assessment, 26*(3), 162–171.

Dafe, F. (2009). *No business like slum business? The political economy of the continued existence of slums: A case study of Nairobi*. Development Studies Institute, London School of Economics and Political Science. London, England, February 2009, pp. 1–35.

European Commission-Humanitarian Aid and Civil Protection. (2011). *Humanitarian implementation plan (HIP) Kenya*. Retrieved May 5, 2011 from http://ec.europa.eu/echo/files/funfing/decisions/2011/HIPs/kenya.pdf.

Gettleman, J. (2008). *VengeanceReignitesKenyanCity*. Retrieved May 5, 2011 from nytimes.com/2008/01/29/world/Africa/29kenya.html.

Goldenberg, T. (2006). *Urban somali refugees call Nairobi's 'little Mogadishu' Home*. Retrieved May 5, 2011 from http://www.monstersandcritics.com/news/africa/features/article_1233394.php/Urban_Somali_refugees_call_Nairobi.html.

Haub, C. (2006). *World population data sheet*. Washington, DC: Population Reference Bureau.

Herz, M. (2008). *Somali refugees in Eastleigh* (pp. 1–4). Black Dog Publishing: In Instant Cities.

Human Rights Watch. (1999). *Spare the child: Corporal punishment in Kenyan schools*. Retrieved March 8, 2011 from http://www.uchr.org/refWorld/docid/45dladbc2.html.retrieved.

Jordani, R. B. (2008). *Translation and validation of the resiliency scales for children and adolescents*. Brazil: Dissertation. CAPES.

Karanja, L. (2010). The educational pursuits and obstacles for urban refugee students in Kenya. *International Journal for Cross-Disciplinary Subjects in Education, 1*(3), 1–9.

Kenya-Ethnic groups. (2010). Retrieved online March 21, 2011 from Nationencyclopedia.com/africa/kenya-ethnic-groups.html.

Library of Congress-Federal Research Division, *Country Profile: Kenya* (2007). Retrieved online January 8, 2007 from http://lcweb2.loc.gov.

Low, U. (1998). *A World of Violence, The Daily Battles of Nairobi's Street Children*, pp. 1–6. Retrieved March 21, 2011 from http://www.europrofem.org/contri/2_04_en/en-viol/20en_vio.htm.

Masten, A. (2001). Ordinary magic: Resilience processes in development. *American Psychologist, 56*(3), 227–238.

Masten, A. S. (2009). Ordinary magic: Lessons from research on resilience in human development. *Education Canada, 49*(3), 28–32.

Mitullah, W. (2003). *The Case of Nairobi, Kenya. Understanding Slums: Case Studies for the Global Report on Human Settlements*. pp. 1–22. http://www.begakwabega.com/document/nairobi-habitatreport2003.pdf.

Mutambo, A. (2011). *Sudanese in Kenya Educated on Vote*. Retrieved March 21, 2011 from http://www.gurtong.net/ECM/Editorial/tabid/124/ctl/articleID/4592/Sudanese-in-Kenya-educa.html.

Mwangi, E. (2003). *Sexual abuse continues unabaited*. Retrieved March 10, 2011 from http://www.newsfromafrica.org/newsfromafrica/articles/art_2622.html.

Oberg, C., & Caselton, D. (2009). Children of Genocide in the 21st Century: Four Case Studies of Sub-Sahara Africa. The Forum on Public Policy, School of Public Health, University of Minnesota, Minneapolis, Minnesota. pp. 1–12.

Obradović, J., Bush, N. R., Stamperdahl, J., Adler, N. E., & Boyce, W. T. (2010). Biological sensitivity to context: The interactive effects of stress reactivity and family adversity on socioemotional behavior and school readiness. *Child Development, 81*(1), 270–289.

Olima, W. (2001). *The dynamics and implications of sustaining urban spatial segregation in Kenya: Experiences from Nairobi metropolis*. Lincoln Institute of land Policy Conference Paper , Lincoln Institute of Land Policy, Nairobi, Kenya. (pp. 1–26).

Prince-Embury, S. (2007). *Resiliency scales for children and adolescents, a profile of personal strengths*. Minneapolis: NCS Pearson, Inc.

Prince-Embury, S., & Courville, T. (2008a). Comparison of a one, two and three factor models of the resiliency scales for children and adolescents. *The Canadian Journal of School Psychology, 23*(1), 11–25.

Prince-Embury, S., & Courville, T. (2008b). Measurement invariance of the resiliency scales for children and adolescents across gender and age cohorts. *The Canadian Journal of School Psychology, 23*(1), 26–40.

Prince-Embury, S., & Steer, R. (2010). Profiles of personal resiliency for normative and clinical samples of children and adolescents using the Resiliency Scales for Children and Adolescents. *Journal of Psychological Assessment, 28*(4), 303–315.

Refugees International. (2010). *Somalis in Kenya: Invest in the Long-Term*. pp. 1–4. Retrieved March 21, 2011 from http://www.refugeesinternational.org/policy/field-report/somalis-kenya-invest-long-term.

The African Child Policy Forum. (2010). *Violence against children in Africa*. Proceedings of the 15th Session of the African Committee of Experts on the Rights and Welfare of the Child, 15–19 March 2010, Addis Ababa, Ethiopia. Self published by the African Child Policy Forum from http://www.africanchildforum.org.

The World Factbook (2009). Washington, DC: Central Intelligence Agency.

Ungar, M. (2008). Resilience across cultures. *British Journal of Social Work, 38*, 218–235.

Ungar, M., & Liebenberg, L. (2005). The International resilience project. In M. Ungar (Ed.), *Handbook for working with children and youth, pathways to resilience across cultures and contexts* (pp. 211–229). California: Sage Publications, Inc.

Ungar, M., Liebenberg, L., Boothroyd, R., Kwong, W., Lee, T., LeBlanc, J., et al. (2008). The study of youth resiliency across cultures: Lessons form a pilot study of measure development. *Research in Human Development, 5*(3), 166–180.

United Nations General Assembly Special Session on HIV and AIDs, Country Report-Kenya, 2010, Published by National AIDS Control Council, pp. 1–96. Retrieved April 13, 2011 from http://www.unaids.org/en/dataanalysis/knowyourresponse/countryprogressreports/2010countries/kenya_2010_country_progress_report_en.pdf.

Van Wyk, H. (2011). *The Relationship between vulnerability factors and life satisfaction in Adolescents: A cross cultural study*. Unpublished Thesis. University of the Free State, South Africa.

Wamwere, K. (2003). *Negative ethnicity, from bias to genocide*. New York: Seven Stories Press.

Warah, R. (2008). *Kenya: Kenyans are fighting inequality, not ethnicity (commentary)*. Daily Nation, 14 January. Retrieved March 16, 2011 from http://www.afrika.no/Detailed/15789.html.

Werner, E. E., & Smith, R. S. (1982). *Vulnerable but invincible: A longitudinal study of resilient children and youth*. New York: McGraw-Hill.

Werner, E. E., & Smith, R. S. (1992). *Overcoming the odds: High risk children from birth to adulthood*. Ithaca: Cornell University Press.

Cultural Considerations for Building Social–Emotional and Academic Resilience in Hispanic Preschool Children

20

Geraldine V. Oades-Sese, Mark Kitzie, Christopher Velderman, Wai-Ling Rubic, Sarah Rutstein, and Miles Waltuck

The number of young immigrant children from Hispanic families is steadily growing in the US (Hernandez, Denton, & Blanchard, 2011). Many of these families experience the adverse effects of adjusting to a new environment with differing cultural and linguistic factors and struggling financially in the context of a host culture, whose systems (e.g., socio-political, educational) are unprepared to address these stressors. Multiple sources of stress (e.g., migration, poverty, language, cultural differences) potentially have a disruptive effect on families and place children at risk for poor developmental outcomes. The transition from home to school for these children brings with it a sudden encounter with cultural and linguistic discontinuities that affect social–emotional and academic adjustment. Schools, however, can have a powerful influence on the developmental trajectories of these children through early interventions that build resilience from a culturally relevant perspective.

This chapter identifies the unique stressors and protective mechanisms experienced by Hispanic preschool children, especially those from low-income families. In particular, acculturation, bilingualism, attachment, social–emotional and academic development will be explored within the theoretical framework of resilience for this population. Culturally based risk and protective factors associated with resilience and their interaction with individual attributes, school, and family systems will be discussed. Finally, ways in which families and schools can foster resilience in children within a culturally relevant manner will be discussed. Despite the likelihood of facing many challenges, young Hispanic children can demonstrate resilience and fare well in the face of adversity with the help of their environment.

G.V. Oades-Sese, Ph.D., (✉)
Institute for the Study of Child Development, Department of Pediatrics, Robert Wood Johnson Medical School, Rutgers University, 89 French Street, Room 1218, New Brunswick, NJ 08854, USA
e-mail: sesege@umdnj.edu

M. Kitzie, Psy.D.
Youth Development Clinic, 500 Broad St., Newark, NJ, USA
e-mail: drkitzie@gmail.com

C. Velderman • S. Rutstein • M. Waltuck
Graduate School of Applied and Professional Psychology, Rutgers University, Piscataway, NJ 08854, USA
e-mail: chrisvelderman@gmail.com; sarah.rutstein45@gmail.com; mrwmusic@gmail.com

W.-L. Rubic, M.S.
Head Start Serving Northern San Diego, Community Development Institute, San Diego, CA 92128, USA
e-mail: wrubic@webkalusugan.org

Overview of Risk and Protective Factors

Resilience originates from multiple sources that are found within the child, family, community, and school. Protective factors that have been

S. Prince-Embury and D.H. Saklofske (eds.), *Resilience in Children, Adolescents, and Adults: Translating Research into Practice*, The Springer Series on Human Exceptionality, DOI 10.1007/978-1-4614-4939-3_20, © Springer Science+Business Media New York 2013

identified in young resilient children from culturally diverse backgrounds include the ability to relate to others, at least average intelligence, good problem-solving and verbal skills, and the ability to control emotional and behavioral responses (Masten & Coatsworth, 1998; Mendez, Fantuzzo, & Cicchetti, 2002; Oades-Sese, Esquivel, Kaliski, & Maniatis, 2011). These are important foundations from which social and academic competencies are derived. Equally important are protective factors that stem from the family which include, but are not limited to, close family relationships, financial stability, a lack of parental psychopathology; and community factors such as access to a social support system, access to a quality education, affordable housing and health care, and living in safe neighborhoods.

Conversely, risk factors can threaten the social–emotional well-being of young Hispanic children. Well-known proximal and distal risk factors such as prejudice, economic hardship, mental health issues, unsafe neighborhoods, family discord and violence, and ineffective schools are associated with negative developmental outcomes. However, caution must be employed when attempting to understand the development of young Hispanic children through the lens of mainstream society. Such a perspective often leads to the characterization of *differences* relative to the mainstream culture as *deficits*. Instruments normed within the mainstream, as well as mainstream interpretations and biases can lead to a "deficit model" of development which may undermine the validity of cross-cultural comparative research (McLoyd & Randolph, 1985).

Demographics of Young Hispanic Children

The Hispanic population is the largest and fastest growing immigrant group in the US (U.S. Census Bureau, 2011). Thirty-one percent of all immigrant children are from Spanish-speaking countries (Hernandez et al., 2011). Of the 4.2 million immigrant children in poverty, Hispanic children make up a disproportionate share. Children of recent immigrants have the highest rates of poverty (78.6%), while even those from established Hispanic families (in the US at least 10 years) account for only slightly less (72%) (Wight, Thampi, & Chau, 2011). Poor Hispanic children are less likely to participate in early childhood education, have limited English proficiency, are more likely to experience academic problems later in life, and are at-risk for developing delinquent behaviors and dropping out of high school (Hernandez et al., 2011; National Center for Educational Statistics, 2001).

Effects of Acculturation

Social hierarchy, prejudice, discrimination, and poverty all contribute to the stressors associated with the process of adjustment to the mainstream culture, known as "acculturation" for immigrants (Collier, Brice, & Oades-Sese, 2007; Szapocznik & Kurtines, 1980). The process of acculturation results in "great stress for child immigrants who have to face the difficult task of adapting to a host culture during a developmental period of rapid change" (Leondari, 2001, p. 36). The Social Science Research Council (1954) defines acculturation as:

> …cultural change that is initiated by the conjunction of two or more autonomous cultural systems. Acculturative change may be the consequence of direct cultural transmission; it may be derived from noncultural causes, such as ecological or demographic modifications induced by an impinging culture; it may be delayed, as with internal adjustments following upon the acceptance of alien traits or patterns; or it may be a reactive adaptation of traditional modes of life. Its dynamics can be seen as the selective adaptation of value systems, the process of integration and differentiation, the generation of developmental sequences, and the operation of role determinants and personality factors (p. 974).

This broad definition of acculturation can be contrasted with acculturation experienced at the individual level, known as *psychological acculturation* (Graves, 1967, as cited in Castro, 2003). Psychological acculturation is characterized by changes in attitudes, beliefs, behaviors, values, and identity within the individual who comes into contact with a host culture.

Generally, immigrant families will progress through multiple phases of acculturation (Berry, 1980). In the *pre-contact* phase, individuals remain within an insular community comprised of their native cultural group. In the *contact* phase, interaction with the host culture begins. This interaction will often lead to *conflict*, in which minority group members vacillate between maintaining their own culture and assimilating to the host culture. This leads to stress in the *crisis* stage and ultimately ends in one of several possible ways: *assimilation* to the host culture (high acculturation), *separation* from the host culture and embracement of the native culture (low acculturation), or *integration* of both cultures (biculturalism). The least adaptive strategy is *marginalization*, which results from failed attempts both to assimilate to the host culture and embrace the new culture, resulting in the rejection of both.

Research findings regarding the effects of acculturation on young Hispanic children's developmental outcomes have been contradictory and mostly limited to adolescents. For instance, once adolescents have assimilated to the host culture, it is typically expected that outcomes will be positive (Grossman, Wirt, & Davids, 1985). However, high acculturation of Hispanic adolescents relative to their parents and other family members has been associated with lower levels of family cohesion higher risk of deviant behaviors, and increased drug use (Brooks, Whiteman, Balka, Win, & Gursen, 1997; Gil, Vega, & Dimas, 1994). In contrast, other studies have indicated that adolescents with low acculturation are more likely to experience anxiety, isolation, stress, and low self-esteem (Castro, 2003). Fourth grade Hispanic children living in high acculturated families were shown to demonstrate a lower incidence of depression (Dumka, Roosa, & Jackson, 1997). An important distinction must be made between the acculturation of children and that of their parents/family as disparate levels of acculturation between them can increase family stress and conflict. Parental level of acculturation may impact parenting practices, which in turn may have an impact on the social–emotional functioning of their children (Brice, 2002; Cardona, Nicholson, & Fox, 2000). Thus, differences in the rate and degree of acculturation of Hispanic children and adolescents relative to their parents may cause stress within the family as their cultural identities diverge.

Research in acculturation of young Hispanic children is limited. In a sample of Hispanic preschool children, parenting behaviors were not found to have a direct effect on children's behaviors. However, negative social–emotional outcomes were found among children of parents with higher levels of acculturation (Ramirez, Oades-Sese, & Bry, 2011). Parents with high levels of acculturation tend to be more assimilated to the dominant culture. They are more likely to forgo their own bicultural identity and bilingualism—a substantial loss of social and human capital available to their children. Inadvertently, their children are often affected by the stressors associated with parental assimilation. Specifically, Hispanic preschool girls from these high acculturated families were identified as being more likely to display externalizing behaviors such as oppositional behaviors and anger problems. In another study, acculturation level did not affect the social–emotional well-being of young Hispanic children (Weiss, Goebel, Page, Wilson, & Warda, 1999). This study, however, discovered different outcomes once country of origin was accounted for, highlighting the importance of examining within-group variability. Such findings speak to the importance of viewing Hispanics as a heterogeneous group consisting of distinct subcultures and acculturative pathways. Variations in sociocultural and sociolinguistic beliefs are important considerations when examining the development of young Hispanic children (Nicoladis, 1997).

In summary, acculturation is a complex, dynamic process that is often difficult to navigate for both children and parents. The process of acculturation has a significant impact on psychological functioning; "virtually everything that an individual knows, does, feels, thinks, believes, or says can be traced to the interactions between the cultural roots of the home, the community, and the society in which the individual is raised" (Rhodes, Ochoa, & Ortiz, 2005 p. 135). Therefore, acculturation is a central factor that needs to be accounted for in order to fully understand resilience within a cultural and developmental context.

Practical Tips for Teachers and Schools to Help Immigrant Families Adjust During the Acculturation Process

- Be aware of where your students and their families are in relation to adjusting to their new environment. Offer strategies to navigate the school system and access resources that may help them acculturate with the least amount of stress.
- Pair up a new immigrant family with a "cultural mediator" to help them navigate the school system and link them to other resources in the community.
- Form family mentorship programs or connect new families together with more acculturated families to develop support networks within the classroom or school to ameliorate feelings of isolation and gain social capital from school–family partnerships.
- Welcome new families to the school by holding meet and greet nights with a potluck dinner and music to develop personal working relationships.
- Schools can offer a time and a place for parents to meet each other and create support groups at school. The school psychologist can begin and maintain these support groups and later designate a parent leader.
- Refer families to school psychologists and family liasons to gain an understanding of the acculturative process.
- Educate parents about their parental rights with respect to their child's education and school expectations.
- Encourage and emphasize the importance of parental involvement in the school. Let parents know that they are the experts of their child (culturally they may not readily accept this because they believe that teachers are the educational experts) and that a partnership between parents and teachers ensures academic success. Suggest volunteering in the classroom or school during school hours to help as extra language support and/or cultural brokers. Parent involvement outside of school hours can include volunteering as the head classroom parent to communicate with non-English speaking parents or helping with classroom activities (e.g., cutting art pieces, making Spanish labels for the classroom).
- Use bilingual parents from the school community to organize and hold orientation sessions, offer native language support, and share their insights into cultural differences regarding the role of parents in the education of their children and the school's expectations of them.
- Work with other staff, school psychologists, parents, and community members to develop a community map of resources and local organizations to share with parents.
- Translate all communication letters and newsletters for families into their native language.
- Invite parents to bring photos of their family from past vacations, parties, family traditions, and performing their favorite activities.
- Invite parents to share their talents and skills with students in the classroom.
- Invite families to bring household materials such as empty boxes of food items and canned foods that they regularly eat for your housekeeping/dramatic play area.
- Invite parents to bring different food such as fruits and vegetables for children to try. Have parents share their recipes with children and other parents in the program.
- Invite parents to bring their child's favorite food. Curriculum-wise: Every child can bring

a bread product they eat at home such as tortillas, pan de sal, pita bread, siopao, etc., to nurture a cosmopolitan palate in children.

- Visit your child's classroom or meet with your child's teacher to gain an understanding of what is expected from you and your child.

Practical Tips for Parents, Grandparents, and Extended Family Members to Help Them Cope During the Acculturation Process

- Seek out extended family members or friends who can act as cultural mediators to access information and resources about your child's school and available services in the community.
- Seek out support groups at schools, churches, or within the community.
- Continue to value and teach your child about your culture, beliefs, and traditions, while also recognizing that children exposed to the mainstream culture are likely to develop different beliefs and behaviors, especially as they enter adolescence.
- Get involved with your child's school and volunteer in your child's classroom to read books in Spanish, teach children Spanish songs, Spanish folktales, or cuentos.
- Volunteer with other parents and partners in the Hispanic community to celebrate Cinco de Mayo, and other holidays in the school so that others who differ in culture can learn about your traditions.
- Help teachers put together activities during Hispanic Heritage Month (September 15th to October 15th) and invite leaders from the community to attend, present, and participate in the celebrations.
- Contact the Family–School Liaison in your school. The Family-School Liaison works together with you and teachers to help your child meet his/her learning goals at school, connects you with community services and agencies, and helps you in any aspects of your child's education to ensure academic success.
- Ask the school administrator or Family-School Liaison about financial assistance and other resources that may help you and your family adjust well to your new environment.

The Power of Bilingualism

Acculturation influences important domains in young children's lives such as language development. In considering the impact of acculturation on language, researchers have found that the shift from one language to another is closely related to the pressures of assimilating to the new environment (Orellana, 1994). Use of the host culture's language may be beneficial in terms of alleviating acculturative stress and assimilating to the host culture. However, when young Hispanic children do not continue to develop skills in their native language before learning a second language, it may negatively affect overall language development and, in turn, the development of social and academic competencies, family relationships, and communication between parents and children (Wong Fillmore, 1991).

Early language development is linked to several factors that are protective for at-risk young Hispanic children. These include positive relationships with peers, secure attachment to significant figures in a child's life, the ability to regulate emotions, and increased autonomy (Oades-Sese et al., 2011; Oades-Sese & Li, 2011). Hispanic children are more likely to encounter obstacles not faced by other children, including competing forces between language usage at home and in the mainstream society. For these children, this often begins with their initial exposure to the language and cultural expectations of school (Berry, 1980; García, 2005). Before entering a classroom for the first time, young Hispanic children have been exposed to years of their native language which has served as a frame by which they have acquired knowledge, basic concepts, and a general understanding of their environment. Although children enter school with a complex social and conceptual framework in their native language and culture, they are likely to be shoehorned into a mainstream culture which is not equipped to build upon these existing strengths. The mismatch between home and school expectations of language and school-readiness (Kayser, 1998) can have detrimental effects on young Hispanic children, compounding existing risk factors for negative psychological and educational outcomes (Lequerica & Hermosa, 1995; National Center for Children in Poverty, 2008). These disparate expectations can affect the development of language acquisition, social–emotional functioning, and academic achievement (Heath, 1983, 1986). Hispanic children entering the education system may, therefore, be seen as "unprepared" or "behind" their same-age peers by educators, when in fact they may have appropriate levels of language ability.

Cultural beliefs about the status and role of children as conversational partners influence the quality of parent–child verbal interactions (Schieffelin & Eisenberg, 1984). For example, Hispanics may not view young children as active conversational partners at an early age and instead take a more passive, rather than active, approach to language development. They may also not work specifically on building school readiness concepts with their children in an active manner (Kayser, 1998). Furthermore, there is often a lack of emphasis on a "question and answer" format during reading and discussions. Rather, the focus may be on narratives and oral stories to communicate information (Heath, 1983, 1986). The complexity and nature of language exposure is of tremendous importance. This is evidenced by studies in which children who are exposed to their native language by family members have better language development than children whose parents are limited English proficient, yet speak English at home, which can result in restricting complex and diverse language use (Dolson, 1984). The amount of language stimulation that parents provide determines language competence in children, regardless of socioeconomic status (Hart & Risely, 1995). Children who do not participate in complex or extended language interactions with caregivers may be at risk for later difficulties upon US school entry (Schieffelin & Eisenberg, 1984). However, older siblings, grandparents, and extended family members may be overlooked in assuming the role of teachers and conversational partners—untapped resources that influence child development in immigrant families.

Children's second language acquisition has been shown to be dependent on mastery of the primary language. For instance, children will often transfer phonological rules from one language to another (Gildersleeve-Neumann, Kester, Davis, & Pena, 2008). As noted previously, young Hispanic bilingual children are an incredibly heterogeneous group. Some children tend to be dominant in one language with functional skills in another (partial bilingualism), fully bilingual (balanced bilingualism), or have limited ability in both languages (negatively referred to as semilingualism). Longitudinal research suggests that mastery in either English or Spanish with functional levels in another language (English or Spanish dominant bilinguals) during early childhood is a predictor of better reading and math skills in first grade (Oades-Sese et al., 2011). There were no significant differences found between English or Spanish dominant children in terms of later English language acquisition and academic achievement. This implies that educators should foster children's dominant language during early childhood, while exposing them to a second language in order to build already mastered skills to a higher level. Young Hispanic children who demonstrated low levels in both languages, or who were monolingual, fared most poorly.

Two general theories have been put forth by Cummins (1979, 1986) regarding the mechanism by which bilingual children acquire a second language. Based on his work with French–English bilingual children in Canada, Cummins posited that a child's development of a second language occurs at a more rapid rate when a child has developed his or her primary language to a "threshold" point. This base level of development of the first language allows the child to transfer more linguistic knowledge to the second language. In this way, the languages children learn are interdependent. The "threshold" levels described by Cummins may be environmentally dependent, based on early language exposure and the linguistic-richness of a child's environment. Furthermore, base-level threshold rather than higher level threshold was found to be enough to reap cognitive and academic benefits in older children (Ardasheva, Tretter, & Kinny, 2011). Therefore, developing proficiency in the first language, regardless of whether or not it is the majority language, is important in future language acquisition (Cummins, 2000; Oades-Sese, Li, & Velderman, 2012) and to the development of a fully bilingual child.

Attending dual-language preschool programs can have a positive impact on both English and Spanish language abilities (Oades-Sese & Li, in preparation, 2011; Thomas & Collier, 2003). For this reason, high-quality bilingual preschool programs have been a significant area of research, as exposure to an effective preschool program can often serve as a protective mechanism against negative social–emotional and academic outcomes for at-risk Hispanic children (Oades-Sese & Li, in preparation, 2011). Children are still developing first-language mastery at preschool age, and, as noted previously, early development of mastery in a primary language is essential in developing later (or concurrent) abilities in a second language. High-quality bilingual preschool programs provide language-rich environments in which significant, numerous, and complex verbal interactions with teachers, teachers aides, and other peers serve as a scaffold for young children's language development. Importantly, complexity of language, which is a key component of native language (and subsequent second language) development, was greater in children who attended dual language preschool programs (Rodríguez, Díaz, Duran, & Espinosa, 1995). Early fluency in either a native or second language has also been shown to be related to more positive parent–child, teacher–student, and peer relationships (Bergin & Bergin, 2009; Dawson & Williams, 2008). This is thought to occur in a reciprocal fashion, by which increases in language development lead to more positive teacher–student interactions, which, in turn, bolsters further language development.

Practical Tips for Teachers to Foster Second Language Acquisition and Bilingualism in Children

- Develop relationships with your students' parents, communicating to them in Spanish or through a translator. Invite them to participate in or contribute to class activities, including those that allow for expression of their heritage.
- Discuss the positive benefits of early education for their children and reassure parents that a good foundation in their native language is important and that their children can learn a second language in the school environment over time.
- Because language is the binding factor in forming social relationships, it is important that teachers learn words and key phrases in Spanish. Using Spanish communicates to children that you value their native language as well as their culture. Learn key phrases such as greetings, statements of praise, commands, feelings vocabulary, and instruction.
- Take a course in Spanish. This will provide you with additional sought-after skills as a teacher and allow you to directly experience the process of acquiring a second language which some of your students are experiencing. This will also enhance your teaching skills and provide you with insights in teaching English.
- Teachers can garner help from their teacher's assistants to learn and practice Spanish by becoming conversational partners in the classroom.
- Extended discourse in both English and Spanish during play, circle time, or small groups offer opportunities to build language skills as well as solidify teacher–student relationships (Dickinson & Tabors, 2001).
- Given that the nature of teacher–student relationships and the quality of verbal interactions have predicted oral language skills and literacy, reading books that represent children's language, culture, ethnic identity, heritage, and interests help teachers better connect with students (Baker, 2001). The combination of nurturing a child students' first language and

access to close teacher–student relationships has the potential to advance students toward bilingualism, which has been shown to have important cognitive advantages such as flexibility and meta-cognitive awareness (Bialystok, 1997).

- Observe the conversation between you and your students. Make a note on who is talking more in your classroom and on the length and quality of verbal responses of your students. Do students in your classroom have enough opportunities to practice their verbal skills? Are children's responses limited to 1–3 word responses?

Practical Tips for Parents, Grandparents, and Extended Family Members to Foster Bilingualism in Children

- Develop your child's native language by speaking Spanish at home and expanding his/her vocabulary. Use expressive and powerful vocabulary words. An eloquently enriched vocabulary in the first language will later help your child become articulate and fluent in the second language.
- Develop early literacy skills by reading books in Spanish to your child and ask him/her who, what, where, and how questions about the story. This will also help prepare your child for school by getting them acclimated to a question and answer format used by the teacher. Practicing these skills will contribute to your child's language and critical thinking skills. Reading books to your child also engages your child's attention and contributes to learning about text by making comments, predicting what is going to happen next in the story, and discussing how the characters are feeling or thinking.
- To promote maintenance of your child's native language and promote oral language skills, have your child make up oral stories in Spanish.
- Have different family members narrate stories to your child, especially abuelos and abuelitas. Use rich vocabulary and complex language even if you feel your child does not understand.
- Form a Spanish workshop with other parents and members of the community to help teachers, staff, and parents learn Spanish and immerse them in your culture.
- Learn English by working with native English speaking parents and school staff in exchange for teaching them Spanish.
- An effective way to teach children new words is by playing with your child and having a fun conversation.
- Enroll your child in a school that offers a dual-language preschool program to foster the development of English and Spanish.
- Create play groups with other parents to support bilingualism.
- Search or develop family language camps, heritage-language Saturday schools, and music and art programs in Spanish (Pearson, 2008).
- Use older adults or retirees in the community to interact bilingually with "adopted children" (Pearson, 2008).

The following sections discuss some of the key protective factors in young children such as attachment, emotion regulation, problem-solving skills, autonomy, and self-efficacy (Masten & Coatsworth, 1998; Mendez et al., 2002). Although, research is limited, the roles of acculturation, bilingualism, and cultural values will be discussed in relation to these protective factors in young Hispanic children.

Attachment: The Foundation of Relatedness and All Other Developmental Competencies

Children develop close bonds with important caregivers which set the stage for future social–emotional development (Ainsworth, 1973; Bowlby, 1969). Early demonstrations of attachment and affection in young children have a tremendous impact on later social and academic development (Caprara, Barbaranelli, Pastorelli, Bandura, & Zimbardo, 2000; Eisenberg et al., 1997) as well as the development of academic oral language skills in English and Spanish

(Oades-Sese & Li, in preparation, 2011). Attachment has historically been categorized as either secure or insecure. When attachment is insecure, children can be avoidant, resistant, or disorganized-disoriented in their attachment style (see Bergin & Bergin, 2009 for a review). Young children who develop secure attachments often have caregivers who are receptive and "tuned in" to their needs. An early secure attachment history is predictive of positive social–emotional and educational development. Children who develop insecure attachments may experience social and academic issues (Kennedy & Kennedy, 2004). Securely-attached children are also more likely to communicate and explore language than insecurely attached children, whose withdrawn and reserved tendencies result in fewer opportunities to build language skills (Van Izendoorn, Dijkstra, & Bus, 1995). Consequently, insecure children display lower levels of verbal ability (Pianta & Harbers, 1996).

It is important to note that within Hispanic families, the mother–child dyad may not serve as the only model for attachment as it does in Western Anglo society (Madding, 2002, p. 73). Within Hispanic families, there is a stronger emphasis on family ties as compared to Anglo culture, known as *familismo*. For young Hispanic children, it is often the case that they will form numerous adult attachment relationships with other extended family members (e.g., aunts, uncles, grandparents). Extended family members frequently engage in conversations and who play an instrumental role in both children's Spanish and English language acquisition. Attachment as a construct is also viewed differently in Hispanic families, where emphasis is placed on issues of respect (*respeto*) and closeness accompanied by physical affection such as hugs and kisses (*abrazos* and *besos*) (Rodriquez, 1999). Western definitions of attachment tend to overlook or deemphasize these components, and as a result, tests designed to measure the construct of attachment might miss these nuances common to Hispanic family culture (Oades-Sese & Li, in preparation, 2011).

Attachment relationships are not exclusive to parents and caregivers, as relationships between teachers and students have been recognized within attachment theory (Justice, Cottone, Mashburn, & Rimm-Kaufman, 2008). Early attachment relationships are predictive of early language ability, and can strengthen parent and teacher–student bonds (Murray & Yingling, 2000). Positive, secure attachments with caregivers are predictive of positive outcomes for children, and similar results have been found for positive attachment relationships with teachers (O'Connor & McCartney, 2007). These relationships have been shown to be particularly important in early childhood and in early school experiences (Birch & Ladd, 1997; Hamre & Pianta, 2001). While the parent–child attachment relationship is often viewed as being solely important to a child's development, Oades-Sese and Li (in preparation, 2011) found teacher–child relationships to be a more significant predictor of preschoolers' English and Spanish language competence. Positive early relationships with teachers may even counteract negative aspects of the educational or community environment. Attachment to teachers can promote a sense of security, enabling the child to explore freely, learn effectively (Bergin & Bergin, 2009), and to foster a sense of autonomy.

High-quality teacher-student relationships are more important in predicting language skills for children who come from ethnic minority backgrounds (Ewing & Taylor, 2009). Close teacher–student relationships have been found to predict better English and Spanish academic oral language skills for Hispanic preschool children from economically disadvantaged backgrounds (Oades-Sese & Li, in preparation, 2011). Furthermore, the effects of teacher–student relationships outweighed those of parental attachment relationships for this sample of children. Such findings emphasize the importance of establishing close relationships between teachers and students in early childhood school settings. Within close teacher–student relationships, conversations tend to be longer and have richer vocabulary. As a result, language flourishes and increases in complexity. However, a central factor in fostering close teacher–student relationships is the ability of preschools to bridge the cultural and linguistic differences between home and school.

Incorporating children's native language in the classroom offers many benefits such as establishing connections by building school–family relationships, cultivating positive teacher–child relationships, fostering positive self-concept and pride for one's heritage, and laying the foundations of bilingualism—all of which contribute to children's resilience. In addition, conversations within close and nurturing relationships with caregivers and teachers set the stage to provide the "linguistic framework for understanding emotions, emotional events, and ways they can be managed" (Cole, Armstrong, & Pemberton, 2010, p. 69).

Preschool settings have the potential to foster resilience in at-risk Hispanic preschool children. However, the early enrollment of 3 year old Hispanic preschoolers are among the lowest ranking groups in the US: only 27% of children from the Dominican Republic, 20% from Central America, and 16% from Mexico enroll in preschool by age 3 (Hernandez et al., 2011). Although the main causes of low enrollment are due to socioeconomic and structural factors such as poverty, unemployment or low-waged jobs, and low parental education, Hernandez et al. (2011) highlight cultural factors that have a major influence on parents' likelihood to enroll their children in preschool. These factors include a preference to care for their children at home rather than at school by non-related adults, limited funding despite being eligible to receive financial assistance, lack of awareness about the importance of early education, limited space in early education programs, and reticence to enroll children in schools where teachers lack proficiency in their native language or cultural competence.

Practical Tips for Teachers to Foster Quality Teacher–Student Relationships

- You can have a powerful influence as a teacher when you form close and warm relationships with students. These relationships provide an important foundation for language, academic, and social development (Ewing & Taylor, 2009; Oades-Sese & Li, in preparation, 2011).
- Provide a warm, friendly, and nurturing learning environment that fosters multiple opportunities to interact with students. Have multiple opportunities to smile and laugh with students in the classroom and playground.
- Communicate how much you value your students' heritage by integrating their culture and language into your daily classroom activities and curriculum—a culturally relevant curriculum.
- Have students teach you words, phrases, rhymes, poems, and songs in their native language.
- Get involved in students playtime and show them how much you enjoy talking to them.
- Create a positive learning and caring environment by using humor and relate personal experiences within the academic context (Roseberry-McKibbin, 2002). Creating a positive and safe environment where students' culture and language is validated promotes self-esteem, competence, and effective learning (Baker, 2001).
- During morning meetings, snack time, or lunch, students can discuss an exciting family event or situation or share something new that they have learned outside of the classroom (Cote, 2001).
- Extended discourse about favorite toys, super heroes, TV shows, and foods during free play or choice time offers opportunities to build language and teacher–student relationships (Dickinson & Tabors, 2001).
- Given that the nature of teacher-student relationships and the quality of verbal interaction predict oral language skills and literacy, reading books that represent students' lives and interests helps teachers connect with their students (Baker, 2001).
- During emotional situations, allow students to express themselves in the language they are most comfortable with. Use clear, expanded and rich language to describe feeling words. Parallel talk using their first language to help students express their emotions.

Practical Tips for Parents, Grandparents, and Extended Family Members to Foster Quality Caregiver–Child Relationships

- Parents can engage in regular discussions with children about events of the day or what was learned in school during mealtime (Beals, 2001), on the way to school or the supermarket, or before bedtime. These discussions should be in the child's home language, which allows him or her to connect emotionally, cognitively, and linguistically with caregivers (Kohnert, Yim, Nett, Kan, & Duran, 2005). The emphasis is on the quality of these verbal interactions such that your child is excited about talking, inquiring, building vocabulary, and expanding their knowledge base (Dickinson & Tabors, 2001). All of these experiences should occur within a "secure base" of positive and caring relationships.
- Set aside 20–30 minutes each day to have a "special time" to connect with your child about what happened in school, what was the best and worst things that happened today, and discuss what your child plans to do tomorrow.
- Share special moments together each day such as drawing, painting, baking, cooking, or watching a special show.
- Play a family game for 15 minutes after dinner.
- Read a story or share a family story before bedtime or during bath time.
- Remind your child how much you love him/her before bedtime and when you drop him/her off to school.
- Show understanding and be empathetic when your child is sad, angry, disappointed, anxious, and frustrated. Validate his/her feelings by actively listening to what they have to say in his/her primary language.
- Support your child's emotions by helping him/her describe his/her emotions in his/her primary language.
- Value your child's opinions, choices, and viewpoints by listening and making positive and thoughtful comments.

Despite its central importance, attachment does not stand alone as a predictor of later success. In fact, attachment exists in a reciprocal relationship with language and several social–emotional factors. The development of secure attachments also underlies the development of many of the social–emotional skills necessary for positive school functioning and peer interactions. These skills are discussed below.

Emotion Regulation: The Product of Attachment Relationships and Language

Emotional regulation is the process of initiating, maintaining, modulating, or changing the occurrence, intensity, or duration of internal feeling states and emotion-related physiological processes, often in the service of accomplishing one's goals (Eisenberg, Fabes, Guthrie, & Reiser, 2000). Development of early emotional regulation is an important component for social–emotional adjustment and resilience in young children (Garmezy, Masten, & Tellegen, 1984). Differences among children in emotional regulation and reactivity can affect a child's popularity with peers, adjustment, development of shyness, sympathy, prosocial behaviors, and externalizing behaviors such as aggression (Doise, 1990; Oades-Sese et al., 2011; Parker & Asher, 1987). The preschool years are crucial in the development of emotional regulation skills as children begin to gain more experience with choice, self-directed behavior, perspective taking, and other executive functions (Bronson, 2000).

Concurrent development of language skills provides children with a framework by which to control their emotions and problem-solve effectively with others in their environment (Bronson, 2000; Cole et al., 2010). Increases in language skills allow children to have an internal dialogue, plan, and consider past and future consequences of actions (Bronowski, 1977). Parent–child emotional communication has been found by Cole et al. (2010) to set the foundation for self-regulation of emotions: "Children's accurate, coherent understanding of their own emotions must benefit from parental input. When parents elaborate about events in emotionally meaningful contexts, children are more engaged in conversation and their narratives are more coherent" (p. 64).

There are cultural considerations in managing, expressing, and displaying emotions. In some cultures, expressing emotions is considered immature and inappropriate while other cultures are more expressive (Mesquita & Albert, 2007). Research on the emotional regulation of Hispanic children is limited. A recent study, however, suggests that language development is highly intertwined with the ability to regulate emotions, especially for a sample of Hispanic preschoolers (Oades-Sese et al., 2011). Hispanic children with a mastery of one language and with functional communication skills in a second language (i.e., English Dominant and Spanish Dominant bilinguals) demonstrated better emotion regulation skills compared to children who had low mastery in one or both languages (Oades-Sese et al., 2011). These children were rated by their teachers as having the ability to respond positively to adults, recover quickly when upset, modulate extreme emotions, verbally express feelings, and transition well from one activity to another without becoming upset or anxious. As a result, these children displayed higher levels of social competence during peer play. Specifically, they were likely to demonstrate prosocial behaviors such as helping, taking turns, sharing, and encouraging others. Possessing better emotional regulation skills in conjunction with language skills in preschool was also associated with higher reading and math performance two years later for this sample of children. These findings are consistent with previous research that shows that language skills predict positive expression of emotions and social competence (Cassidy, Werner, Rourke, Zubernis, & Balarman, 2003; Schultz, Izard, Ackerman, & Youngston, 2001).

Practical Tips for Teachers, Parents, Grandparents, and Extended Family Members to Promote Emotion Regulation in Children

- Teach children a feelings vocabulary to express how they feel in English and in Spanish.
- Read books that explore different feelings in different situations (e.g., birthday, holiday, sibling rivalry, moving, attending a new school) that elicits different emotions among the characters of the story. Select stories that demonstrate ways children can cope with their feelings in a positive manner.
- Cut out pictures from a magazine and discuss how each person is feeling in a given situation. Discuss how a child might feel and ways he/she can deal with each situation.
- When you see that your child is feeling frustrated because he/she cannot complete a task, verbalize and validate how the child is feeling and suggest ways that the child can cope with his/her feelings (Landy, 2009).
- Acknowledge your child's feelings (e.g., disappointment, anger, anxiety) and rephrase the situation in a positive way (Landy, 2009).
- Use puppets and stuffed animals to play out different situations and discuss feelings and other people's points of view (Landy, 2009). Role-play different ways to deal with a given situation.
- Help your child cope with his/her anger by teaching breathing techniques, methods to calm down, and verbalizing feelings.
- Set aside at least 30 minutes a day, without distractions from the TV, cell phone, or computers, to discuss your child's day, how he or she felt about the events of the day, and how he/she coped with it.

In summary, emotional and linguistic development serve as a basis for the development of the social and academic competencies essential to developing resilience. An important subset of social–emotional and social problem-solving skills are considered next.

Social Problem-Solving Skills

Early language development and social–emotional competencies have implications for children's later ability to solve cognitive and social problems. Children with poor verbal and social skills are more likely to exhibit aggression and externalizing behaviors in the classroom (Shure, 1994). The early onset and lack of amelioration of aggression and externalizing behaviors can have serious implications for young children that can lead to a variety of negative life outcomes (Campbell, Shaw, & Gilliom, 2000). A study by Hill et al. (2006) found that risk factors common in low-income, bilingual, immigrant children are predictive of externalizing behaviors in the classroom such as the inability to regulate emotions and inattention.

Children with poor ability to solve social problems are more likely to experience peer rejection and later negative emotional and psychological outcomes. This is a particular concern for preschoolers, as it has been found that aggression and peer rejection in early development are predictive of both internalizing and externalizing disorders in adolescence (Coie, Lochman, Terry, & Hyman, 1992). Such a trajectory highlights the importance of the early development of problem-solving skills in at-risk preschoolers.

A number of programs exist to teach problem-solving skills to elementary school-age children. However, there are only a few manualized, evidence-based interventions. Interventions that focus on teaching emotion and problem-solving language, as well as teaching young children how to recognize, regulate, understand, and cope with negative emotions, have been shown to be effective in reducing social withdrawal, frustration, and aggression in low-SES minority school populations (Shure, 1994; Shure & Spivack, 1982). The problem-solving language developed by these programs involves both basic and higher-level linguistic concepts. For instance, basic concepts focus on labeling and teaching emotion words, followed by children progressing to more complex language concepts such as "if-then" and "maybe." For Hispanic preschool children, it is particularly important that they develop problem-solving skills in both their native and second languages in order to apply problem-solving techniques and strategies in both the host and native cultural environment.

Practical Tips for Teachers, Parents, and Caregivers to Teach Social Problem-Solving Skills to Children

- Teach children how to solve problems or resolve conflicts (in English and in Spanish) at home or in the classroom by providing them with the steps for identifying the problem, assessing feelings, brainstorming solutions, and evaluating consequences.
- Teach children the process of solving everyday problems such as asking for help, going to the bathroom, or wanting a toy that another child has.
- Use any problem that arises in the classroom or at home (e.g., sharing one toy, waiting for another child to finish using the computer) as a teachable moment to reinforce problem solving skills.
- Create and sing a song about the problem-solving steps in English and in Spanish to reinforce learning.
- Read storybooks and watch digital media of characters facing a problem and have children come up with possible solutions.
- Help children realize that there are many possible solutions to a problem. Foster creativity and flexible thinking.
- Structure the situation to scaffold and support the children's problem-solving skills. Stay within close proximity to children and be available, if needed (Landy, 2009).
- Celebrate or praise children's successes and discuss how problems were solved during circle time so other children can benefit vicariously from the experience.
- Teach children sequences of events and routines to understand how planning can help things run smoothly.
- Allow children to experience consequences (if not dangerous or harmful) as a result of their actions in a given situation. Discuss what happened and why it happened (both positive and negative consequences) (Landy, 2009).
- Allow the child to come up with solutions first and have them try it even if the solutions are not your first choice. This allows the child to discover which solutions work as well as foster independent thinking. If the child is stuck, provide an example that may help him or her.
- Encourage children to try again or try another solution if the first solution does not work. Perseverance is key to success.

Autonomy in Young Children

Rooted in the parent–child relationship, autonomy evolves into characteristics such as initiative, agency, and self-determinism (Deci & Ryan, 1985) and fosters the development of guilt, shame, and pride (Sroufe, 1996). Autonomy is considered to be instrumental in the development and maintenance of childhood resilience and social and academic competencies of Hispanic preschool children (Oades-Sese et al., 2011). *Autonomy* refers to a child's ability to act independently and to exert control over his or her environment, including a sense of task mastery, internal locus of control, and self-efficacy (Benard, 1995, p. 2). Independence is considered fundamental to the development of social competence in preschool children, and autonomy is a necessary condition for its development (Cicchetti, 1990; Crockenberg & Litman, 1990). Autonomy is also reflected in the child's ability to initiate decisions and actions without direct guidance from a teacher or caregiver. *Initiative* refers to a child's capacity and propensity to begin an action or task by his/her own volition, without first being prompted to do so. Both initiative and autonomy influence one another, and are necessary in developing a stronger sense of self.

Teachers in Western societies tend to value these traits as children with higher levels of autonomy require less supervision from teachers, make efforts to resolve conflicts on their own, and approach tasks with a positive attitude (LaFreniere & Dumas, 1995). However, cross-cultural research has shown that the importance of autonomy in child rearing tends to be de-emphasized by Puerto Rican mothers of preschool children. Respectfulness, obedience, loyalty, and affection were found to be of higher importance as compared to autonomy for these Puerto Rican mothers. By comparison, non-Hispanic mothers were found to place more emphasis on autonomy, creativity, assertiveness, and individualism in raising their children (Gonzalez-Ramos, Zayas, & Cohen, 1998; Quirk et al., 1986). Puerto Rican mothers tended to define autonomy in terms of how the child's self-sufficiency was helpful to the parent (interdependency), rather than a sign of independence from the parent (i.e., psychological and physical separation) as interpreted by Anglo culture (Gonzalez-Ramos et al., 1998). Individualist ideals reflected in Western culture, such as personal achievement and success, appear to make independence a more culturally desirable trait. Cultural differences in how autonomy is defined as a construct are an important consideration in the interpretation of such findings. For collectivistic cultures such as for Hispanics, interdependence and harmonious relations between family members are more highly valued than independence (Mesquita & Albert, 2007).

Depending on the levels of language mastery, degree of bilingualism can promote or hinder the development of autonomy and self-efficacy (Oades-Sese et al., 2011). Bilingual skills have been found to have numerous cognitive benefits (Bialystok, 2001), including the ability of children to solve problems and think more flexibly (Oades-Sese et al., 2011). Children who have confidence and view themselves as self-determining agents are more likely to persist and display resilience in response to life's challenges and tribulations. Children's confidence, or "self-efficacy" follows closely from the development of autonomy.

Self-Efficacy in Young Children

Self-efficacy is a broader psychological construct which refers to children's confidence in performing a particular behavior and overcoming any obstacles (Bandura, 1994). Children's self-efficacy beliefs will influence how they think and feel about themselves, which in turn, affects both behavior and motivation. Children with strong self-efficacy beliefs are more successful in managing their schoolwork, and are better able to avoid potentially negative outcomes (i.e., delinquency). These children are more likely to succeed in school, highlighting the important link between developing strong self-efficacy beliefs in childhood, and later academic and occupational success (Bandura, Barbaranelli, Caprara,

& Pastorelli, 2001). Thus, fostering a strong sense of self-efficacy in young Hispanic children is paramount in helping them cope and overcome the many stressors that they are likely to encounter in their environment. To date, research in the areas of autonomy and self-efficacy of young, Hispanic children is scarce.

Practical Tips for Teachers, Parents, and Extended Family Members to Promote the Development of Autonomy and Self-Efficacy

- Provide children with multiple opportunities to demonstrate success by allowing children to try new things on their own with you as their coach or cheerleader. Structure the situation so you are able to provide support and monitor the situation, if needed.
- Although you would like to help your child solve problems and offer him/her solutions, your child needs to think for himself/herself in order to function successfully in schools and in the community. Allow your child time to independently make decisions and solve everyday problems through trial and error to foster critical thinking skills and to practice developing alternative solutions. You can offer your child support if he/she has tried multiple attempts to solve a problem and when he/she asks for your assistance.
- Teachers need to help children make choices in their everyday play and activities. As making choices may not be a norm in the child's family culture, teachers need to scaffold and nurture this skill. Explain to parents that this is an expectation and that will help their child succeed in school.
- Instill in children perseverance and task persistence by encouraging them to keep trying even though their first few attempts were unsuccessful. Emphasizing effort or hard work is important.
- Allocate chores and responsibilities at home to develop life skills and develop a sense of self by being an active contributor to the family.
- The National Association for School Psychologists (2010) suggests that parents should use *process praise*. "Praising children for their efforts and the strategies they used to bring about success (e.g., "You did well because you kept at it and tried different ways to solve the problem.") can lead to greater mastery, persistence, and achievement than simply praising children for being smart (e.g., "You did well because you're just so smart!"). Emphasizing effort and strategy helps children focus their attention on variables they can control: how hard they try and the strategies used" (p. 2). Positive acknowledgment draws attention to children's awareness of what they are doing and allows them to judge their performance on their own thus promoting internal motivation and rewards rather than extrinsic or external rewards (Kohn, 1999).

Conclusion

Despite adversity and major life challenges, many young Hispanic children demonstrate competence and achieve positive social and academic outcomes (Oades-Sese et al., 2011). However, it is important to examine how structural and sociopolitical factors influence the environment in which children develop, and whether these factors promote or hinder success (Garcia Coll et al., 1996). Differences in language, cultural beliefs, values, and traditions need to be accounted for when educating Hispanic children who come into classrooms with unique experiences. For example, Hispanic cultures have different perceptions of autonomy, and attachment relationships that may include a broader range of family members. Such differences between the native and mainstream cultures can be further exacerbated for children who come from impoverished home environments (Lequerica & Hermosa, 1995; National Center for Children in Poverty, 2008). When monolingual, middle-class, Anglo children are used as a reference for understanding Hispanic children or as a basis for applying current developmental theories that do not reflect Hispanic children's unique experiences, they will always appear to be "less than."

Hispanic children, and developing bilingual children in general, must master one language before they can attain mastery in a second, unless they are simultaneously acquiring both languages since birth. This recommendation comes from research conducted by the first author who has found that the majority of Hispanic bilingual preschool children in her studies have not developed adequate mastery in any language leading to poorer academic achievement in grade school two years later. Hispanic bilingual children with a solid linguistic foundation have an advantage in regard to their social–emotional and academic skills which enhance resilience. Therefore, continuing to support native language development is important for Hispanic children, particularly those from low socioeconomic families. This chapter focused on how acculturation and language have an impact on key developmental attributes within the context of the school and home settings. Language mastery potentiates social–emotional and self-efficacy which, in turn, reinforces language development. In this sense, language begets language, and this is true regardless of socioeconomic status (Hart & Risely, 1995).

The development of social–emotional skills such as emotion regulation, social problem-solving and academic competencies are intertwined with the development of a strong language foundation and early attachment experiences. In many ways, each of these factors are mutually reinforcing, resulting in the strong scaffolding of development which underlies resilience. We have discussed how a preschool environment which addresses the cultural and linguistic needs of Hispanic preschool children can have a significant effect on multiple aspects of development that underline resilience. The importance of high-quality teacher–student relationships is a central factor for children's success. It is therefore essential to understand and address the factors associated with low preschool enrollment rates for Hispanic preschool children within their cultural and social context and to design culturally informed interventions to increase enrollment rates.

The United Nations General Assembly's (1989) Convention on the Rights of the Child (CRC) was the first to incorporate a comprehensive enumeration of human rights for children (e.g., civil, cultural, economic, political, social rights). It states that a child—regardless of race, color, sex, language, religion, political or other opinion, national, ethnic, or social origin, property, disability, birth or other status—has the right to an adequate standard of living, access to education that promotes the *fullest potential* of the child, quality healthcare, and the *preservation of their cultural identity and language.* Hopefully, the research findings and recommendations described in this chapter can move us closer to meeting these goals.

References

Ainsworth, M. (1973). The development of infant–mother attachment. In B. Caldwell & H. Ricciuti (Eds.), *Review of child development research* (Vol. 3, pp. 1–94). Chicago, IL: University of Chicago Press.

Ardrasheva, Y., Tretter, T. R., & Kinny, M. (2011). English language learners and academic achievement: Revisiting the threshold hypothesis. *Language Learning Online First.* doi:10.1111/j.1467-9922.2011.00652.x.

Baker, C. (2001). *Foundations of bilingual education and bilingualism.* Toronto: Multilingual Matters LTD.

Bandura, A. (1994). Self-efficacy. In V. S. Ramachaudran (Ed.), *Encyclopedia of human behavior* (Vol. 4, pp. 71–81). New York, NY: Academic.

Bandura, A., Barbaranelli, C., Caprara, G. V., & Pastorelli, C. (2001). Self-efficacy beliefs as shapers of children's aspirations and career trajectories. *Child Development, 72*, 187–206.

Beals, D. E. (2001). Eating and reading: Links with family conversation with preschoolers and later language and literacy. In D. K. Dickenson & P. O. Tabors (Eds.), *Beginning literacy with language: Young children learning at home and school* (pp. 75–92). Baltimore, MD: Paul H. Brookes.

Benard, B. (1995). *Fostering resilience in children (ED386327).* Urbana, IL: ERIC Clearinghouse on Elementary and Early Childhood Education.

Bergin, C., & Bergin, D. (2009). Attachment in the classroom. *Educational Psychology Review, 21*, 141–170.

Berry, J. W. (1980). Acculturation as varieties of adaptation. In A. Padilla (Ed.), *Acculturation: Theory, models, and some new findings* (pp. 9–27). Boulder, CO: Westview.

Bialystok, E. (1997). Effects of bilingualism and biliteracy on children's emerging concepts of print. *Developmental Psychology, 33*, 429–440.
Bialystok, E. (2001). *Bilingualism in development: Language, literacy, and cognition*. New York, NY: Cambridge University Press.
Birch, S. H., & Ladd, G. W. (1997). The teacher–child relationship and children's early school adjustment. *Journal of School Psychology, 35*, 61–79.
Bowlby, J. (1969). *Attachment and loss I: Attachment*. London: Hogarth.
Brice, A. E. (2002). *The Hispanic child: Speech, language, culture, and education*. Boston, MA: Allyn & Bacon.
Bronowski, J. (1977). *A sense of the future*. Cambridge, MA: M.I.T. Press.
Bronson, M. B. (2000). *Self-regulation in early childhood: Nature and nurture*. New York, NY: Guildford.
Brooks, J. S., Whiteman, M., Balka, E. B., Win, P. E., & Gursen, M. D. (1997). African American and Puerto Rican drug use: A longitudinal study. *Journal of the American Academy of Child Adolescent Psychiatry, 36*, 1260–1268.
Campbell, S. B., Shaw, D. S., & Gilliom, M. (2000). Early externalizing behavior problems: Toddlers and preschoolers at risk for later maladjustment. *Development and Psychopathology, 12*, 467–488.
Caprara, G. V., Barbaranelli, C., Pastorelli, C., Bandura, A., & Zimbardo, P. G. (2000). Prosocial foundations of academic achievement. *Psychological Science, 11*, 302–306. doi:10.1111/1467-9280.00260.
Cardona, P. G., Nicholson, B. C., & Fox, R. A. (2000). Parenting among Hispanic and Anglo-American mothers with young children. *The Journal of Social Psychology, 140*, 357–365.
Cassidy, K. W., Werner, R. S., Rourke, M., Zubernis, L. S., & Balarman, G. (2003). The relationship between psychological understanding and positive social behaviors. *Social Development, 12*, 198–221.
Castro, V. S. (2003). *Acculturation and psychological adaptation*. Westport, CT: Greenwood.
Cicchetti, D. (1990). Perspectives on the interface between normal and atypical development. *Development and Psychopathology, 2*, 329–333. doi:10.1017/S0954579400005757.
Coie, J. D., Lochman, J. E., Terry, R., & Hyman, C. (1992). Predicting early adolescent disorder from childhood aggression and peer rejection. *Journal of Counseling and Clinical Psychology, 60*(5), 783–792.
Cole, P. M., Armstrong, L. M., & Pemberton, C. K. (2010). The role of language in the development of emotion regulation. In S. D. Calkins & M. A. Bell (Eds.), *Child development at the intersection of emotion and cognition* (pp. 59–77). Washington, DC: American Psychological Association.
Collier, C., Brice, A. E., & Oades-Sese, G. V. (2007). Assessment of acculturation. In G. B. Esquivel, E. Lopez, & S. Nahari (Eds.), *Handbook of multicultural school psychology: An interdisciplinary perspective*. Hillside, NJ: Lawrence Erlbaum Associates.
Cote, L. R. (2001). Language opportunities during mealtimes in preschool classrooms. In D. K. Dickenson & P. O. Tabors (Eds.), Beginning literacy with language: Young children learning at home and school (pp. 205–221). Baltimore: Paul H. Brookes.
Crockenberg, S., & Litman, C. (1990). Autonomy as competence in 2-yearolds: Maternal correlates of child defiance, compliance, and self assertion. *Developmental Psychology, 26*, 961971. doi:10.1037/0012-!649.26.6.961.
Cummins, J. (1979). Linguistic interdependence and the educational development of bilingual children. *Review of Educational Research, 49*, 222–251.
Cummins, J. (1984). *Bilingualism and special education: Issues in assessment and pedagogy*. Clevedon: Multilingual Matters.
Cummins, J. (1986). Empowering minority students: A framework for intervention. *Harvard Educational Review, 56*, 18–36.
Cummins, J. (2000). *Language, power, and pedagogy: Bilingual children in the crossfire*. England: Multilingual Matters.
Dawson, B. A., & Williams, S. A. (2008). The impact of language status as an acculturative stressor on internalizing and externalizing behaviors among Latino/a children: A longitudinal analysis from school entry through third grade. *Journal of Youth and Adolescence, 37*, 399–411.
Deci, E. L., & Ryan, R. M. (1985). The General Causality Orientations Scale: Self-determination in personality. *Journal of Research in Personality, 19*, 109–134. doi:10.1016/0092-6566(85)90023-6.
Dickinson, D. K., & Tabors, P. O. (2001). *Beginning literacy with language: Young children learning at home and school*. Baltimore, MD: Brookes Publishing.
Doise, W. (1990). The development of individual competencies through social interaction. In H. Foot, M. Morgan, & R. Shute (Eds.), *Children helping children*. Chichester: Wiley.
Dolson, D. P. (1984). *The influence of various home bilingual environments on the academic achievement, language development, and psychosocial adjustment of fifth and sixth grade Hispanic students*. Unpublished doctoral dissertation, University of San Francisco.
Dumka, L. E., Roosa, M. W., & Jackson, K. M. (1997). Risk, conflict, mothers' parenting, and children's adjustment in low-income, Mexican immigrant, and Mexican American families. *Journal of Marriage and the Family, 59*, 309–323.
Eisenberg, N., Fabes, R., Guthrie, I. K., & Reiser, M. (2000). Dispositional emotionality and regulation: Their role in predicting quality of social functioning. *Journal of Personality and Social Psychology, 78*, 136–157.
Eisenberg, N., Fabes, R. A., Shepard, S. A., Murphy, B. C., Guthrie, I. K., Jones, S., et al. (1997). Contemporaneous and longitudinal prediction of children's social functioning from regulation and emotionality. *Child Development, 68*, 642–664.
Ewing, A. R., & Taylor, A. R. (2009). The role of child gender and ethnicity in teacher–child relationship

quality and children's behavioral adjustment in preschool. *Early Childhood Research Quarterly, 24*, 92–105.

Garcia, E. E. (2005). *Teaching and learning in two languages: Bilingualism & schooling in the United States*. New York, NY: Teacher College Press.

Garcia Coll, C., Lamberty, G., Jenkins, R., McAdoo, H., Crnic, K., Wasik, B., et al. (1996). An integrative model for the study of developmental competencies in minority children. *Child Development, 67*, 1891–1914.

Garmezy, N., Masten, A. S., & Tellegen, A. (1984). The study of stress and competence in children: A building block for developmental psychopathology. *Child Development, 55*, 97–111. doi:10.2307/1129837.

Gil, A. G., Vega, W. A., & Dimas, J. M. (1994). Acculturative stress and personal adjustment among Hispanic adolescent boys. *Journal of Community Psychology, 22*(1), 43–54.

Gildersleeve-Neumann, C. E., Kester, E. S., Davis, B. L., & Peña, E. D. (2008). English speech sound development in preschool-aged children from bilingual English-Spanish environments. *Language, Speech, and Hearing Services in Schools, 39*, 314–328.

Gonzalez-Ramos, G., Zayas, L. H., & Cohen, E. V. (1998). Child-rearing values of low-income, urban Puerto Rican mothers of preschool children. *Professional Psychology: Research and Practice, 29*, 377–382. doi:10.1037/0735-7028.29.4.377.

Grossman, B., Wirt, T., & Davids, A. (1985). Self-esteem, ethnic identity, and behavioral adjustment among Anglo and Chicano adolescents in West Texas. *Journal of Adolescence, 8*, 57–68.

Hamre, B. K., & Pianta, R. C. (2001). Early teacher–child relationships and the trajectory of children's school outcomes through eighth grade. *Child Development, 72*, 625–638.

Hart, B., & Risely, T. (1995). *Meaningful differences in everyday experiences of young American children*. Baltimore, MD: Paul H. Brooks.

Heath, S. B. (1983). *Ways with words: Language, life and work in communities and classrooms*. Cambridge: Cambridge University Press.

Heath, S. B. (1986). Separating "things of the imagination" from life learning to read and write. In W. Tesle & E. Sulzby (Eds.), *Emergent literacy* (pp. 156–172). Norwood, NJ: Able.

Hernandez, D. J., Denton, N. A., & Blanchard, V. L. (2011). Children in the United States of America: A statistical portrait by race-ethnicity, immigrant origins, and language. *The Annals of the American Academy of Political and Social Science, 633*, 102–127. doi:10.1177/0002716210383205.

Hill, A., Degnan, K., Calkins, S. D., & Keane, S. P. (2006). Profiles of externalizing behavior problems for boys and girls across preschool: The roles of emotion regulation and inattention. *Developmental Psychology, 42*, 913–928.

Justice, L. M., Cottone, E. A., Masburn, A., & Rimm-Kaufman, S. E. (2008). Relationships between teachers and preschoolers who are at risk: Contribution of children's language skills, temperamentally based attributes, and gender. *Early Education & Development, 19*, 600–621.

Kayser, H. (1998). *Assessment and intervention resource for Hispanic children*. San Diego, CA: Singular Publishing.

Kennedy, J. H., & Kennedy, C. E. (2004). Attachment theory: Implications for school psychology. *Psychology in the Schools, 41*(2), 247–259.

Kohn, A. (1999). *Punished by rewards: The trouble with gold stars, incentive plans, A's, praise, and other bribes*. New York, NY: Houghton Mifflin.

Kohnert, K., Yim, D., Nett, K., Kan, P. F., & Duran, L. (2005). Intervention with linguistically diverse preschool children: A focus on developing home language(s). *Language, Speech, and Hearing Services in Schools, 36*, 251–263.

Ladd, G. W., & Burgess, K. (2001). Do relational risks and protective factors moderate the linkages between childhood aggression and early psychological and school adjustment? *Child Development, 72*(5), 1579–1601.

LaFreniere, P., & Dumas, J. (1995). *Social competence and behaviour evaluation, preschool evaluation*. Los Angeles, CA: Western Psychological Services.

Landy, S. (2009). *Pathways to competence: Encouraging healthy social and emotional development in young children* (2nd ed.). Baltimore, MD: Paul H. Brookes.

Lequerica, M., & Hermosa, B. (1995). Maternal reports of behavioral problems in preschool Hispanic children: An exploratory study in preventive pediatrics. *Journal of National Medical Association, 87*, 861–868.

Madding, C. C. (2002). Socialization practices of Latinos. In A. E. Brice (Ed.), *The Hispanic child: Speech, language, culture, and education* (pp. 68–84). Boston, MA: Allyn & Bacon.

Masten, A. S., & Coatsworth, J. D. (1998). The development of competence in favorable and unfavorable environments: Lessons from research of successful children. *American Psychologist, 53*, 205–220.

McLoyd, V. C., & Randolph, S. M. (1985). Secular trends in the study of Afro-American children: A review of "Child Development", 1936–1980. In *Monographs of the society for research in child development* (Vol. 50, (4/5), pp. 78–92). History and research in child development.

Mendez, J. L., Fantuzzo, J., & Cicchetti, D. (2002). Profiles of social competence among low-income African American preschool children. *Child Development, 73*, 1085–1100.

Mesquita, B., & Albert, D. (2007). The cultural regulation of emotions. In J. J. Gross (Ed.), *Handbook of emotional regulation* (pp. 485–503). New York, NY: Guilford.

Murray, A. D., & Yingling, J. L. (2000). Competence in language at 24 months: Relations with attachment security and home stimulation. *The Journal of Genetic Psychology, 161*(2), 133–140.

National Association for School Psychologists (2010). Self-Efficacy: Helping children believe they can succeed. Communique, 39(3), 1–4.

National Center for Children in Poverty. (2008). *United States early childhood profile: U.S.A.* Retrieved May 21, 2010, from http://www.nccp.org/profiles/pdf/profile_early_childhood_U.S..pdf

National Center for Educational Statistics. (2001). *Digest of education statistics.* Retrieved February 4, 2004, from http://nces.ed.gov/pubs2002/2002130.pdf

Nicoladis, E. (1997). Language development in preschool bilingual children. *Journal of Speech-Language Pathology and Audiology, 21*(4), 258–270.

O'Connor, E., & McCartney, K. (2007). Examining teacher–child relationships and achievement as part of an ecological model of development. *American Educational Research Journal, 44*(2), 340–369.

Oades-Sese, G. V., Esquivel, G. B., Kaliski, P. K., & Maniatis, L. (2011). A longitudinal study of the social and academic competence of economically disadvantaged bilingual preschool children. *Developmental Psychology, 47*, 747–764. doi:10.1037/a0021380.

Oades-Sese, G. V., & Li, S. (in preparation) Effects of dual language programs on preschool children's bilingual language skills.

Oades-Sese, G. V., & Li, Y. (2011). Attachment relationships as predictors of language skills for at-risk bilingual preschool children. *Psychology in the Schools.* doi:10.1002/pits.20583.

Oades-Sese, G. V., Li, S., & Velderman, C. (submitted for publication). The effects of cognitive abilities on bilingual skills of at-risk Hispanic American preschool children.

Ochoa, S. H., & Ortiz, S. O. (2005). Language proficiency assessment: The foundation for psychoeducational assessment of second-language learners. In R. Rhodes, S. H. Ochoa, & S. O. Ortiz (Eds.), *Assessing culturally and linguistically diverse students: A practical guide.* New York: Guilford Press.

Orellana, M. F. (1994). Appropriating the voice of the superheroes: Three preschoolers' bilingual language uses in play. *Early Childhood Research Quarterly, 9*, 171–193.

Parker, J. G., & Asher, S. R. (1987). Peer relations and later personal adjustment: Are low-accepted children "at risk"? *Psychological Bulletin, 102*, 357–389.

Pearson, B. Z. (2008). *A step-by-step guide for parents raising a bilingual child.* New York, NY: Living Language.

Pianta, R. C., & Harbers, K. (1996). Observing mother and child behavior in problem-solving situation at school entry: Relations with academic achievement. *Journal of School Psychology, 67*, 307–322.

Quirk, M., Ciottone, R., Minami, J., Wapner, S., Yamamoto, S., Ishii, S., et al. (1986). Values mothers hold for handicapped and nonhandicapped preschool children in Japan, Puerto Rico, and the United States Mainland. *International Journal of Psychology, 21*, 463–485. doi:10.1080/00207598608247602.

Ramirez, V., Oades-Sese, G. V., & Bry, B. (submitted for publication). The effects of parental acculturation and parenting behaviors on the social–emotional functioning of young Hispanic children.

Rodríguez, J. L., Díaz, R. M., Duran, D., & Espinosa, L. (1995). The impact of bilingual preschool education on the language development of Spanish-speaking children. *Early Childhood Research Quarterly, 10*, 475–490.

Rodriquez, G. (1999). *Raising nuestros ninos: Bring up children in a bicultural world.* New York, NY: Fireside.

Roseberry-McKibbin, C. (2002). Principles and strategies in intervention. In A. E. Brice, The Hispanic child: Speech, language, culture, and education (pp. 199–233). Boston: Allyn & Bacon.

Schieffelin, B. B., & Eisenberg, A. R. (1984). Cultural variation in children's conversations. In R. L. Schiefelbusch & A. Pickar (Eds.), *The development of communicative competence* (pp. 237–266). Baltimore, MD: University Park Press.

Schultz, D., Izard, C. E., Ackerman, B. P., & Youngstrom, E. A. (2001). Emotion knowledge in economically disadvantaged children: Self-regulatory antecedents and relations to social difficulties and withdrawal. *Development & Psychopathology, 13*, 53–67.

Shure, M. B. (1994, October). *I can problem solve (ICPS): A cognitive approach to preventing early high risk behaviors.* Presented at Safe Schools, Safe Students Conference, Washington, DC.

Shure, M. B., & Spivack, G. (1982). Interpersonal problem-solving in young children: A cognitive approach to prevention. *American Journal of Community Psychology, 10*(3), 341–356.

Social Science Research Council. (1954). Acculturation: An exploratory formulation. *American Anthropologist, 56*, 973–1002.

Sroufe, L. A. (1996). *Emotional development: The organization of emotional life in the early years.* New York, NY: Cambridge University Press.

Szapocznik, J., & Kurtines, W. M. (1980). Acculturation, biculturalism, and adjustment among Cuban Americans. In A. Padilla (Ed.), *Recent advances in acculturation research: Theory, models, and some new findings* (pp. 139–157). New York, NY: Westview.

Thomas, W. P., & Collier, V. P. (2003). The multiple benefits of dual language. *Educational Leadership, 61*(2), 61–64.

U.S. Census Bureau. (2011). *The Hispanic population: 2010.* Retrieved from, http://www.census.gov/prod/cen2010/briefs/c2010br-04.pdf

United Nations General Assembly. (1989). *On the Rights of the Child 44/25.* New York: United Nations. Retrieved from http://www2.ohchr.org/english/law/crc.htm

Van IJzendoorn, M. H., Dijkstra, J., & Bus, A. G. (1995). Attachment, intelligence, and language: A meta-analysis. *Social Development, 4*(2), 115–128.

Weiss, S. J., Goebel, P., Page, A., Wilson, P., & Warda, M. (1999). The impact of cultural and familial context on behavioral and emotional problems of preschool Latino children. *Child Psychiatry and Human Development, 29*, 287–301.

Wight, V. R., Thampi, K., & Chau, M. (2011). http://nccp.org/publications/pub_1006.html. Poor children by parents' nativity: What do we know?. National Center for Children in Poverty, Columbia University Mailman School of Public Health.

Wong Fillmore, L. (1991). When learning a second language means losing the first. *Early Childhood Research Quarterly, 6*, 323–346.

A Strengths-Based Social Psychological Approach to Resiliency: Cultural Diversity, Ecological, and Life Span Issues

21

Phillip J. Bowman

..."But still, like dust...like hopes spring high... like air, I'll rise...Bringing the gifts that my ancestors gave...I rise."—from STILL I RISE by Maya Angelou, 1986.

Over the past 50 years, the study of resiliency continues to evolve with a theoretical focus on related psychosocial issues—psychopathology, vulnerability, risk, protection, and strengths—and their implications for preventive intervention and assessment (e.g., Cicchetti & Cohen, 1995; Erikson, 1968, 1980; Fergus & Zimmerman, 2005; Garmezy, 1971, 1984, 1991; Luthar, 1991, 2003; Masten, 1994, 2001; Prince-Embury, 2007, 2010; Rutter, 1987, 1993; Werner & Smith, 1992). Studies continue to investigate these psychosocial issues to deepen our understanding of *resiliency* or why some people bounce back and thrive in the face of adversity while the less adaptive experience more negative outcomes. A major challenge for future research is to develop integrative theoretical frameworks to further clarify complex resiliency processes among marginalized racial/ethnic[1] populations faced with chronic adversity within the USA and other diversifying nations in the twenty-first century (e.g. Bowman, 2006, 2011; Bowman & Betancur, 2010; Feagin & Feagin, 1999; Jackson, 2000; Marger, 2000; Rowley & Bowman, 2009).

To provide a better foundation for such inquiry, this chapter critically reviews major research perspectives in existing literature and presents an integrative strengths-based social psychological approach to resiliency theory, intervention, and related assessment. With a particular focus on marginalized racial–ethnic populations, this chapter begins with an analysis of the complex *resiliency*

P.J. Bowman, Ph.D. (✉)
National Center for Institutional Diversity (NCID), The University of Michigan, 3338 Education Building, 610 East University Avenue, Ann Arbor, MI 48109-1259, USA
e-mail: pjbowman@umich.edu

[1]Throughout this chapter we link the terms "racial/ethnic" because of the complex interplay between these two diversity constructs—especially in the USA. Generally, ethnic groups of all national origins within the USA are also racially classified as either *white* (European phenotype) or *black* (African phenotype) *or* increasingly as another *racialized category*—Native American/Indian, Hispanic/Latino, Asian/Pacific, Middle Eastern/Arab, etc. At other times, we use these two terms separately when greater conceptual specificity and clarity are needed to amplify the discussion. Hence, ethnic refers to the national, social, and/or cultural heritage of a group. In contrast, the increasingly contested construct of race has less to do with biology and more to do with racialized systems of social stratification, caste-like inequality, and related group ideologies, interests, and policies.

S. Prince-Embury and D.H. Saklofske (eds.), *Resilience in Children, Adolescents, and Adults: Translating Research into Practice*, The Springer Series on Human Exceptionality, DOI 10.1007/978-1-4614-4939-3_21, © Springer Science+Business Media New York 2013

concept and related research perspectives that focus on the effects of psychosocial risk, vulnerability, protection, and strengths on psychopathology and resilient outcomes. Second, major theoretical propositions in a *strengths-based social psychological approach* to resiliency are highlighted along with related conceptual, assessment, and preventive intervention issues. Third, this integrative strengths-based framework is employed to help better understand the socio-cultural context of resiliency including *cultural diversity*, *ecological*, and *life span development considerations*. Finally, a *reciprocal-translation model* is presented to promote the importance of bridging strengths-based resiliency scholarship with more policy-relevant preventive intervention research and assessment systems.

Resiliency Research Perspectives

Conceptual Issues and Evolving Psychosocial Themes

The resiliency concept derives from the Latin word meaning to jump or bounce back. With an emphasis on human agency, the psychological literature on resiliency has focused on critical life stress, psychosocial adaptation, and developmental processes (e.g. Brooks & Goldstein, 2005; Katz, 1997; Kersting, 2003; Masten & Reed, 2002; McCubbin et al., 1993; Smith, 2006a, 2006b). The psychosocial concept of resiliency refers to an individual's adaptation and healthy development in the face of life stressors or strains that can be severe (Hetherington & Blechman, 1996; Katz, 1997; Kersting, 2003; Masten, 2001). The evolving literature on this rather complex construct has begun to make clearer distinctions between resilience, resiliency, and resilient outcomes. For example, some researchers refer to resiliency as personal attributes and resilience as person and environment interaction (e.g. Prince-Embury, 2007; Prince-Embury & Courville, 2008a, 2008b). Others view *resiliency* as the *process* of persisting in the face of adversity with a focus on how an individual successfully struggles rather than the end goal or *resilient outcome* (Masten & Reed, 2002; McCubbin et al., 1993). In this process, *resilience* can occur when a person shows strength rather than vulnerability in response to adversity or risk exposure. A related *adversity paradox* is noted when a person becomes stronger by confronting or mastering adversity rather than by denying or distorting it (Affleck & Tenneen, 1996; Smith, 2006a, 2006b). Hence, the resilient person becomes stronger and achieves positive outcomes while confronting adversity. However, the other side of the paradox is that chronic exposure to adversity can also erode resources, produce psychosocial harm, and increase vulnerability rather than strength.

Early research on resiliency focused on why some children and adolescents managed to thrive despite adversity while others developed psychopathology (e.g., Erikson, 1968; Garmezy, 1971, 1984, 1991; Garmezy, Masten, & Tellegen, 1989; Luthar, 1991; Rutter, 1987, 1993; Werner & Smith, 1992). As illustrated in Table 21.1, four sets of explanatory factors are highlighted in the expanding resiliency literature—*environmental risk factors*, *personal vulnerability*, *environmental protective factors*, and *personal strengths* (Evans, 2004; Brooks & Goldstein, 2005; Lightsey, 2006; Luthar, 2003; Luthar, Cicchetti, & Becker, 2000; Masten, 2001; Prince-Embury, 2007; Reich, Zautra, & Hall, 2010; Smith, 2006a, 2006b; Zimmerman & Brenner, 2010). These *four evolving resiliency research perspectives* differ in the degree to which they emphasize *internal* or *external causal factors* in the study of *negative risks* or *positive adaptation* patterns in the psychosocial stress-coping process.

Table 21.1 Evolving resiliency research perspectives

Psychosocial stress-coping process				
		Negative risks		Positive adaptation
Causal Factors	External	*Environmental risk factors*	×	*Environmental protective factors*
		↓		↓
	Internal	*Personal vulnerabilities*	×	*personal strengths*
		↓		↓
		Psychopathology	vs.	resilient outcomes

The evolving literature continues to clarify the pivotal factors—both environmental and personal—in the lives of people who somehow thrive in the face of adversity rather than fall victim to distress with less adaptive psychosocial outcomes (e.g. Garmezy, 1984, 1991; Luthar, 2003; Prince-Embury, 2007; Rutter, 1987). In the context of environmental risks, resiliency studies may focus on the effects of personal vulnerabilities, personal strengths, or external protective factors in adaptive outcomes. Resiliency research may also consider the complex interactions between *external risk factors* and *personal vulnerabilities* on the one hand and *external protective factors* and *personal strengths* on the other.

As suggested in Table 21.1, one direction for future resiliency theory and research is to provide further insight into two interrelated psychosocial strain-adaptation hypotheses. First, the *psychosocial strain hypothesis* is that chronic environmental risk factors increase personal vulnerabilities which, in turn, reduce psychological wellbeing and resilient outcomes. This first hypothesis is based on growing evidence in the psychosocial stress literature that chronic role-related strains rooted in systemic inequalities elevate psychopathological symptoms more than short-term life events (e.g. Kahn, Wolfe, Quinn, Snoek, & Rosenthal, 1964; Kaplan, 1996; Kessler, 1979; Pearlin, 1983; Pearlin, Menaghan, Lieberman, & Mullan, 1981). Second, the *psychosocial adaptation hypothesis* is that, despite chronic environmental risks and vulnerabilities, protective socio-cultural factors can reinforce personal strengths which, in turn, promote resilient outcomes (e.g. Bowman, 1989, 2006, 2011; Bronfenbrenner, 1979, 1996; Masten, 1994; Pearlin & Schooler, 1978). This second hypothesis supports the importance of a strengths-based approach to resiliency among marginalized racial/ethnic populations.

Resiliency Research on Marginalized Populations: A Challenge for the Twenty-First Century

Guided by these two interrelated psychosocial strain-adaptation hypotheses, future research can help to further clarify critical resiliency processes within the context of marginalized racial–ethnic populations faced with intergenerational inequalities and chronic adversity in major life roles (e.g. Bowman, 2006, 2011; Bowman & Betancur, 2010; Marger, 2000; Wilson, 1978, 1987, 1996). In the USA and beyond, such resiliency challenges are increasingly exacerbated as historical inequities combine with globalization, immigration, and growing intergroup disparities. Moreover, a conservative color-blind discourse in the twenty-first century continues to make these unique resiliency challenges both controversial and ill understood. Globalization, race, ethnicity, and class interact in complex ways to place marginalized group members at disturbing risks for persistent school failure, underemployment, family poverty, stress-related illness, and other psychosocial problems. However, despite such risks, many defy the odds and excel in student, work, family, community, and national leadership roles.

Because of the unique history of the USA, there is a substantial literature on risk and resiliency issues among marginalized racial–ethnic populations—especially African Americans (e.g. Berry & Blassingame, 1985; Billingsley, 1992; Bowman, 1989; Hill, 1998; Jackson, 1991, 2000; Johnson & Bowman, 2003; Neighbors, Jackson, Bowman, & Gurin, 1983; Rowley & Bowman, 2009). For example, Hill (1998) documented how African American families have promoted resilience by empowering individuals to show strength rather than vulnerability in the face of chronic risk exposure and role-related adversity. Such studies also provide unique insight into the *adversity paradox* that people can become stronger by confronting or mastering adversity especially when supported by strong family, community, and cultural support systems (Affleck & Tenneen, 1996; Smith, 2006a, 2006b).

Similar to the USA, a growing body of research on marginalized immigrant and ethnic–racial groups in other diversifying nations also supports the importance of better understanding how resiliency operates within a variety of socio-cultural contexts (Bowman & Betancur, 2010; Janssens, Bechtoldt, Ruijter, Pinelli, Prarolo, & Stenius, 2010; Marger, 2000). For example, Janssens et al. (2010) presents several cross-national studies of cultural diversity with a focus on concepts such as social exclusion, segregation, institutional barriers, and concentrated poverty which help clarify the global context of chronic environmental risks, problematic outcomes, and resiliency challenges among marginalized groups. These cross-national studies strongly suggest that cultural diversity policies can promote multilevel interventions including strategies that reinforce resiliency among individuals in marginalized populations despite personal adversity associated with systemic inequalities, chronic poverty, environmental threats, and globalization.

Cross-national resiliency studies can further clarify how institutionalized barriers and discriminatory organizational practices, especially in economic and educational contexts, pose major resiliency challenges for marginalized racial–ethnic group members. Across a range of national settings, systemic barriers can impose chronic psychosocial strains, pressures and frustrations in major social roles. The socio-cultural contexts may differ, but the basic focus on chronic environmental risks, vulnerabilities, and the desirability of resilience over problematic outcomes remains a central challenge for individuals from all marginalized populations. Within diversifying socio-cultural contexts, resiliency research is needed to better clarify pivotal factors that mitigate deleterious links between chronic environmental risks, personal vulnerabilities, and problematic outcomes. To guide such research on marginalized populations, critical resiliency issues in the two psychosocial stain-adaptation hypotheses are discussed in greater detail below along with related conceptual, theoretical, and empirical literature.

Psychosocial Strain and Resiliency: Beyond Risks, Vulnerabilities, and Psychopathology

Generally, a *risk factor* is any aspect of the person or the environment that increases the likelihood of a negative outcome (e.g., Dryfoos, 1990; Garbarino, 1991; Rhodes & Brown, 1991; Rowley & Bowman, 2009; Sanders, 2000). Despite some conceptual confusion in existing literature, Table 21.1 makes a clear distinction between *external or environmental risks* and *internal or personal vulnerabilities* that increase the probability of a negative outcome. Based on this distinction, resiliency-related research seeks to clarify the relationships between modifiable environmental risks, personal vulnerabilities, and problematic outcomes. For example, research on African Americans has helped to clarify how multilevel race-related risks—societal, institutional, community, and familial—tend to erode one's personal sense of efficacy and increase psychosocial distress (e.g. Bowman, 1989; Bowman, Jackson, Hatchett, & Gurin, 1982; Gary & Leashore, 1982; Miller & Dreger, 1973; Williams, Neighbors, & Jackson, 2003).

Risks, Vulnerabilities, and Resiliency: Going beyond the *psychosocial strain hypothesis*, future research needs to further clarify conditions under which chronic risk factors result in resilient outcomes—*rather than* increase personal vulnerabilities and result in psychopathological symptoms. In the face of such chronic risks, future resiliency research can help to further clarify specific socio-cultural factors that reinforce a sense of mastery, psychological well-being, and resilient outcomes. A growing number of studies on African Americans in high-risk circumstances have already begun to clarify such sources of resiliency despite chronic risks and personal vulnerabilities (e.g. Byrd & Chavous, 2009; Bowman, 1989; Caldwell, Kohn-Wood, Schmeelk-Cone, Chavous, & Zimmerman, 2004; Fergus & Zimmerman, 2005; Jackson, 1991, 2000; Neighbors et al., 1983; Rowley & Bowman, 2009; Spencer, Cole, DuPree, & Glymp, 1993; Zimmerman & Brenner, 2010). In the public health tradition, future research can also further clarify how such resiliency factors function, and design interventions to prevent, reduce, or eliminate problematic outcomes (e.g. psychosocial distress, health disparities, social role achievement gaps, etc).

Beyond Psychopathology to Resiliency: Despite advances in research on resiliency, traditional studies on racial–ethnic groups in high-risk environments continue to focus disproportionately on psychopathology rather than resiliency processes (Bowman, 1989; Jackson, 1991; Miller & Dreger, 1973). Rather than external barriers, traditional theory-driven pathology studies among African Americans have tended to view their own internal psychological and cultural deficits as primary causal factors. Moreover, despite larger samples, pathology-oriented statistics on US racial–ethnic minorities are too often framed in denigrating cross-racial comparisons and used to reinforce mainstream stereotypes or victim-blaming ideologies. Ryan (1972) and others have documented how such pathology-oriented statistics have too often been utilized to "blame the victim" and frame a bleak portrait of racial–ethnic minorities as essentially deviant or pathological.

Traditional studies of marginalized populations that narrowly focus on psychopathology rather than resiliency are often restricted by both conceptual and methodological problems (e.g. Auletta, 1982; Bowman, 1989; Jackson, 1991; Ryan, 1972). For example, critical questions should be raised about studies of subordinate racial–ethnic groups that not only focus narrowly on psychopathology but also over-generalize from small samples with rather extreme psychosocial symptoms. Moreover, archival studies on racial–ethnic minorities based on the decennial census, institutional records, and qualitative data sources often de-contextualize what is interpreted as widespread patterns of personal vulnerability and psychopathology. Rather than clarify systemic or social determinants, epidemiological studies too often "characterize" and "pathologize" racial–ethnic populations with descriptive profiles or patterns of severe emotional disorder and psychopathological symptoms.

Future resiliency studies on marginalized populations can go beyond the conventional focus on psychological or cultural pathology to further clarify risks created by external societal barriers as the major causal factors in problematic outcomes (Glasgow, 1980). Guided by a resiliency framework, research on marginalized racial–ethnic populations can avoid the pejorative tone of pathology studies and further clarify factors that empower many to overcome adversity associated with systemic race, ethnic, and class barriers. The complexity of resiliency research on marginalized groups calls for the culturally appropriate use of multiple methods including epidemiological analyses, theory-driven scholarship, and intervention studies that combine quasi-experimental, psychometric, and qualitative methods.

Epidemiological and national survey studies on marginalized groups cannot only document the incidence and prevalence of psychopathology but also provide very helpful estimates of both risk and protective factors associated with resilient outcomes (Georges-Abeyie, 1984; Heckler et al., 1985; Jackson, 1991; Kessler, 1979; Neighbors et al., 1983; Williams et al., 2003). More detailed risk, vulnerability, and protective factor analyses can also help to clarify their relationships to both problematic and resilient outcomes. Furthermore, policy-relevant analysis of national data can also monitor change in social determinants of inter-group disparities over time, identify subgroups at greatest risks for various problems, isolate specific etiologic patterns and protective factors, and aid in the design, evaluation, and improvement of preventive interventions.

Psychosocial Adaptation: Protection, Strengths, and Resiliency

In general, a *protective factor* is any aspect of a person or the environment that increases the likelihood of a positive outcome or decreases the likelihood of a problematic outcome despite exposure to risk factors (e.g., Bowman, 2006; Caldwell et al., 2004; Hurd, Zimmerman, & Xue, 2009; Rhodes & Brown, 1991; Rowley & Bowman, 2009; Rutter 1985; Smith, 2006a, 2006b; Werner & Smith, 1992). Although existing literature is more equivocal, Table 21.1 makes a clear distinction between *external or environmental protective factors* and *internal or personal strengths* that increase the probability of positive and resilient outcomes. The resiliency literature increasingly emphasizes the importance of identifying modifiable environmental protective factors, and there is also growing emphasis on better understanding the relationship between multilevel environmental protective factors and personal strengths. Moreover, similar to literature on risks, research on multilevel protection and strengths seeks to clearly identify specific factors, determine how they function, and guide preventive interventions designed to promote resilient outcomes.

Linking Environmental Protection and Personal Strengths: In addition to the operation of risks and vulnerabilities, future resiliency studies also need to further clarify how environmental protective factors combine with personal strengths to promote specific resilient outcomes (psychosocial wellbeing, health, role achievement, etc.). Guided by the *psychosocial adaptation hypothesis*, multilevel research on marginalized populations can further clarify how various socio-cultural protective factors might reinforce specific personal strengths which, in turn, promote more resilient outcomes. Hence, *protection* implies an external process to either support what is vulnerable, shield from injury, or guard against harm. In contrast, *personal strength* is more consistent with an internal quality of being strong, tough, or able to do, endure, or resist something. We need to better understand how the effects of protective factors at multiple levels—family, community, societal—on resilient outcomes might be mediated by personal strengths. For example, multilevel protective factors within marginalized populations may reinforce pivotal personal strengths—sense of mastery, sense of relatedness, and emotional reactivity—in specific ways in the resiliency process (e.g. Prince-Embury, 2007).

Strengths-Based Approaches: Cultural Protection, Strengths and Resiliency

Future resiliency research on marginalized populations can also build on insights from strengths-based approaches to further clarify the operation of both external protective factors and personal strengths on resilient outcomes (e.g., Bowman, 1989, 2006, 2011; Bowman & Howard, 1985; Chavous et al., 2007; Hurd et al., 2009; Neblett, Chavous, Nguyen, & Sellers, 2009; Ostaszewski & Zimmerman, 2006; Rowley & Bowman, 2009; Sellers, Chavous, & Cooke, 1998; Smith, 2006a). This growing strengths-based literature is part of a broader paradigm shift away from the traditional pathology model towards a more positive focus on human development in psychology and related fields (positive psychology, cultural psychology, youth development, prevention research, public health, social work, positive education, positive organizational scholarship, etc.). In the tradition of resiliency research, this strengths-based movement looks beyond pathology or deficit approaches that tend to divert attention away from human agency and those who manage adaptive outcomes despite adversity. Strengths-based researchers can help to further understand the resiliency process through which protective factors reinforce personal strengths to enable those faced with chronic risk exposure to avoid devastation, to struggle against the odds, and to even excel despite adversity.

In high-risk environments, strengths-based approaches have particular virtues for cross-cultural research on the importance of cultural strengths in resilient outcomes within diverse populations (Bowman, 1989, 2006, 2011; Smith, 2006a, 2006b). For example, Smith (2006a) reviews the strengths-based paradigm and highlights the need for new theoretical frameworks to better clarify the operation of cultural strengths in resiliency. She encourages

> …cross-cultural researchers to begin identifying the cultural strengths that have permitted members of various ethnic groups to survive and flourish. We might begin to learn what strengths are universally valued and which are valued only by some cultures (p. 17).

She also notes that "each ethnic group and culture has its own strengths, which serve as protective factors during times of crisis." A major limitation in current strengths-based research on resiliency issues is the failure to clearly distinguish between *ethnic-specific (emic)* and *universal (etic)* cultural factors—at multiple levels—that facilitate personal resilience and resilient outcomes (e.g., Bowman, 1989, 1990a, 1990b, 2006, 2011; Smith, 2006b). Guided by a cross-cultural perspective, future resiliency research on marginalized populations can help to further clarify how multilevel *emic factors—protective and personal cultural strengths*—operate to promote resilient outcomes (Berry, Poortinga, Segall, & Dasen, 1992; Brislin, 1993; Triandis et al., 1980–1981).

Ethnic Sources of Resiliency: The *ethnic studies movement* in the USA continues to expand literature that helps to clarify the unique emic protective factors and cultural strengths within diverse racial–ethnic groups including African American, Latina/o, Asian/Pacific, and Native American communities (Feagin & Feagin, 1999; Karenga, 1993; Nagel, 1996; Suarez-Orozco & Paez, 2002; Takaki, 1989, 2008). As one example, African American studies go beyond a focus on positive "reactions" and emphasize the cultural origins of authentic and "proactive" adaptations to inequality and adversity in major life roles (Billingsley, 1992; Bowman, 1989, 1990b; Drake & Cayton, 1964; DuBois, 1903; Herskovits, 1935; Jones, 2005; McAdoo, 1997). Rather than material culture, multidisciplinary studies emphasize the adaptive value of unique *social*, *expressive*, and *subjective* aspects of African American culture. Emphasis is placed on the adaptive value of indigenous extended family, religious, and other social institutional patterns within African American communities (Berry & Blassingame, 1985; Billingsley, 1992; Hill, 1998; Layng, 1978; Sudarkasa, 1981). In addition, the adaptive value of African American music, language, literature, psychological belief systems, and other distinctive modes of cultural expression are also emphasized (Baratz, 1973; DuBois, 1903; Herskovits, 1955; Jones, 2005).

Among ethnic researchers, a sharp divergence exists on the origins of distinct ethnic or cultural strengths among black people in America. The traditional view is that African American ethnic patterns are devoid of African origins and basically reactions to racial oppression in America (e.g. Frazier, 1939; Hannerz, 1969). In contrast, others view these patterns as distinctly African adaptations to American circumstances rather than mere reactions to oppressive institutional barriers (e.g., Herskovits, 1935, 1941; Jones, 2005; Karenga, 1993; Sudarkasa, 1981). These more African-centered scholars focus on the unique African-American cultural heritage as the primary source of adaptive emic or ethnic cultural strengths. Such ethnic-centered perspectives may help to further clarify how indigenous ethnic patterns promote resiliency and facilitate adaptive over pathological responses to oppressive role barriers. Ethnic institutions, community organizations, extended families, and cultural belief systems may be crucial sources of personal strengths and resiliency for African Americans as they struggle with discouraging barriers in major roles (Berry & Blassingame, 1985; Billingsley, 1992; Hill, 1998; Levine, 1977; McAdoo, 1997; Morris, 1984; Nobles, 1974; Yearwood, 1980).

A major impediment to strengths-based research among African Americans to further clarify cultural strengths in the resiliency process is pejorative mainstream scholarship which concludes that the most unique thing about African Americans is their lack of indigenous ethnic culture (Glazier & Moynihan, 1975; Myrdal, 1964). For example, Hannerz (1969, p. 195) notes in an early critique of this invidious but persistent mainstream perspective:

> To them, black people are only Americans, without values and culture of their own to guard and protect, and without an opportunity to view themselves as other ethnic groups do. Thus they would be less likely to organize themselves to take care of their own social problems.

In contrast to pathology and assimilation scholars, ethnic researchers focus on both protective socio-cultural factors (e.g. extended family strengths) and subjective cultural strengths (e.g. racial–ethnic identity) among African Americans that differ in style and/or substance from mainstream European-American, middle class cultural forms (e.g. Bowman & Howard, 1985; Billingsley, 1992; Hill, 1998; Sellers et al., 1998).

As with any ethnic group, African Americans systematically transmit core cultural strengths across generations through ethnic socialization processes—but often adapt specific strategies to more effectively respond to changing social, economic, political, and ecological circumstances (e.g. Bowman & Howard, 1985). In the context of globalization, strengths-based studies need to explore both emic and cross-cultural sources of adaptive strengths that foster resiliency and successful outcomes despite discouraging barriers in major life roles. We need to better understand how resilient individuals may achieve resilient outcomes by mobilizing their own group's emic strengths, and by possibly borrowing adaptive emic strengths through exposure to other ethnic groups. In the twenty-first century, marginalized group members might mobilize a range of cross-cultural strengths in high-risk circumstances to promote resiliency and adaptive coping as globalization, immigration, urbanization, and related public policies result in greater intergroup interaction within diversifying nations, communities, and organizations.

An Integrative Social Psychological Approach

Theoretical, Assessment and Socio-cultural Considerations

Building on insights from the evolving resiliency literature, we need an integrative strengths-based approach to further clarify complex resiliency processes among marginalized racial–ethnic populations in diversifying socio-cultural contexts. To be most viable in the twenty-first century, an integrative strengths-based resiliency paradigm should have at least three features. First, it must provide a comprehensive theoretical framework that incorporates insights from the *four major research perspectives* in the evolving literature on resiliency—vulnerability, risk, protection, and strengths. As highlighted earlier in Table 21.1, this integrative framework should systematically consider how *complex interactions* between such pivotal variables result in resilient rather than pathological outcomes. Secondly, a viable approach must not only inform *basic resiliency scholarship* but also the development of policy-relevant *intervention and assessment systems*. Finally, a viable approach must help to clarify the socio-cultural context of resiliency including critical *cultural diversity*, *multilevel*, and *life span issues* among high-risk populations, especially those faced with systemic inequalities, chronic poverty, environmental stressors, and adversity in major social roles.

Role Strain and Adaptation Model: A Strengths-Based Approach to Resiliency

As a theoretical foundation, an integrative *role strain and adaptation model* provides one viable approach to resiliency scholarship, assessment, and preventive intervention on marginalized populations (e.g. Bowman, 1989, 2006, 2011). As illustrated in Fig. 21.1, this strengths-based social psychological approach integrates critical insights from resiliency research perspectives with an emphasis on the concepts of chronic role strain and role adaptation. *Chronic role strain* refers to *persistent objective* adversity (systemic role barriers, difficulty or repeated failure) and related *cognitive* appraisals (role discouragement, attributions, or conflicts) that increase multilevel risks, risky coping, vulnerability, and impede resilient outcomes. Despite role strain, *role adaptation* is the related process through which *resilient individuals* mobilize *multilevel strengths* to enable more adaptive coping, resiliency, and successful outcomes.

As highlighted in Fig. 21.1, this integrative model focuses on the nature, antecedents, context, moderators, and consequences of chronic role strain faced by individuals in major life roles (education, economic, family, civic, etc.). Hence, chronic role strains are not only rooted in intergroup inequalities (e.g. class, race, gender), but their deleterious effects can be exacerbated by *multilevel risk factors* (institutional barriers, poverty, stressors). However, despite chronic role strains, *preventive intervention* can promote more resilient outcomes by reinforcing multilevel protective factors (institutional opportunities, resources) and personal strengths.

This strengths-based model not only has particular relevance for understanding resiliency

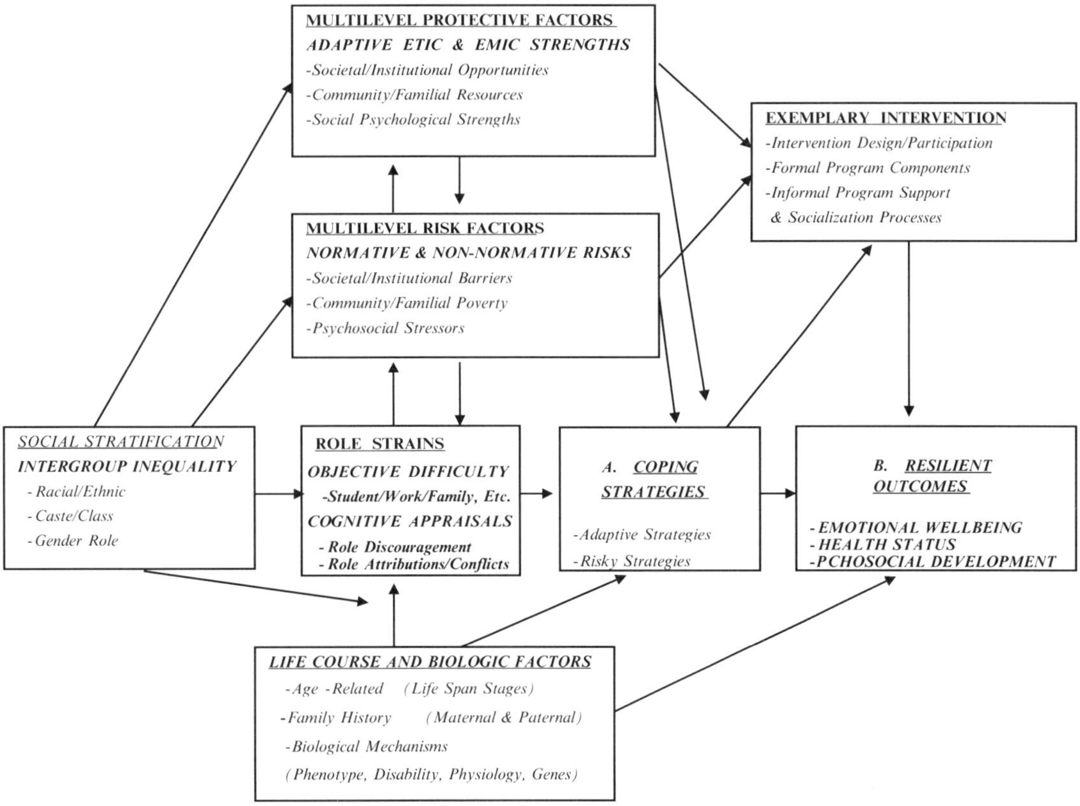

Fig. 21.1 A strengths-based role strain and adaptation model: toward a comprehensive social psychological approach to resiliency. Adapted from Bowman (2006)

issues facing marginalized groups, but the core social psychological propositions also have deep theoretical roots—in *role theories* that focus on person-environment fit issues (Allen & Vande Vliert, 1981; Barnett & Baruch, 1985; Barnett, Biener, & Baruch, 1987; Kahn et al., 1964; Sarbin & Allen, 1968), *expectancy-value theories* in psychology (Bandura, 1986; 1997 Bowman, 1977, 1996b; Feather, 1982), and *blocked opportunity theories* in sociology (Goode, 1960; Merton, 1968; Pearlin, 1983). In a social psychological sense, the central focus on roles is important because our cultural values, personal goals, and self-identities are centered in the major roles we play in life. Our self-evaluations, socio-emotional well-being, and even our health may depend heavily on success or failure in playing the major life roles we most cherish. Despite the strong values and high stakes all people place in major life roles, the resiliency process becomes more challenging for marginalized group members whose role success is systematically threatened by chronic role adversity rooted in intergroup inequalities and institutionalized barriers.

This social psychological approach to resiliency has begun to provide valuable insight into how individuals from marginalized populations cope with adversity in highly valued life roles—student, work, family, civic, etc. For example, a growing role strain and adaptation literature on African Americans has focused on resiliency issues in the face of *student role adversity* (Bowman, 1977, 1996a; Bowman & Howard, 1985; McAdams, Reynolds, Lewis, Patten, & Bowman, 2001; Orellana & Bowman, 2003; Rowley & Bowman, 2009), *work role adversity* (Bowman, 1984, 1990a, 1991a, 1991b; Bowman et al., 1982), *family role adversity* (Bowman, 1988, 1990b, 1993, 1995; Bowman & Forman, 1997; Bowman & Sanders, 1998; Gadsden & Bowman, 1999), and *intergroup status-based role adversity* (Bowman, 1996b; Bowman & Betancur, 2010; Bowman & Smith, 2002; Jackson, 1991; Johnson & Bowman, 2003; McAdams & Bowman, 2001; Neighbors et al., 1983).

Preventive Intervention and Strengths-Based Assessment: A Social Psychological Approach

Beyond basic theoretical contributions, this strengths-based social psychological approach to resiliency also has important practical implications for preventive intervention and related assessment. As suggested in Fig. 21.1, in the context of *exemplary intervention*, a better understanding of role strain-adaptation mechanisms can *inform innovative support strategies* to boost resilient outcomes. Related role strain and adaptation studies suggest that the *efficacy of exemplary interventions* designed to promote resilient outcomes might be *impeded by role strain variables* but *enhanced by adaptive social psychological strengths* (e.g. Bowman, 1977, 1984, 1989, 1990a, 1990b, 1996a, 1996b, 2006, 2011; Bowman & Howard, 1985; Bowman & Sanders, 1998).

This integrative social psychological approach can also build on insights from the resiliency literature to further develop more comprehensive strengths-based assessment systems. As outlined in Table 21.2, a viable strengths-based assessment system can help to clarify the relationship between *policy-relevant intervention*, *role strain-adaptation mechanisms*, and *resilient outcomes*. For preventive interventions in high-risk contexts, there are *two basic propositions*. These propositions are based on hypothesized pathways between inequality, chronic role strain, protective factors, coping processes, and resilience outcomes. First, the efficacy of *preventive intervention is often impeded* when inequalities exacerbate chronic role strains, multilevel risks, and risky coping strategies to reduce resilient outcomes. Second, despite chronic role strains, *intervention efficacy can be enhanced* if innovative support strategies reinforce social psychological strengths, mobilize multilevel protection, and promote adaptive coping to boost resilient outcomes. For example, supportive intervention strategies might reinforce pivotal social psychological strengths that help to mobilize multilevel protective factors (e.g. opportunities, resources), promote adaptive coping, and boost resilient outcomes.

Table 21.2 Exemplary intervention, role stain-adaptation, and resilient outcomes: foundations for a comprehensive strengths-based assessment system

I. Exemplary preventive interventions
- A. Intervention design and participation
- B. Formal intervention components and activities

II. Major role strain-adaptation variables
- A. Chronic role strains: Objective adversity and cognitive appraisals
  1. *Objective role strain*: Role barriers and adversity
     - Student role barriers: Education adversity
     - Work role barriers: Economic adversity
     - Parental role barriers: Family adversity
  2. Subjective role strain: Risky cognitive appraisals
     - Role expectancy: Discouragement
     - Role attributions: Self-blame
     - Role stress: Ambiguity, conflict, overload
- B. Adaptive social psychological strengths
  1. Perceived informal support
     - Intervention support: Mentors and staff
     - Peer support: Program and non-program
     - Extended family support: Kin and Para-Kin
  2. Social-cognitive motivational orientations
     - Path-goal beliefs
     - Academic self-efficacy
     - Career-related efficacy
     - Resilient problem-solving efficacy
  3. Multilevel engagement orientations
     - Leadership commitment
     - Service commitment
     - Diversity commitment

III. Resilient outcomes
- A. Emotional wellbeing
- B. Health status
- C. Psychosocial development
- D. Successful role achievements

Preventive Interventions—Formal Activities, Informal Support and Outcomes: As suggested in Table 21.2, a growing literature continues to document the importance of research on preventive interventions that show efficacy in promoting more resilient outcomes among children, youth, and adults faced with adversity (e.g. Comer, 1996; Hogan, Linden, & Najarian, 2002; Holden & Zimmerman, 2009; Kohn & Chavous, 2002; Maton, Schellenback, Leadbetter, & Solarz, 2004; Price et al., 1980; Price, Cowen, Lorion, & Ramos-McKay, 1988; Rappaport, 1990; Smith, 2006a, 2006b; Weissberg, Kumpfer, & Seligman, 2003). With a focus on high-risk populations, this literature highlights a growing array of exemplary interventions with demonstrated efficacy for promoting a range of resilient outcomes—well-being, healthy development, and role success.

Governmental agencies such as the National Institutes for Health (NIH), National Science Foundation (NSF), and the Department of Education, along with non-profit foundations currently sponsor a range of preventive pipeline interventions. Evaluation studies have begun to identify *exemplary pipeline interventions* with demonstrated *efficacy* in promoting successful outcomes among marginalized students who excel in K-12 public schools, enroll in college, pursue advanced degrees, and achieve competitive careers often against great odds. Despite the efficacy of exemplary pipeline interventions, there is a growing interest in better understanding *why* some participants benefit from formal intervention activities more than others. A growing collaboration among NIH, NSF, and other stakeholders has begun to provide additional insight into factors associated with pipeline intervention efficacy and differential benefits (e.g., Chubin, DePass, & Blockus, 2009; DePass & Chubin, 2008; Olson & Fagen, 2007). *Rigorous outcome evaluation* studies show clear *average benefits* for intervention participants over control groups—but *do not* explain *differential benefits* among participants within intervention groups.

As highlighted in Table 21.2, in addition to role strain measures, more comprehensive strengths-based assessment can help to clarify how *formal support components of* exemplary interventions combine with *perceived informal support* and other *social psychological strengths*—to further explain resilient outcomes. *Exemplary preventive interventions* often provide participants with *access* to facilities and *formal activities* that include *program staff* to implement structured strategies. For example, NIH-National Institute for General Medicine has developed a bold new initiative to study *exemplary educational and career pipeline interventions* for underrepresented groups based on *two core assumptions* regarding program success: (1) when participants are provided the opportunity to engage in state-of-the-art research with supportive mentors, appropriate facilities, and structured activities, their career-related motivation is strengthened; and (2) once focused, participants will be more resilient and strive for educational and career success at various developmental stages.

Toward A Viable Assessment System: Adaptive Social Psychological Strengths: *Objective aspects* of chronic role strain or adversity (i.e. systemic role barriers or repeated failure) can be directly assessed and *cognitive aspects* (i.e. role discouragement, attributions, or stress) can be measured with standard social psychological indicators (e.g. Bowman, 2011; King & King, 1990). Moreover, resiliency researchers have also developed viable assessment systems with valid and reliable measures of *social psychological strengths* to guide interventions that promote resilient outcomes (Prince-Embury, 2007, 2009, 2010; Prince-Embury & Courville, 2008a, 2008b; Sedlacek, 2004; Seligman & Csikszentmihalyi, 2000). As highlighted in Table 21.3, Prince-Embury (2007) has developed an especially promising *Resiliency Scales for Children and Adolescents* (*RSCA*) which provides psychometrically sound measures of three strengths-based constructs—*Sense of Mastery*, *Sense of Relatedness*, and *Emotional Reactivity*.

As noted in Table 21.3, Sedlacek (2004) has developed a *Noncognitive Questionnaire* (*NCQ*) to assess eight noncognitive strengths which appear to be convergent with a *sense of mastery* (*long term goals*, *positive self concept*, and *knowledge in a field*), sense of relatedness (*strong support person*, *leadership experience*), and *emotional reactivity* (*realistic self-appraisal and*

Table 21.3 Comparison of major concepts in three strengths-based assessment systems

RSCA—*Prince-Embury*	NCQ—*Sedlacek*	Social psychological strengths—*Bowman*
Sense of mastery	Long term goals	Path-goal motivation
	Positive self-concept	Salient role self-efficacy
	Knowledge in a field	Career-related efficacy
Sense of relatedness	A strong support person	Perceived social support
	Leadership experience	Leadership commitment
	Community involvement	Service commitment
Emotional reactivity	Realistic self-appraisal	Resilient problem-solving
	Handling the system	Diversity commitment

handling the system). Both the RSCA and NCQ are increasingly employed to assess personal strengths and guide innovative support strategies to enhance resiliency in a wide range of intervention settings. Future resiliency research on marginalized racial–ethnic groups should further clarify how the three core RSCA measures converge with the eight NCQ variables and related social psychological strengths within Bowman's (2011) comprehensive role strain and adaptation approach. For example, a *general sense of mastery* (i.e., optimism, adaptability, self-efficacy) may well be associated with a positive self-concept, long-range goals, knowledge in a chosen field, as well as path-goal motivation, academic self-efficacy, and career-efficacy. Moreover, *sense of relatedness* (i.e., support, trust, social tolerance) may be associated with having a strong support person, leadership/community involvement, as well as informal support, and leadership/service/diversity commitments. Finally, *emotional reactivity* (i.e., sensitivity, recovery, impairment) is a physiologically based process which may impede emotional self-regulation, realistic self-appraisal, handling the system, and resilient problem-solving.

Future resiliency research should build on a better understanding of the interrelationships between RSCA concepts, NCQ variables and high quality measures of related social psychological strengths to develop a comprehensive *Strengths-based Assessment System* (*SAS*). In addition to basic research on resiliency, a viable SAS could also further clarify the process through which exemplary preventive interventions promote resilient outcomes among high-risk populations. A growing literature supports the idea that a SAS with more specific measures of social psychological strengths may be especially useful in preventive interventions to promote resiliency among marginalized populations with chronic role adversity exacerbated by systematic class, racial, ethnic, or gender role barriers (Bernhard, 1997; Bowman, 1977, 1989, 2006, 2011; Ebreo, 1998; Feldman, 1999; McAdams et al., 2001; McNeil, 1999; Reyes, 2002; Rowley & Bowman, 2009; Orellana & Bowman, 2003; Sanders, 1997; Shiraishi, 2000). Therefore, a viable SAS with theory-driven measures of chronic role strains and social psychological strengths could provide unique insight into the operation of related RSCA and NCQ measures within preventive interventions that promote resilient outcomes.

Guided by a role strain and adaptation framework, the specific SAS variables outlined in Table 21.2 can also inform future research to better understand intervention efficacy including differential intervention benefits (e.g. Chubin et al., 2009; DePass & Chubin, 2008; Olson & Fagen, 2007). A SAS with high quality measures of these social psychological variables can help clarify pivotal mechanisms that *impede* or *enhance efficacy of exemplary interventions*. More specifically, SAS measures can help clarify: (1) how *role strain and related risk processes* may reduce intervention benefits among participants and *impede* intervention efficacy, and (2) how *social psychological strengths and related resiliency processes* may enhance benefits among intervention participants and *improve* intervention efficacy. Bowman (2011) reviews a growing literature on these role strain and adaptation concepts that shows how a more coherent, reliable and valid SAS could guide innovative support strategies to further enhance intervention efficacy. In addition to formal intervention activities, development of informal support strategies might further enhance efficacy and resilient outcomes by reinforcing social psychological strengths, mobilizing multilevel resources, and empowering individuals to successfully strive toward their valued goals despite chronic adversity in major life roles.

Socio-cultural Considerations: Diversity, Ecological, and Life Span Issues

A growing literature shows how the basic strengths-based role strain and adaptation approach can be further extended to provide greater insight into the complex socio-cultural context of resiliency (e.g. Bowman, 1989, 1990a, 1990b, 2006; Bowman & Sanders, 1998; Orellana & Bowman, 2003; Rowley & Bowman, 2009). This literature supports the importance of a *Role Strain and Adaptation (RSA)-extension* that systematically considers the socio-cultural context of resiliency processes including *cultural diversity*, *ecological*, and *life span issues*. More systematic consideration of such socio-cultural and human development issues in resiliency research will become increasingly critical in the twenty-first century as marginalized groups face racial–ethnic inequalities, environmental threats, and chronic role strains within diversifying nations.

Cultural Diversity Issues—Racial and Ethnic Considerations: Guided by cross-cultural studies, a RSA-extension can further clarify cultural diversity issues in strength-based scholarship and interventions (Berry et al., 1992; Bowman, 1989, 2006, 2011; Brislin, 1993; Sue & Sue, 2008; Triandis et al., 1980–1981). As suggested in Fig. 21.1, the RSA-extension considers three culturally relevant propositions: (1) both *group-specific* (*emic*) and *universal* (*etic*) cultural strengths promote resilient outcomes; (2) emic and etic cultural strengths can buffer the deleterious effects of objective role strain (e.g. systemic barriers, repeated failure) on resilient outcomes; and (3) emic and etic cultural strengths can also promote resilient outcomes by reducing cognitive aspects of role strain (discouragement, self-blame, distress, etc.).

A growing number of role strain and adaptation studies on African Americans provide basic support for these three cultural diversity propositions (e.g. Bowman, 1989, 1990b, 1998, 2006, 2011; Bowman & Howard, 1985; Bowman & Sanders, 1998; Orellana & Bowman, 2003; Rowley & Bowman, 2009). Related cross-ethnic studies also suggest that racial/ethnic socialization and social support may reinforce a person's cultural strengths which, in turn, can reduce their risky cognitive appraisals and boost resilient outcomes (Ebreo, 1998; Feldman, 1999; McNeil, 1999; Reyes, 2002; Sanders, 1997; Shiraishi, 2000). Despite role adversity, multilevel cultural strengths may help to explain why more resilient people manage to maintain a sense of hope, vitality, mastery, and persistence and excel against discouraging odds. Cultural strengths may reduce vulnerable feelings of being discouraged, overwhelmed, cut off or dispirited due to gaps between highly valued life goals and objective role obstacles.

Bowman and Betancur (2010) review literature showing how cultural diversity issues are especially critical in policy-relevant interventions to promote resilient outcomes among caste-like racial and ethnic groups in the USA such as African Americans, American Indians, and Chicanos who continue to face resiliency challenges associated with deeply-rooted historical inequalities and status hierarchies. In the context of globalization, similar status-based resiliency challenges also face growing numbers of marginalized immigrants in the USA and other nations (e.g. Chirkov, Ryan, & Wilness, 2005; Janssens, Bechtold, Prarolo, & Stenius, 2010). In the USA and beyond, resiliency challenges facing marginalized groups from diverse backgrounds are rooted in their elevated risk of chronic adversity in major life roles and related environmental threats, chronic poverty, and intergroup inequalities.

Ecological Contexts: Multilevel Micro, Meso, and Micro Issues: From an *ecological perspective*, Fig. 21.1 highlights how both risk factors and protective factors operate at multiple levels—*micro* (e.g. personal stress and strengths), *meso* (e.g. family/community poverty and resources), and *macro* (e.g. institutional/societal barriers and opportunities) to affect resiliency processes (e.g., Bronfenbrenner, 1979, 1986, 1996). In social-ecological terms, a viable RSA-extension can better clarify how micro or *individual-level* resiliency processes operate among at-risk populations within a broader *multilevel context* that also considers pressing family, community, and public policy issues (Bowman, 1988, 1989, 1993, 1995; Bowman & Forman, 1997; Rowley & Bowman, 2009).

This RSA-extension can also draw on a growing literature that supports the importance of multilevel ecological or environmental factors in risk and resiliency studies (Brodsky, 1996; Bronfenbrenner, 1986, 1996; Fitzpatrick & LaGory, 2000; Garbarino, 1995; Kessler, Price, & Wortman, 1985; Leventhal & Brooks-Gunn, 2000; Marsella, 1998; McLoyd & Flanagan, 1990; Moen, Elder, & Luscher, 1995; Ogbu, 1981; Spencer et al., 1993; Steele, 1997; Taylor, 1996; Vera & Shin, 2006). Although specific findings vary, these studies help to clarify environmental risks and show how *macro-level risks* within societies and institutions combine with *meso-level risks* within communities and families to increase *micro-level personal vulnerability* for negative rather than resilient outcomes. In this tradition, several role strain studies among African Americans suggest that *macro-level inequalities* produce a set of *meso-level family role strains*—among fathers, mothers, and children—which, in turn, result in *micro-level personal vulnerabilities* for negative rather than resilient outcomes (e.g. Bowman, 1984, 1988, 1990a, 1991a, 1991b, 1993, 1995; Bowman & Forman, 1997; Bowman et al., 1982; McLoyd & Wilson, 1990; Rowley & Bowman, 2009).

As suggested in Fig. 21.1, role strain and adaptation studies among African Americans also suggests that multilevel macro, meso, and micro protective factors might combine to better explain the predominance of resilient over negative outcomes despite systemic barriers (e.g. Bowman, 1989, 1990b, 2006, 2011; Bowman & Howard, 1985; Bowman & Sanders, 1998; Rowley & Bowman, 2009). Related African American studies have long argued that successful individual and collective empowerment strategies often depend on the mobilization of ethnic strengths at multiple levels—community, family, and personal (i.e. Berry & Blassingame, 1985; Billingsley, 1992; Dawson, 1994; DuBois, 1903; Gurin, Hatchett, & Jackson, 1989; Hill, 1998; Jones, 2005; Morris, 1984; Taylor, Chatters, & Levin, 2005).

Life Span Issues: Stages of Adult Development: A *life span framework* can help clarify how critical factors in the resiliency process operate as individuals move through various developmental stages over the life course—from childhood, adolescence, and through adulthood. As highlighted in Table 21.4, a RSA-extension can build on the life span literature to further clarify critical adult development issues in the resiliency process among African Americans and other marginalized populations. As noted earlier, because of the emphasis on children and adolescents by developmental psychopathologists, there is an extensive literature on resiliency processes in early, middle, and later childhood. However, chronic risk exposure and resiliency remain a major challenge for individuals across the life span. Resiliency challenges are critical for *children born* to a mentally ill parent (Garmezy, 1993, 1987), for *young children* in poverty (Werner 1995), for *adolescents* attending schools in distressed communities (Dryfoos, 1990; Zimmerman & Brenner, 2010), for *young adults* faced with chronic work role strains (Bowman, 1984, 1990a, 1991a, 1991b; Bowman et al., 1982), for *middle-aged adults* faced with family role adversity (Barnett, Biener, & Baruch, 1987; Baruch & Barnett 1986; Bowman & Forman, 1997), and for *older adults* with chronic health problems (Jackson, 1991).

To go beyond the early focus on children, future resiliency research can further extrapolate from a growing literature on life span and adult development issues (e.g., Baltes, Lindenberger, & Staudinger, 1998; Bowman, 1989, Bowman & Sanders, 1998; Elder, George, & Shanahan, 1996;

Table 21.4 Life span development issues in role stain and adaptation

	Salient goals	Persistent barriers	Resiliency challenges
(A) Chronic role strain and resiliency challenges			
Adolescence			
Student role strain	Educational preparation	Ineffective public schools	Student role discouragement vs. educational achievement
Early adulthood			
Worker role strain	Career consolidation	Global economic dislocations	Worker role discouragement vs. career attainment
Middle adulthood			
Provider role strain	Familial fulfillment	Chronic employment problems	Provider role discouragement vs. spouse/parent success
Older adulthood			
Elder role strain	Dignified aging	Inadequate retirement policies	Elder role discouragement vs. functional health
	Community	Extended family	Personal belief systems
(B) Protective emic cultural strengths			
Adolescence	Rites-of-passage rituals	Ethnic/race-related socialization	Ethnic achievement orientations
Early adulthood	Para-Kin friendships	Flexible family roles	Ethnic/racial identity and consciousness
Middle adulthood	Work-related ethnic groups	Extended family households	Religious beliefs
Older adulthood	Ethnic institutions	Intergenerational family bonds	Spirituality

Adapted from Bowman (2006)

Jones, 1989a, 1989b; Kail & Cavanaugh, 2000; Lerner, 2002; McAdams & de St. Aubin, 1998; McAdams et al., 1993). Building on the classic work by Erikson (1966, 1968, 1980), these life span researchers have provided valuable insights into *normative* psychosocial and resiliency challenges at four distinct stages of adulthood—*adolescence, early adulthood, middle adulthood,* and *older adulthood*. However, future resiliency research on marginalized racial–ethnic populations should also consider the operation of *non-normative* role strain and adaptation issues during each stage of adulthood.

With a particular emphasis on African Americans, Table 21.4 highlights two critical non-normative resiliency issues that provide the basis for a more coherent adult development approach to role strain and adaptation: (a) *chronic role strain and related resiliency challenges*, and (b) the *operation of protective emic cultural strengths* (Bowman, 1989, 1990a, 1990b, 1996b, 2006; Bowman & Sanders, 1998; Bowman & Rowley 2000). Within a life span framework, future inquiry on these non-normative resiliency issues at different stages of adulthood can help to further clarify complex role strain and adaptation challenges. What are the pivotal non-normative resiliency issues for individuals from marginalized groups during adulthood as they face greater risks for chronic student, work, family, and elderly role strains? Does the psychosocial significance of these specific role strains and various cultural strengths in the resiliency process shift systematically as people move from early to middle to older adulthood? How is the successful adaptation to salient role strains at earlier stages of adulthood related to successful navigation of role barriers during later stages?

Chronic Role Strain and Resiliency Challenges Across Adult Stages: Going beyond normative life span paradigms, Table 21.4A highlights three chronic role strain concepts which can help to explain the non-normative psychosocial risk and resiliency challenges faced by marginalized populations during various stages of adulthood. The focus on *salient role performance goals, persistent barriers*, and *critical role conflicts* at each stage of adulthood provides a conceptual basis to better understand non-normative resiliency challenges.

A "perceived gap" between salient goals and systemic barriers in a major life role may pose a critical resiliency challenge during each adult stage. In an early review of related literature, Bowman (1989) notes that:

> student, work, family, and elderly role conflicts have special developmental effects during the pre, early, middle and older adult years respectively… From late adolescence to old age salient goals typically shift from educational preparation, to career consolidation, to familial/social fulfillment and dignified aging…during each period, extreme discouragement…may severely test the strength of motivation and value commitment in major life roles (pp. 126–128).

During each adult stage, a salient role strain and resiliency challenge can occur when persistent barriers (e.g. ineffective schools, joblessness, chronic poverty, inadequate healthcare) result in extreme discouragement. These systemic barriers can result in a series of resiliency-related conflicts as a person develops from adolescence (*student role discouragement* vs. *educational achievement*), to early adulthood (*worker role discouragement* vs. *career attainment*), to middle adulthood (*provider role discouragement* vs. *spouse/parent success*), to old age (*elder role discouragement* vs. *functional health*). Student role discouragement is especially critical because it not only threatens a sense of mastery, but may also generate identity confusion, erode social commitments, and produce problematic adult psychosocial trajectories. By contrast, student role resiliency can afford at-risk youth the opportunity to proceed into adulthood without serious educational handicaps and with a sense of mastery or empowerment. More resilient youth who successfully prepare for college can shift their salient goals during adulthood to career success, familial fulfillment, and finally to dignified aging. However, such student resiliency can be severely tested for marginalized students when educational barriers and related risk factors elevate *chronic role strain trajectories* as workers, parents, and elders.

Protective Emic Cultural Strengths Across Adult Stages: A RSA-extension can also guide future research on how members of marginalized racial–ethnic populations somehow manage to overcome discouraging role barriers and achieve more resilient outcomes across the life span. As Table 21.4B illustrates, members of marginalized racial–ethnic populations may mobilize a range of unique cultural strengths to promote resilient responses to chronic role strains across adult life stages. With a focus on African Americans, Bowman (1989) explains why the mobilization of ethnic-specific cultural strengths may be especially critical for resilient responses to chronic role strains during each stage of adulthood:

> In all cultures, indigenous ethnic resources are transmitted across generations to facilitate coping with normative role strains as individuals progress through adult life stages. However, African Americans face the additional challenge of devising cultural strategies to overcome race and class barriers which dramatically reduce the odds of excelling as students, workers, and family providers (p. 128).

To guide future inquiry, the analysis in Table 21.4B suggests that we need to better understand how ethnic-specific cultural strengths at the community, familial, and personal levels promote resilient responses to chronic role strains at each stage of adult life. Future research on life span issues in the operation of cultural strengths can further clarify critical sources of resiliency as members of diverse cultural groups struggle with normative and non-normative adult role demands. For example, related studies on African Americans suggest that the efficacy of various cultural strengths in promoting resilient outcomes may shift systematically along with salient role strains as one moves from adolescence through early, middle, and older adulthood (Bowman, 1989, 1990a, 1990b, 2006, 2011; Bowman & Howard, 1985; Rowley & Bowman, 2009; Bowman & Sanders, 1998).

Ethnic-specific rites of passage rituals, race-ethnic socialization, and ethnic achievement orientations may promote resilient outcomes better for students during adolescence than for workers, family providers, or elders during later adult years (e.g., Bowman, 1989; Hill, 1998; Stevenson, 2005). There is growing evidence that African American youth who participate in formal passage rituals may experience less role discouragement, identity confusion and distress in the

Table 21.5 Life span analysis of unmarried African American fathers

	Salient role strains	Cultural strengths	Resilient outcomes
Early adulthood (18–34 years)	Joblessness/ father role	Para-Kin peer relationships	Sense of personal efficacy
Middle adulthood (35–54 years)	Low income/ primary provider	Religiosity	Self-esteem
Older adulthood (55 years and over)	Underemployment/ primary provider	Extended family closeness	Perceived life quality

transition to adulthood (Boyd-Franklin & Franklin, 2000; Brookins, 2005; Jones, 1989a, 1989b, 2005; Williams, 2004). Racial–ethnic socialization has also been found to be an especially critical emic strength during the adolescent-to-adult transition (Bowman & Howard, 1985; Hughes & Chen, 1999; McNeil, 1999; Miller, 1999; Phinney & Chavira, 1995; Phinney & Rotheram, 1987; Stevenson, 2005).

Racial–ethnic socialization may function by promoting adaptive ethnic achievement orientations and, in turn, more resilient student outcomes (e.g., Sellers et al., 1998; Spencer et al., 1993; Stevenson, 2005). For example, in an early study of race-related socialization, Bowman and Howard (1985) found that 64% of males and 59% of females in a national sample of African American youth revealed that their parents had transmitted some message to them about their racial/ethnic status. These African American parents transmitted proactive messages regarding the virtues of racial pride, ethnic achievement, strategic responses to racism, racial egalitarianism, and self-development. African American youth who could not recall such parental messages were found to have less efficacious and resilient outcomes. Those whose parents emphasized self-development messages reported a higher sense of personal mastery and efficacy, while strategic responses to racism were linked to more successful academic outcomes in the student role.

Compared to adolescence, there is less literature on the operation of ethnic-specific cultural strengths as sources of resiliency during the early, middle, and older adult years. However, as summarized in Table 21.5, findings from a national study of unmarried African American fathers by Bowman and Sanders (1998) can help to guide future research. This study also provides one example of how both salient role strains and cultural strengths might promote resilient outcomes for especially high-risk individuals at different stages of adult development.

During the early adult years, unmarried African American fathers depended more heavily on para-kin (family-like) friendships to reduce the deleterious effects of joblessness and father role discouragement on a sense of personal efficacy. In contrast, during the middle adult years, such unmarried fathers relied more on religiosity than peers to offset the adverse effects of low income and primary provider role discouragement on self-esteem. Later, during the older adult years, these high-risk fathers relied most heavily on extended family closeness to counter negative effects of underemployment on perceived life quality. As suggested in Table 21.4B, future studies can also build on related studies among African Americans to further clarify life span variations in the operation of multilevel cultural strengths as sources of resiliency. For example, *community-level* resources such as para-kin peer relationships, work-related ethnic groups, and ethnic institutions may differentially effect empowerment and resiliency at different life stages (e.g., Dawson, 1994; Jackson, 1991, 2000; Milburn & Bowman, 1991; Taylor et al., 2005). At the *family level*, flexible family roles, extended family households, and intergenerational bonds may also effect resilient outcomes differentially from one life stage to the next (Billingsley, 1992; Bowman & Sanders, 1998; Hill, 1998; McAdoo, 1997; Taylor, Jackson, & Chatters, 1997). Finally, *personal belief systems* such as racial identity, religiosity, and spirituality may also have differential effects on resilient outcomes during the early, middle, and older adult years (Bowman,

Muhammad, & Ifatunji, 2004; Jones, 2005; Sellers et al., 1998; Taylor et al., 2005).

Conclusions and Implications

Bridging Resiliency Scholarship with Policy-Relevant Intervention

This chapter has highlighted the complexity of the resiliency concept and supported the importance of strengths-based resiliency scholarship and intervention research on marginalized racial–ethnic populations in diversifying nations, communities, and organizations. Building on basic social psychological theory, an integrative role strain and adaptation approach to resiliency incorporates insights from existing studies on psychosocial risk, vulnerability, protection, and strengths. To better address twenty-first century challenges, this comprehensive strengths-based theoretical framework can also be extended to further clarify the complex socio-cultural context of resiliency including critical *cultural diversity*, *ecological*, and *life span development issues*.

Beyond the theoretical contributions, strengths-based scholarship on resiliency also has important practical implications for policy-relevant intervention and assessment systems. As noted throughout this volume, a growing number of scholars are translating innovative resiliency scholarship for applications with children, youth, and adults. Toward this end, translational strengths-based scholarship on resiliency can help to further *understand and improve the efficacy of exemplary preventive interventions* to promote resilient outcomes. Such translational scholarship is especially critical for members of marginalized racial–ethnic groups whose pathways to life goals are often obstructed by systematic barriers, adversity, and discouragement.

As illustrated in Fig. 21.2, *Reciprocal Translation* is an especially promising approach to more systematically bridging basic scholarship

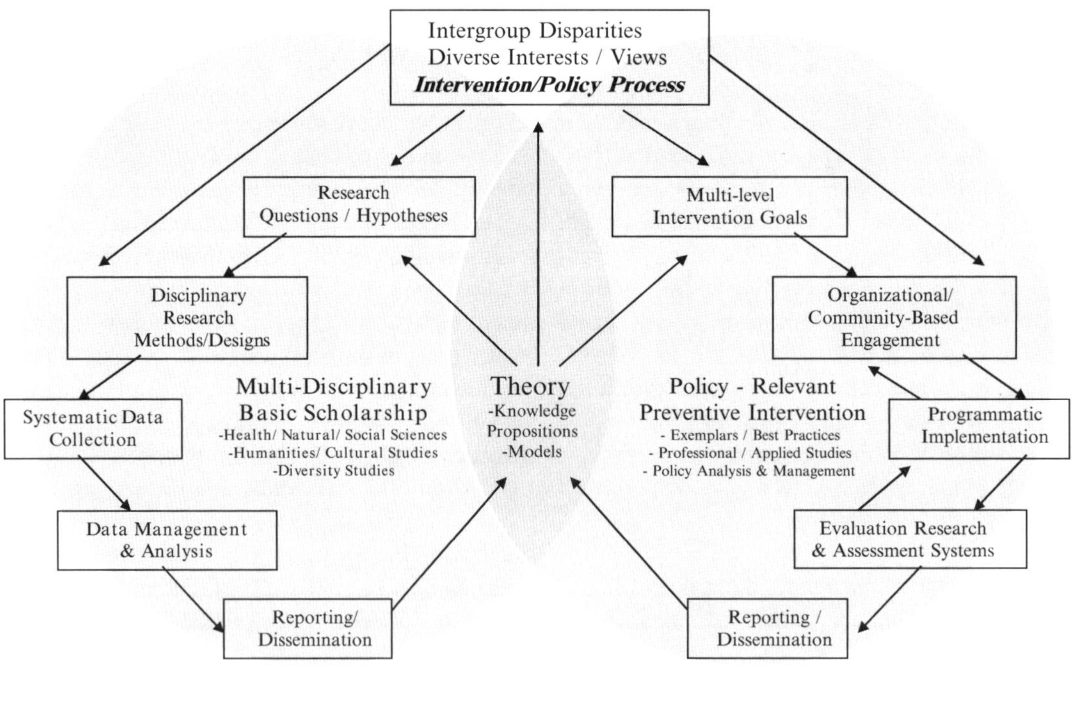

Fig. 21.2 National Center for Institutional Diversity. Bridging basic scholarship with Preventive Intervention Research. Reciprocal translation model: scholarship ↔ intervention

on resiliency with more policy-relevant intervention research and assessment systems. This unique translational approach was developed at the University of Michigan's National Center for Institutional Diversity to promote the *reciprocal benefits* of *basic scholarship* and *policy-relevant intervention research* to address the challenges and opportunities of diversity in the twenty-first century. Figure 21.2 highlights how the reciprocal translation of "basic scholarship" ↔ "intervention research" focuses on both: (a) the "*traditional translation*" of basic scholarship to guide the innovative design and improvement of exemplary interventions (left oval), and (b) the "*reverse translation*" of policy-relevant intervention research to not only institutionalize best practices but also to generate new hypotheses, stimulate basic scholarship and further promote theory-development (right oval).

Traditional Translation: From Scholarship-to-Intervention: In the classic deductive tradition, the conventional translation of basic scholarship-to-intervention reflects the foundational pillar for evidence-based professional practice. For example, resiliency scholarship is deeply rooted in basic developmental, personality, and social psychology theory—but is also applied and translated into innovative interventions within clinical, counseling, family, community, and educational psychology as well as public health, social work, and related professions. In addition to the conventional application of theory-to-practice, translational science can also help to further build basic theory by systematically testing core theoretical propositions through interventions within a wider range of natural settings (e.g. Price et al., 1980; Prince-Embury, 2008; Seligman, et al. 2005.

Reverse Translation: From Intervention-to-Scholarship: As suggested in Fig. 21.2, *policy-relevant intervention* research is primarily designed to evaluate best practices and to inform policy-makers, administrators, and professionals. Policy-relevant intervention research provides very useful assessment systems as well as formative and outcome evaluation data to systematically plan, monitor, develop, and institutionalize exemplary intervention strategies. However, in addition to such practical benefits, exemplary intervention research also has heuristic value for generating new hypotheses to guide basic scholarship and to further test, validate, develop, extend, or reformulate basic theory. Therefore, as a heuristic device, reverse translation can promote both *formative evaluation* of interventions to increase resiliency and *scholarly translation* of intervention research findings into new hypotheses and basic research for theory-development.

Reciprocal Translation and Strengths-Based Assessment: Reciprocal translation ("basic scholarship" ↔ "intervention research") also depend on the development of viable strengths-based assessment systems for use in both basic resiliency studies and policy-relevant intervention research that promote resilient outcomes (Prince-Embury, 2007; Prince-Embury & Courville, 2008a, 2008b; Sedlacek, 2004; Seligman & Csikszentmihalyi, 2000). Bowman (2011) suggests that future resiliency research on marginalized populations should adapt existing strengths-based systems to more fully consider critical life span and cross-cultural issues. With a focus on life span issues, assessment systems should be expanded to also consider the operation of critical role strain and adaptation issues in resilient outcomes at specific stages of development. Developmentally relevant assessment systems that further clarify how role strain, adaptation, and resilient outcomes may operate in unique ways at different life course stages (childhood, adolescence, adulthood) have both theoretical and practical implications.

A growing cross-cultural literature also supports the importance of viable strengths-based assessment systems in translational research to further clarify and reinforce the operation of adaptive cultural strengths in resilient outcomes (i.e., Banks, 2004; Berry et al., 1992; Bowman, 2011; Brislin, 1993; Gonzalez, Moll, & Amantqi, 2005; Gutiérrez, 2006; Hill, 1998; Jones, 1989a, 1989b, 2005; Lee, 2003; Orellana & Bowman, 2003). A strengths-based focus on the systematic assessment and understanding of cultural strengths both across and within diverse groups goes beyond the traditional emphasis in resiliency research on vulnerability and psychopathology. Strengths-based assessment can inform the design of innovative informal support strategies within intervention settings to systematically mobilize cultural strengths and, in turn, promote more resilient outcomes. In the twenty-first century, strengths-based translational research is especially critical to address the resiliency challenges faced by marginalized populations within diversifying socio-cultural ecologies. By promoting more resilient outcomes, such policy-relevant translational research can also promote social justice goals by reducing the often devastating consequences of chronic adversity in major life roles which are deeply rooted in growing inequalities within diversifying nations, communities, and organizations.

References

Affleck, G., & Tenneen, H. (1996). Construing benefits from adversity: Adaptational significance and dispositional underpinnings. *Journal of Personality, 64*, 899–922.

Allen, V., & Vande Vliert, E. (1981). *Role transitions*. New York, NY: Plenum.

Angelou, M. (1986). In Maya Angelou poems (PP. 154–155). New York: Bantam Books

Auletta, K. (1982). *The underclass*. New York, NY: Vintage.

Baltes, B. P., Lindenberger, U., & Staudinger, U. M. (1998). Life-span theory in developmental psychology. In R. M. Lerner (Ed.), *Handbook of child psychology: Vol. 1. Theoretical models of human development* (5th ed., pp. 1029–1143). New York, NY: Wiley.

Bandura, A. (1986). *Social foundations of thought and action: A social cognitive theory*. Englewood Cliffs, NJ: Prentice Hall.

Bandura, A. (1997). *The exercise of control*. New York, NY: Freeman.

Banks, J. A. (2004). *Handbook of research on multicultural education* (2nd ed.). San Francisco, CA: Jossey Bass.

Baratz, J. C. (1973). Language abilities of Black Americans. In K. S. Miller & R. M. Dreger (Eds.), *Comparative studies of Blacks and Whites in the United States* (pp. 127–184). New York, NY: Seminar Press.

Barnett, R. C., & Baruch, G. K. (1985). Women's involvement in multiple roles, role strain, and psychological distress. *Journal of Personality Social Psychology, 49*, 135–145.

Barnett, R. C., Biener, L., & Baruch, G. K. (1987). *Gender and stress*. New York, NY: Free Press.

Baruch, G. K., & Barnett, R. C. (1986). Consequences of fathers' participation in family work: Parents, role strain and well-being. *Journal of Personality and Social Psychology, 51*, 983–992.

Bernhard, E. (1997). *Gender differences in role stress: Role ambiguity, conflict and overload during the college transition*. Unpublished dissertation, Northwestern University.

Berry, M. F., & Blassingame, J. W. (1985). *Long memory: The Black experience in America*. New York, NY: Academic.

Berry, J. W., Poortinga, Y. H., Segall, M. H., & Dasen, P. R. (1992). *Cross-cultural psychology: Research and application*. New York, NY: Cambridge University Press.

Billingsley, A. (1992). *Climbing Jacob's ladder: The enduring legacy of African American families*. New York, NY: Simon & Schuster.

Bowman, P. J. (1977). *Motivational dynamics and achievement among urban community college students: A situationally-oriented path goal expectancy approach*. Unpublished doctoral dissertation, University of Michigan.

Bowman, P. J. (1984). A discouragement-centered approach to studying unemployment among Black youth: Hopelessness, attributions and psychological distress. *International Journal of Mental Health, 13*, 68–91.

Bowman, P. J. (1988). Post-industrial displacement and family role strains: Challenges to the Black family. In P. Voydanoff & L. C. Majka (Eds.), *Families and economic distress* (pp. 75–99). Beverly Hills, CA: Sage Publications.

Bowman, P. J. (1989). Research perspectives on Black man: Role strain and adaptation across the adult life cycle. In R. L. Jones (Ed.), *Black adult development and aging* (pp. 117–150). Berkeley, CA: Cobbs & Henry.

Bowman, P. J. (1990a). The adolescent to adult transition: Discouragement among jobless Black youth. In V. C. McLoyd & C. Flanagan (Eds.), *New directions in child development* (pp. 87–105). San Francisco, CA: Jossey-Bass.

Bowman, P. J. (1990b). Cultural resources among Black husband-fathers. *Journal of Black Psychology, 16*, 1–22.

Bowman, P. J. (1991a). Joblessness. In J. S. Jackson (Ed.), *Life in Black America* (pp. 156–178). Newbury Park, CA: Sage Publications.

Bowman, P. J. (1991b). Work life. In J. S. Jackson (Ed.), *Life in Black America* (pp. 124–155). Newbury Park, CA: Sage Publications.

Bowman, P. J. (1993). Impact of economic marginality among African American husbands and fathers. In H. P. McAdoo (Ed.), *Family ethnicity: Strength in diversity* (pp. 120–137). Newbury Park, CA: Sage Publications.

Bowman, P. J. (1995). Family structure and marginalization of Black men: Policy implications/commentary.

In M. B. Tucker & C. Mitchell-Kernan (Eds.), *The decline of marriage among African Americans: Causes, consequences and policy implications* (pp. 309–323). New York, NY: Russell Sage.

Bowman, P. J. (1996a). Naturally occurring psychological expectancies: Theory and measurement among African Americans. In R. L. Jones (Ed.), *Handbook of tests and measurements for Black populations* (pp. 553–578). Berkeley, CA: Cobbs & Henry.

Bowman, P. J. (1996b). Education and responsible fatherhood among African Americans: Socialization, mobilization, and allocation challenges. In V. L. Gadsden & W. Trent (Eds.), *Transitions in the life course of African American males* (pp. 13–52). Philadelphia, PA: National Center for Fathers and Families.

Bowman, P. J. (2006). Role strain and adaptation in the strength-based model: Diversity, multilevel, and life span considerations. *The Counseling Psychologist, 34*(1), 118–133.

Bowman, P. J. (2011). Toward a comprehensive strength-based assessment system: A social psychological approach. In P. J. Bowman & E. St. John (Eds.), *Diversity, merit, and higher education (readings on equal education, Vol. 25)*. New York, NY: AMS.

Bowman, P. J., & Betancur, J. J. (2010). Sustainable diversity and inequality: Race in the USA and beyond. In M. Janssens, M. Bechtold, G. Prarolo, & V. Stenius (Eds.), *Sustainability of cultural diversity: Nations, cities & organizations*. Cheltenham: Edward Elger.

Bowman, P. J., & Forman, T. (1997). Instrumental and expressive family roles among African American. In R. J. Taylor, J. S. Jackson, & L. M. Chatters (Eds.), *Family life in Black America fathers* (pp. 216–247). Newbury Park, CA: Sage.

Bowman, P. J., & Howard, C. S. (1985). Race-related socialization, motivation and academic achievement: A study of Black youth in three generation families. *Journal of the American Academy of Child Psychiatry, 24*, 134–141.

Bowman, P. J., Jackson, J. S., Hatchett, S. J., & Gurin, G. (1982). Joblessness and discouragement among Black Americans. *Economic Outlook USA, Autumn*, 85–88.

Bowman, P. J., Muhammad, R., & Ifatunji, M. (2004). Skin tone, class and racial attitudes among African Americans. In C. Herring, V. Keith, & H. Horton (Eds.), *Skin deep: How race and complexion matters in the "color-blind" era*. Urbana, IL: University of Illinois Press.

Bowman, P. J., & Sanders, R. (1998). Unmarried African American fathers: A comparative life span analysis. *Journal of Comparative Family Studies, XXIX*, 39–56.

Bowman, P. J., & Smith, W. A. (2002). Racial ideology in the campus community. In W. A. Smith, P. G. Altbach, & K. Lomotey (Eds.), *The racial crisis in higher education: Continuing challenges for the 21st century* (pp. 103–120). Albany, NY: State University of New York Press.

Boyd-Franklin, N., & Franklin, A. J. (2000). *Boys into men: Raising our African American sons*. New York, NY: Dutton.

Brislin, R. (1993). *Understanding culture's influence on behavior*. New York, NY: Harcourt Brace.

Brodsky, A. E. (1996). Resilient single mothers in risky neighborhoods: Negative psychological sense of community. *Journal of Community Psychology, 24*, 347–363.

Bronfenbrenner, U. (1979). *The ecology of human development*. Cambridge, MA: Harvard University Press.

Bronfenbrenner, U. (1986). Ecology of the family as a context for human development. *Developmental Psychology, 22*, 723–742.

Bronfenbrenner, U. (1996). Ecological systems theory. *Annals of Child Development, 6*, 185–246.

Brookins, C. (2005). Promoting ethnic identity development in African American youth: The role of rites-of-passage. In R. L. Jones (Ed.), *Black psychology*. Hampton, VA: Cobb & Henry.

Brooks, R. B., & Goldstein, S. (2005). *Handbook of resilience in children*. New York, NY: Kluwer Academic/Plenum.

Byrd, C., & Chavous, T. M. (2009). Racial identity in the neighborhood context: A multilevel analysis. *Journal of Youth and Adolescence, 38*(4), 544–559.

Caldwell, C. H., Kohn-Wood, L. P., Schmeelk-Cone, K., Chavous, T., & Zimmerman, M. (2004). Racial discrimination and racial identity as risk or protective factors for violent behaviors in African American young adults. *American Journal of Community Psychology, 33*, 91–105.

Chavous, T., Branch, L., Cogburn, C., Griffin, T., Maddox, J., & Sellers, R. M. (2007). Achievement motivation among African American college students at predominantly White institutions: Risk and protective processes related to group identity and contextual experiences. In F. Salili & R. Hoosain (Eds.), *Culture, motivation, and learning: A multicultural perspective*. Charlotte, NC: Information Age Publishing.

Chirkov, V. I., Ryan, R. M., & Wilness, C. (2005). Cultural context and psychological needs in Canada and Brazil: Testing a self-determination approach to the internalization of cultural practices, identity, and wellbeing. *Journal of Cross-Cultural Psychology, 36*, 423–443.

Chubin, D. E., DePass, A. L., & Blockus, L. (2009). *Understanding interventions that broaden participation in research careers: Embracing the breadth of purpose* (Vol. III). Washington, DC: American Association for the Advancement of Science.

Cicchetti, D., & Cohen, D. (1995). *Developmental psychopathology: Risk, disorder, and adaptation* (Vol. 2). New York, NY: Wiley.

Comer, J. P. (1996). *Rally the whole village: The Comer process for reforming education*. New York, NY: Teachers College Press.

Dawson, M. C. (1994). *Behind the mule: Race and class in African-American politics*. Princeton, NJ: Princeton University Press.

DePass, A. L., & Chubin, D. E. (2008). *Understanding interventions that encourage minorities to pursue research careers: Building a community of research and practice*. Bethesda, MD: American Society of Cell Biology.

Drake, S., & Cayton, H. (1964). *Black metropolis*. New York, NY: Harper Tourchbooks.

Dryfoos, J. G. (1990). *Adolescents at risk: Prevalence and prevention*. New York, NY: Oxford University Press.

DuBois, W. E. B. (1903). *Souls of Black folk*. New York, NY: Penguin.

Ebreo, A. (1998). *Subjective culture, perceived social support, and adaptive coping: A multi-ethnic study of the transition to college*. Unpublished doctoral dissertation, University of Illinois at Urbana-Champaign.

Elder, G., George, L., & Shanahan, M. (1996). Psychosocial stress over the life course. In H. B. Kaplan (Ed.), *Psychosocial stress: Perspectives on structure theory life course & methods* (pp. 247–292). San Diego, CA: Academic Press.

Erikson, E. H. (1966). The concept of identity in race relations. In T. Parsons & K. B. Clark (Eds.), *The Negro American* (pp. 227–253). Boston, MA: Beacon Press.

Erikson, E. H. (1968). *Identity, youth, and crisis*. New York, NY: Norton.

Erikson, E. H. (1980). *Identity and the life cycle*. New York, NY: Norton.

Evans, G. W. (2004). The environment of poverty. *American Psychologist, 59*, 77–92.

Feagin, J. R., & Feagin, C. B. (1999). *Racial and ethnic relations*. Upper Saddle River, NJ: Prentice Hall.

Feather, N. T. (1982). *Expectations and actions: Expectancy-value models in psychology*. Hildale, NJ: Erlbaum.

Feldman, G. S. (1999). *Self-efficacy and outcome expectancies in successful student development: A multi-ethnic study of the college transition*. Unpublished doctoral dissertation, Northwestern University.

Fergus, S., & Zimmerman, M. (2005). Adolescent resilience: A framework for understanding healthy development in the face of risk. *Annual Review of Public Health, 26*, 399–419.

Fitzpatrick, K. M., & LaGory, M. (2000). *Unhealthy places: The ecology of risk in the urban landscape*. New York, NY: Routledge.

Frazier, E. F., (1939). *The negro family in the United States*. Chicago: University of Chicago Press.

Gadsden, V., & Bowman, P. J. (1999). African American males and the struggle toward responsible fatherhood. In V. C. Polite & E. W. Gordon (Eds.), *African American males in school and society* (pp. 166–183). New York, NY: Teachers College Press.

Garbarino, J. (1991). The human ecology of early risk. In S. J. Meisels & J. Shankoff (Eds.), *Handbook of early child intervention* (pp. 78–96). New York, NY: Cambridge University Press.

Garbarino, J. (1995). *Raising children in a socially toxic environment*. San Francisco, CA: Jossey Bass.

Garmezy, N. (1971). Vulnerability research and the issue of primary prevention. *American Journal of Orthopsychiatry, 57*, 101–116.

Garmezy, N., Masten, A., & Tellegen, A. (1984). The study of stress and competence in children: A building block for developmental psychopathology. *Child Development, 55*, 97–111.

Garmezy, N. (1987). Stress, competence, and development continuities in the study of schizophrenic adults, children vulnerable to psychopathology, and the search for stress resistant children. *American Journal of Orthopsychiatry, 57*, 159–174.

Garmezy, N. (1991). Resilience and vulnerability to adverse developmental outcomes associated with poverty. *American Behavioral Scientist, 34*, 416–430.

Garmezy, N. (1993). Children in poverty: Resilience despite risk. *Psychiatry, 56*, 127–136.

Garmezy, N., Masten, A., & Tellegen, A. (1984). The study of stress and competence in children: A building block for developmental psychopathology. *Child Development, 55*, 97–111.

Gary, L., & Leashore, B. (1982). High-risk status of Black men. *Social Work, 27*, 45–54.

Georges-Abeyie, D. (1984). *Criminal justice system and Blacks*. New York, NY: Clark Roardman.

Glasgow, D. G. (1980). *The Black underclass*. San Francisco, CA: Jossey-Bass.

Glazer, N., & Moynihan, D. P. (1975). *Beyond the melting pot*. Cambridge, MA: Massachusetts Institute of Technology Press.

Gonzalez, N., Moll, L., & Amantqi, C. (2005). *Funds of knowledge: Theorizing practices in households, communities, and classrooms*. Mahwah, NJ: Erlbaum.

Goode, W. J. (1960). A theory of role strain. *American Sociological Review, 11*, 483–496.

Gurin, P., Hatchett, S., & Jackson, J. (1989). *Hope and independence: Blacks' response to electoral and party politics*. New York, NY: Russell Sage.

Gutiérrez, K. (2006). *Culture matters: Rethinking educational equity*. New York, NY: Carnegie Foundation.

Hannerz, U. (1969). *Soulside: Inquires into ghetto culture and community*. N.Y.: Columbia Unversity Press.

Heckler, M. H., et al. (1985). *Report of the Secretary's task force on Black and minority health*. Washington, DC: U. S. Department of Health and Human Services.

Herskovits, M. J. (1935). Social history of the Negro. In C. Murchinson (Ed.), *A handbook of social psychology* (pp. 207–267). Worchester, MA: Clark University Press.

Herskovits, M. J. (1941). *The myth of the Negro past*. New York, NY: Harper & Brothers.

Herskovits, M. J. (1955). *Cultural anthropology*. New York, NY: Knopf.

Hetherington, E. M., & Blechman, E. (1996). *Stress, coping and resilience in children and families*. Mahwah, NJ: Lawrence Erlbaum.

Hill, R. B. (1998). *Strengths of African American families: 25 years later*. New York, NY: R&B Press.

Hogan, B. F., Linden, W. M., & Najarian, B. (2002). Social support interventions: Do they work? *Clinical Psychology Review, 22*, 381–440.

Holden, D. J., & Zimmerman, M. A. (2009). *A practical guide to program evaluation planning: Theory and case examples*. University of Michigan: School of Public Health.

Hughes, D., & Chen, L. (1999). The nature of parents' race-related communications to children: A developmental perspective. In L. Barber & C. Tamis-LeMonda (Eds.), *Child psychology: A handbook of contemporary issues*. Philadelphia, PA: Taylor & Francis.

Hurd, N., Zimmerman, M., & Xue, Y. (2009). Negative adult influences and the protective effects of role models: Study with urban adolescents. *Journal of Youth & Adolescence, 6*, 777–789.

Jackson, J. S. (1991). *Life in Black America*. Newbury Park, CA: Sage.

Jackson, J. S. (2000). *New directions: African Americans in a diversifying nation*. Washington, DC: National Policy Association.

Janssens, M., Bechtold, M., Ruijter, A., Pinelli, D., Prarolo, G., & Stenius, V. (2010). *Sustainability of cultural diversity: Nations, cities, and organizations*. Cheltenham: Edward Elger.

Johnson, T. P., & Bowman, P. J. (2003). Cross-cultural sources of measurement error in substance use surveys. *Substance Use and Misuse, 38*(10), 1447–1490.

Jones, R. L. (1989a). *Black adolescents*. Hampton, VA: Cobb & Henry.

Jones, R. L. (1989b). *Black adult development and aging*. Hampton, VA: Cobb & Henry.

Jones, R. L. (2005). *Black psychology*. Hampton, VA: Cobb & Henry.

Kahn, R. L., Wolfe, D. M., Quinn, R., Snoek, J. D., & Rosenthal, R. A. (1964). *Organizational stress*. New York, NY: Wiley.

Kail, R. V., & Cavanaugh, J. C. (2000). *Human development: A life span view*. Belmont, CA: Wadsworth.

Kaplan, H. B. (1996). *Psychosocial stress: Perspectives on structure, theory, life course, and methods*. New York, NY: Academic.

Karenga, M. (1993). *Introduction to Black studies*. Los Angeles, CA: University of Sankore Press.

Katz, M. (1997). *On playing a poor hand well*. New York, NY: Norton.

Kersting, K. (2003). Lessons in resilience. *APA Monitor on Psychology, 32*(8), 30–31. Retrieved from http://www.apa.org/monitor/sep03/lessons.html.

Kessler, R. C. (1979). A strategy for studying differential vulnerability to the psychological consequences of stress. *Journal of Health and Social Behavior, 20*, 100–108.

Kessler, R. C., Price, R., & Wortman, C. (1985). Social factors in psychopathology: Stress, social support, and coping processes. *Annual Review of Psychology, 36*, 531–572.

King, L. A., & King, D. W. (1990). Role conflict and ambiguity: A critical assessment of construct validity. *Psychological Bulletin, 107*, 48–64.

Kohn, L. P., & Chavous, T. M. (2002). How far have we come—Where should we go? Representatives of the next generation of prevention researchers respond to Biglan, Eddy, Ialongo, Roosa, and Sandler. *Prevention & Treatment, 5*(7).

Layng, A. (1978). Voluntary associations and Black ethnic identity. *Phylon, 39*, 171–179.

Lee, C. (2003). Guest Editor: Reconceptualizing race and ethnicity in educational research. *Educational Researcher, 32*(5), 3–5.

Lerner, R. M. (2002). *Concepts and theories of human development* (3rd ed.). Mahwah, NJ: Lawrence Erlbaum.

Leventhal, T., & Brooks-Gunn, J. (2000). The neighborhood they live in: Effects of neighborhood residence on child and adolescent outcomes. *Psychological Bulletin, 126*, 309–337.

Levine, L. (1977). *Black culture and Black consciousness*. New York, NY: Oxford University Press.

Lightsey, O. (2006). Resilience, meaning, and wellbeing. *Counseling Psychologist, 34*, 96–107.

Luthar, S. S. (1991). Vulnerability and resilience: A study of high-risk adolescents. *Child Development, 62*, 600–606.

Luthar, S. S. (2003). *Resilience and vulnerability: Adaptation in the context of childhood adversities*. New York, NY: Cambridge University Press.

Luthar, S. S., Cicchetti, D. C., & Becker, B. (2000). The construct of resilience: A critical evaluation and guidelines for future work. *Child Development, 71*, 543–562.

Marger, M. N. (2000). *Race and ethnic relations: American and global perspectives*. Belmont, CA: Wadsworth.

Marsella, A. J. (1998). Urbanization, mental health, and social deviancy: A review of issues and research. *American Psychologist, 53*, 624–634.

Masten, A. S. (1994). Resilience in individual development: Successful adaptation despite risk and adversity. In M. Wang & E. Gordon (Eds.), *Educational resilience in inner-city America* (pp. 3–25). Hillsdale, NJ: Lawrence Erlbaum.

Masten, A. S. (2001). Ordinary magic: Resiliency processes in development. *American Psychologist, 56*, 227–238.

Masten, A. S., & Reed, M. (2002). Resilience in development. In C. Snyder & S. Lopez (Eds.), *Handbook of positive psychology* (pp. 74–88). New York, NY: Oxford University Press.

Maton, K. I., Schellenback, C. J., Leadbetter, B. J., & Solarz, A. L. (2004). *Investing in children, youth, families, and communities: Strengths-based research and policy*. Washington, DC: American Psychological Association.

McAdams, D. P., & Bowman, P. J. (2001). Narrating life's turning points: Redemption and contamination. In D. P. McAdams, R. Josselson, & A. Lieblich (Eds.), *Turns in the road: Narrative studies of lives in transition* (pp. 3–34). Washington, DC: American Psychological Association.

McAdams, D., & de St. Aubin, E. (1998). *Generativity and adult development: How and why we care for the next generation*. Washington, DC: American Psychological Association.

McAdams, D., de St. Aubin, E., & Logan, R. (1993). Generativity among young, midlife, and older adults. *Psychology and Aging, 8*, 221–230.

McAdams, D. P., Reynolds, J., Lewis, M., Patten, A., & Bowman, P. J. (2001). When bad things turn good and good things turn bad: Sequences of redemption and contamination in life narrative and their relation to psychosocial adaptation in midlife adults and students. *Personality & Social Psychology Bulletin, 27*, 486–496.

McAdoo, H. (1997). *Black families*. Newbury Park, CA: Sage.

McCubbin, H. I., McCubbin, M. A., & Thompson, A. I. (1993). Resiliency in families: The role of family schema and appraisal in family adaptation to crisis. In T. T. H. Brubaker (Ed.), *Family relations: Challenges for the future*. Beverly Hills, CA: Sage.

McLoyd, V. C., & Flanagan, C. (1990). *New directions in child development*. San Francisco, CA: Jossey-Bass.

McLoyd, V. C., & Wilson, L. (1990). Maternal behavior, social support, and economic conditions as predictors of distress in children. In V. C. McLoyd & C. Flanagan (Eds.), *New directions in child development* (pp. 49–69). San Francisco, CA: Jossey-Bass.

McNeil, J. D. (1999). *Racial and ethnic socialization among college students: A multi-ethnic family ecology approach*. Unpublished doctoral dissertation, Northwestern University.

Merton, R. (1968). *Social theory and social structure*. New York, NY: Free Press.

Milburn, N., & Bowman, P. J. (1991). Neighborhood life. In J. S. Jackson (Ed.), *Life in Black America* (pp. 31–45). Newbury Park, CA: Sage Publications.

Miller, D. B. (1999). Racial socialization and racial identity: Can they promote resiliency for African American adolescents? *Adolescence, 34*, 493–501.

Miller, K. S., & Dreger, R. M. (1973). *Comparative studies of Blacks and whites in the United States*. New York, NY: Seminar Press.

Moen, P., Elder, G., & Luscher, K. (1995). *Examining lives in context: Perspectives on the ecology of human development*. Washington, DC: American Psychological Association.

Morris, A. (1984). *Origins of the civil rights movement: Black communities organizing for change*. New York, NY: Free Press.

Myrdal, G. (1964). *An American dilemma: The Negro problem and modern democracy* (Vol. I–III). New York, NY: Harper.

Nagel, J. (1996). *American Indian ethnic renewal: Red power and the resurgence of identity and culture*. New York, NY: Oxford University Press.

Neblett, E. W., Chavous, T. M., Nguyen, H. X., & Sellers, R. M. (2009). 'Say it loud—I'm Black and I'm proud': Parents messages about race, racial discrimination, and academic achievement in African American boys. *Journal of Negro Education, 78*, 246–259.

Neighbors, H., Jackson, J. S., Bowman, P. J., & Gurin, G. (1983). Stress, coping and Black mental health. *Journal of Prevention in Human Service, 2*, 5–9.

Nobles, W. (1974). American fruit: The Black family. *Journal Social & Behavioral Sciences, 20*, 52–64.

Ogbu, J. U. (1981). Origins of human competence: A cultural-ecological perspective. *Child Development, 52*, 413–429.

Olson, S., & Fagen, A. P. (2007). *Understanding interventions that encourage minorities to pursue research careers: Summary of a Workshop*. Washington, DC: National Academies Press.

Orellana, M., & Bowman, P. J. (2003). Cultural diversity issues in learning and development. Conceptual, methodological and strategic considerations. *Educational Researcher, 32*(5), 26–33.

Ostaszewski, K., & Zimmerman, M. A. (2006). The effects of cumulative risks and promotive factors on urban adolescent alcohol and other drug use: A longitudinal study of resiliency. *American Journal of Community Psychology, 38*(3), 237–249.

Pearlin, L. I. (1983). Role strains and personal stress. In H. B. Kaplan (Ed.), *Psychosocial stress: Trends in theory and research* (pp. 3–32). New York, NY: Academic.

Pearlin, L. I., Menaghan, M. A., Lieberman, E. G., & Mullan, J. T. (1981). The stress process. *Journal of Health and Social Behavior, 22*, 337–356.

Pearlin, L. I., & Schooler, C. (1978). The structure of coping. *Journal of Health and Social Behavior, 19*, 2–22.

Phinney, J. S., & Chavira, V. (1995). Parental ethnic socialization and adolescent coping with problems related to ethnicity. *Journal of Research on Adolescence, 5*, 31–53.

Phinney, J. S., & Rotheram, M. J. (1987). *Children's ethnic socialization: Pluralism and development*. Newbury Park, CA: Sage.

Price, R. H., Cowen, E. L., Lorion, R. P., & Ramos-McKay, J. (1988). *14 ounces of prevention: A casebook for practitioners*. Washington, DC: American Psychological Association.

Price, R. H., Ketterer, R. F., Bader, B. C., & Monahan, J. (1980). *Prevention in community mental health: Research, policy and practice*. Beverly Hills, CA: Sage.

Prince-Embury, S. (2007). *Resiliency Scale for adolescents: Profiles of personal strengths*. San Antonio, TX: Pearson Education, Inc.

Prince-Embury, S. (2008). Translating resiliency theory into application with children and adolescents. *The Canadian Journal of School Psychology, 23*(1), 4–10.

Prince-Embury, S. (2009). The Resiliency Scales for children and adolescents as related to parent education and race/ethnicity in children. *The Canadian Journal of School Psychology, 24*(2), 167–182.

Prince-Embury, S. (2010). Assessment for integrated screening and prevention using the Resiliency Scales for children and adolescents. In B. Doll, W. Pfohl, & J. Yoon (Eds.), *Handbook of youth prevention science* (pp. 141–162). New York, NY: Routledge (Chapter 7).

Prince-Embury, S., & Courville, T. (2008a). Comparison of a one, two and three factor models of the Resiliency Scales for children and adolescents. *The Canadian Journal of School Psychology, 23*(1), 11–25.

Prince-Embury, S., & Courville, T. (2008b). Measurement invariance of the Resiliency Scales for children and adolescents across gender and age cohorts. *The Canadian Journal of School Psychology, 23*(1), 26–40.
Rappaport, J. (1990). Research methods and the empowerment social agenda. In P. Tolan, C. Keys, F. Chertak, & L. Jason (Eds.), *Researching community psychology* (pp. 51–63). Washington, DC: American Psychological Association.
Reich, J., Zautra, A., & Hall, J. (2010). *Handbook of adult resilience*. New York, NY: Guilford Press.
Reyes, E. A. (2002). *Extended family support as a protective factor among college students: An exploratory multi-ethnic study*. Unpublished doctoral dissertation.
Rhodes, W., & Brown, W. (1991). *Why some children succeed despite the odds*. Westport, CT: Greenwood.
Rowley, L., & Bowman, P. J. (2009). Risk, protection, and achievement disparities among African American males: Cross-generation theory, research and comprehensive intervention. *Journal of Negro Education, 78*(3), 305–320.
Rutter, M. (1985). Resilience in the face of adversity: Protective factors and resistance to psychiatric disorder. *British Journal of Psychiatry, 147*, 5598–5611.
Rutter, M. (1987). Psychosocial resilience and protective mechanisms. *American Journal of Orthopsychiatry, 57*, 316–333.
Rutter, M. (1993). Resilience: Some conceptual considerations. *Journal of Adolescent Health, 14*, 626–631.
Ryan, W. (1972). *Blaming the victim*. New York: Random House.
Sanders, R. T. (1997). *Intellectual and psychosocial predictors of success in the college transition: A multiethnic study of freshmen students on a predominantly white campus*. Unpublished doctoral dissertation, University of Illinois at Urbana-Champaign.
Sanders, M. G. (2000). *Schooling students placed at risk: Research, policy, and practice in the education of poor and minority adolescents*. Mahwah, NJ: Lawrence Erlbaum.
Sarbin, T. R., & Allen, V. L. (1968). Role theory. In G. Lindzey & E. Aronson (Eds.), *Handbook of social psychology* (pp. 488–568). Reading, MA: Addison-Wesley.
Sedlacek, W. E. (2004). *Beyond the big test: Noncognitive assessment in higher education*. San Francisco, CA: Jossey-Bass Publishers.
Seligman, M. E. P., Sten, T., Park, N., & Peterson, C. (2005). Positive psychology progress: Empirical validation of interventions. *American Psychologist, 60*, 410–421.
Sellers, R., Chavous, T. M., & Cooke, D. Y. (1998). Racial ideology and centrality as predictors of African American college students' academic performance. *Journal of Black Psychology, 24*(1), 8–27.
Seligman, M. E., & Csikszentmihalyi, M. (2000). Positive psychology: An introduction. American Psychologist, *55*, 5–14.
Shiraishi, Y. (2000). *Attributional patterns and adjustment in the college transition: A cross-cultural study*. Unpublished doctoral dissertation, Northwestern University.
Smith, E. J. (2006a). The strength-based counseling model. *Counseling Psychologist, 34*, 13–79.
Smith, E. J. (2006b). The strength-based counseling model: A paradigm shift in psychology. *Counseling Psychologist, 34*, 134–144.
Spencer, M. B., Cole, S. P., DuPree, D., & Glymp, A. (1993). Self-efficacy among urban African American early adolescents: Exploring issues of risk, vulnerability, and resilience. *Development and Psychopathology, 5*(4), 719–739.
Steele, C. (1997). A threat in the air: How stereotypes shape intellectual identity and performance. *American Psychologist, 52*, 613–629.
Stevenson, H. (2005). Racial socialization. In R. L. Jones (Ed.), *Black psychology* (pp. 353–381). Hampton, VA: Cobb & Henry.
Suarez-Orozco, M. M., & Paez, M. M. (2002). *Latinos: Remaking America*. Berkeley, CA: University of California Press.
Sudarkasa, N. (1981). Interpreting the African heritage in Afro-American family organization. In H. McAdoo (Ed.), *Black families*. Beverly Hills, CA: Sage Publications.
Sue, D. W., & Sue, D. (2008). *Counseling the culturally diverse*. New York, NY: Wiley.
Takaki, R. (1989). *Strangers from a different shore: A history of Asian Americans*. Boston, MA: Little Brown.
Takaki, R. (2008). *A different mirror: A history of multicultural America*. Boston, MA: Little Brown.
Taylor, S. (1996). Mediating and moderating processes in psychosocial stress. In H. B. Kaplan (Ed.), *Psychosocial stress: Perspectives on structure, theory, life course, and methods* (pp. 71–110). New York, NY: Academic.
Taylor, R. J., Chatters, L., & Levin, J. (2005). *Religion in the lives of African Americans: Social, psychological, and health perspectives*. Newbury Park, CA: Sage.
Taylor, R. J., Jackson, J. S., & Chatters, L. (1997). *Family life in Black America*. Thousand Oaks, CA: Sage.
Triandis, H. C., Lambert, W., Berry, J., Lonner, W., Hernon, A., Brislin, R., et al. (1980–1981). *Handbook of cross-cultural psychology* (pp. 1–6). Boston, MA: Allyn & Bacon.
Vera, E. M., & Shin, R. (2006). Promoting strengths in a socially toxic world: Supporting resiliency with systemic interventions. *Counseling Psychologist, 34*(1), 80–89.
Weissberg, R. P., Kumpfer, K. L., & Seligman, M. P. E. (2003). Special issue: Prevention that works for children and youth. *American Psychologist, 58*, 425–432.
Werner, E. E. (1995). Resilience in development: Current directions. *Psychological Science, 4*, 81–82.

Werner, E. E., & Smith, R. S. (1992). *Overcoming the odds: High risk children from birth to adulthood*. Ithaca, NY: Cornell University Press.

Williams, L. (2004). *Cultural intervention and perceptions of violence-related behavior among adolescents: A role strain and adaptation approach*. Unpublished doctoral dissertation, University of Illinois at Chicago.

Williams, D. R., Neighbors, H. W., & Jackson, J. S. (2003). Racial/ethnic discrimination and health: Findings from community studies. *American Journal of Public Health, 93*, 7–15.

Wilson, W. J. (1978). *The declining significance of race*. Chicago, IL: University of Chicago Press.

Wilson, W. J. (1987). *The truly disadvantaged: The inner city, the underclass, and public policy*. Chicago, IL: University of Chicago.

Wilson, W. J. (1996). *When work disappears*. New York, NY: Alfred A. Knopf.

Yearwood, L. (1980). *Black organizations: Issues and survival techniques*. Lanham, MD: University Press of America.

Zimmerman, M. A., & Brenner, A. (2010). Resilience in adolescence: Overcoming neighborhood disadvantage. In J. W. Reich, A. J. Zautra, & J. S. Hall (Eds.), *Handbook of adult resilience* (pp. 282–308). New York, NY: Guilford Press.

22 Bowen Systems Theory Applied to Systemic Resilience Versus Vulnerability

Sandra Prince-Embury

This chapter explores a conceptual framework for the potential linking of different levels of resilience in human functioning. For this purpose "family systems theory," originally proposed by Murray Bowen (1978), is introduced and briefly discussed. Bowen's theory has not formally been discussed within the context of resilience theory partly because the theory and constructs were developed and applied in clinical populations manifesting severe pathology. Also, Bowen's theory has generally stayed within the purview of practice and training for family therapy. Nonetheless, Bowen's theory presents conceptual principles that warrant its inclusion in a discussion of resilience. As with many principles of human functioning it is easier to observe severe dysfunction than to observe normal functioning. We might say that observation of normal human functioning is as difficult to observe as "a fish examining wetness." Thus, this chapter endeavors to apply principles of Bowen theory to the understanding of resilient human functioning.

S. Prince-Embury, Ph.D. (✉)
Resiliency Institute of Allenhurst, LLC,
625 North Edgemere Drive, West Allenhurst,
NJ 07711, USA
e-mail: sandraprince-embury@earthlink.net

Systems Theories

Bowen's theory is one of a number of systems theories that are characterized by certain common assumptions. Systems theories assume the interrelatedness of events and processes. The term originates from Bertalanffy's General System Theory (GST) (1950, 1955, 1974, 1968). System theory generally assume that there are different levels of analysis pertaining to processes that operate simultaneously and that these different levels are interrelated. These levels might include the following: physiological, individual, dyad, triad, nuclear family, extended family, multigenerational family, community, culture, social, economic, and political environment. Focus of attention or intervention may shift from one level to another, but one level is not necessarily considered as inherently more important than the others. System theories search for the existence of underlying principles that account for some degree of regularity, redundancy, and possible predictability in the interrelatedness of events and processes.

Murray Bowen

Murray Bowen, considered one of the founders of family therapy, was a psychiatrist who treated families, conducted research, and trained many family therapists while developing his

S. Prince-Embury and D.H. Saklofske (eds.), *Resilience in Children, Adolescents, and Adults: Translating Research into Practice*, The Springer Series on Human Exceptionality,
DOI 10.1007/978-1-4614-4939-3_22, © Springer Science+Business Media New York 2013

comprehensive theory. Bowen's psychiatric training was obtained at the Menninger Foundation in Topeka, Kansas, beginning in 1946. He became a staff member upon completion of his formal training and remained at Menninger's until 1954. He then embarked on a unique 5-year research project at the National Institute of Mental Health in Bethesda, Maryland. The project involved families with an adult schizophrenic child living on a research ward for long periods of time. Bowen left N.I.M.H. in 1959 to become a half-time faculty member in the Department of Psychiatry at Georgetown University Medical Center. He became a Clinical Professor, was Director of Family Programs, and in 1975 founded the Georgetown Family Center. Dr. Bowen was the Director of the Family Center until his death.

Bowen's theory suggests that individuals with higher levels of differentiation would be capable of better functioning over the life course because they would not experience the disruption in the achievement of goals and the maintenance of relationships that would characterize individuals with lower levels of differentiation. Herein we find the essential definition of resilience as the ability to continue functioning in the face of adversity or to quickly return to functioning. Within this framework, highly differentiated, resilient individuals would be capable of maintaining functioning in the face of everyday adversity or emotional upset and would recover more quickly in the face of more extreme adversity. The rest of this chapter introduces Bowen's concept of differentiation and how it manifests as a protective factor at different levels of human systems.

Bowen's Systems Theory

Bowen's theory involves two main underlying factors that are presumed to influence functioning at multiple levels. One factor is the degree of anxiety present in the system. There are several variables having to do with this anxiety or emotional tension. Among these are intensity, duration, and source of the anxiety. From the perspective of traditional resilience theory, whether internally or externally generated, anxiety would represent the condition of adversity and potential disruption of functioning in the system. Bowen acknowledged that low levels of anxiety or temporary increases of anxiety are more easily managed by most systems. On the other hand, Bowen's theory assumed that extreme levels of anxiety or chronically elevated anxiety present a potentially disruptive force at multiple levels of human systems: physiological, individual, family, community, and society.

The other major factor and cornerstone of Bowen theory is *level of differentiation,* which is the set of mechanisms that protect human systems from disruption due to extreme or chronic anxiety. From the perspective of resilience theory *level of differentiation* represents a protective factor which operates across multiple levels of analysis.

Differentiation of Thinking Versus Emotional Process

At the physiological level, Bowen defined *differentiation* as the ability of the individual to differentiate between intellectual functioning and the emotional process. According to Bowen, this level of *differentiation* is related to the individual's ability to choose between a life guided by feelings or thoughts. According to Bowen, those individuals with the greatest fusion between the intellectual and emotional processes do not have this choice, are driven by the more primitive, reflexive emotional process, are more likely to be at the mercy of involuntary emotional reactions and tend to become dysfunctional even under low levels of stress. For example, an individual who strikes out at others when upset, later feeling bad about his or her actions, might be operating at a lower level of differentiation. Bowen suggested that fusion between intellectual functioning and emotional process could be intensified under conditions of severe stress even among those with average degrees of differentiation. Such conditions of extreme and or chronic stress could lower resilience in those with higher levels of differentiation as a result of emotional impairment of cognitive functioning.

Extending this concept to the consideration of resilience we would suggest that those who are less differentiated or unable to separate cognitive functioning and emotional processes would be less resilient and more vulnerable to everyday difficulties as well as more severe adversities. On the other hand, those with more differentiation between these processes would be more resilient in their functioning in everyday living and would be better prepared to cope resiliently with more extreme adversities should they occur.

Among children, lower differentiation might be manifested as problems with emotional regulation whereby they are unable to appropriately inhibit or control their emotional reactions resulting in learning difficulties or behavior problems at school. Among adolescents lower levels of differentiation might result in being overwhelmed by emotion, reacting emotionally or reflexively and by an inability to exercise good judgment when under stress. Those who work with adolescents are often puzzled at how some teens will repeatedly react emotionally, getting themselves in trouble even though they are well aware of the consequences. A more differentiated adolescent might become very upset, but would also be able to delay, process, and consider the consequences of various actions.

Differentiation and Ego-Resiliency

Block's definition of ego-resilience (1980) as flexibility of emotional control is compatible with Bowen's concept of "differentiation" at this level. Someone who is resilient and capable of deciding how much to control emotion would likely be able to distinguish between cognition and emotion. Bowen might suggest that lack of flexibility in emotional control is due to lack of differentiation between cognitive and emotional processes. Thinking that is emotion driven might be recognized as being rigid, more simplistic, polarized, characterized as "good versus bad" or "all versus nothing," manifesting few if any shades of gray. Emotion driven, truncated thinking may appear to provide expediency but may limit the quality of problem solving. Some of these characteristics are similar to Block's description of individuals with lower "ego-resiliency."

Physiological Aspects of Differentiation

Although Bowen's thinking about differentiation was informed by observations in clinical practice, there has been a significant body of research exploring the relationship between cognition, executive functioning, and emotional process. Researchers have attempted to identify specific brain systems responsible for links between cognition and emotion although specific physiological mechanisms are still unknown. The anterior cingulate cortex (ACC) has been identified as involved in emotional drives, experience, and integration. Associated cognitive functions include inhibition of inappropriate responses, decision making, and motivated behaviors. Bush, Luu, and Posner (2000) suggest the involvement of the cingulate cortex, a network that integrates input from various sources and contributes to the modulation of processing in other brain regions. Dolcos and McCarthy (2006) provided functional neuroimaging evidence that impaired performance in the presence of emotional distracters is associated with disrupted activity in the brain regions responsible for active maintenance of goal relevant information in the WM (dorsal system) and enhanced activity in the brain regions responsible for emotional processing (ventral system). Consistent with models of hemispheric asymmetry in emotional processing, the Dolcos and McCarthy's study also provided evidence for a right-lateralization of the observed effects.

Dolcos and McCarthy have also identified individual differences concerning the relationship between brain activity and behavioral responses in the presence of emotional distraction. These results shed light on the neural mechanisms underlying the impairing effect of emotional distraction on working memory and extend the evidence concerning the neural mechanisms underlying the modulatory effect of emotion on executive functions (Gray, Braver, & Raichle, 2002; Yamasaki, LaBar, & McCarthy,

2002; Bishop, Duncan, Brett, & Lawrence, 2004; Simon-Thomas, Role, & Knight, 2005; Wang, McCarthy, Song, & Labar, 2005; Mather et al., 2006).

Differentiation of Self in Relation to Others

An important aspect of human functioning addressed by Bowen was the relationship between self and others. Bowen's theory was consistent with those of developmental theorist stating that human development proceeds from a state in which the infant is undifferentiated, symbiotic, or unable to distinguish between self and parent to increasingly differentiated states. Human development involves increased ability to distinguish self from others as well as increased balancing of need for autonomy or separateness and need for attachment or closeness with others.

According to Bowen, a person with a well-differentiated "self" recognizes his or her realistic dependence on others, but can stay calm and clear headed enough in the face of conflict, criticism, and rejection. A well-differentiated person can distinguish thinking rooted in a careful assessment of the facts from thinking clouded by the emotionality of his or her relationship or family. The decisions and behaviors of a well-differentiated person are based on cognitive processing informed by rationally derived guiding principles as opposed to reflexive emotional reactions or the need to be in agreement with and accepted by others. These individuals would be capable of accepting assistance from and considering the opinions of others while rationally making their own decisions. They would be capable of maintaining communication and commitments to others in times of increased tension when there were "bad feelings between them." Thus, those who are more differentiated in relation to others might be more capable of sustaining long-term, supportive relationships.

One can infer that level of differentiation between thought and feeling provides the underpinning for level of differentiation at the relational level. An individual who is incapable of differentiating thought from feeling might find him or herself highly sensitive to opinions, behaviors, and emotional reactions of others. This heightened interpersonal sensitivity could result in significant volatility in relationships, and frequently disrupted functioning in these volatile relationships.

Bowen referred to low levels of differentiation in relatedness as enmeshment or in extreme circumstances, fusion. These individuals may be so enmeshed with others that they are incapable of using their own judgment when needed in times of heightened anxiety. Lower levels of differentiation can alternatively lead to high defensiveness or emotional cutoff, in which the individual tries to shut off contact with others in an attempt to avoid being emotionally triggered and overwhelmed. Less differentiated individuals may be so cut off from others that they are unable to ask for support when needed in times of heightened anxiety. Emotional cutoff is not an effective mechanism for avoiding anxiety in that it may ultimately lead to isolation. We can presume that individuals employing emotional cutoff to control emotional reactivity may be less capable of sustaining long-term supportive relationships.

Level of Differentiation in the Nuclear Family

According to Bowen, families vary as do individuals along a continuum of differentiation with some families having fairly high levels and others having relatively low levels of differentiation. Adequately differentiated family systems may serve as protective units for handling stress/anxiety in reaction to life transitions, adversities, and traumas. Within this framework, the level of differentiation of a particular family would determine the family's resilience in handling stress associated with adversity. Bowen suggested that families characterized by low differentiation manifested lives with much instability and crisis. He theorized that negative events that impact all families would set off a disabling emotional process in enmeshed families, resulting in poor collective functioning. In an undifferentiated or enmeshed family, distress in one member would spread rapidly to other members potentially impairing the ability of everyone in the family to think clearly, thus impairing the ability of the family or individual family members to cope with the adversity. Thinking in enmeshed families might be characterized as rigid, polarized, right or wrong, with little room for disagreement, discussion, and compromise, resulting in more conflict and less realistic resolution of presenting problems. We might characterize such families as manifesting low resilience to adversity.

On the other hand, Bowen suggested that negative life events would have less impact on families characterized by higher levels of differentiation because more of these family members could engage in clear thinking and problem solving. These families might be characterized as resilient in that life transitions or traumas might be handled more calmly settling differences and making decisions in spite of heightened stress. In a differentiated family, stress would be experienced but it would not disrupt the thinking and functioning of family members. If one member was temporarily overwhelmed other family members would be supportive but remain calm assisting the distressed family members return to functioning.

Level of differentiation in families may manifest when children reach adolescence. A developmental task for adolescence is the development of psychological independence from parental control. For teens in families characterized by lower levels of differentiation this can be a difficult process resulting in acting out and rebellion on the part of the adolescent. Teens in families with higher levels of differentiation are more capable of less conflicting negotiating with their families on issues of importance to them.

Mechanisms of Family Emotional Process

Bowen introduced several mechanisms by which families handle anxiety; the *family projection process*, *triangulation* and *under-functioning* versus *over-functioning*. Since Bowen's theory was developed while observing impaired families, his description of mechanisms tended to focus on description of dysfunctional forms of these processes..

The Family Projection Process

The emotional projection process is a process by which emotional reactivity in one person can be transmitted to another by nonverbal, behavioral, and largely subconscious methods. To some extent transmission of anxiety is a natural function, developed with evolutional significance. Expression such as "feeling the tension in the room," expresses such a process as an everyday occurrence. An example of the projection process in family life may be illustrated by the following example. A man is yelled at by his boss at work. He does not respond but when he returns home he is sulking and irritable with his wife without telling her about the incident at work. The wife senses that something is wrong and feels that it is her fault. She in turn becomes sad and is irritable with one of her children. The child in turn yells at his younger brother. Thus, the emotional upset has been passed among family members without awareness of or discussion of the original event. The prevalence of this process across species is exemplified by the popularity of "the dog whisperer" and the "horse whisperer" in highlighting the result of animals detecting fear in others.

Under circumstances of adequate differentiation, anxiety may be communicated among families along with rational communication about the source of the anxiety and in a rational and conscious manner. In this way the source of the anxiety is "owned" and rational processes among family members may be utilized to address and alleviate the anxiety. Bowen as a psychiatrist became aware of the process in its more dysfunctional form. According to Bowen, in families that are low in differentiation, the family projection process describes the transmission of anxiety in parents to their child. For example, a parent may be highly anxious but not be aware of the source of the anxiety or in more severe cases not be aware that the heighted anxiety resides within them.

This parent may unintentionally transmit nonverbal, behavioral, and verbal cues of this anxiety to their child. The parent may also be hypervigilant to signs of anxiety in the child and frequently question the child implying that the source of the anxiety is in the child. The child, picking up the nonverbal cues of the anxious parent may become more anxious. In addition, frequent concerned questioning by the parent may convince the child that the source of the anxiety resides in him, thus making him feel responsible for the parent's anxiety. This projection process undermines the family's ability to function more resiliently in resolving the actual sources of anxiety but instead leaves a symptom bearer in its wake.

Triangulation

Bowen identified triangulation as a mechanism used under conditions of lower differentiation to manage anxiety in a system. Triangulation consists of three family members where two members are communicating about a third. The triangle according to Bowen is a mechanism for releasing tension between two people by releasing it to a third person. Although this is a basic mechanism in family systems it could potentially be dysfunctional to the degree that it disrupts communication. In triangulation, anxiety between two individuals is released by one of the two venting to a third person. The venting of tension to a third person does not necessarily lead to the resolution of the original problem. In a differentiated family system, family members would resolve conflict directly with each other instead of having to spread heightened emotionality to previously uninvolved family members. In such families, differences in dyads could be tolerated and dealt with rationally and would not generate the stress that leads to triangulation.

Another example of triangulation is the following. Consider a family in which one member is seriously ill. Other family members may release their anxiety by discussing the ill family member without communicating with the ill member, which can result in the ill family member feeling isolated. In addition this mode of communication can deprive the ill family member with important information needed for involvement in decision making about recovery.

Over-Functioning Versus Under-Functioning

Another anxiety driven mechanism under conditions of lower differentiation is called over-functioning versus under-functioning; a process of imbalance of functioning between two family members. This is a process in which one family member assumes more worry driven responsibility for another family member in ways that the other family member is capable of functioning for him or herself. Although over-functioning is often well intentioned, it sometimes has an undermining effect on the under-functioning family member who learns to have lower and lower expectations for him or herself. This process has been observed in families with substance abuse problems and is referred to as "co-dependency" or "enabling" the individual with a substance abuse problem. Counseling with family members will frequently involve identifying this process and helping the "enabling" family members to back off in the hopes that the dysfunctional family member can recover and increase functioning with respect to him or herself.

This process is also seen in families with special needs children in which parents become emotionally overprotective of the child, anticipating his or her every need. This process can inadvertently prevent the child from increasing his or her ability to function for him or herself. Alternatively, a differentiated family with a special needs child would be capable of allowing the child to function for him or herself to maximum capacity even when doing so might involve some struggle on the part of the child and patience on the part of the parent.

Societal Regression

Bowen expanded his thinking on differentiation to apply to more complex social groupings including organizations, communities and societies. His notion was that underlying principles of differentiation versus fusion or enmeshment are reflected at different levels of analysis. Societal regression referred to a more complex level of analysis whereby an entire society could manifest fluctuating degrees of enmeshment versus differentiation. The symptoms of societal regression would vary depending on the period of history, level of anxiety, and zeitgeist of the times and might best be recognized in retrospect. Hypothetically, a society confronted by increased threat and/or diminished resources would experience an increase in collective anxiety. Increased anxiety would in turn interfere with many aspects of collective societal functioning. For example, societal discourse would become more polarized, truncated with few nuanced exchanges of information or areas of compromise. There might be more occasions of "group thinking," or "mob mentality." Opinions might be presented as all right or all wrong. Polarization might take the form of "us against them" with no room for positions of objectivity or neutrality. Societal regression would be associated with more reactive responding aimed at immediate relief or feeling better and less on principle based problem solving and long-term consequences. Exchanges between polarized groups would consist of reciprocal triggering of predetermined emotional prejudices with predetermined ideological explanations as opposed to more differentiated listening and cognitive processing. One might speculate that financial difficulties stemming from spending and debt exceeding productivity is such a symptom of decision making based on relieving anxiety as opposed to objective, differentiated problem solving and consideration of long-term consequences.

Implications for Enhancing Resilience in Human Functioning

Having introduced Bowen theory briefly as a framework for considering resiliency in human functioning, what are more general implications for enhancing resilient functioning? First we can consider that Bowen theory continues since the time of its inception as a basis for training clinicians, treating families, and providing consultation to organizations. The Bowen Family Center originally founded by Bowen continues to train clinicians to this day. There are publications describing various applications of Bowen theory in clinical practice (Kerr, 1994; Gilbert, 1992; Friedman 1991).

Bowen Family Therapy

Bowen family therapists may work with one or more family members to lower emotional reactivity clarify boundaries and appropriate areas of functioning by members of the family. Family therapy may sometimes focus on one family member helping him or her to function calmly in a differentiated manner while remaining in contact with other family members. It is often the case that the presence of one family member manifesting a higher level of differentiation can raise the functional level of differentiation in the family.

Recognizing and Lowering Emotional Reactivity

Bowen family therapy often begins with managing emotional reactivity as the first line of defense. Various methods are employed for this purpose including relaxation techniques, meditation, and training in bio-feedback. When clinically appropriate, psychotropic medication may be used to reduce the level of emotional reactivity. As demonstrated by Connor and Davidson (2003), psychotropic medication, particularly antidepressant, has been shown to lower levels of symptoms of PTSD and raise levels of resiliency as assessed by the CD-RISC. It has been the experience of this author that patients who have started serotonin uptake inhibitors may report that their reactivity to events that would have formerly triggered an extreme emotional reaction is lowered after beginning the medication. This awareness of their own reactivity and its impact on functioning is useful to patients even when they have stopped taking the medication.

Assessment and Research of Emotional Reactivity

Given the significance and potential disruptive effect of emotional reactivity for human functioning, it makes sense to systematically identify this process and research the relationship of emotional reactivity with other aspects of human functioning such as mastery and relatedness. The Emotional Reactivity Scale of the Resiliency Scale for Children and Adolescents (Prince-Embury, 2007) was designed to tap emotional reactivity at the individual level. Consistent with Bowen's notion, providing a measure of one's emotional reactivity relative to others would provide a tool by which the individual can observe and evaluate his or her own emotional reactivity as well as efforts to modify this reactivity. Bowen's proposal that emotional reactivity is disruptive of individual functioning is supported by consistent negative relationships between the RSCA Emotional Reactivity Scale and both the RSCA Sense of Mastery and Sense of Relatedness Scales (Prince-Embury, 2007). Furthermore, Bowen's proposal that emotional reactivity is related to the development of psychopathology is supported by comparisons of RSCA Emotional Reactivity Scale scores of clinical groups and matched controls (Prince-Embury, 2007). Clinical practice also suggests that in children and adolescents, sense of mastery and sense of relatedness consistently improve with decreases in emotional reactivity (see Chap. 3 of this volume).

Conclusion

Remembering that Bowen theory is a systems theory we would assume that intervention and change at one level might have impact for change at other levels of the interrelated system. The assumption would be that lowering ones base line of emotional reactivity would make the likelihood of emotional interference of cognitive functioning less likely, allowing the individual to exercise a higher level of cognitive control. It might be suggested that lowered emotional reactivity at the individual level allows more differentiation in relation to others and may in turn lower reactivity at the family level, allowing more rational problem solving. Lowered emotional reactivity and more differentiated functioning at the family level may in turn allow more community stability and so on.

There are many other possible applications of Bowen Theory for enhancing resilience that are beyond the scope of this chapter. The Family Health Tree (Prince-Embury, 1984) was designed for use by family physicians to help them understand and identify patterns of symptoms in families as possible indications of the family emotional process and distribution of stress. At the community level, one might consider the Information Series discussed in Chap. 17 of this volume as an application of Bowen theory designed to increase resilience of a community by decreasing polarization through interjecting emotionally neutral purveyors of information.

In closing, the purpose of this chapter is to introduce Bowen theory as a framework for considering interventions to enhance resilience at multiple levels.

References

Bertalanffy, L. V. (1950). An outline of general system theory. *British Journal for the Philosophy of Science, 1*(2), 134–165. retrieved 24 October 2010.

Bertalanffy, L. V. (1955). An essay on the relativity of categories. *Philosophy of Science, 22*(4), 243–263.

Bertalanffy, Ludwig Von. (1974). *Perspectives on general system theory*. Edited by Edgar Taschdjian. George Braziller. New York.

Bishop, S., Duncan, J., Brett, M., & Lawrence, A. D. (2004). Prefrontal cortical function and anxiety: Controlling attention to threat-related stimuli. *Nature Neuroscience, 7*, 184–188.

Block, J. H., & Block, J. (1980). The role of ego-control and ego-resiliency in the origination of behavior. In W. A. Collings (Ed.), *The Minnesota symposia on child psychology* (Vol. 13, pp. 39–101). Hillsdale: Erlbaum.

Bowen, M. (1978). *Family therapy in clinical practice*. Northvale: Jason Aronson.

Bush, G., Luu, P., & Posner, M. I. (2000). Cognitive and emotional influences in anterior cingulate cortex. *Trends in Cognitive Science, 4*(6), 217–222.

Connor, K. M., & Davidson, J. R. (2003). Development of a new resilience scale: The Connor-Davidson Resilience Scale (CD-RISC). *Depression and Anxiety, 18*, 76–82.

Dolcos, F., & McCarthy, G. (2006). Brain systems mediating cognitive interference by emotional distraction. *The Journal of Neuroscience, 26*(7), 2072–2092.

Friedman, E. H. (1991). Bowen theory and therapy. In A. S. Gurman & D. P. Kniskern (Eds.), *Handbook of family therapy* (Vol. 2, pp. 134–170). Philadelphia: Brunner/Mazel.

Gilbert, R. M. (1992). *Extraordinary relationships: A new way of thinking about human interactions*. Minneapolis: Chronimed Publishing.

Gray, J. R., Braver, T. S., & Raichle, M. E. (2002). Integration of emotion and cognition in the lateral prefrontal cortex. *Proceedings of the National Academy of Sciences USA, 99*, 4115–4120.

Mather, M., Mitchell, K. J., Raye, C. L., Novak, D. L., Greene, E. J., & Johnson, M. K. (2006). Emotional arousal can impair feature binding in working memory. *Journal of Cognitive Neuroscience, 18*(4), 614–625.

Prince-Embury, S. (1984). The family health tree: A form for identifying physical symptom patterns with the family. *The Journal of Family Practice, 1*, 75–84.

Prince-Embury, S. (2007). *The resiliency scales for children and adolescents*. San Antonio: The Psychological Corporation.

Simon-Thomas, E. R., Role, K. O., & Knight, R. T. (2005). Behavioral and electrophysiological evidence of a right hemisphere bias for the influence of negative emotion on higher cognition. *Journal of Cognitive Neuroscience, 17*, 518–529.

von Bertalanffy, L. V. (1968). *Organismic psychology and systems theory*. Worchester: Clark University Press.

Wang, L., McCarthy, G., Song, A. W., & Labar, K. S. (2005). Amygdala activation to sad pictures during high-field (4 tesla) functional magnetic resonance imaging. *Emotion, 5*, 12–22.

Yamasaki, H., LaBar, K. S., & McCarthy, G. (2002). Dissociable prefrontal brain systems for attention and emotion. *Proceedings of the National Academy of Sciences USA, 99*, 11447–11451.

Epilogue

23

Sandra Prince-Embury and Donald H. Saklofske

The chapters in this book have variously considered resilience within the individual as a state, trait, or combination of competencies. Also addressed have been the contexts such as family or educational environments, as well as social and cultural contexts, within which resilience may be manifested, fostered, and assessed. Useful constructs have been identified as central to resiliency including sense of mastery, initiation, self-efficacy, problem solving, sense of relatedness, attachment, social support, meaning and emotion regulation. Psychometrically sound instruments have been identified to assess various combinations of resiliency competencies at different stages of development.

At the onset in the chapter focusing on conceptual issues, we acknowledged the lack of consensus on definitions of the construct of resilience as well as criteria to assert its presence. It has been the intention of this volume to provide a variety of definitions, assessments, and applications allowing the reader the opportunity to critically evaluate the degree of consistency, transparency, and practical utility of specific translations. Such diverse exposure informed by conceptual concerns provides a context within which clinicians and researchers may make informed choices on how best to view and use the resilience/resiliency constructs.

In reviewing the chapters in this volume we may identify some areas of consensus in defining personal resiliency.

1. Personal resiliency is based in core developmental systems of human functioning.
2. Personal resiliency is most likely multifaceted, competency based, and modifiable.
3. Personal resiliency is not necessarily an enduring trait, although there is overlap between aspects of resiliency and the personality traits of extraversion and emotional stability.

Assessment of resiliency varies depending on the age of the individual and purpose of the assessment. For example, assessment of resiliency in children tends to be strength or assets based: sense of mastery, sense of relatedness, emotional reactivity; initiative, self-control/self-regulation, and attachment; self-efficacy, self-determination, behavioral self-control. Child assessments presented in this volume suggest consensus on the importance of attachment/relatedness, emotional reactivity/self-control/self-regulation, sense of mastery/initiative/self-efficacy/self-determination.

Some assessments of resilience in adults have focused on specific purposes such as assessing changes in response to the pharmacological treatment of PTSD and assessing quick recovery

S. Prince-Embury, Ph.D. (✉)
Resiliency Institute of Allenhurst, LLC, 625 North Edgemere Drive, West Allenhurst, NJ 07711, USA
e-mail: sandraprince-embury@earthlink.net

D.H. Saklofske, Ph.D.
Department of Psychology, Social Science Centre, The University of Western Ontario, 7th Floor, London, ON, Canada N6A 5C2
e-mail: dsaklofs@uwo.ca

S. Prince-Embury and D.H. Saklofske (eds.), *Resilience in Children, Adolescents, and Adults: Translating Research into Practice*, The Springer Series on Human Exceptionality,
DOI 10.1007/978-1-4614-4939-3_23, © Springer Science+Business Media New York 2013

in the face of adversity. Other assessments of resiliency in adults have proposed more complex constructs such as ego-resiliency, commitment, sense of purpose, existential aloneness, or positive self-evaluation. The relative value of these varied approaches most likely depends on the population with which they are being employed and the purpose.

Other chapters presented in this volume demonstrate that resilience constructs may be integrated into other theoretical constructs for the purpose of considering cultural, social-psychological, and systemic issues and for possible inclusion in policy decisions.

While we hope this book will have immediate relevance and application to social scientists and the helping professions, we also very much want to encourage further research into resilience and resiliency. Human kind has always been faced with challenges, whether from each other, the social and economic worlds we have created, or nature itself. But the challenges we face today and our capacity to meet and even conquer them are being tested as never before. For humanity to psychologically and physically thrive is the quest we must confront and one which brings resilience to the forefront. This is no where better captured than the question by Stephen Hawking, mathematics professor at Cambridge University, and famous for his work in theoretical physics, who posted this question on *Yahoo Answers* "**Ask the Planet**" campaign (July, 2006): "In a world that is in chaos politically, socially and environmentally, how can the human race sustain another 100 years?"

Index

S. Prince-Embury and D.H. Saklofske (eds.), *Resilience in Children, Adolescents, and Adults: Translating Research into Practice*, The Springer Series on Human Exceptionality,
DOI 10.1007/978-1-4614-4939-3, © Springer Science+Business Media New York 2013

Printed by Printforce, the Netherlands